Matthijs Oudkerk · Edwin J. R. van Beek · Jan W. ten Cate (Eds.)

Pulmonary Embolism
Epidemiology, Diagnosis and Treatment

Matthijs Oudkerk · Edwin J. R. van Beek · Jan W. ten Cate (Eds.)

Pulmonary Embolism
Epidemiology, Diagnosis and Treatment

With more than 450 illustrations and 78 tables

Blackwell Science
Berlin · Vienna · Oxford · Edinburgh · Boston · London · Melbourne · Tokyo

Blackwell Science Ltd
Editorial Offices:
Osney Mead, Oxford OX2 0EL
25 John Street, London WC1N 2BL
23 Ainslie Place, Edinburgh EH3 6AJ
Commerce Place, 350 Main Street,
Malden, MA 02148 5018, USA
54 University Street, Carlton,
Victoria 3053, Australia

Other Editorial Offices:
Blackwell Wissenschafts-Verlag GmbH
Kurfürstendamm 57, 10707 Berlin, Germany
Zehetnergasse 6, 1140 Vienna, Austria

Blackwell Science KK
MG Kodemmacho Building, 3F
7–10 Kodemmacho Nihonbashi
Chuo-ku, Tokyo 104, Japan

Editors' addresses:
M. Oudkerk, MD, PhD
Head Department of Radiology
Daniel den Hoed Center/University Hospital
Rotterdam
Groene Hilledijk 301
3075 EA Rotterdam
The Netherlands

E. J. R. van Beek, MD, PhD
Academic Department of Radiology
Department of Radiology, Floor C
Royal Hallamshire Hospital
Glossop Road
Sheffield S10 2JF
United Kingdom

Prof. J. W. ten Cate, MD, PhD
Academic Medical Center
Department of Hematology
Meibergdreef 9
1105 AZ Amsterdam
The Netherlands

© 1999 by Blackwell Wissenschaft Berlin · Vienna
A catalogue record for this title is available from
the British Library

Set by SATZFABRIK 1035, Berlin
Printed and bound by GAMMedia, Berlin

The Blackwell Science Logo is a trade mark of
Blackwell Science Ltd, registered at the United
Kingdom Trade Marks Registry
ISBN 0-632-04223-0
Printed in Germany

DISTRIBUTORS
Marston Book Services Ltd
PO Box 269
Abingdon, Oxon OX14 4YN
(Orders: Tel: 01235 465500
                Fax: 01235 465555)
USA
Blackwell Science, Inc.
Commerce Place
350 Main Street
Malden, MA 02148 5018
(Orders: Tel: 800 759–6102
                781 388–8250
                Fax: 781 388–8255)
Canada
Copp Clark Professional
200 Adelaide St West, 3rd Floor
Toronto, Ontario, M5H 1W7
(Orders: Tel.:   416 597–1616
                 800 815–9417
                 Fax: 416 597–1617)
Australia
Blackwell Science Asia Pty Ltd
54 University Street
Carlton, Victoria 3053
(Orders: Tel: 3 9347–0300
                Fax: 3 9347–5001)

Preface

Pulmonary embolism is a major cause of morbidity and mortality which is no longer confined to the western world. Traditionally, most emboli originated from the lower extremities, but the more frequent use of indwelling catheters has shown an increasing number of emboli originating from the upper extremities.

The clinical management of thromboembolism has shown major developments in recent years.

This implies diagnostic and treatment strategies for both acute and chronic pulmonary thromboembolism. These developments could only be achieved by a global multidisciplinary scientific approach to this serious disorder, involving epidemiologists, radiologists, cardiologists, pulmonologists, surgeons, physicians and laboratory scientists. Therefore, this book provides, for the first time, a fully integrated management approach to patients suspected of having pulmonary embolism and/or deep vein thrombosis. This is well reflected in the multidisciplinary origin of the authors contributing to this textbook.

The chapters have been arranged according to specific issues related to the diagnosis and treatment of thromboembolism. The final part of the book is dedicated to evidence-based synthesis of these chapters into a full-scope integrated management strategy. Thus, the book provides strategies for solving medical problems tailored to the individual patient in each clinical setting.

In the last decade, cost-effectiveness has become a major issue in medicine. Recent calculations show that the current diagnosis and treatment of pulmonary embolism is associated with considerable costs. This book offers an approach designed to minimize these costs through optimal use of diagnostic test characteristics and correct assignment of patients to treatment.

Moreover, this book offers insight into the latest developments in imaging techniques and gives indications of their potential setting within the diagnostic process.

The editors gratefully acknowledge the privilege of collaborating with such distinguished authors. Furthermore, we are grateful to all those who offered their expert technical assistance in planning, preparing and writing this extensive work.

M. Oudkerk
E. J. R. van Beek
J. W. ten Cate

V

Table of contents

Chapter V

Vena Cava Filter Devices

Chapter VI

Conservative and Surgical Treatment

Chapter VII

Management Strategies

Contributors

Editors

M. Oudkerk, MD, PhD
Head, Department of Radiology
Daniel den Hoed Center
University Hospital Rotterdam
Groene Hilledijk 301
3075 EA Rotterdam
The Netherlands

E. J. R. van Beek, MD, PhD
Academic Department of Radiology
Department of Radiology, Floor C
Royal Hallamshire Hospital
Glossop Road
Sheffield S10 2JF
United Kingdom

Prof. J. W. ten Cate, MD, PhD
Academic Medical Center
Department of Vascular Medicine
Meibergdreef 9
1105 AZ Amsterdam
The Netherlands

Authors

Prof G. Agnelli
Università di Perugia
Instituto di Medicina Interna e Vascolare
Via Enrico Dal Pozzo
06126 Perugia
Italy

M. Andrew, MD
Henderson General Hospital
Hamilton Civic Hospital Research Center
711 Concession Street
Hamilton, Ontario L8V 1C3
Canada

H. J. Baarslag, MD
Academic Medical Center
Department of Radiology
Meibergdreef 9
1105 AZ Amsterdam
The Netherlands

E. J. R. van Beek, MD, PhD
Academic Department of Radiology
Department of Radiology, Floor C
Royal Hallamshire Hospital
Glossop Road
Sheffield S10 2JF
United Kingdom

A. G. M. van den Belt, MD
Academic Medical Center
Department of Clinical Epidemiology
and Biostatistics
Meibergdreef 9
1105 AZ Amsterdam
The Netherlands

A. H. H. Bongaerts, MD
Department of Radiology
Daniel den Hoed Cancer Center
University Hospital Rotterdam
Groene Hilledijk 301
3075 EA Rotterdam
The Netherlands

S. R. Brennan, MD, FRCP
Respiratory Medicine, Clinical Sciences Division
Northern General Hospital NHS Trust
Herrios Road
Sheffield S5 7AU
United Kingdom

Ch. Bruch, MD
Klinikum der Universität – GSH Essen
Abteilung für Kardiologie
Hufelandstraße 55
45122 Essen
Germany

Prof. H. R. Büller, MD, PhD
Academic Medical Center
Department of Vascular Medicine F4–209
Meibergdreef 9
1105 AZ Amsterdam
The Netherlands

Prof. J. W. ten Cate, MD, PhD
Academic Medical Center
Department of Vascular Medicine
Meibergdreef 9
1105 AZ Amsterdam
The Netherlands

W. S. Chan, MD
Department of Medicine,
Women's College Campus
Sunnybrook and Women's College Health
Sciences Centre
76 Grenville Street
Toronto, Ontario, M5S 1B2
Canada

Direktor Univ.- Prof. Dr. R. Erbel
Universität-Gesamthochschule Essen
Abteilung für Kardiologie
Hufelandstraße 55
45122 Essen
Germany

J. S. Ginsberg, MD
Director, Associate Professor
Department of Medicine,
Thromboembolism Service
McMaster University
1200 Main Street West, HSC-3W11
Hamilton, Ontario L8N 3Z5
Canada

S. Z. Goldhaber, MD
Department of Medicine
Cardiovascular Division
Brigham and Womens
Harvard Medical School
75 Francis Street
Boston, MA 02115

Priv.-Doz. Dr.med. G. Görge
Director of the
Department of Heart and Lung Disease,
Medical Intensive Care and Angiology
Saarbrücker Winterbergkliniken GmbH
Academic Teaching Hospital
P. O. Box 102629
66026 Saarbrücken
Germany

H. W. Gray, MD, FRCP
Dept. of Nuclear Medicine
Royal Infirmary
University NHS Trust
16 Alexandra Parade
Glasgow G31 2ER
Scotland

Prof. Dr. med. R. W. Günther
Medizinische Fakultät der RWTH Aachen
Radiologische Abteilung
Pauwelsstrasse 30
D-52057 Aachen
Germany

H. Harmsen, MD
Academic Medical Center
Department of Radiology
Meibergdreef 9
1105 AZ Amsterdam
The Netherlands

Prof. T. W. Higenbottam, BSc, MD, MA, FRCP
Clinical Sciences Division (CSUH Trust)
Section of Respiratory Medicine
University of Sheffield
Floor F, The Medical School
Sheffield S10 2RX
United Kingdom

Prof. J. Hirsh
Director, Hamilton Civic Hospitals
Research Center
Henderson General Division
711 Concession Street
Hamilton, Ontario L8V 1 C3
Canada

Y. L. Hoogeveen, PhD
Clinical Research
Cordis Endovascular
Roden
The Netherlands

S. W. Jamieson, MB, FRCS
Professor and Head,
Division of Cardiothoracic Surgery
Department of Surgery
University of California Medical Center
200 West Arbor Drive
San Diego, California 92103–8892
USA

D. P. Kapelanski, MD
Division of Cardiothoracic Surgery
University of California Medical Center
200 West Arbor Drive
San Diego, California 92103–8892
USA

R. Kraaijenhagen, MD
Academic Medical Center
Department of Vascular Medicine
and Thrombosis F4–209
Meibergdreef 9
1105 AZ Amsterdam
The Netherlands

A. W. A. Lensing, MD, PhD
Academic Medical Center
Department of Neurology
Meibergdreef 9
1105 AZ Amsterdam

J. A. Macoviak, MD
Division of Cardiothoracic Surgery
University of California Medical Center
200 West Arbor Drive
San Diego, California 92103–8892
USA

M. W. Mewissen, MD
Director, Vascular/Interventional Radiology
Froedtert Memorial Lutheran Hospital,
Room 2803
9200 West Wisconsin Avenue
Milwaukee, Wisconsin 53226
USA

P. Monagle, MBBS
Department of Hematopathology
Royal Children's Hospital
Flemington Road
Parkville, Victoria
Australia 3052

M. Monreal, MD, PhD
Facultat de Medicina
Hospital Universitari Germans Trias i Pujol
Carretera del Canyet, S/N
08916 Badalona, Barcelona
Spain

J. B. Neilly, MD, FRCP
Dept. of Nuclear Medicine
Royal Infirmary
University NHS Trust
16 Alexandra Parade
Glasgow G31 2ER
Scotland

C. H. van Ommen MD
Emma Children's Hospital AMC
Department of Pediatrics
PO Box 22700
1100 DE Amsterdam
The Netherlands

P. M. A. van Ooijen, MSc
Department of Radiology
Daniel den Hoed Clinic
University Hospital Rotterdam
Groene Hilledijk 301
3075 EA Rotterdam
The Netherlands

M. Oudkerk, MD, PhD, FACA
Head, Radiology Department
Daniel den Hoed Center
University Hospital Rotterdam
Groene Hilledijk 301
3075 EA Rotterdam
The Netherlands

M. Peters, MD, PhD
Emma Children's Hospital AMC
Department of Pediatrics
PO Box 22700
1100 DE Amsterdam
The Netherlands

P. Prandoni, MD, PhD
Institute of Medical Semeiotics
University of Padua Medical School
Via Ospedale Civile, 105
35128 Padua
Italy

M. H. Prins, MD, PhD
Department of Clinical Epidemiology &
Biostatistics
Academic Medical Center
Room J2–221
Meibergdreef 9
1105 AZ Amsterdam
The Netherlands

W. L. J. van Putten
Department of Statistics
Daniel den Hoed Cancer Center
University Hospital Rotterdam
Groene Hilledijk 301
3075 EA Rotterdam
The Netherlands

J. A. Reekers, MD, PhD
Academic Medical Center
Department of Radiology
Meibergdreef 9
1105 AZ Amsterdam
The Netherlands

S. A. Renshaw, MD, MA, MRCP (UK)
Division of Molecular and Genetic Medicine
Respiratory Cell and Molecular Biology
Royal Hallamshire Hospital
Glossop Road
Sheffield, S10 2JF
United Kingdom

A. B. van Rossum, MD
Catharina Hospital
Department of Radiology
Michelangelolaan 2
5623 EJ Eindhoven
The Netherlands

F. F. H. Rutten, PhD
Professor, Institute for
Medical Technology Assessment
Erasmus University, L. Building
P.O. Box 1738
3000 DR Rotterdam
The Netherlands

P. F. Sheedy II, MD
Mayo Clinic, Dept. of Diagnostic Radiology
200 First Street SW
Rochester, Minnesota 55905
USA

T. P. Smith, MD
Professor of Radiology
Chief Division of Vascular and Interventional
Radiology
Duke University Medical Center
Department of Radiology
Erwin Road, Room 1502
Durham, North Carolina 27710
USA

P. A. Wielopolski, MD, PhD
Department of Radiology
Daniel den Hoed Cancer Center
University Hospital Rotterdam
Groene Hilledijk 301
3075 EA Rotterdam
The Netherlands

P. K. Woodard, MD
Assistant Professor, Division of Chest Radiology
Cardiovascular Imaging Laboratory
Mallinckrodt Institute of Radiology
510 South Kingshighway Boulevard
St. Louis, Missouri 63110
USA

Chapter 1
Introduction

1 Epidemiology, risk factors, and natural history of venous thromboembolism

P. Prandoni, J. W. ten Cate

Epidemiology

For many years, deep vein thrombosis (DVT) of the limbs and pulmonary embolism (PE) have been regarded as separate entities. It is now well established that about 70% of patients with confirmed PE have thrombosis in their deep leg veins [1, 2], and about 50% of patients with confirmed DVT of both lower and upper extremities have (asymptomatic) PE [3–9]. Post-mortem studies have shown a strong association between PE and the presence of venous thrombosis in the lower limbs [10]. Moreover, similarities in the clinical outcome of patients with DVT or PE have been revealed during long-term follow-up [11, 12]. For these reasons, PE and DVT should be regarded as a single clinico-pathological entity, i. e. venous thromboembolism [13].

DVT and PE most often complicate the course of severely ill, hospitalised patients but may also affect ambulatory and otherwise healthy people [14]. Even if the importance of venous thromboembolic disorders as a major cause of morbidity and mortality has been gaining attention in the past two decades, the true incidence of venous thromboembolism in the general population remains difficult to determine. Unlike in hospitalised patients, most population-based studies were conducted without the use of objective diagnostic tests. Since both DVT and PE may produce no symptoms or symptoms that are non-specific and compatible with many other disease conditions, epidemiological data based on subjective symptoms and physical findings are less reliable.

Data from Vital Statistics and from the National Hospital Discharge Survey in the United States from 1970 to 1985 revealed an age-adjusted rate for PE of 51 per 100,000 and for phlebitis and thrombophlebitis of 79 per 100,000 inhabitants [15]. In the Tecumseh Community Health Study, using data provided by history and physical examination, the age-adjusted prevalence of post-phlebitic sequelae was estimated to be 5% [16]. The incidence of DVT was 14.8 per 10,000 per year in men aged from 40 to 49 years, increasing to 49.9 in men aged from 70 to 79 years. The corresponding incidence rates for women were 31.0 and 10.0 per 10,000 per year, respectively. In a retrospective survey of a defined community, Anderson et al. found an average annual incidence of 48 initial cases and 36 recurrent cases of DVT (confirmed objectively in 86%) plus 23 cases of pulmonary emboli (confirmed objectively in 54%) per 100,000 inhabitants [17]. Extrapolation from their data yields an estimated total of 170,000 initial episodes and 90,000 recurrent episodes of venous thromboembolism in the United States each year [18]. Corresponding figures have been reported in European countries. In order to determine the incidence of DVT in a well-defined population, all abnormal venograms within the city of Malmö during 1987 were studied [19]. The incidence was found to be equal for both sexes, i. e. 1.6 per 1,000 inhabitants and year. The median age for men was 66 years, compared to 72 years for women.

The introduction of thromboprophylactic measures, particularly in the perioperative time, in addition to changes in hospital practice, have most likely affected the pattern of venous thromboembolic disease in the last decade. In a series of 14,667 necropsy reports reviewed from 1965 to 1990 and of 6,436 diagnostic venograms performed between 1976 and 1990, undertaken at a single teaching hospital in London, a progressive reduction in the percentage of fatal PE (from 6.1 to 2.1% over the 25-year period), as well as a remarkable reduction in the rate of venographically diagnosed postoperative DVT from 50 to 25 per 100,000 population was observed, which was in marked contrast to the constant rate of non-postoperative DVT [20]. To evaluate the effect of the progression in the intensity of prevention and quality of treatment of PE, Soskolne et al. investigated the death rates from PE in Canada between 1965–87 and compared them with those for the United States between 1962–84 [21]. In both countries the annual death rates increased until 1977–80 (reaching the value of approximately 3.5 per 100,000) and then decreased, although the changes in the Canadian rates occurred later and were less pronounced than those in the US rates. A corresponding decline in the PE discharge rate was reported by Lilienfeld et al. by investigating hospital discharge data for all acute care facilities in the Minneapolis-St. Paul metropolitan area from 1979 to 1984 [22]. It is interesting to note, however, that the hospital case-fatality for PE appeared to be constant over years.

Because of the silent nature of this disease, its highly aspecific clinical presentation, and the costs and inconveniences of the standard diagnostic tools (ascending phlebography and pulmonary angiography), the total incidence, prevalence, and mortality rates of venous thromboembolism remain elusive, in particular for PE. Contemporary autopsy studies reveal that PE continues to be under or overdiagnosed among hospitalised patients [23]. They show that PE is particularly difficult to diagnose among elderly patients and among subjects with underlying cardiopulmonary disease [24, 25]. The frequency of unsuspected PE in patients at autopsy has not diminished over the last three decades [23].

Because of the persisting underestimation of the diagnosis of venous thromboembolism, it is reasonable to hypothesise that in the United States up to five million patients each year suffer from an episode of venous thrombosis, a prevalence about five-fold more than that of malignant disease. A total of 10 % of these patients have a pulmonary embolic event, and about 10 % of those who develop embolism die within the first hour [26].

Conditions at risk

A first step in determining the epidemiology of venous thromboembolism is to assess the demographic groups and the clinical conditions that are associated with the greatest risk of developing the disease.

Old age

Considerable evidence lends consistent support to the association between increasing age and venous thromboembolism. In the Framingham study, advanced age was significantly associated with fatal PE, when comparing all participants at entry into the study versus those with major PE at autopsy [27]. In the general community study by Coon et al. there was evidence of increasing rates of venous thrombosis with age among males [16]. In their study of out-of-hospital patients, Anderson et al. reported an association between advancing age and thrombosis [17]. In keeping with these studies, Nordström et al. in their community-base study in the Malmö area observed a strong age-dependency of thrombosis [19].

Based on discharge summary diagnoses, an increase was noted in the rate of PE in hospitalised patients in the United States (1985) from 12 per 100,000 in the group aged 15 to 44 years to 265 per 100,000 in those aged 65 years and over. Corresponding rates for phlebitis and thrombophlebitis were 35 and 289 per 100,000 respectively. Intermediate rates were found for individuals aged 45 to 65 years [15].

Kniffin et al., by analysing a random 5 % sample of all US Medicare claims from 1986 till 1989, found that the annual incidence rates per 1,000 for PE and DVT increased steadily with age [28]. At the age of 65 to 69 years they were 1.3 and 1.8, respectively. Corresponding figures reached 2.8 and 3.1 by the age of 85 to 89 years. By extracting data from the Medicare population Siddique et al. also found that the 30-day case-fatality rates in patients with PE increased steadily with age both in patients in whom PE was indicated as the primary diagnosis and in those in whom PE was indicated as a comorbid condition [29]. With nonmultivariate techniques, increasing age has shown a consistently positive association with postoperative DVT that is independent of the type of surgery [30]. Multivariate analysis confirmed this association [31]. In a case-control study performed at Padua University in a large series of consecutive outpatients with clinically suspected DVT, the occurrence of venography proven DVT was significantly associated with old age (>60 years) [32]. Finally, in virtually all studies recruiting consecutive patients with documented venous thromboembolism for scientific purposes, old patients formed the large majority of the entire cohort.

A recent case-control study, which requires confirmation, suggests that low to moderate alcohol consumption is associated with a decreased risk of venous thromboembolism in older persons [33].

Previous venous thromboembolism

Results of studies conducted in surgical and in out-of-hospital patients support the view that previous venous thromboembolism is an important independent risk factor for venous thromboembolic disorders. It is to be specified, however, that in many cases recurrence is most likely determined by the persistence of risk factors (such as cancer or thrombophilia) accounting for the first episode rather than by residual anatomic changes, as recurrent venous thromboembolism involves the contralateral leg as frequently as the ipsilateral one [11]. This seems confirmed by the striking difference in the rate of recurrences between patients with idiopathic thrombosis or thrombosis related to persisting risk factors versus patients in whom the thrombotic episode is triggered by reversible risk factors, such as recent trauma or surgery [11, 34, 35].
A clinical history of previous DVT or PE has been shown in three surgical studies using radiofibrinogen leg scanning for detection of DVT to be associated with an increased frequency of postoperative DVT [31, 36, 37].
In a case-control study, Coon and Willis found that the risk of recurrent DVT after an index episode was higher at all stages of follow-up for patients with a history of venous thromboembolism compared with those who did not report a previous episode [38].
In two studies in out-of-hospital patients presenting with symptomatic DVT, previous venous thrombosis was a strong predictive factor [17, 39]. The Malmö study, in which 14% of the cases had a previous documentation of an earlier venous thrombosis episode, is probably the strongest community-based evidence for previous thrombosis as a risk factor [19].
It is common experience that a previous thrombotic episode places patients at a particularly high risk of recurrent episodes when they undergo surgical procedures, become pregnant, or are confined to bed for a variety of medical disorders. This is especially true in carriers of thrombophilia and in those with underlying malignancies [40].

Prolonged immobilisation

Immobility represents a convincing risk factor for venous thromboembolism. The association between lack of mobility and venous thrombosis has been confirmed in a number of autopsy and clinical studies [10, 41]. Although it might be argued that the underlying condition is the principal determinant of the development of venous thrombosis, the consistency of the pattern of thrombosis observed in diverse groups with different causes of limb inactivity supports the concept that prolonged immobilisation is an independent risk factor in the development of venous thrombosis.
Furthermore, the contribution of immobilisation as an independent risk factor for venous thromboembolism emerged in a study in hemiplegic patients, in which the non-paralysed leg served as control [42]. Warlow et al. found evidence of DVT, using the radiofibrinogen leg scanning technique, in 60% of paralysed limbs compared with only 7% in the nonparalysed limbs. Finally, immobilisation was significantly and independently associated with the occurrence of thrombosis, as shown by phlebography, in a case-control study performed by Cogo et al. in a large series of consecutive outpatients presenting with the clinical suspicion of DVT [32].

Surgery and trauma

Patients who sustain major trauma or undergo prolonged surgical procedures are at risk of developing venous thromboembolism. The risk continues after discharge from hospital. The degree of risk is increased by age, obesity, malignancy, prior history of venous thromboembolism, varicose veins, recent operative procedures and thrombophilic states [10, 31, 32, 40, 41, 43–46]. The thrombi in these patients are usually asymptomatic, small and non-occlusive. Most of them are confined to the calf vein system [47]. This is especially true for thrombi developing after general (abdominal, urologic or gynaecologic) surgery, whereas in patients undergoing major orthopedic procedures, thrombi more often involve the proximal veins (Table 1). Even when occult, these thrombi have the potential to cause PE. Furthermore, unrecognised and untreated DVT may also lead to long-term morbidity from the postphlebitic syndrome as well as predispose patients to future episodes of recurrent venous thromboembolism [11].

Table 1. Risk categories in surgical and trauma patients.

	Calf DVT	Proximal DVT	Fatal PE
High risk – general and urological surgery in pts > 40 yrs with recent history of DVT or PE – extensive pelvic or abdominal surgery for malignant disease – major orthopedic surgery of lower limbs – major trauma	40–80%	10–30%	> 1%
Moderate risk – general surgery in pts > 40 yrs lasting 30 min or more, and in pts < 40 yrs on oral contraceptives – neurosurgery	10–40%	1–10%	0.1–1%
Low risk – Uncomplicated surgery in pts < 40 yrs without additional risk factors – Minor surgery (i. e., less than 30 min) in pts > 40 yrs without additional risk factors	< 10%	< 1%	< 0.1%

Abdominal and pelvic surgery

The study of the incidence of DVT associated with abdominal surgery was greatly facilitated by the development of the radiofibrinogen uptake test. The two best-studied areas have been urologic and gynaecologic surgery [30]. The overall incidence of DVT as assessed by radiofibrinogen leg scanning is consistently around 25% in patients without anticoagulant prophylaxis [49]. The rate of proximal DVT is 6 to 7%, and that of fatal PE approximately 0.8%. Interestingly, in pooled data from North American trials, the incidence is about one half of the incidence of European trials.

In surgical patients with malignant disease, the incidence of DVT is approximately 30%. PE is a leading cause of death following gynaecological cancer surgery [50] and accounts for approximately 20% of perioperative hysterectomy deaths [51].

Pooled data from trials based on radiofibrinogen leg scanning indicate that low-molecular-weight-heparin (LMWH) at low doses reduces the incidence of postoperative DVT in general surgery by 80%, low-dose heparin by 68%, intermittent pneumatic compression (IPC) and oral anticoagulants by 60% [49].

Major orthopedic surgery

In the absence of a proper anticoagulant prophylaxis, the incidence of DVT, as shown by phlebography, ranges from 50 to 60% in elective hip surgery [52–56], from 40 to 80% in emergency hip surgery [57–59], and from 50 to 80% in major knee surgery [60–62]. About one in 20 patients will have a clinically recognisable PE; however, objective findings suggestive of (asymptomatic) PE are detectable in more than 20% of patients [63].

DVT and PE are both more likely after surgery for a fractured hip [40, 49, 64, 65]. An observation of interest is that in fractured hips the site, and by association the extent of trauma, seems to be an important variable. Peritrochanteric fractures are associated with more thrombi than subcapital fractures [30]. Thrombi are most commonly seen in the operated limb, however an appreciable incidence of thrombosis of the non-operated limb has been consistently found in all series. Bilateral venous thrombosis occurs in at least 25% of cases.

Pooled data from trials employing ascending venography indicate that LMWH, at doses which on average were twice as high as those recommended for DVT prevention in general surgery, reduces the incidence of postoperative DVT in elective hip surgery by 71%, in elective knee surgery by 49%, and by 44% following hip fracture surgery; corresponding figures for oral anticoagulants are 61%, 25% and 50%, respectively [66]. It is interesting to note that the incidence of venous thromboembolic complications remains disappointingly high in patients undergoing major knee surgery despite adequate measures of prophylaxis, approaching one third of operated patients [67–69].

Elective neurosurgery

Venous thromboembolism is a common complication in patients who have undergone neurosurgery. Without thromboprophylaxis, the incidence of symptomless DVT ranges between 20 and 50%, and fatal PE is reported to occur in 1.5 to 5% of patients [70]. In the vast majority of studies, the diagnostic standard was radiofibrinogen leg scanning, supplemented in some studies by venography or impedance plethysmography. Recently,

5

Nurmohamed et al. performed a prospective double-blind trial in a large series of patients who were to undergo elective neurosurgery, randomising them to receive prophylactic doses of an LMWH or placebo [71]. All patients wore elastic compression stockings. DVT was detected by bilateral phlebography. The overall incidence of DVT in the placebo group was 26.3%, as compared to 18.7% in the LMWH group. The respective rates for proximal-vein thrombosis were 11.5 and 6.9%.

Other surgical interventions

Studies in other types of surgery are limited. In one thoracotomy study a thrombosis incidence of 50% was noted [72]. In reconstructive arterial vascular surgery, DVT rates between 10 and 40% have been reported [30]. Recently, the incidence of proximal-vein thrombosis, as assessed by postoperative duplex scan, has been reported as low as 2% in aortic surgery in the absence of thromboprophylaxis [73].

Major trauma

The frequency of venous thromboembolic complications after major trauma has been recently investigated with systematic phlebography in a large cohort of consecutive patients admitted to a regional trauma unit [59]. Although most patients were asymptomatic, overall DVT was found in 58% of patients, and proximal-vein thrombosis in 18%. In detail, DVT complicated 50% of patients with major injuries involving the face, chest, or abdomen; 54% of patients with major head injuries; 62% of patients with spinal injuries; and 69% of patients with lower-extremity orthopedic injuries. Data are impressive, and underscore the need for effective prophylactic regimens in these conditions. A recent trial suggests that LMWH at doses comparable to those adopted for major orthopedic surgery is more effective than low-dose heparin, resulting in a 30% reduction in the risk of venous thromboembolism [74].

Malignant diseases

After the initial observation by Armand Trousseau in 1865, numerous studies have addressed the relationship between cancer and thrombosis. Postmortem studies have demonstrated a markedly increased incidence of thromboembolic disease in patients who died of cancer, particularly those with mucinous carcinomas of the pancreas, lung, and gastrointestinal tract [75, 76]. Cohort studies of surgical patients showed that the incidence of venous thrombosis was markedly higher in patients with malignant disorders than in patients with other (non-malignant) diseases [36, 77–82]. Subclinical activation of the coagulation system is often seen in non-surgical patients with cancer [83–85]. The relationship between cancer and thrombosis is further supported by the high risk of developing overt malignancy in patients with idiopathic venous thromboembolism when compared with patients whose thrombotic episode is associated with a well recognised risk factor [86–89].

The most common and well-demonstrated conditions that make patients with cancer susceptible to thrombosis are the following: prolonged immobilisation from any cause, surgical intervention, chemotherapy, and the insertion of indwelling central venous catheters.

Prolonged immobilisation

Patients with cancer during their hospital stay are at a higher risk of developing fatal PE. This was shown by a study conducted by Shen and Pollak in 1979 [90]. They reported that as many as 14% of patients with cancer admitted to a hospital department died of PE (confirmed by autopsy), as compared to 8% of patients without malignant diseases (P < 0.05).

Surgical intervention

Patients with cancer are at a markedly high risk of developing postoperative DVT. The overall incidence of postoperative DVT in patients with cancer is about twice as high as that of patients free of malignancy [36, 77–82] (Table 2). As recently

Table 2. Post-operative DVT in cancer patients.

Series (General Surgery)	Postoperative DVT	
	Cancer pts	Non-cancer pts
Kakkar, 1970 [36]	24/59 (41%)	38/144 (26%)
Hills, 1972 [77]	8/16 (50%)	7/34 (21%)
Walsh, 1974 [78]	16/45 (35%)	22/217 (10%)
Rosemberg, 1975 [80]	28/66 (42%)	29/128 (23%)
Sue-Ling, 1986 [79]	12/23 (52%)	16/62 (26%)
Allan, 1983 [81]	31/100 (31%)	21/100 (21%)
Multicentre Trial, 1984 [82]	9/37 (22%)	13/53 (24.5%)
Total	128/343 (37%)	146/738 (20%)*

* = statistically significant

demonstrated by Huber and associates, the incidence of postoperative PE is remarkably higher in patients with cancer than those without cancer [91].

According to the degree of risk of venous thrombosis, the European Consensus Statement, recently held in London, has established that to reduce the risk of thromboembolism, patients with cancer, when undergoing low-risk surgical procedures, require low-dose heparin, LMWH at low doses, or physical measures [40]. Extensive abdominal or pelvic surgery places patients with cancer at a remarkably high risk for developing post-operative DVT and PE. Therefore, these patients require prophylactic measures comparable to those usually recommended for major orthopedic surgery. These measures include adjusted-dose heparin, higher doses of LMWH (average twice as high as those suggested for general surgery), or oral anticoagulants [40]. As compared to the standard heparin regimen that is used in the prevention of thromboembolism in patients with cancer who undergo surgery, no selective advantage has yet been shown with LMWHs [92]. A recent study compared two doses of an LMWH (dalteparin, 5,000 and 2,500 units once daily) for thromboprophylaxis in 2,070 patients undergoing elective general surgery for abdominal diseases, 63 % of whom had malignant disease [93]. The higher dosage schedule reduced the incidence of DVT from 12.6 to 6.7 % at the expense of more hemorrhagic complications (4.7 versus 2.7 %). This higher rate of bleeding was not seen among patients undergoing operation for cancer.

Chemotherapy

Patients with cancer are at a significantly increased risk of developing both venous and arterial thrombosis when they receive chemotherapeutic drugs [94 – 97] (Table 3). A recent trial randomised a wide series of women with breast cancer to receive tamoxifen only (30 mg/d for 2 years, N = 352) or associated with a 6-month course of chemotherapy (N = 353) [98]. During the study period, 54 thromboembolic events were observed among 48 women (15.3 %) allocated to receive the chemotherapy, most of whom were actually receiving the chemotherapeutic treatment, as compared to only 9 events in the women allocated to tamoxifen only (2.6 %; P < 0.0001). Local reactions and superficial phlebitis were inappropriately included among thromboembolic complications. However, even confining the evaluation to serious events (venous thromboembolism, arterial events), the difference remains highly statistically significant and clinically relevant. Thromboembo-

Table 3. Venous and arterial thrombosis in cancer patients during chemotherapy.

Series	No pts	Type of cancer	Thrombosis during chemotherapy	after
Weiss, 1981 [94]	433	Breast st II	22 (5 %)	0*
Goodnough, 1984 [95]	159	Breast st IV	24 (15 %)	4 (2.5 %)*
Levine, 1988 [96]	205	Breast st II	14 (7 %)	0*
Saphner, 1991 [97]	2352	Breast	128 (5 %)	0*

* = statistically significant

Table 4. Central venous catheters-related upper extremity DVT in cancer patients.

Series	Cancer patients	Upper limb DVT
Lokich, 1983 [100]	53	22 (42 %)
Bern, 1990 [102]	40	15 (37.5 %)
Monreal, 1996 [103]	13	8 (62 %)

lism related to chemotherapy represents, therefore, a relatively common and serious complication that may outweigh any benefits by this additional therapy. This risk, at least for patients with breast cancer, appears significantly reduced with the use of fixed low doses of warfarin (1 mg/day) [99].

Central venous catheters

A few studies using venography demonstrated an unexpectedly high incidence of upper limb venous thrombosis following the insertion of indwelling central venous catheters in patients with cancer (Table 4) [100, 101]. This risk appears significantly reduced with the use of fixed low doses of warfarin (1 mg/day) [101, 102] or low doses of LMWH [103]. This topic is more extensively discussed in chapter III.2.

Before concluding this section, it is worth mentioning that patients with active cancer, after developing an episode of venous thromboembolism, remain at a high risk of recurrent thromboembolism after discontinuation of warfarin therapy [11]. Therefore, they require prolongation of the anticoagulant strategy for as long as the cancer is active. Furthermore, they are often resistant to usual intensities of warfarin [104, 105], making it highly desirable to explore the benefit-to-risk of alternative modalities of anticoagulation.

Puerperium

The postpartum period has consistently been found to be a higher-risk condition for the development of venous thromboembolism than the antepartum period. Unfortunately, clinical grounds alone were used to diagnose DVT and PE in most studies. Therefore, data on the epidemiology of venous thromboembolism in the puerperium should be interpreted with caution [10, 41]. In an extensive summary of clinically diagnosed thrombosis in pregnancy, the reported monthly incidence of postpartum thrombosis per 1,000 pregnancies ranged from 2.7 to 20: these figures were significantly higher than those observed in the antepartum period and in non-pregnant women of childbearing age [106]. It is reasonable to assume that in women who are free from underlying disorders predisposing to thrombosis, the relative risk of venous thromboembolism in the postpartum period is in excess of 20-fold when compared to the antepartum period [10, 41].

No comprehensive studies exist using objective diagnostic techniques to investigate the additional thrombotic risk that may be associated with caesarean section versus normal delivery.

Oral contraceptives and hormone replacement therapy

One of the most controversial and extensively studied risk factors for venous thromboembolism is oral contraceptive (OC) use and hormone-replacement therapy. Unfortunately, most studies published until the end of '80s lacked the methodological criteria to reliably detect differences between thrombotic rates in users and non-users.

Koster et al. performed a meta-analysis of controlled studies published until 1993 on the risk for venous thromboembolism of users of OCs [107]. The review revealed serious methodological flaws in both cohort and case-control studies, although both types consistently showed an association between OC use and venous thromboembolism. OC were associated with almost three-fold increase in risk of venous thrombosis (RR = 2.9; 95% CI = 0.5 – 17). The pooled summary estimate of case-control studies (RR = 4.2) was higher than the pooled summary estimate of follow-up studies (RR = 2.1). The risk of venous thromboembolism rose with increasing oestrogen dose, being higher

for formulations containing more than 50 µg per pill. The consistency of these findings strongly supports the validity of the association, but the conclusions are significantly weakened by the fact that in all studies objective diagnostic methods were either not performed at all, or were only performed in some of the patients. Women with leg symptoms who are using OC are more likely to be diagnosed as having venous thrombosis on clinical grounds, resulting in an over-estimation of the relative risk.

The WHO Collaborative Study of Cardiovascular Disease and Steroid Hormone Contraception investigated the risk of idiopathic venous thromboembolism associated with the use of combined OCs [108]. This analysis, which involved 1,143 cases and 2,998 age-matched controls in 17 countries, revealed a 3 – 4-fold increased risk among OC users compared with non-users. The increased risk was apparent within 4 months of starting OCs, and disappeared within 3 months of stopping OCs. Relative risk estimates were unaffected by age, by a history of hypertension, or by smoking. Odds ratios associated with the use of third-generation progestagens were slightly higher than those observed with progestagens of the first and second generation.

This unexpected observation prompted a detailed analysis of the risk of venous thromboembolism associated with the use of low oestrogen OCs containing levonorgestrel or two of the newer third-generation progestagens, gestodene and desogestrel. This analysis of data from 9 countries involved 769 cases and 2,225 age-matched controls [109]. Risk estimates were 3.4, 7.3, and 10.2 for levonorgestrel, desogestrel, and gestodene, respectively, compared with non-users, and 2.2 and 3 for desogestrel and gestodene, respectively, compared with levonorgestrel. In two other large case-control analyses, low-oestrogen OCs containing third-generation progestagens were associated with a risk for venous thromboembolism which was on average twice as high as that observed in users of second generation products [110, 111]. The association persisted after adjustment for several risk factors for venous thromboembolism that could have influenced the choice of the preparation (e. g. age, weight, smoking, parity, and varicose veins). The increased risk of venous thromboembolic disease attributable to use of a third-generation OC, beyond the risk associated with use of an earlier OC, appeared to be about 10 – 15 per 100,000 woman-years of use [111]. If the typical case-fatality was about 1%, the increased rate of fatal venous thromboembolism would be 1 – 1.5 per million woman-years [112].

The absolute risk of DVT associated with the third-generation OC seems to be especially high among carriers of the factor V Leiden mutation and among women with a strong family history of thrombosis [113].

Until recently, hormone-replacement therapy was reputed to carry a small risk for venous thromboembolism, if any [10, 114]. In order to explore the relation between use of postmenopausal oestrogen hormone-replacement therapy and venous thromboembolism, four hospital or population-based case-control studies have been carried out recently [115 – 118]. Each of the four studies showed a two-fold to four-fold relative risk of venous thromboembolism with oestrogen-only as well as with combined oestrogen-progestagen hormone-replacement therapy. However, the absolute risk was small: 16 – 23 excess cases per 100,000 women per year for VTE and 6 per 100,000 women per year for PE [115 – 118]. The risk was higher following the start of therapy (as with OC), and disappeared after hormone-replacement therapy was stopped.

The underlying mechanism by which oestrogens alone or in combination with progestagens may contribute to thrombosis is unknown [119]. The changes in hemostatic parameters in women using OC are minor and generally remain within the normal range. In a recent investigation, women who used OC exhibited a significantly decreased sensitivity to APC when compared with non-OC users, independent of the kind of drug used [120].

In addition, women who used third-generation monophasic OC were significantly less sensitive to APC than women using second-generation OC, and had an APC ratio that did not significantly differ from heterozygous female carriers of factor V Leiden who did not use OC [120]. Thus, acquired APC resistance may explain the epidemiological observation of increased risk for venous thrombosis in OC users, especially in women using third-generation OC [120]. As epidemiological evidence accumulates supporting a role for these widely diffused drugs in thrombotic disorders, there is a greater need for studies of the mechanism of action.

Medical conditions requiring hospitalisation

The incidence of thromboembolic disease in hospitalised medical patients varies widely according to the disease. The risk ranges from 3 % in patients without pre-existing risk factors to 50 % in patients with predisposing factors, such as prior thromboembolism or thrombophilia [121]. The importance of thromboembolic disease arising in the medical wards is confirmed by the fact that three quarters of patients presenting with PE are presently non-surgical patients [122]. Massive PE is responsible for 4 – 8 % of hospital mortality in medical wards [123, 124].

The Thromboembolic Risk Factors Consensus Group has agreed to divide medical patients into three different levels, according to their risk of thrombosis following hospitalisation (Table 5) [121].

Certain diseases, especially neurologic and cardiac diseases, place patients at a particularly high risk of venous thromboembolism following hospitalisation.

Neurologic diseases

Leg swelling in the paralysed limb in hemiplegia is a common finding. The advent of the radiofibrinogen leg scanning and associated phlebography showed that the majority of post-stroke swollen legs were the results of DVT. Venous thromboembolic complications can complicate the clinical course of a patient with stroke in up to 60 % of cases [40]. These rates are similar to those observed in major orthopedic surgery or trauma [30]. PE accounts for a significant incidence of fatality rates in stroke patients [125]. The overall incidence of leg DVT is 42 % from the untreated control arm of randomised studies [126 – 128]. The risk is particularly high when the neurologic disease results in a paralysed leg [49]. The throm-

Table 5. Risk categories in medical patients requiring hospitalisation (Thromboembolic Risk Factors Consensus Group, 1992).

	DVT	PE
High risk – major medical disease in pts with prior thromboembolism or thrombophilia – lower-limb paralysis	~ 40 %	1 – 10 %
Moderate risk – minor medical disease in pts with prior thromboembolism or thrombophilia – heart or respiratory failure, cancer, inflammatory gastrointestinal disease, severe sepsis	20 – 40 %	0 – 1 %
Low risk – minor medical conditions in pts without prior thromboembolism or thrombophilia	< 10 %	< 0.1 %

bosis rate is up to 10 times higher in the paralysed side [30].

The systematic use of preventive doses of LMWH or danaparoid for as long as immobilisation persists is associated with a considerable reduction in the risk of venous thromboembolism in patients with ischemic stroke [129–133].

In patients with acute spinal cord injury, the radioisotopic or venographic incidence of DVT has been reported as 18 to 100%, with an average incidence of 40% [49]. In a multicenter review of 1,419 patients with acute spinal cord injury, Waring and Karunas reported a 14.5 and 4.6 incidence of clinically recognised DVT and PE, respectively [134]. The period of greatest risk appeared to be during the first two weeks following injury. There is no evidence from (small) available studies that low-dose heparin provides adequate protection from DVT in this category of patients [49]. Although large well-conducted studies in this field are lacking, patients appear better protected by adjusted-dose of heparin, LMWH, or a combination of low-dose heparin with physical measures [135–137].

Heart diseases

Congestive heart failure and acute myocardial infarction pose a particularly high risk of venous thromboembolism. Venous thromboembolic complications can complicate the clinical course of a hospitalised patient with congestive heart failure in up to 70% of cases [138–140], and with acute myocardial infarction in up to 30% [141–145]. The risk is particularly high when the two clinical conditions are combined [142, 144, 146]. PE accounts for a significant incidence of fatality rates in patients with congestive heart failure [147] or myocardial infarction [148–150].

The current incidence of venous thromboembolism following acute myocardial infarction is probably lower than in the past, because patients are much more rapidly mobilised. Cardiac failure is more efficiently treated, and most patients now receive some form of thrombolytic or anticoagulant treatment [30]. The systematic use of preventive doses of heparin for as long as the medical disease requires hospitalisation is associated with a strong reduction in the risk of venous thromboembolism in both myocardial infarction and congestive heart failure [140–142, 146, 151].

Other medical diseases requiring hospitalisation

There are relatively few studies on venous thromboembolism prevalence in medical patients admitted to hospitals without acute myocardial infarction or stroke. The heterogeneity of diseases, and therefore the wide variability of thrombotic risk, precludes extrapolation of the results of studies conducted in a well-defined medical population to hospitalised medical patients as a whole [152].

In patients with pulmonary or cardiopulmonary failure, the prevalence of leg scan detected DVT ranges from 13 to 26% [140, 153, 154], and is considerably reduced by low-dose heparin [140, 154].

Among patients admitted to medical intensive care units, the prevalence of DVT was reported to be 29% by Cade with the use of radiofibrinogen leg scanning [155]) and, more recently, 33% by Hirsch et al. in a consecutive series of 100 patients investigated with colour-Doppler [156].

The true incidence of venous thromboembolism in ordinary bedridden patients has been poorly investigated. Controlled trials evaluating the impact of low doses of LMWH for prevention of overall or PE-related death in patients hospitalised in internal medicine suggest that the risk of venous thrombosis causing fatal PE in these conditions is low [157, 158]. In a recent trial, Gärdlund et al. reported on the rate of necropsy-verified PE in a wide series of consecutive patients admitted to six departments of infectious diseases in Sweden [159]. In the absence of prophylactic measures during hospital stay they were able to record only 16 episodes of fatal PE among 5,917 patients (0.27%). The rate of PE-related death did not differ from that observed in patients randomised to receive low-dose heparin (15/5776, 0.43%). The overall mortality was similarly low in both groups. Dahan et al. randomised 262 medical patients older than 65 years to either LMWH or placebo [160]. The rate of leg scan-detected DVT was 9.1% in the placebo-treated patients, compared with 3% in the LMWH-treated patients. In two recent studies comparing low doses of standard versus LMWH for prevention of venous thromboembolism in wide series of internal-medicine bedridden patients, the rate of objectively documented venous thromboembolism was similarly low in both groups of treatment [152, 161].

Other diseases

Some evidence exists that other diseases are associated with the risk of venous thromboembolic complications: among them, systemic lupus erythematosus [32, 162, 163] inflammatory bowel diseases [165–167], nephrotic syndrome [168, 169], paroxysmal nocturnal hemoglobinuria [170–172], myeloproliferative disorders [173–177], Behçet disease [178], Cushing syndrome

[179], and sickle cell disease [180–182]. These conditions contribute a small number of cases of DVT to the general population, although the case frequency in conditions such as lupus erythematosus can be quite high [30]. For most of them only observational studies exist, that lack control groups. Therefore, incidence, prevalence and patterns of venous thromboembolic disorders in these conditions remain unclear.

Uncertain association

For a few factors, limited, weak, or controversial evidence exists suggesting an association with venous thromboembolism. They include pregnancy, obesity, varicose veins, ethnicity, and blood group.

Pregnancy
Most information on the epidemiology of pregnancy-related thrombosis is based on descriptive studies that utilised suboptimal diagnostic techniques. Although pregnancy exposes women to many of the known risk factors for venous thromboembolism (enlarged uterus-related venous stasis, increased levels of many clotting factors and of markers of thrombin generation, such as fibrinopeptide-A, transitory reduction of APC response connected to factor VIII elevation [183]), an extensive summary of clinically diagnosed thrombosis in pregnancy compiled by Drill and Calhoun failed to show differences in the rate of thrombosis between pregnant women in the antepartum period (0.08–0.15 : 1,000) and that of non-pregnant women of childbearing age (0.07–0.25 : 1,000) [106]. A retrospective venography-based series from Sweden documented only 2 cases of DVT over a 5-year study of 15,000 pregnant women in the antepartum period [184]. A notable feature was the low rate of positive venograms (2 of 17 suspected cases), suggesting that the earlier clinical reports described an incidence of thrombosis that is no longer accurate for the present day [30]. Thus, in the absence of underlying factors predisposing to thrombosis, the antepartum period does not appear to be associated with excess risk of venous thrombosis. Hereditary deficiencies of clotting inhibitors, particularly antithrombin deficiency and resistance to activated protein C considerably increase the thrombotic risk [185–188]. DVT in pregnancy electively affects the left lower limb (probably due to the anatomic stenosis of the left iliac vein by the branching of the right femoral artery), and is uniformly distributed along the three trimesters [189].

Obesity
The association of obesity with an increased risk of postoperative DVT was shown by univariate analysis in a few studies using radiofibrinogen leg scanning [31, 36, 190, 191]. Furthermore, in two prospective studies obesity was significantly and independently associated with PE among women [27, 192]. However, this association could not be confirmed by others [31, 193]. Further studies are needed to provide a definite evidence that increase of body weight is a risk factor for venous thromboembolic disorders [10, 30, 41].

Varicose veins
Varicosity has been considered as a risk factor for venous thromboembolism for half a century. A few studies using leg scan-detected DVT showed a significant increase in postoperative DVT among patients with varicose veins [31, 36]. However, it is well known that varicosis, as well as superficial thrombophlebitis, may produce false-positive scans [194].

Recently, Jorgensen et al. performed a Duplex ultrasound study in a consecutive series of 44 patients presenting with clinical and ultrasound manifestations of superficial thrombophlebitis, and were able to detect DVT in 10 of them (23%) [195]. All cases were clinically occult. Six of these were in continuity with the superficial thrombus. None of the known risk factors for venous thrombosis were helpful in identifying patients at risk for DVT. Since it is well known that varicose veins predispose affected people to the risk of superficial thrombophlebitis, this and other similar observations [196–198] lend new support to the association of varicose veins with venous thromboembolism. Further studies are needed to properly address this relationship. They should include both in- and outpatients.

Ethnicity
Many studies in which investigators attempted to define ethnic differences in the incidence of venous thromboembolism have been severely limited methodologically. In many, objective testing was not carried out. Few studies included direct comparisons of different ethnic groups living in the same geographic location [41]. Joffe found a similar incidence of leg scan-detected DVT in Europeans, Coloureds, Bantus, and Indians living in Cape Town [199]. Post-mortem studies showed no difference in the incidence of venous thromboembolism among ethnic groups in the same location [10]. Nonetheless, some evidence suggests that a few Asiatic populations (i.e. Thai, Korean, Indian, Chinese) exhibit a lower thrombotic risk than West-

ern populations following major surgery [200–203]. It is presently impossible to say whether these findings reflect genetic or environmental variations.

Blood group

Similarly controversial is the question whether people with different blood group exhibit a different thrombotic risk. Limited and conflicting information suggests that carriers of blood group O have a lower thrombotic risk than the remaining population [10, 19]. Proper studies are indicated to answer this potentially important issue.

Antiphospholipid antibody syndrome

Antiphospholipid antibodies (APA) are a heterogeneous group of immunoglobulins directed against negatively charged phospholipids, protein-phospholipid complexes, or plasma proteins such as beta-2-glycoprotein I [162, 204]. APA include anticardiolipin (ACA) and lupus anticoagulant (LAC) antibodies. Both LAC and ACA are characteristically found in patients with systemic lupus erythematosus, but can be observed in other auto-immune diseases, and even in the absence of any underlying disease [162, 205, 206]. The presence of these antibodies has been associated with the clinical features of the so-called "antiphospholipid antibody syndrome" (APS), including arterial and venous thrombosis, recurrent foetal loss, and thrombocytopenia [162, 207–211].

The underlying mechanism by which APA may contribute to thrombosis is unknown. It is likely that endothelial and/or platelet activation initiates thrombus formation. Whether antiphospholipid antibody is an activator, a toxic response to endothelial/platelet injury, or a protective response is not yet clear, nor is it certain whether antiphospholipid antibody is germ-line encoded or antigen-driven, but the latter is likely [212]. An attractive hypothesis to explain venous thrombosis is that the APA interfere with the protein C system [213]. As epidemiological evidence accumulates supporting a role for APA in thrombotic disorders, there is a greater need for studies of the mechanism of action.

APA have been estimated to occur in 2% of the general population [214]. Their frequency in systemic lupus erythematosus varies between 30 and 40% [204]. In a recent review of the literature comprising over 1,000 patients, the frequency of thrombosis in APA-positive patients with systemic lupus erythematosus was 42%, versus 13% in patients without these antibodies [205].

In contrast to the extensive documentation on the risk for both arterial and venous thrombosis in patients with APA and systemic lupus erythematosus [162, 205, 215, 216], no definite evidence in favour of an association of venous thromboembolism with APA in patients free from lupus erythematosus has been available until recently. Two recent case-control studies of patients with suspected venous thromboembolism showed a strong association of venous thromboembolism with LAC [217, 218]. In both studies, the prevalence of LAC in unselected patients with the first episode of venous thromboembolism was unexpectedly high, ranging from 8.5 to 14% [217, 218]. In contrast, available reports on the association of ACA with venous thromboembolism yielded conflicting results [208, 217, 219]. In a recent multicentre prospective investigation, an IgG ACA titer above 40 units was significantly associated with the development of thrombotic events [220]. However, there are presently no standardised methods for the detection of ACA and no standardised criteria for the expression and interpretation of results [221]. Therefore, further investigations are needed to establish whether different antiphospholipid antibodies are differently associated with thrombosis.

The true clinical relevance of APA in patients suffering an episode of venous thromboembolism is still unknown. APA persist for many years, possibly a lifetime [222]. Our experience and that of other centres suggest that the risk of thromboembolic recurrences after interruption of oral anticoagulants in patients with (both primary and secondary) APA syndrome suffering an episode of DVT is almost three times as high as that observed in patients free from these antibodies [223–225]. New thrombotic events are to be expected at any time following cessation of warfarin. Even if a recent retrospective investigation suggests that patients with APA are resistant to usual intensities of warfarin [223], in our experience the recurrence rate per patient-year under conventional low-dose warfarin was low (0.0038) and fully comparable to that observed in patients without APA [11, 224, 226].

Inherited thrombophilia

Inherited thrombophilia is a genetically determined tendency to venous thromboembolism. The true prevalence of inherited thrombophilia in the general population is presently unknown, since we most likely do not know all genetic abnormalities causing a tendency to venous thrombosis. Indirect evidence suggests that it might be much higher than estimates from prevalence studies on the known genetic defects.

The more frequent and well-established thrombophilic syndromes are antithrombin (AT) deficiency, protein C (PC) deficiency, protein S (PS) deficiency, resistance to activated protein C (APC resistance), and hyperhomocysteinemia. Other causes of inherited thrombophilia are much rarer, such as dysfibrinogenemia, abnormalities of the fibrinolytic system, of heparin cofactor II, and of thrombomodulin, or only recently established, such as prothrombin 20 210 GrA [227]. They will not be discussed in the present chapter.

For all of the well-known thrombophilic syndromes, a true association with venous thromboembolism has been firmly established by comparing the prevalence of thrombosis in the population of interest with an appropriately matched control group, using either a cross-sectional analysis, a case-control study, or a prospective cohort study design [228]. The prevalence of these abnormalities varies widely according to the population investigated [229, 230]. The prevalence observed in selected patients who experienced recurrent thrombotic events, developed thrombosis in unusual sites or at a young age, presented in the absence of any of the known risk factors for venous thrombosis, or exhibit a positive family history is (on average) twice as high as that observed in unselected patients with objectively confirmed DVT. The latter, in turn, is much higher than in healthy individuals.

Until recently, inherited thrombophilia was considered a rare finding, and most authorities questioned the need for a systematic screening in patients with venous thromboembolism [10, 228]. It is now widely accepted that underlying abnormalities (isolated or in various association) are recognisable in almost 50 % of patients experiencing an episode of DVT or PE [231]. Patients with spontaneous episodes of venous thromboembolism are as likely to exhibit one or more of these abnormalities as are patients whose thrombotic episode is triggered by acquired risk factors [228, 229, 231]. The relative risk of developing further thrombotic events following the first episode of DVT in carriers of hereditary defects, once anticoagulant treatment is interrupted, is approximately twice as high as that of patients free from these abnormalities; this risk is similarly high in patients with idiopathic and in those with secondary DVT [11, 232]. Accordingly, screening of patients with thromboembolic events, irrespective of the modality of presentation, has the potential to identify patients requiring a prolonged course of anticoagulation. Finally, among family members of sympto-

matic patients with an established hereditary deficiency, a statistically significant and clinically important difference exists in the risk of both spontaneous and risk-related venous thromboembolic events between subjects with and without clotting inhibitory defects [233]. Accordingly, screening of family members of index cases has the potential to identify asymptomatic individuals who might benefit from vigorous prophylactic measures during exposure to circumstantial risk factors.

Antithrombin deficiency

AT is a single-chain glycoprotein, synthesised by the liver. It is the primary inhibitor of thrombin and also inhibits most of the other activated serine proteases involved in the intrinsic clotting system, i. e. factor Xa, IXa, XIa, XIIa, and kallikrein [234–240]. Protease inactivation by AT involves the formation of a complex between the active site of the protease and the reactive centre of AT, formed by Arg^{393} and Ser^{394} [241]. Inhibition of most of the blood coagulation proteinases is relatively slow, but is markedly accelerated by the binding of heparin and heparin-like compounds to AT. The interaction between heparin and AT results in a conformational change of the molecule, which facilitates its interaction with the proteinases [242, 243].

AT defects are currently classified as follows: *type I AT deficiency*, identified by concordant reduction of both functional and immunological AT; and *type II AT deficiency*, identified by a variant AT molecule, which has a defect in the reactive site (II RS), a defect affecting the heparin binding site (II HBS) or multiple functional defects (II PE). The pattern of inheritance is autosomal dominant. The majority of affected individuals are heterozygotes, with AT levels between 40 and 70 % of normal. Homozygotes are extremely rare [229, 231].

In the general population the frequency of symptomatic AT deficiency has been estimated to be between 1 : 2,000 and 1 : 5,000, and that of asymptomatic deficiency approximately 1 : 600. In unselected patients presenting with the first episode of venous thromboembolism, the frequency is approximately 1 %, in selected patients 2.5 % [229, 231].

Although it is difficult to obtain exact figures on the risk of thrombosis in affected persons, review of the literature indicates that more than 50 % of affected persons develop thromboembolic events before the age of 50 years. In most cases, patients develop DVT and/or PE; there are also occasional reports of thrombosis in unusual sites and in the arterial circulation [10, 228]. Anyway, a recent analysis of causes of death in 58 carriers of antithrombin deficiency belonging to 14 families, who died

13

between 1940 and 1994, showed that this abnormality is associated with a normal survival and a low risk of fatal thromboembolic events, when compared with mortality rates from the general population adjusted for age, sex and calendar period [244].

AT deficiency confers a higher risk of thrombosis than deficiencies of PC and PS. This is confirmed by the fifty-fold difference in the prevalence among patients with a first event of DVT and the prevalence in a healthy population [245–247]. Moreover, AT deficiency is associated with a much higher risk of thrombosis in pregnancy than deficiencies of PC or PS [248].

Protein C deficiency

PC is a vitamin K-dependent glycoprotein, which is the precursor of the serine proteinase activated PC (APC). It is synthesised by the liver as a single-chain molecule, and then converted into a two-chain molecule [229, 231]. During coagulation PC is activated slowly by thrombin via cleavage of the Arg^{169}-Leu^{170} bond. This reaction is markedly accelerated by the binding of thrombin with an endothelial receptor, thrombomodulin. The high-affinity binding of thrombin to thrombomodulin produces a 20,000-fold increase in the rate of PC activation. To do this efficiently, APC needs to form a complex with PS on a suitable membrane surface. The APC, thus formed, inactivates the cofactors, factor Va and VIIIa, by selective proteolytic cleavages. APC also has antifibrinolytic activity [249–251].

Two types of protein C deficiency have been described: *type I PC deficiency* is caused by a genetic defect that results in an absolute decrease in PC antigen levels and a normal ratio of PC activity to PC antigen, while *in type II PC deficiency* there is evidence for the presence of an abnormal PC molecule (reduced PC activity, normal PC antigen) [252, 253].

In the general population the frequency of symptomatic PC deficiency has been estimated to be between 1 : 16,000 and 1 : 36,000, and that of asymptomatic deficiency between 1 : 200 and 1 : 300. In unselected patients presenting with the first episode of venous thromboembolism, the frequency is 3.2 %, and 3.8 % in selected patients [229, 231, 245].

Since the first demonstration of an association of PC deficiency with thrombosis in 1981 [254], heterozygous PC deficiency has been described frequently in association with recurrent venous thromboembolism, cerebral venous thrombosis, and coumarin-induced skin necrosis [255, 256]. The risk of thrombosis appears similar for the different

types of PC deficiency [252]. The thrombotic risk increases as the PC levels decrease [257]. The homozygous form is associated with neonatal purpura fulminans and massive fatal thrombosis in new-borns [258].

Recent studies indicate that PC deficiency can be expressed clinically as either an autosomal dominant or an autosomal recessive trait [228, 259]. The deficiency of PC appears to be identical in both forms of deficiency, but for reasons that are obscure, their clinical manifestations are markedly different. When PC deficiency is expressed as an autosomal dominant trait, the cross-sectional studies indicate that over 70 % of affected subjects will develop venous thromboembolism during their lifetime. In contrast, when PC deficiency is expressed clinically as an autosomal recessive trait, venous thrombosis is extremely uncommon unless the disorder occurs in the homozygous or double heterozygous state [228, 229, 231]. This most likely accounts for the low frequency of thrombosis among asymptomatic blood donors who were identified as carriers of PC deficiency [260].

Protein S deficiency

The principal cofactor of APC is PS, a vitamin K-dependent glycoprotein, which is produced by the liver, but also in endothelial cells, megakaryocytes and Leydig cells in the testis. PS circulates in plasma as a free form (40 %) and as a non-covalent complex with C4b-binding protein (60 %). PS acts by enhancing the affinity of APC for negatively charged phospholipids, forming a membrane-bound APC-PS complex that renders factors Va and VIIIa more easily accessible to APC-mediated cleavage. Only the free form of PS has APC cofactor activity [229, 231].

According to the classification proposed by the ISTH in 1992, *type I PS deficiency* results in a reduction of total PS antigen (and of free PS antigen and PS activity), whereas *type II PS deficiency* defines the presence of a functionally abnormal PS molecule (total PS antigen normal, free PS antigen normal but PS activity reduced), and *type III PS deficiency* is defined by normal total PS antigen but reduced free PS antigen and activity [229, 231, 261, 262].

The frequency of PS deficiency in the general population is unknown. In unselected and selected patients, presenting with the first episode of venous thrombosis, the frequency averages 2.2 % and 3 %, respectively [229, 231]. However, in a recent report the prevalence of PS deficiency was found to be as high as 7.3 % in a wide cohort of unselected patients with venous thromboembolism [244].

Since 1984 [263, 264], many families have been reported with venous thrombophilia and PS deficiency, either alone or associated with PC deficiency. It is not clear whether the three different subtypes confer similar risks of thrombosis [229]. Moreover, from an epidemiologist's point of view the risk of venous thromboembolism in deficient individuals has yet to be elucidated. Although the available evidence generally leads to the conclusion that PS deficiency increases the risk of thrombosis, this evidence is much less solid than for PC deficiency [265, 266]. Homozygous PS deficiency has been reported, and while extremely rare, appears to be as severe as homozygous PC deficiency [229].

Resistance to activated PC (APC-R)

APC-R is by far the most common cause of inherited thrombosis. In more than 90% of cases it is caused by a single point mutation in the factor V gene [267, 268]. The mutation is a guanine-to-adenine substitution at nucleotide position 1691 of the factor V gene, resulting in the substitution of arginine by glutamine at position 506 of the polypeptide chain of factor V (factor V Leiden) [269–271]. The mechanism by which the mutation leads to the phenotype of APC-R is still to be elucidated [229]. However, it is clear that the replacement of Arg^{506} by Gln will prevent cleavage of factor V(a) at this site by APC and by that delay the inactivation of factor Va either by preventing the conformational change necessary for the inhibitory cleavage at Arg^{306}, or by preventing the kinetically more favourable inhibitory cleavage at Arg_{506} [272, 273].

The surprisingly high prevalence of APC-R in the general population, ranging from 3 to 10% [274–276], suggests that a positive genetic selection has occurred conferring an evolutionary advantage in such situations as traumatic injury and pregnancy [275]. The mutation is most common among Caucasians, while it is virtually absent in other races [277, 278]. APC-R is, therefore, likely to be the major cause of the high incidence of venous thrombosis in Western countries as compared to the incidence of thrombosis in African and Asian countries [277, 278]. The penetrance of thrombosis in APC resistant individuals is highly variable: some individuals never develop thrombosis, whereas others develop recurrent, severe thrombotic events at a young age [277]. Owing to its high prevalence, APC-R occasionally occurs in individuals with other genetic risk factors for thrombosis [279–281]. In general, individuals with combined defects are characterised by a more severe thrombotic picture than are individuals with a single-gene defect.

Correlation between APC-R and an increased risk of thrombosis was demonstrated by case-control studies [282–286]. In an extended family study, the APC-R phenotype was found in approximately 50% of the family members, which is consistent with an autosomal dominant mode of inheritance [284]. Homozygous carriers of APG-R are not uncommon. The homozygous abnormality appears much less severe than homozygous PC deficiency [287, 288].

The prevalence of APC-R in patients with the first episode of venous thromboembolism is much higher than that of the other inherited abnormalities together, ranging from 15 to 40% [232, 281–286]. Moreover, the risk for recurrent thromboembolism in carriers of this abnormality is clinically and significantly higher than in patients without this abnormality, as shown by a recent prospective cohort study in a wide series of consecutive outpatients suffering the first episode of DVT and followed over years [232]. The cumulative incidence of recurrent thromboembolism in carriers of factor V Leiden mutation after eight years was 39.7% versus 18.3% in patients free from this abnormality (RR, 2.4).

Risk for venous thromboembolism in heterozygous carriers of factor V Leiden mutation increases with age at a rate significantly greater than that in non-carriers. In a recent prospective cohort study, incidence rate differences (per 1,000 person-years of observation) between affected and unaffected men increased significantly from 1.23 for those aged 50 to 59 years to 1.61 for those aged 60 to 69 years of age to 5.97 for those aged 70 years or older [289]. These findings indicate that determination of this abnormality in patients suffering an episode of venous thromboembolism should not be limited to young patients.

The risk of thrombosis is greatly increased among carriers of APC-R during pregnancy and when using oral contraceptives [113, 187, 290]. In a retrospective study, the APC-resistance phenotype was found in 60% of women with thromboembolic complications during pregnancy and in 30% of women with thrombosis occurring during oral contraceptive usage [290]. It has been calculated that women with heterozygosity for the factor V Leiden mutation who use oral contraceptives have a 35 to 50-fold increased risk of thrombosis, whereas homozygous women taking oral contraceptives have a several hundred-fold increased risk of thrombosis [291, 292]. The risk is reported to vary with the type of progestagen used, being higher if the oral contraceptives contain desoges-

15

trel or gestodene [113]. In addition, carriers of factor V Leiden have an increased risk of foetal loss (miscarriage or stillbirth) [293, 294].

Hyperhomocysteinemia

Homocysteine is a sulfydryl amino acid derived from metabolic conversion of methionine. Its intracellular metabolism occurs through remethylation to methionine or transulfuration to cysteine. In the transulfuration pathway, homocysteine is transformed by cystathionine-β-synthase into cystathionine, with pyridoxine acting as a cofactor [231, 295]. Severe hyperhomocysteinemia is usually the result of homozygous cystathionine-β-synthase deficiency, which has a frequency in the general population of 1:200,000 to 1:335,000 [295]. Patients who are homozygotes for cystathionine-β-synthase deficiency develop the classic syndrome of homocystinuria, including premature vascular disease and thrombosis, mental retardation, ectopic lens, and skeletal abnormalities [295].

In recent years, it has been found that inheriting only one functional cystathionine-β-synthase gene can also result in hyperhomocysteinemia, although to a moderate degree. Heterozygous deficiency results in about 50 % of normal enzyme activity, which appears to be adequate to protect against neurologic defects. Recently, it has been shown that individuals who are homozygous for the thermolabile variant of the methylene tetrahydrofolate reductase gene, which results from a common mutation Ala^{677}-Val, also have significantly elevated plasma homocysteine levels [296]. Hyperhomocysteinemia may be the consequence of a hereditary defect in the enzymes involved in methionine metabolism or may result from vitamin deficiency, such as nutritional deficiencies of cobalamin, folate, or pyridoxine. The incidence of mild-to-moderate hyperhomocysteinemia is estimated to be between 0.3 and 1.4 % in the general population [297].

The underlying mechanism by which hyperhomocysteinemia may contribute to thrombosis is unknown. In tissue culture studies, high levels of homocysteine contribute to endothelial damage, but the concentration required for this effect is much higher than that usually observed in vivo [298 – 300]. Recent observations suggest that homocysteine downregulates the endothelial thrombomodulin-protein C pathway and enhances factor V dependent activation of coagulation on the surface of endothelial cells [301, 302]. As epidemiological evidence accumulates supporting a role for homocysteine in circulatory diseases, there is a greater need for studies of the mechanism of action.

In contrast to the extensive documentation available on the risk for arterial disease in patients affected by hyperhomocysteinemia [303 – 305], the association between high levels of homocysteine and occurrence of venous thromboembolism has remained unclear until recently [306 – 308]. Two recent case-control studies have showed a strong association of high plasma homocysteine levels with the occurrence of DVT [309, 310]. In addition, individuals with hyperhomocysteinemia who also carry factor V Leiden are at significantly increased risk of developing thromboembolic events compared with those with neither or only one of these abnormalities. In a recent prospective cohort of initially healthy men, the risk of developing idiopathic venous thromboembolism was 20 times higher among hyperhomocysteinemic patients with factor V Leiden than among individuals without either defect [281].

The prevalence of hyperhomocysteinemia in young patients with venous thromboembolism is unexpectedly high, ranging from 13 to 19 % [311, 312]. Finally, this disorder is associated with the risk of recurrent venous thromboembolism [313, 314].

Natural history of venous thromboembolism

The classic study of the epidemiology of a disease is closely linked to the natural history of the condition. Natural history refers to the evolution of disease in the absence of medical intervention. In the field of venous thromboembolism, these observational aspects are often compromised by interventions. Thus, the definition "clinical course" is likely more appropriate for the description of long-term outcomes of venous thromboembolic disorders.

For practical purposes, we will discuss separately the clinical course of PE, that of isolated calf vein thrombosis and, finally, the clinical course of thrombosis involving the proximal-vein system.

Clinical course of pulmonary embolism

The natural course of acute PE depends primarily on whether the embolism has been detected and (appropriately) treated. Among factors effecting the natural course of acute PE, the most important are the extent of embolic obstruction, the degree of hemodynamic severity, the previous state of the cardiopulmonary system, the age of the embolus, and the degree of spontaneous thrombolytic activity of the patient's pulmonary vasculature endothelium [315].

Mortality

Treatment exerts a major effect on thrombosis. It is generally acknowledged that most patients with PE who are adequately anticoagulated survive the acute episode [10, 316, 317]. It is, however, to be specified that most information comes from studies that have evaluated patients who survived at least a couple of hours after the onset of symptoms. Thus, currently available mortality rates are likely to underestimate the true incidence of PE-related death [10, 316, 317]. Mean mortality (one month) rates of treated and untreated PE are 8 and 30%, respectively [318]. Acute mortality is correlated with hypotension and right ventricular failure [319, 320]. In the absence of shock, the size of the PE as demonstrated by pulmonary angiography is not an independent predictor of mortality [320]. These data suggest the right ventricular pump response to acute PE (regardless of embolus size) is most important in determining acute survival [316]. Patients with pre-existing cardiac disease may not have sufficient right pump reserve to sustain an adequate cardiac output in the face of even a relatively small clot burden [321]. Thus, therapeutic measures that rapidly remove clot burden may restore right heart pump function acutely and improve acute survival [13, 322].

In a recent prospective cohort study, addressing 1-year follow-up of a wide series of patients with angiographically proven PE, Carson et al. observed a mortality rate of 24%, most deaths being observed in an early phase (22% within a week) [12]. The conditions associated with these deaths were cancer (RR = 3.8), left-sided congestive heart failure (RR = 2.7), and chronic lung disease (RR = 2.2). The most frequent causes of death were cancer (35%), infection (22%), and cardiac disease (17%), whereas only 2.5% of patients deceased because of PE.

Resolution and recurrences

Data regarding the degree and rate of PE resolution are conflicting. PE resolves by at least three principal mechanisms: fragmentation, dissolution by endogenous fibrinolytic mechanism, and recanalisation. The processes of dissolution and recanalisation are probably responsible for the late removal of embolic material, occurring within a few weeks following the acute episode [317].

Several studies using serial perfusion lung scans have documented progressive improvement in non-perfused lung segments with time, though the improvement rate is highly variable [319, 321, 323–325]. The rate of improvement of perfusion scans is influenced by the severity of the embolic event, the type of the pharmacological treatment, and the presence or the absence of underlying cardiopulmonary disorders. Most patients with PE show an improvement during the first month of treatment [323]. Approximately 50% of patients with submassive PE have a normal perfusion scan after three months of therapy, the remaining usually show significant improvement [325]. Patients with large emboli or cardiopulmonary disorders exhibit a slower rate of scintigraphic recovery and, sometimes, the perfusion scan never returns to normal [326].

Hemodynamic parameters, usually altered in the acute phase, revert progressively to normal. The improvement rate is greatly influenced by the severity of PE, by the presence of underlying cardiopulmonary disorders, and by delay of treatment [318, 321, 327]. The sooner the therapy is initiated, the faster is the regression of pulmonary hypertension in acute PE [315].

PE tends to recur in some treated patients. The UPET and USPET studies revealed that 15% of patients with acute massive PE had two or more previous minor attacks before a massive attack, and 20 % of treated patients were found to have signs of recurrent PE within the first two weeks [320, 328]. In their prospective follow-up study, Carson et al. showed that as many as 33 among 399 patients (8.3 %) experienced a new pulmonary thromboembolism in the first year following the initial episode [12]. Of them, 45 % died.

Development of chronic thromboembolic pulmonary hypertension

Chronic thromboembolic pulmonary hypertension is the result of single or recurrent pulmonary emboli arising from sites of venous thrombosis. The natural history of most emboli is to undergo total resolution, or resolution leaving minimal residua, with restoration of normal pulmonary hemodynamics [319, 329–332]. For reasons still unclear, the emboli in very few patients do not resolve completely; rather, they follow an aberrant path of organisation and recanalisation, leaving endothelialised residua that obstruct or significantly narrow major pulmonary arteries [333].

It has been estimated that less than 2 % of patients with PE develop chronic pulmonary hypertension [333]. Most acute pulmonary emboli involve the muscular pulmonary arteries at the lobular to third-order level (diameter, 0.3 to 1 mm). For chronic pulmonary hypertension to result, it has been estimated that 16,000 emboli of this size would need to permanently occlude the pulmonary vascular bed to a sufficient degree to raise the resting pulmonary artery pressure [334]. Thus, chronic pulmonary hypertension from acute pulmonary emboli is understandably rare.

Available data indicate that each year in the United States, approximately 600,000 individuals suffer a pulmonary embolic event. Approximately 150,000 of these patients die, leaving 450,000 patients a year a potential denominator. Assuming that 1–2 % of these patients fail to resolve appropriately, then 450–900 new individuals per year develop a chronic thromboembolic pulmonary hypertension [329, 335]. Prior to current surgical techniques, the prognosis of chronic thromboembolic pulmonary hypertension was related to the degree of pulmonary hypertension, being extremely serious in all patients with mean pulmonary artery pressure > 30 mm Hg [324]. Currently, thromboarteriectomy in selected patients has made this condition a potentially remediable one [333]. That is why this condition is probably suspected and recognised more frequently today than in the past. For a more extensive overview of this spectrum the reader is referred to chapter IV.3.

Clinical course of isolated calf-vein thrombosis

Calf vein thrombosis is usually asymptomatic. Calf vein thrombi are encountered regularly in hospitalised patients undergoing radiofibrinogen uptake test [36] and in asymptomatic postoperative orthopedic patients who undergo venography before discharge from the hospital [66]. The incidence of asymptomatic calf vein thrombi varies widely depending on the patient groups: it ranges from 5 to 30 % in general surgery, approximates 50 % in patients with paralytic stroke, and ranges from 40 to 70 % in major orthopedic surgery [336]. Most of these thrombi form at or soon after operation, but many disappear because they undergo spontaneous lysis [337] or embolise into the pulmonary circulation where they undergo spontaneous lysis. Contrary to popular opinion, calf vein thrombi are associated with pulmonary embolism that is detected postoperatively by pulmonary perfusion scanning in 20 % to 30 % of asymptomatic patients who have a positive leg scan of the calf veins [338, 339]. These emboli are small, almost always asymptomatic, and clinically unimportant. The long-term consequences of asymptomatic calf vein thrombosis are unknown but may not be entirely benign [336]. Thus a number of studies have investigated this problem and identified a history of hospital admission over the preceding 6 months as a major risk factor for the occurrence of DVT and PE in ambulatory patients who are seen at the emergency department with confirmed symptomatic venous thromboembolism [17]. It is possible that some of these patients have asymptomatic calf vein thrombosis when discharged from the hospital which then extends and becomes symptomatic during convalescence at home [336]. Whether untreated asymptomatic venous thrombi predispose to the postphlebitic syndrome is also debated. Recently, Anderson and Willie-Jorgensen, using plethysmography to assess venous function 5 to 8 years after operation in patients who had undergone postoperative radioactive fibrinogen leg scanning, found a significantly higher prevalence of impaired venous function in those patients who had asymptomatic venous thrombosis than in those who were free of thrombosis [340]. It is likely, however, that minimal calf vein thrombosis does not precipitate the post-thrombotic syndrome unless the thrombus extends into the large axial calf veins or into the proximal venous segment [336].

Symptomatic calf vein thrombi are usually larger than asymptomatic ones and are important because they occur in 10 to 45 % of symptomatic patients with proven venous thrombosis [341–343].

The fate of symptomatic isolated calf DVT is most likely not different from that observed in symptomatic patients with proximal DVT [344]. A 29% rate of symptomatic extension or recurrence has been reported for patients with symptomatic calf vein thrombosis if treated with an inadequate course of anticoagulants [345]. This recurrence rate was prevented by a 3-month course of anticoagulant therapy [345]. Therefore, patients with symptomatic calf vein thrombosis should be managed as usually recommended for those with proximal DVT. Irrespective of the adequacy of the initial treatment, up to 30% of patients with symptomatic calf vein thrombosis will develop thromboembolic recurrences and post-thrombotic sequelae over a 5-year follow-up period [11]. This rate does not differ from that observed in patients with proximal DVT [11].

Clinical course of thrombosis involving the proximal-vein system

Thrombosis involving the proximal-vein system is usually symptomatic. Patients with proximal-vein thrombosis are usually treated with an initial course of heparin or low-molecular-weight heparin (5 to 10 days) followed by three to six months of oral anticoagulant therapy [346]. This treatment regimen reduces the risk for short-term thromboembolic complications to approximately 5% [347–353].

In contrast with the extensive and uniform documentation on the short-term outcome of DVT, sparse and conflicting results are available about the long-term clinical course of this disease. Recurrent thromboembolism and the post-thrombotic syndrome (PTS) are the most important complications of DVT. The cost implications of such complications are relevant [354].

Long-term recurrent thromboembolism

In a recent large randomised clinical trial comparing six weeks of oral anticoagulant therapy with six months of therapy, patients with symptomatic DVT were followed for two years for recurrences and death [34]. This trial showed a substantial reduction in the risk for recurrent thromboembolism among patients in the 6-month group. However, there was no difference in the incidence of recurrent events in the two groups from six to 24 months after the initial episode. In both groups, there was a linear increase in the cumulative risk, corresponding to 5 to 6% annually. Furthermore, the overall rate of recurrence after two years was much lower among patients with temporary risk

factors than among those with permanent risk factors (6.6% vs. 18%), although there was a trend toward a higher rate of recurrent disease in patients with temporary risk factors in the 6-week group compared to the 6-month group (8.6% vs. 4.8%).

In a small prospective 12-year follow-up study in patients with symptomatic DVT (Zürich Study), venous thromboembolic recurrent events were observed in 14 (24%) of 58 patients [355]. None of these patients had a malignancy or other risk factors for venous thrombosis.

The long-term incidence of recurrent venous thromboembolism was determined in 355 consecutive patients with a first episode of venography confirmed DVT [11]. Patients were followed-up over a period of eight years. Potential risk factors associated with these outcomes were also assessed. A high risk of recurrent venous thromboembolic disease that persisted after the period of (anticoagulant) treatment was found, resulting in a cumulative incidence of 30% after eight years of follow-up. One of every five recurrent episodes was PE (which was fatal in more than half of them), and approximately one-third of the recurrent leg vein thromboses were in the previously asymptomatic leg. Patients with underlying malignancy or with defects that impaired coagulation inhibition were at a significantly higher risk for recurrences than patients without these features. As expected, a considerable number of patients had their initial DVT following surgery or trauma. The finding that these patients were at a significantly lower risk for recurrent venous thromboembolism indicates that these conditions are transient risk factors for DVT.

Post-thrombotic syndrome

The PTS is probably caused by a combination of venous hypertension, resulting from persisting venous obstruction and venous valves damage, and abnormal microcirculation [356]. The precise incidence of the PTS following confirmed DVT is unknown, but has varied between 20% and 100% in the published studies [357–367]. Thus far, most studies have been limited to small or retrospective series of patients. The lack of objective diagnostic criteria for the assessment of the PTS makes comparison of the studies difficult. Furthermore, in all studies the potential for bias was high due to either the selection of patients with extensive thrombotic disease or to failure to distinguish post-thrombotic sequelae from recurrent vein thrombosis.

Recently, the results of a prospective randomised Dutch study on the prevention of the PTS in patients with DVT have become available [368].

One hundred and ninety-four consecutive patients with confirmed proximal-vein thrombosis were randomly allocated to wear elastic compression stockings or not. The study was designed to have at least five years of follow-up. A predefined scoring system was used to classify two categories of patients: mild-to-moderate PTS and severe PTS. Median follow-up was 76 months in both groups. Mild-to-moderate PTS occurred in 19 (20%) of the 96 patients with stockings, and in 46 (47%) of the 98 patients without stockings (P < 0.001). Eleven (11.5%) patients in the stocking group developed the severe PTS while this occurred in 23 (23.5%) patients without stockings (P < 0.001). In both groups, the majority of this syndrome was documented within the first 24 months after the thrombotic event. The extent of the initial thrombus on venography was not related with the development of the PTS.

In 1996, data from the long-term follow-up of 355 consecutive symptomatic patients with a first episode of venography-proven DVT were published [11]. All patients were treated with full-dose (low-molecular-weight)heparin followed by at least three months of oral anticoagulation, and were instructed to wear elastic compression stockings as soon as possible after hospital discharge for at least two years. At each follow-up visit, the presence and severity of post-thrombotic signs and symptoms were scored using a standardised scale. Of the 355 patients, a total of 84 developed the PTS. Of these, 25 (30%) had severe post-thrombotic manifestations. The cumulative incidence of the PTS was 18% after one year and 24.5% after two years of follow-up. Hereafter, the incidence of the PTS increased gradually until 29.6% after five years. Subsequently, the incidence of the PTS did not increase substantially. Considering only severe post-thrombotic manifestations, a slightly different pattern was seen: the cumulative incidence increased gradually from 2.7% after one year to 8.1% after five years. Thereafter, severe PTS did not increase substantially. In the large majority of patients, post-thrombotic manifestations became apparent within the first two years following the acute episode of DVT. These findings, which challenge the general view that the PTS requires a long time to become manifest, are in agreement with those of the Dutch study [368].

The results of these studies also suggest that severe post-thrombotic manifestations are relatively rare following an episode of venous thrombosis in patients wearing elastic compression stockings and who are adequately treated with anticoagulants [11, 368]. These conclusions are supported by the findings of another recent study in which a cohort of 58 consecutive patients with DVT were prospectively followed up for a period of 12 years [355]. During this long follow-up period only 1 patient developed a severe PTS, while 37 patients had both clinical and hemodynamic normal findings.

Although it was expected that the extent of the initial thrombosis and the degree of thrombus occlusiveness would be associated with the risk of developing the PTS, this could not be demonstrated [11, 368]. Among factors associated with the development of the PTS, the strongest seems to be the development of ipsilateral recurrent DVT [11].

Mortality

The short-term mortality (three to six months) of patients suffering an episode of DVT is reported to range between 7 and 15% [347–353]. Causes of death include cancer, PE and major bleeding. Cancer accounts for the large majority of patients who die within the first months after DVT [347–353].

Recently, data from the long-term follow-up of 355 consecutive symptomatic patients with a first episode of DVT were published [11]. Out of the 355 patients, 90 died during follow-up. The causes of death in the patients who died included malignancy (n = 52), PE (n = 9), acute myocardial infarction or heart failure (n = 5), ischemic stroke (n = 10), anticoagulant-related hemorrhage (n = 2), miscellaneous (n = 6). In 6 patients, who died suddenly, a definite diagnosis could not be made.

Survival was 83.3% after one year and 80.1% after two years of follow-up. After 5 and 8 years the survival was 74.6 and 70.2%, respectively. The presence of malignancy increased the risk of death remarkably (RR = 8.1). Other clinical features showed no associations with mortality.

Mortality occurred mainly during the first year in patients with underlying malignancy. In fact, most patients who died did so because of a neoplastic disorder which was already known at the time of patient's presentation or which subsequently became manifest. These results are fully consistent with those of a similar study in patients with PE [12], and suggest that the occurrence of venous thromboembolism is strongly related to a bad prognosis in patients with cancer. Furthermore, 26 patients (most of them presenting with spontaneous DVT) died because of a neoplastic disease which became manifest after referral for venous thrombosis. These findings support previous observations, and suggest that a clinically relevant association exists between idiopathic vein thrombosis and subsequent overt malignant disease [86].

References

1. Kruit WHJ, de Boer AC, Sing AK, van Roon F. The significance of venography in the management of patients with clinically suspected pulmonary embolism. J Intern Med 1991; 230: 333–339

2. Hull RD, Hirsh J, Carter CJ, et al. Pulmonary angiography, ventilation lung scanning and venography for clinically suspected pulmonary embolism with abnormal perfusion lung scan. Ann Intern Med 1983; 98: 891–899

3. Dorfman GS, Cronan JJ, Tupper TB. Occult pulmonary embolism: a common occurrence in deep venous thrombosis. Am J Roentgenol 1987; 148: 263–266

4. Huisman MV, Büller HR, ten Cate JW, et al. Unexpected high prevalence of silent pulmonary embolism in patients with deep-vein thrombosis. Chest 1989; 95: 498–502

5. Kriemer Nielsen H, Husted SE, Krusell LR, Fasting H, Charles P, Hansen HH. Silent pulmonary embolism in patients with deep venous thrombosis. Incidence and fate in a randomized, controlled trial of anticoagulation versus no anticoagulation. J Int Med 1994; 235: 457–461

6. Moser KM, Fedullo PF, LitteJohn JK, Crawford R. Frequent asymptomatic pulmonary embolism in patients with deep venous thrombosis. JAMA 1994; 271: 223–225

7. Prandoni P, Polistena P, Bernanrdi E, et al. Upper-extremity deep vein thrombosis. Risk factors, diagnosis, and complications. Arch Intern Med 1997; 157: 57–62

8. Monreal M, Raventos A, Lerma R, et al. Pulmonary embolism in patients with upper extremity deep venous thrombosis associated to central venous lines: a prospective study. Thromb Haemost 1994; 72: 548–550

9. Monreal M, Lafoz E, Ruiz J, Valls R, Alasstrue A. Upper extremity deep venous thrombosis and pulmonary embolism: a prospective study. Chest 1991; 99: 280–283

10. Salzman EW, Hirsh J. The epidemiology, pathogenesis, and natural history of venous thrombosis. In: Colman RW, Hirsh J, Marder V, Salzman EW (eds): Thrombosis and Haemostasis. Basic principles and clinical practice. JB Lippincott, Philadelphia, 1993: 1275–1296

11. Prandoni P, Lensing AWA, Cogo A, et al. The long-term clinical course of acute deep venous thrombosis. Ann Intern Med 1996; 125: 1–7

12. Carson JL, Kelley MA, Duff A, et al. The clinical course of pulmonary embolism. N Engl J Med 1992; 326: 1240–1245

13. Ten Cate JW. Thrombolytic treatment of pulmonary embolism. Lancet 1993; 341: 1315–1316

14. Hirsh H, Hoak J. Management of deep vein thrombosis and pulmonary embolism. A statement for healthcare professionals. Circulation 1996; 93: 2212–2245

15. Gillum RF. Pulmonary embolism and thrombophlebitis in the United States, 1970–1985. Am Heart J 1987; 114: 1262–1264

16. Coon WW, Willis PW, Keller JB. Venous thromboembolism and other venous diseases in the Tecumseh Community Health Study. Circulation 1973; 48: 839–846

17. Anderson FA, Wheeler HB, Goldberg RJ, et al. A population-based perspective of the hospital incidence and case-fatality rates of deep vein thrombosis and pulmonary embolism. The Worcester DVT study. Arch Intern Med 1991; 151: 933–938

18. Weinman EE, Salzman EW. Deep-vein thrombosis. N Engl J Med 1994; 31: 1630–1641

19. Nordström M, Lindbläd B, Bergqvist D, Kjellström T. A prospective study of the incidence of deep-vein thrombosis within a defined urban population. J Intern Med 1992; 232: 155–160

20. Cohen AT, Edmondson RA, Phillips MJ, Ward VP, Kakkar VV. The changing pattern of venous thromboembolic disease. Haemostasis 1996; 26: 65–71

21. Soskolne CL, Wong AW, Lilienfeld DE. Trends in pulmonary embolism death rates fro Canada and the United States, 1962–87. Can Med Assoc 1990; 142: 321–324

22. Lilienfeld DE, Godbold JH, Burke GL, Sprafka JM, Pham DL, Baxter J. Hospitalization and case fatality for pulmonary embolism in the twin cities: 1979–1984. Am Heart J 1990; 120: 392–395

23. Stein PD, Henry JW. Prevalence of acute pulmonary embolism among patients in a general hospital and at autopsy. Chest 1995; 108: 978–981

24. Karwinski B, Svendsen E. Comparison of clinical and post-mortem diagnosis of pulmonary embolism. J Clin Pathol 1989; 42: 135–139

25. Bussani R, Cosatti C. L'embolia polmonare: analisi epidemiologica su 27 410 soggetti sottoposti ad autopsia nel corso di 10 anni. Medicina 1990; 10: 40–43

26. Moser KM. Venous Thromboembolism. Am Rev Respir Dis 1990; 141: 235–249

27. Goldhaber SZ, Savage DD, Garrison RJ, et al. Risk factors for pulmonary embolism. The Framingham Study. Am J Med 1983; 74: 1023–1028

28. Kniffin WD, Baron JA, Barrett J, Birkmeyer JD, Anderson FA. The epidemiology of diagnosed pulmonary embolism and deep venous thrombosis in the elderly. Arch Intern Med 1994; 154: 861–866

29. Siddique RM, Siddique MI, Connors AF, Rimm AA. Thirty-day case-fatality rates for pulmonary embolism in the elderly. Arch Intern Med 1996; 156: 2343–2347

30. Carter CJ. Epidemiology of venous thromboembolism. In: Hull R, Pineo GF (eds). Disorders of thrombosis. WB Saunders Company, Philadelphia, 1996: 159–174

31. Nicolaides AN, Irving D. Clinical factors and the risk of deep venous thrombosis. In: Nicolaides AN (ed). Thromboembolism: Aetiology, advances in prevention and management. MTP Press, Lancaster, 1975: 193–204

32. Cogo A, Bernardi E, Prandoni P, et al. Acquired risk factors for deep-vein thrombosis. Arch Intern Med 1994; 154: 164–168

33. Pahor M, Guralnik JM, Havlik RJ, et al. Alcohol consumption and risk of deep venous thrombosis and pulmonary embolism in older persons. J Am Geriatr Soc 1996; 44: 1030–1037

34. Schulman S, Rhedin AS, Lindmarker P, et al. A comparison of six weeks with six months of oral anticoagulant therapy after a first episode of venous thromboembolism. N Engl J Med 1995; 332: 1661–1665

35. Levine MN, Hirsh J, Gent M, et al. Optimal duration of oral anticoagulant therapy: a randomized trial comparing four weeks with three months of warfarin in patients with proximal deep vein thrombosis. Thromb Haemost 1995; 74: 606–611

36. Kakkar VV, Howe CT, Nicolaides AN, Renney JTG, Clarke MB. Deep vein thrombosis of the leg. Is there a "high risk group"? Am J Surg 1970; 120: 527–530

37. Flordal PA, Bergqvist D, Burmark US, Ljungström KG, Törngren S. Risk factors for major thromboembolism and bleeding tendency after elective general surgical operations. Eur J Surg 1996; 162: 783–789

38. Coon WW, Willis W. Recurrency of venous thromboembolism. Surgery 1973; 73: 823–827

39. Scurr JH, Coleridge-Smith PD, Hasty JH. Deep venous thrombosis: a continuing problem. Br Med J 1988; 297: 28–30

40. European Consensus Statement. Prevention of venous thromboembolism. Intern Angiol 1997; 16: 3–38

41. Paltiel O. Epidemiology of venous thromboembolism. In: Leclerc JR (ed): Venous thromboembolic disorders. Fea & Febiger, Philadelphia 1991: 141–165

42. Warlow C, Ogston D, Douglas AS. Venous thrombosis following strokes. Lancet 1972; 1: 1305–1306

43. Anderson FA, Wheeler HB, Goldberg RJ, Hosmer DW, Forcier A. The prevalence of risk factors for venous thromboembolism among hospital patients. Arch Intern Med 1992; 152: 1660–1664

44. De Boer K, Büller HR, ten Cate JW, Levi M. Deep vein thrombosis in obstetric patients: diagnosis and risk factors. Thromb Haemost 1992; 67: 4–7

45. Janssen HF, Schachner J, Hubbard J, Hartman JT. The risk of deep venous thrombosis: a computerized epidemiologic approach. Surgery 1986; 101: 205–212

46. Sigel B, Ipsen J, Felix WR Jr: The epidemiology of lower extremity deep venous thrombosis in surgical patients. Ann Surg 1974; 179: 278–290

47. Büller HR, Lensing AWA, Hirsh J, ten Cate JW. Deep vein thrombosis: new non-invasive diagnostic tests. Thromb Haemost 1991; 66: 133–137

48. Bounameaux H, Huber O, Khabiri E, Schneider PA, Didier D, Rohner A. Unexpectedly high rate of phlebographic deep venous thrombosis following elective general abdominal surgery among patients given prophylaxis with low-molecular-weight heparin. Arch Surg 1993; 128: 326–328

49. Clagett GP, Anderson FA, Heit J, Levine MN, Salzman EW, Wheeler HB. Prevention of venous thromboembolism. Chest 1995; 108 (Suppl. 4): 312–334

50. Creasman WT, Weed JC. Radical hysterectomy. In: Schaefer G, Graber EA, Hagerstown MD (eds). Complications in obstetrics and gynecologic surgery. Harper and Row, 1981: 389–400

51. Report of the National Confidential Enquiry into Perioperative Deaths. 1991/92. London: HMSO, 1993

52. Harris WH, Athanasoulis CA, Waltman AC, Salzman EW. Prophylaxis of deep-vein thrombosis after total hip replacement. J Bone Joint Surg 1985; 7A: 57–62

53. Turpie AGG, Levine MN, Hirsh J, et al. A randomized controlled trial of a low-molecular-weight-heparin (enoxaparin) to prevent deep-vein thrombosis in patients undergoing elective hip surgery. N Engl J Med 1986; 315: 925–929

54. Sautter RD, Koch EL, Myers WO, et al. Aspirin-sulfinpyrazone in prophylaxis of deep venous thrombosis in total hip replacement. JAMA 1983; 250: 2649–2654

55. Hull RD, Raskob GE, Gent M, et al. Effectiveness of intermittent pneumatic leg compression for preventing deep-vein thrombosis after total hip replacement. JAMA 1990; 263: 2313–2317

56. Hoek JA, Nurmohamed MT, Hamelynck KJ, et al. Prevention of deep vein thrombosis following total hip replacement by low molecular weight heparinoid. Thromb Haemost 1992; 67: 28–32

57. Powers PJ, Gent M, Jay RM, et al. A randomized trial of less intensive postoperative warfarin or aspirin therapy in the prevention of venous thromboembolism after surgery for fractured hip. Arch Intern Med 1989; 149: 771–774

58. Agnelli G, Volpato R, Radicchia S, et al. Accuracy of real-time B-mode ultrasonography in the diagnosis of asymptomatic deep vein thrombosis in hip surgery patients. Thromb Haemost 1991; 65: 17–28

59. Geerts W, Code KI, Jay RM, Chen E, Szalai JP. A prospective study of venous thromboembolism after major trauma. N Engl J Med 1994; 331: 1601–1606

60. Hull RD, Delmore TJ, Hirsh J, et al. Effectiveness of intermittent pulsatile stockings for the prevention of calf and thigh vein thrombosis in patients undergoing elective knee surgery. Thromb Res 1979; 16: 37–45

61. Francis CW, Marder VJ, McCollister EC, Yaukoolbodi S. Two-step warfarin therapy. Prevention of postoperative venous thrombosis without excessive bleeding. JAMA 1983; 249: 374–378

62. Stulberg BN, Insall JN, Williams GW, et al. Deep-vein thrombosis following total knee replacement. J Bone Joint Surg 1984; 66: 194–200

63. Williams JW, Eikman EA, Greenberg S. Asymptomatic pulmonary embolism. Ann Surg 1982; 195: 323–327

64. Gallus AS, Salzman EW, Hirsh J. Prevention of venous thromboembolism. In: Colman RW, Hirsh J, Marder VJ, Salzman EW (eds). Hemostasis and Thrombosis. Basic principles and clinical practice. JH Lippincott Company, Philadelphia, 1993: 1331–1345

65. Turpie AGG, Leclerc JR. Prophylaxis of venous thromboembolism. In: Leclerc JR (ed). Venous thromboembolic disorders. Lea & Febiger, Philadelphia, 1991: 303–345

66. Prandoni P, Goldhaber SZ, Piccioli A, Girolami A. Prevention of venous thromboembolism in major orthopedic surgery. Clin Appl Thromb/Haemost 1996; 3: 153–157

67. Hull R, Raskob G, Pineo G, et al. A comparison of subcutaneous low-molecular-weight heparin with warfarin sodium for prophylaxis against deep-vein thrombosis after hip or knee implantation. N Engl J Med 1993; 329: 1370–1376

68. Leclerc JR, Geerts WH, Desjardins L, et al. Prevention of venous thromboembolism after knee arthroplasty. A randomized, double-blind trial comparing enoxaparin with warfarin. Ann Intern Med 1996; 124: 619–626

69. Hamulyak K, Lensing AWA, van der Meer J, Smid WM, van Ooy A, Hoek JA. Subcutaneous low-molecular-weight heparin or oral anticoagulants for the prevention of deep-vein thrombosis in elective hip and knee replacement. Thromb Haemost 1995; 74: 1428–1431

70. Hamilton MG, Hull RD, Pineo GF. Venous thromboembolism in neurosurgery and neurology patients: a review. Neurosurgery 1994; 34: 280–296

71. Nurmohamed MT, van Riel AM, Henkens C, et al. Low molecular weight heparin and compression stockings in the prevention of venous thromboembolism in neurosurgery. Thromb Haemost 1996; 75: 233–238

72. Jackman FR, Perry BJ, Siddons H. Deep vein thrombosis after thoracotomy. Thorax 1978; 33: 761–765

73. Killewich LA, Aswad MA, Sandager RN, Lilly MP, Flinn WR. A randomized, prospective trial of deep venous thrombosis prophylaxis in aortic surgery. Arch Surg 1997; 132: 499–504

74. Geerts WH, Jay RM, Code KI, et al. A comparison of low-dose heparin with low-molecular-weight heparin as prophylaxis against venous thromboembolism after major trauma. N Engl J Med 1996; 335: 701–707

75. Sproul EE. Carcinoma and venous thrombosis: the frequency of association of carcinoma in the body or tail of the pancreas with multiple venous thrombosis. Am J Cancer 1938; 34: 566–585

76. Ambrus JL, Ambrus CM, Mink IB, Pickren JW. Causes of death in cancer patients. J Med 1975; 6: 61–64

77. Hills NH, Pflug JJ, Jeyasingh K, Boardman L, Calnan JS. Prevention of deep vein thrombosis by intermittent pneumatic compression of calf. Br Med J 1972; 1: 131–135

78. Walsh JJ, Bonnar J, Wright FW. A study of pulmonary embolism and deep vein thrombosis after major gynaecological surgery using labelled fibrinogen-phlebography and lung scanning. J Obstet Gynaecol Br Commonw 1974; 81: 311–316

79. Sue-Ling HM, Johnston D, McMahon MU, Philips PR, Davies JA. Preoperative identification of patients at high risk of deep venous thrombosis after elective major abdominal surgery. Lancet 1986; 1: 1173–1176

80. Rosemberg IL, Evans M, Pollock AV. Prophylaxis of postoperative leg vein thrombosis by low-dose subcutaneous heparin or peroperative calf muscle stimulation: a controlled clinical trial. Br Med J 1975; 1: 649–651

81. Allan A, Williams JT, Bolton JP, Le Quesne LP. The use of graduated compression stockings in the prevention of postoperative deep vein thrombosis. Br J Surg 1983; 70: 172–174

82. Multicentre Trial. Dihydroergotamine-heparin prophylaxis of postoperative deep vein thrombosis. JAMA 1984; 251: 2960–2966

83. Nand S, Fischer SG, Salgia R, Fisher RI. Hemostatic abnormalities in untreated cancer: incidence and correlation with thrombotic and hemorrhagic complications. J Clin Oncol 1987; 5: 1998–2003

84. Nanninga PB, van Teunenbroek A, Veenhof CHN, Büller HR, ten Cate JW. Low prevalence of coagulation and fibrinolytic activation in patients with primary untreated cancer. Thromb Haemost 1990; 64: 361–364

85. Luzzatto G, Schafer AI. The prethrombotic state in cancer. Semin Oncol 1990; 17: 147–159

86. Prandoni P, Lensing AWA, Büller HR, et al. Deep-vein thrombosis and the incidence of subsequent symptomatic cancer. N Engl J Med 1992; 327: 1128–1133

87. Baron JA, Gridley G, Weiderpass E, et al. Venous thromboembolism and cancer. Lancet 1998; 351: 1077–1080

88. Sørensen HT, Mellemkjaer L, Steffensen FM, et al. The risk of a diagnosis of cancer after primary deep venous thrombosis or pulmonary embolism. N Eng J Med 1998; 338: 1169–1173

89. Büller H, Ten Cate JW. Primary venous thromboembolism and cancer screening (Editorial). N Engl J Med 1998; 338: 1221–1222

90. Shen VS, Pollak EW. Fatal pulmonary embolism in cancer patients: is heparin prophylaxis justified? South Med J 1980; 73: 841–843

91. Huber O, Bounameaux H, Borst F, Rohner A. Postoperative pulmonary embolism after hospital discharge. An underestimated risk. Arch Surg 1992; 127: 310–313

92. Godwin J. Use of low molecular weight heparins in malignancy-related thromboembolic disorders: a clinical review. Clin Appl Thromb/Haemost 1996; 2 (Suppl.1): 28–34

93. Bergqvist D, Burmark US, Flordal PA, et al. Low molecular weight heparin started before surgery as prophylaxis against deep vein thrombosis: 2500 versus 5000 XaI units in 2070 patients. Br J Surg 1995; 82: 496–501

94. Weiss RB, Tormey DC, Holland JF, Weinberg VE. Venous thrombosis during multimodal treatment of primary breast carcinoma. Cancer Treat Rep 1981; 65: 677–679

95. Goodnough LT, Saito H, Manni A, Jones PK, Pearson OH. Increased incidence of thromboembolism in stage IV breast cancer patients treated with a five-drug chemotherapy regimen: a study of 159 patients. Cancer 1984; 54: 1264–1268

96. Levine MN, Gent M, Hirsh J, et al. The thrombogenic effect of anticancer drug therapy in women with stage II breast cancer. N Engl J Med 1988; 318: 404–407

97. Saphner T, Tormey DC, Gray R. Venous and arterial thrombosis in patients who received adjuvant therapy for breast cancer. J Clin Oncol 1991; 9: 286–294

98. Pritchard KI, Paterson AHG, Paul NA, Zee B, Fine S, Pater J. Increased thromboembolic complications with concurrent tamoxifen and chemotherapy in a randomized trial of adjuvant therapy for women with breast cancer. J Clin Oncol 1996; 14: 2731–2737

99. Levine MN, Hirsh J, Gent M, et al. Double-blind randomized trial of very-low-dose warfarin for prevention of thromboembolism in stage IV breast cancer. Lancet 1994; 343: 886–889

100. Lokich JJ, Becker B. Subclavian vein thrombosis in patients treated with infusion chemotherapy for advanced malignancy. Cancer 1983; 52: 1586–1589

101. Bern MM, Bothe ARJr, Bistrian B, Champagne CD, Keane MS, Blackburn GL. Prophylaxis against central vein thrombosis with low-dose warfarin. Surgery 1986; 99: 216–221

102. Bern MM, Lokich JJ, Wallach SR, et al. Very low doses of warfarin can prevent thrombosis in central venous catheters. Ann Intern Med 1990; 112: 423–428

103. Monreal M, Alastrue A, Rull M, et al. Upper extremity deep venous thrombosis in cancer patients with venous access devices. Prophylaxis with a low molecular weight heparin (Fragmin). Thromb Haemost 1996; 75: 251–253

104. Prandoni P. Antithrombotic strategies in patients with cancer. Thromb Haemost 1997; 78: 141–144

105. The Columbus Investigators. Low molecular weight heparin in the treatment of patients with venous thromboembolism. N Engl J Med 1997; 337: 657–662

106. Drill VA, Calhoun DW. Oral contraceptives and thromboembolic disease. JAMA 1968; 206: 77–84

107. Koster T, Small RA, Rosendaal FR, Helmerhorst FM. Oral contraceptives and venous thromboembolism: a quantitative discussion of the uncertainties. J Intern Med 1995; 238: 31–37

108. World Health Organization Collaborative Study of Cardiovascular Disease and Steroid Hormone Contraception. Venous thromboembolic disease and combined oral contraceptives: results of international multicentre case-control study. Lancet 1995; 346: 1575–1582

109. World Health Organization Collaborative Study of Cardiovascular Disease and Steroid Hormone Contraception. Effect of different progestagens in low oestrogen oral contraceptives on venous thromboembolic disease. Lancet 1995; 346: 1582–1588

110. Spitzer WO, Lewis MA, Heinemann LAJ, Thorogood M, MacRae KD. Third generation oral contraceptives and risk of venous thromboembolic disorders: an international case-control study. Br Med J 1996; 312: 83–88

111. Jick H, Jick SS, Gurewich V, Myers MW, Vasilakis C. Risk of idiopathic cardiovascular death and non fatal venous thromboembolism in women using oral contraceptives with different progestagen components. Lancet 1995; 346: 1589–1593

112. Weiss N. Third-generation oral contraceptives: how risky? Lancet 1995; 346: 1570

113. Bloemenkamp KWM, Rosendaal FR, Helmerhorst FM, Büller HR, Vandenbroucke JP. Enhancement by factor V Leiden mutation of risk of deep-vein thrombosis associated with oral contraceptives containing a third-generation progestagen. Lancet 1995; 346: 1593–1596

114. Goldhaber SZ. Epidemiology of pulmonary embolism and deep vein thrombosis. In: Bloom AL, Forbes CD, Thomas DP, Tuddenham EGD (eds). Haemostasis and Thrombosis. Churchill Livingstone, Edinburgh, 1994: 1275–1296

115. Daly E, Vessey MP, Hawkins MM, Carson JL, Gough P, Marsh S. Risk of venous thromboembolism in users of hormone replacement therapy. Lancet 1996; 348: 977–980

116. Jick H, Derby LE, Myers MW, Vasilakis C, Newton KM. Risk of hospital admission for idiopathic venous thromboembolism among users of postmenopausal oestrogens. Lancet 1996; 348: 981–983

117. Grodstein F, Stampfer MJ, Goldhaber SZ, et al. Prospective study of exogenous hormones and risk of pulmonary embolism in women. Lancet 1996; 348: 983–987

118. Pérez Gutthann S, García Rodríguez LA, Castellsague J, Duque Oliart A. Hormone replacement therapy and risk of venous thromboembolism: population based case-control study. Br Med J 1997; 314: 796–800

119. Vandenbroucke JP, Helmerhorst FM. Risk of venous thrombosis with hormone-replacement therapy. Lancet 1996; 348: 972

120. Rosing J, Tans G, Nicolaes AF, et al. Oral contraceptives and venous thrombosis: different sensitivities to activated protein C in women using second- and third-generation oral contraceptives. Br J Haematol 1997; 97: 233–238

121. Thromboembolic Risk Factors Consensus Group: Risk of and prophylaxis for venous thromboembolism in hospital patients. Br Med J 1992; 79: 1–17

122. Bergmann JF, Elkharrat D. Prevention of venous thromboembolic risk in non-surgical patients. Haemostasis 1996; 26 (Suppl. 2): 16–23

123. Gross JS, Neufeld RR, Libow LS, Gerber I, Rodstein M. Autopsy study of the elderly institutionalised patients. Arch Intern Med 1988; 48: 173–176

124. Rubinstein I, Murray D, Hoffstein V. Fatal pulmonary emboli in hospitalized patients. An autopsy study. Arch Intern Med 1988; 148: 1425–1426

125. Brown M, Glassenberg M. Mortality factors in patients with acute stroke. JAMA 1973; 224: 1493–1495

126. McCarthy ST, Turner JJ, Robertson D, et al. Low dose heparin as a prophylaxis against deep vein thrombosis after acute stroke. Lancet 1977; 2: 800–801

127. Prins MH, den Ottolander GJH, Gelsema R, et al. Prophylaxis of deep venous thrombosis with a low molecular weight heparin (Kabi 2165) in stroke patients. Haemostasis 1989; 19: 245–250

128. Sandset PM, Dahl T, Stiris M, Rostad B, Scheel B, Abildgaard U. A double-blind and randomized placebo-controlled trial of low molecular weight heparin once daily to prevent deep-vein thrombosis in acute ischemic stroke. Semin Thromb Haemost 1990; 16 (Suppl.): 25–33

129. Dumas R, Woitinas F, Kutnowski M, et al. A multicentre, double-blind, randomized study to compare the safety and efficacy of once-daily ORG 10172 and twice-daily low-dose heparin in preventing deep-vein thrombosis in patients with acute ischaemic stroke. Age Ageing 1994: 23: 512–516

130. McCarthy ST, Turner J. Low-dose subcutaneous heparin in the prevention of deep-vein thrombosis and pulmonary emboli following acute stroke. Age Ageing 1986; 15: 84–88

131. Turpie AGG. Orgaran in the prevention of deep vein thrombosis in stroke patients. Haemostasis 1992; 22: 92–98

132. Turpie AGG, Gent M, Côte R, et al. A low molecular weight heparinoid compared with unfractionated heparin in the prevention of deep vein thrombosis in patients with acute ischemic stroke. Ann Intern Med 1992; 117: 353–357

133. Turpie AGG, Levine MN, Hirsh J, et al. A double-blind randomized trial of ORG 10172 low molecular weight heparinoid in the prevention of deep vein thrombosis in thrombotic stroke. Lancet 1987; 1: 523–526

134. Waring WP, Karunas RS. Acute spinal cord injury and the incidence of clinically occurring thromboembolic disease. Paraplegia 1991; 29: 8–16

135. Green D, Lee MY, Ito VY, et al. Fixed- vs adjusted-dose heparin in the prophylaxis of thromboembolism in spinal cord injury. JAMA 1988; 260: 1255–1258

136. Green D, Lee MY, Lim AC, et al. Prevention of thromboembolism after spinal cord injury using low-molecular weight heparin. JAMA 1990; 113: 571–574

137. Merli GJ, Crabbe S, Doyle L, et al. Mechanical plus pharmacological prophylaxis for deep vein thrombosis in acute spinal cord injury. Paraplegia 1992; 30: 558–562

138. Anderson GM, Hull E: The effect of Dicumarol upon the mortality and incidence of thromboembolic complications in congestive heart failure. Am Heart J 1950; 39: 697–702

139. Harvey WP, Finch CA. Dicumarol prophylaxis in thromboembolic disease in congestive heart failure. N Engl J Med 1950; 242: 208–211

140. Belch JJ, Lowe GDO, Ward AG, et al. Prevention of deep venous thrombosis in medical patients by low-dose heparin. Scott Med J 1981; 26: 115–117

141. Emerson PA, Marks P. Prevention of thromboembolism after myocardial infarction: effect of low-dose heparin or smoking. Br Med J 1977; 1: 18–20

142. Marks P, Teather D. Subcutaneous heparin: a logical prophylaxis for deep-vein thrombosis after myocardial infarction. Practitioner 1978; 220: 425–429

143. Murray TS, Lorimer AR, Cox FC, Lawrie TDV. Leg vein thrombosis following myocardial infarction. Lancet 1970; 2: 792–793

144. Simmons AV, Sheppard MA, Cox AF. Deep venous thrombosis after myocardial infarction. Predisposing factors. Br Heart J 1973; 35: 623–625

145. Warlow C, Beattie AG, Terry G, Ogston D, Kenmure AC, Douglas AS. A double-blind trial of low doses of subcutaneous heparin in the prevention of deep-vein thrombosis after myocardial infarction. Lancet 1973; 2: 934–936

146. Pitt A, Anderson ST, Habersberger PG, Rosengarten DS. Low-dose heparin in the prevention of deep-vein thromboses in patients with acute myocardial infarction. Am Heart J 1980; 99: 574–579

147. Harvey WP, Finch CA. Dicumarol prophylaxis of thromboembolic disease in congestive heart failure. N Engl J Med 1950; 242: 208–211

148. Medical Research Council. Assessment of short-term anticoagulant administration after cardiac infarction. Br Med J 1969; 1: 335–342

149. Drapkin A, Merskey C. Anticoagulant therapy after acute myocardial infarction. JAMA 1972; 222: 541–548

150. Veterans Administration. Anticoagulants in acute myocardial infarction. JAMA 1973; 225: 724–729

151. Gallus AS, Hirsh J, Tuttle RJ, et al. Small subcutaneous doses of heparin in prevention of venous thrombosis. N Engl J Med 1973; 288: 545–551

152. Bergmann JF, Neuhart E. A multicenter randomized double-blind study of enoxaparin compared with unfractionated heparin in the prevention of venous thromboembolic disease in elderly in-patients bedridden for an acute medical illness. Thromb Haemost 1996; 76: 529–534

153. Moser KM, LeMoine JR, Nachtwey FJ, Spragg RG. Deep venous thrombosis and pulmonary embolism. Frequency in a respiratory intensive care unit. JAMA 1981; 246: 1422–1424

154. Ibarra-Perez C, Lau-Cortes E, Colmenero-Zubiate S, et al. Prevalence and prevention of deep venous thrombosis of the lower extremities in high-risk pulmonary patients. Angiology 1988; 39: 505–513

155. Cade JF. High risk of the critically ill for venous thromboembolism. Crit Care Med 1982; 10: 448–450

156. Hirsch DR, Ingenito EP, Goldhaber SZ. Prevalence of deep venous thrombosis among patients in medical intensive care. JAMA 1995; 274: 335–337

157. Halkin H, Goldberg J, Modan M, Modan B. Reduction of mortality in general medical in-patients by low-dose heparin prophylaxis. Ann Intern Med 1982; 6: 561–565

158. Caulin C. The influence of CY216 administration on hospital mortality of general medical in-patients. In: Breddin K, Fareed J, Samama M (eds). Fraxiparine. First International Symposium. Schattauer, Stuttgart, 1989: 149–154

159. Gärdlund B. Randomised, controlled trial of low-dose heparin for prevention of fatal pulmonary embolism in patients with infectious diseases. Lancet 1996; 347: 1357–1361

160. Dahan R, Houlbert D, Caulin C, et al. Prevention of deep-vein thrombosis in elderly patients by a low-molecular-weight heparin: a randomized double-blind trial. Haemostasis 1986; 16: 159–164

161. Harenberg J, Roebruck P, Heene DL. Subcutaneous low-molecular-weight heparin versus standard heparin and the prevention of thromboembolism in medical inpatients. Haemostasis 1996; 26: 127–139

162. Triplett DA. Antiphospholipid-protein antibodies: laboratory detection and clinical relevance. Thromb Res 1995; 78: 1–31

163. Long AA, Ginsberg JS, Brill-Edwards P, et al. The relationship of antiphospholipid antibodies to thromboembolic disease in systemic lupus erythematosus: a cross-sectional study. Thromb Haemost 1991, 66: 520–524

164. Graef V, Baggenstoss AH, Sauer WG, Spittell JA Jr. Venous thrombosis occurring in nonspecific ulcerative colitis. Arch Intern Med 1966; 117: 377–382

165. Lambrecht L, Baele G, Barbier F. Hemostatic alterations in Crohn's disease. Acta Clin Belg 1987; 42: 5–11

166. Talbot RW, Hepell J, Dozois RR, Beart RW. Vascular complications of inflammatory bowel disease. Mayo Clin Proc 1986; 61: 140–145

167. Jackson LM, O'Gorman PJ, O'Connell J, Cronin CC, Cotter KP, Shanahan. Thrombosis in inflammatory bowel disease: clinical setting, procoagulant profile and factor V Leiden. Q J Med 1997; 90: 183–188

168. Llach F. Hypercoagulability, renal vein thrombosis, and other thrombotic complications of nephrotic syndrome. Kidney Internat 1985; 28: 429–434

169. Llach F, Arieff AI, Massry SG. Renal vein thrombosis and nephrotic syndrome. A prospective study of 36 adult patients. Ann Intern Med 1975; 83: 8–13

170. Hartmann RC, Luther AB, Jenkins DE Jr, et al. Fulminant hepatic venous thrombosis (Budd-Chiari syndrome) in paroxysmal nocturnal hemoglobinuria: definition of a medical emergency. Johns Hopkins Med J 1980; 146: 247–250

171. Mitchell MC, Boitnott JK, Kaufman S, Cameron JL, Maddrey WC. Budd-Chiari syndrome: etiology, diagnosis, and management. Medicine (Baltimore) 1982; 61: 199–210

172. Wozniak AJ, Kitchens CS. Prospective hemostatic studies in a patient having paroxismal nocturnal hemoglobinuria, pregnancy, and cerebral venous thrombosis. Am J Obstet Gynecol 1982; 142: 591–594

173. Chievitz E, Thiede T. Complications and causes of death in polycythaemia vera. Acta Med Scand 1962; 172: 513–523

174. Dawson AA, Ogston D. The influence of the platelet count on the incidence of thrombotic and haemorrhagic complications in polycythaemia vera. Postgrad Med J 1970; 46: 76–78

175. Jabaily J, Iland HJ, Laszlo J, et al. Neurologic manifestations of essential thrombocythaemia. Ann Intern Med 1983; 99: 513–518

176. Singh AK, Wetherley-Mein G. Microvascular occlusive lesions in primary thrombocythaemia. Br J Haematol 1977; 36: 553–558

177. Van Genderen PJJ, Mulder PGH, Waleboer M, van de Moesdijk D, Michiels JJ. Prevention and treatment of thrombotic complications in essential thrombocythaemia: efficacy and safety of aspirin. Br J Haematol 1997; 97: 179–184

178. Wechsler B, Piette JC, Conard J, Le Thi Huong Du, Blétry O, Godeau P. Les thromboses veineuses profondes dans la maladie de Behçet. 106 localisations sur une série de 177 malades. Presse Méd 1987; 16: 661–664

179. Sjoberg HE, Blomback M, Granberg PO. Thromboembolic complications, heparin treatment and increase in coagulation factors in Cushing's syndrome. Acta Med Scand 1976; 199: 95–100

180. Kitchens CS. Concept of hypercoagulability: a review of its development, clinical application, and recent progress. Sem Thromb Haemost 1985; 11: 293–315

181. Rickles FR, O'Leary DS. Role of coagulation system in pathophysiology of sickle cell disease. Arch Intern Med 1974; 133: 635–639

182. Ballas SK, Saidi P. Thrombosis, megaloblastic anaemia, and sickle cell disease: a unified hypothesis. Br J Haematol 1997; 96: 872–873

183. Bokarewa MI, Wramsby M, Bremme K, Blombäck M. Variability of the response to activated protein C during normal pregnancy. Blood Coagul Fibrinolysis 1977; 8: 239–244

184. Kierkegaard A. Incidence and diagnosis of deep vein thrombosis associated with pregnancy. Acta Obstet Gynecol Scand 1983; 62: 239–244

185. Friederich PW, Sanson BJ, Simioni P, et al. Frequency of pregnancy-related venous thromboembolism in anticoagulant factor-deficient women: implications for prophylaxis. Ann Intern Med 1996; 125: 955–960

186. Conard J, Horellou MH, van Dreden P, Lecompte T, Samama M. Thrombosis and pregnancy in congenital deficiencies in AT, protein C or protein S. Study of 78 women. Thromb Haemost 1990; 63: 319–324

187. Cook G, Walker ID, McCall F, Conkie JA, Greer IA. Familial thrombophilia and activated protein C resistance: thrombotic risk in pregnancy? Br J Haematol 1994; 87: 873–875

188. Pabinger I, Schneider B. Thrombotic risk of women with hereditary antithrombin III, protein C and protein S deficiency taking oral contraceptive medication. Thromb Haemost 1994; 71: 548–552

189. Ginsberg JS, Brill-Edwards P, Prandoni P, et al. Venous thrombosis during pregnancy: leg and trimester of presentation. Thromb Haemost 1992; 67: 519–520

190. Clayton JK, Anderson JA, McNicol GP. Effect of smoking on subsequent postoperative thromboembolic disease in gynaecological patients. Br Med J 1978; 2: 402–403

191. Kerstein MD, Mcswain NE, O'Connell RC, Webb WR, Brennan LA. Obesity: is it really a risk factor in thrombophlebitis? South Med J 1987; 80: 1236–1238

192. Goldhaber SZ, Grodstein F, Stampfer MJ, et al. A prospective study on risk factors for pulmonary embolism in women. JAMA 1997; 277: 642–645

193. Flordal PA, Berqvist D, Burmark US, Ljungström KG, Törngren S. Risk factors for major thromboembolism and bleeding tendency after elective general surgical operations. Eur J Surg 1996; 162: 783–789

194. De Nardo GL, De Nardo SJ. Thrombosis detection: fibrinogen counting and radionuclide venography. Clin Nucl Med 1981; 6: P37–P45

195. Jorgensen JO, Hanel KC, Morgan AM, Hunt JM. The incidence of deep venous thrombosis in patients with superficial thrombophlebitis of the lower limbs. J Vasc Surg 1993; 18: 70–73

196. Lutter KS, Rerr TM, Roedersheimer R, Lohr JM, Sampson MG, Cranley JJ. Superficial thrombophlebitis diagnosed by duplex scanning. Surgery 1991; 100: 42–46

197. Skilman J, Kent KC, Porter DH, Kim D. Simultaneous occurrence of superficial and deep thrombophlebitis in the lower extremity. J Vasc Surg 1990; 11: 818–822

198. Bergqvist D, Jaroszewski H. Deep vein thrombosis in patients with superficial thrombophlebitis of the leg. Br Med J 1985; 292: 658–659

199. Joffe SN. Racial incidence of post-operative deep vein thrombosis in South Africa. Br J Surg 1974; 61: 982–983

200. Chumnijarakij T, Poshyachinda V. Postoperative thrombosis in Thai women. Lancet 1975; 2: 1357–1358

201. Kim YH, Suh JS. Low incidence of deep vein thrombosis after cementless total hip replacement. J Bone Joint Surg 1988; 70A: 878–881

202. Datta BN, Ramesh K, Bhusnurmath B. Autopsy incidence of pulmonary vascular episodes. A study of 218 cases. Angiology 1986; 37: 744–750

203. Chau KY, Yuen ST, Wong MP. Seasonal variation in the necropsy incidence of pulmonary thromboembolism in Hong Kong. J Clin Pathol 1995; 48: 578–579

204. De Groot PG, Derksen RHWM. Specificity and clinical relevance of lupus anticoagulant. Vessels 1995; 1: 22–26

205. Love PE, Santoro SA. Antiphospholipid antibodies: anticardiolipin and the lupus anticoagulant in the systemic lupus erythematosus (SLE) and in non-SLE disorders. Ann Intern Med 1990; 112: 682–698

206. Vila P, Hernandez MC, Lopez-Fernandez MF, Battle J. Prevalence, follow-up and clinical significance of the anticardiolipin antibodies in normal subjects. Thromb Haemost 1994; 72: 209–213

207. Elias M, Eldor A. Thromboembolism in patients with the "lupus"-type circulating anticoagulant. Arch Intern Med 1984; 144: 510–515

208. Ginsburg KS, Liang MH, Newcomer L, et al. Anticardiolipin antibodies and the risk for ischemic stroke and venous thrombosis. Ann Intern Med 1992; 117: 997–1002

209. Hughson MD, McCarty GA, Sholer CM, Brumback RA. Thrombotic cerebral arteriopathy in patients with the antiphospholipid syndrome. Modern Pathol 1993; 6: 644–653

210. Lechner K. In: Verstraete M, et al. (eds). Lupus anticoagulant and thrombosis. Leuven 1987: 525–531

211. Ondi-Ros J, Pérez-Pemàa P, Monasterio J. Clinical and therapeutic aspects associated to phospholipid binding antibodies (lupus anticoagulant and anticardiolipin antibodies). Haemostasis 1994; 24: 165–174

212. Lockshin MD. Pathogenesis of the antiphospholipid antibody syndrome. Lupus 1996; 5: 404–408

213. De Groot PG, Horbach DA, Derksen RHWM. Protein C and other cofactors involved in the binding of antiphospholipid antibodies: relation to the pathogenesis of thrombosis. Lupus 1996; 5: 488–493

214. Gharavi AE, Wilson WA. The syndrome of thrombosis, thrombocytopenia, and recurrent spontaneous abortions associated with antiphospholipid antibodies: Hughes syndrome. Lupus 1996; 5: 343–344

215. Long AA, Ginsberg JS, Brill-Edwards P, et al. The relationship of antiphospholipid antibodies to thromboembolic disease in systemic lupus erythematosus: a cross-sectional study. Thromb Haemost 1991; 66: 520–524

216. Abu-Shakra M, Gladman DD, Urowitz MB, Farewell V. Anticardiolipin antibodies in systemic lupus erythematosus: clinical and laboratory correlations. Am J Med 1995; 99: 624–628

217. Ginsberg JS, Wells PS, Brill-Edwards P, et al. Antiphospholipid antibodies and venous thromboembolism. Blood 1995; 86: 3685–3691

218. Simioni P, Prandoni P, Zanon E, et al. Deep venous thrombosis and lupus anticoagulant. A case-control study. Thromb Haemost 1996; 76: 187–189

219. Finazzi; Bongard O, Reber G, Bounameaux H, de Moerloose P. Anticardiolipin antibodies in acute venous thromboembolism. Thromb Haemost 1992; 67: 724

220. Finazzi G, Brancaccio V, Moia M, et al. Natural history and risk factors for thrombosis in 360 patients with antiphospholipid antibodies: a four-year prospective study from the Italian registry. Am J Med 1996; 100: 530–536

221. Reber G, Arvieux J, Comby E, et al. Multicenter evaluation of nine commercial kits for the quantitation of anticardiolipin antibodies. Thromb Haemost 1995; 73: 444–452

222. Khamashta MA. Management of thrombosis in the antiphospholipid syndrome. Lupus 1996; 5: 463–466

223. Khamashta MA, Cuadrado MJ, Mujic F, Taub NA, Hunt BJ, Hughes GRV. The management of thrombosis in the antiphospholipid-antibody syndrome. N Engl J Med 1995; 332: 993–997

224. Prandoni P, Simioni P, Girolami A. Antiphospholipid antibodies, recurrent thromboembolism, and intensity of warfarin anticoagulation. Thromb Haemost 1996; 75: 859

225. Rance A, Emmerich J, Fiessinger JN. Anticardiolipin antibodies and recurrent thromboembolism. Thromb Haemost 1997; 77: 221–222

226. Schulman S, Svenungsson E, Granqvist S, the Durae Study Group. Anticardiolipin antibodies predict early recurrence of thromboembolism and death among patients with venous thromboembolism following anticoagulant therapy. Am J Med 1998; 104: 332–338

227. Poort SR, Rosendaal FR, Reitsma PH, Bertina RM. A common genetic variation in the 3'-untranslated region of the prothrombin gene is associated with elevated plasma prothrombin levels and increase in venous thrombosis. Blood 1996; 88: 3698–3703

228. Hirsh J, Prins MH, Samama M. Approach to the thrombophilic patient for hemostasis and thrombosis: basic principles and clinical practice. In: Colman RW, Hirsh J, Marder VJ, Salzman EW (eds). Hemostasis and Thrombosis. Basic principles and clinical practice. JB Lippincott, Philadelphia, 1993, 1543–1561

229. Lane DA, Mannucci PM, Bauer KA, et al. Inherited thrombophilia: part 1. Thromb Haemost 1996; 76: 651–662

230. Lensen RPM, Rosendaal FR, Koster T, et al. Apparent different thrombotic tendency in patients with factor V Leiden and protein C deficiency due to selection of patients. Blood 1996; 88: 4205–4208

231. De Stefano V, Finazzi G, Mannucci G. Inherited thrombophilia: pathogenesis, clinical syndromes, and management. Blood 1996; 87: 3531–3544

232. Simioni P, Prandoni P, Lensing AWA, et al. The risk of recurrent venous thromboembolism in patients with an Arg^{506}-Gln mutation in the gene for factor V (factor V Leiden). N Engl J Med 1997; 336: 399–403

233. Simioni P, Sanson BJ, Prandoni P, et al. Incidence of venous thromboembolism with inherited thrombophilia. Thromb Haemost 1999; 82: 198–202

234. Demers C, Ginsberg JS, Hirsh J, Henderson P, Blajchman MA. Thrombosis in antithrombin-III-deficient persons. Ann Intern Med 1992; 116: 754–761

235. Egeberg O. Inherited antithrombin deficiency causing thrombophilia. Thromb Diath Haemorrh 1965; 13: 516–530

236. Girolami A, Cappellato MG, Vicarioto M, et al. Antithrombin III deficiency: a report of 14 cases belonging to three different kindreds. Folia Haematol 1985; 112: 594–606

237. Hirsh J, Piovella F, Pini M. Congenital antithrombin III deficiency. Am J Med 1989; 87 (Suppl. 3B): 34S–38S

238. Marciniak E, Farley CH, De Simone PA. Familial thrombosis due to antithrombin III deficiency. Blood 1974; 43: 219–231

239. Rodgers GM, Shuman MA. Congenital thrombotic disorders. Am J Hematol 1986; 21: 419–424

240. Miller N, Hulutin MB, Gounder M, Zarrabi MH. Hereditary antithrombin III deficiency: case report and review of recent therapeutic advances. Am J Hematol 1986; 21: 215–219

241. Bjork I, Danielsson A, Fenton JW, Jornwall H. The site in human antithrombin for functional proteolytic cleavage by human thrombin. FEBS 1981; 126: 257

242. Blajchman M, Austin R, Fernandez-Rachubinski F, Sheffield W. Molecular basis of inherited antithrombin deficiency. Blood 1992; 80: 2159–2171

243. Olds RJ, Lane DA, Mille B, Chowdhury V, Thein SL. Antithrombin: the principal inhibitor of thrombin. Semin Thromb Haemost 1994; 20: 353–372

244. Van Boven HH, Vandenbroucke JP, Westendorp RGJ, Rosendaal FR. Mortality and causes of death in inherited antithrombin deficiency. Thromb Haemost 1997; 77: 452–455

245. Mateo J, Oliver A, Borrell M, Sala N, Fontcuberta J. Laboratory evaluation and clinical characteristics of 2,132 consecutive unselected patients with venous thromboembolism – Results of the Spanish Multicentric Study on Thrombophilia. Thromb Haemost 1997; 77: 444–451

246. Heijboer H, Brandjes DPM, Büller HR, Sturk A, ten Cate JW. Deficiencies of coagulation-inhibiting and fibrinolytic proteins in outpatients with deep-vein thrombosis. N Engl J Med 1990; 323: 1512–1515

247. Tait RC, Walker ID, Perry DJ, et al. Prevalence of antithrombin III deficiency subtypes in 4000 healthy blood donors. Thromb Haemost 1991; 65: 839

248. Conard J, Horellou MH, van Dreden P, Lecompte T, Samama M. Thrombosis and pregnancy in congenital deficiencies in AT, protein C or protein S. Study of 78 women. Thromb Haemost 1990; 63: 319–324

249. Esmon CT. The protein C anticoagulant pathway. Arterioscl Thromb 1992; 12: 135–145

250. Esmon CT. Molecular events that control the protein C anticoagulant pathway. Thromb Haemost 1993; 70: 29–35

251. Dahlbäck B. The protein C anticoagulant system: inherited defects as basis for venous thrombosis. Thromb Res 1995; 77: 1–43

252. Reitsma PH, Bernadi F, Doig RG, et al. Protein C deficiency: a database of mutations, 1995 update. Thromb Haemost 1995; 73: 876–889

253. Aiach M, Gandrille S, Emmerich J. A review of mutations causing deficiencies of antithrombin, protein C and protein S. Thromb Haemost 1995; 74: 81–89

254. Griffin JH, Evatt B, Zimmerman TS, Kleiss AJ, Wideman C. Deficiency of protein C in congenital thrombotic disease. J Clin Invest 1981; 68: 1370–1373

255. Cloues LH, Comp PC. The regulation of hemostasis. The protein C system. N Engl J Med 1986; 314: 1298–1304

256. Esmon CT. Protein C: Biochemistry, physiology, and clinical implications. Blood 1983; 62: 1155–1158

257. Koster T, Rosendaal FR, Briet E, et al. Protein C deficiency in a controlled series of unselected outpatients: an infrequent but clear risk factor for venous thrombosis (Leiden Thrombophilia Study). Blood 1995; 85: 2756–2761

258. Seligsohn U, Berger A, Abend M, et al. Homozygous protein C deficiency manifested by massive venous thrombosis in the newborn. N Engl J Med 1984; 310: 559–562

259. Kitchens CS. Thrombophilia and thrombosis in unusual sites. In Colman RW, Hirsh J, Marder VJ, Salzman EW (eds): Hemostasis and Thrombosis. Basic principles and clinical practice. JB Lippincott, Philadelphia, 1993: 1255–1274

260. Miletich J, Sherman L, Broze G Jr. Absence of thrombosis in subjects with heterozygous protein C deficiency. N Engl J Med 1987; 317: 991–996

261. Zöller B, Garcia de Frutos P, Dahlbäck B. Evaluation of the relationship between protein S and C4b-binding protein isoforms in hereditary protein S deficiency demonstrating type I and type III deficiencies to be phenotypic variants of the same genetic disease. Blood 1995; 85: 3524–3531

262. Dahlbäck B, Stenflo J. A natural anticoagulant pathway: protein C, S, C4b-binding protein and thrombomodulin. In: Bloom AL, Forbes CD, Thomas DP, Tuddenham EGD (eds). Haemostasis and Thrombosis. Churchill Livingstone, Edinburgh, 1994: 671–698

263. Schwarz HP, Fischer M, Hopmeier P, Batard MA, Griffin JH. Plasma protein S deficiency in familial thrombotic disease. Blood 1984; 64: 1297–1300

264. Broekmans AW, Bertina RM, Reinalda Poot J, et al. Hereditary protein S deficiency and venous thromboembolism. A study in three Dutch families. Thromb Haemost 1985; 53: 273–277

265. Koster T, Rosendaal FR, Briet E, et al. Protein C deficiency in a controlled series of unselected outpatients: an infrequent but clear risk factor for venous thrombosis (Leiden Thrombophilia Study). Blood 1995; 85: 2756–2761

266. Van den Belt AGM, Prins MH, Huisman MV, Hirsh J. Familial Thrombophilia: A review analysis. Clin Appl Thromb/Haemost 1996; 2: 227–236

267. Hillarp A, Zöller B, Dahlbäck B. Activated protein C resistance as a basis for venous thrombosis. Am J Med 1996; 101: 534–540

268. Dahlbäck B. Inherited thrombophilia: resistance to activated protein C as a pathogenetic factor of venous thromboembolism. Blood 1995; 85: 607–614

269. Bertina RM, Koeleman BPC, Koster T, et al. Mutation in blood coagulation factor V associated with resistance to activated protein C. Nature 1994; 369: 64–67

270. Voorberg J, Roelse J, Koopman R, et al. Association of idiopathic venous thromboembolism with single pointmutation at Arg^{906} of factor V. Lancet 1994; 343: 1535–1536

271. Zöller B, Dahlbäck B. Linkage between inherited resistance to activated protein C and factor V gene mutation in venous thrombosis. Lancet 1994; 343: 1536–1538

272. Griffin JH, Heeb MJ, Kojima Y, Fernandez JA, Hackeng TM, Greengard JS. Activated protein C resistance: molecular mechanisms. Thromb Haemost 1995; 74: 444–448

273. Kalafatis M, Bertina RM, Rand MD, Mann KG. Characterization of the molecular defect in factor VR506Q. J Biol Chem 1995; 270: 4053–4057

274. Beauchamp NJ, Daly ME, Hampton KK, Cooper PC, Preston FE, Peake IR. High prevalence of a mutation in the factor V gene within the U.K. population: relationship to activated protein C resistance and familial thrombosis. Br J Haematol 1994; 88: 219–222

275. Dahlbäck B. Inherited thrombophilia: resistance to activated protein C as a pathogenetic factor of venous thromboembolism. Blood 1995; 85: 607–614

276. Koopman MMW, Voorberg J, Büller HR, et al. Prevalence of factor V Arg-Gln mutation, hyperhomocysteinemia, and hyperlipoproteinemia(a) in patients with venous thromboembolism. Arch Intern Med

277. Zöller B, Hillarp A, Dahlbäck B. Activated protein C resistance: clinical implications. Clin Appl Thromb/Haemost 1997; 3: 25–32

278. Ridker PM, Miletich JP, Hennekens CH, Buring JE. Ethnic distribution of factor V Leiden in 4047 men and women. Implications for venous thromboembolism screening. JAMA 1997; 277: 1305–1307

279. Koeleman BPC, Reitsma PH, Allaart CF, Bertina RM. Activated protein C resistance as an additional risk factor for thrombosis in protein C-deficient families. Blood 1994; 84: 1031–1035

280. Koeleman BPC, van Rumpt D, Hamulyak K, Reitsma PH, Bertina RM. Factor V Leiden: an additional risk factor for thrombosis in protein S deficient families? Thromb Haemostas 1995; 74: 580–583

281. Ridker PM, Hennekens CH, Selhub J, Miletich JP, Malinow MR, Stampfer MJ. Interrelation of hyperhomocyst(e)inemia, factor V Leiden, and risk of future venous thromboembolism. Circulation 1997; 95: 1777–1782

282. Koster T, Rosendaal F, de Ronde H, Briet E, Bertina RM. Venous thrombosis due to poor anticoagulant response to activated protein C: Leiden Thrombophilia Study. Lancet 1993; 342: 1503–1506

283. Ridker PM, Hennekens CH, Lindpaintner K, Stampfer MJ, Lisenberg PR, Miletich JP. Mutation in the gene coding for coagulation factor V and the risk of myocardial infarction, stroke, and venous thrombosis in apparently healthy men. N Engl J Med 1995; 332: 912–917

284. Svensson PJ, Dahlback B. Resistance to activated protein C as a basis for venous thrombosis. N Engl J Med 1994; 330: 517–522

285. Svensson PJ, Zöller B, Mattiasson I, Dahlbäck B. The factor VR506Q mutation causing APC resistance is highly prevalent amongst unselected outpatients with clinically suspected deep venous thrombosis. J Int Med 1997; 241: 379–385

286. Hainaut P, Azerad MA, Lehmann F, et al. Prevalence of activated protein C resistance and analysis of clinical profile in thromboembolic patients. A Belgian prospective study. J Int Med 1997; 241: 427–433

287. Grengard JS, Eichinger S, Griffin JH, Bauer KA. Brief report: variability of thrombosis among homozygous siblings with resistance to activated protein C due to an Arg-Gln mutation in the gene for factor V. N Engl J Med 1994; 331: 1559–1562

288. Rosendaal FR, Koster T, Vandenbroucke JP, Reitsma PH. High risk of thrombosis in patients homozygous for factor V Leiden (activated protein C resistance). Blood 1995; 85: 1504–1508

289. Ridker PM, Glynn RJ, Miletich JP, Goldhaber SZ, Stampfer MJ, Hennekens CH. Age-specific incidence rates of venous thromboembolism among heterozygous carriers of factor V Leiden mutation. Ann Intern Med 1997; 126: 528–531

290. Hellgren M, Svensson PJ, Dahlbäck B. Resistance to activated protein C as a basis for venous thromboembolism associated with pregnancy and oral contraceptives. Am J Obstet Gynecol 1995; 173: 210–213

291. Rosendaal FR, Koster T, Vanderbroucke JP, Reitsma PH. High risk of thrombosis in patients homozygous for factor V Leiden (activated protein C Resistance). Blood 1995; 85: 1504–1508

292. Vanderbroucke JP, Koster T, Brièt E, Reitsma PH, Bertina RM, Rosendaal FR. Increased risk of venous thrombosis in oral-contraceptive users who are carriers of factor V Leiden mutation. Lancet 1994; 344: 1453–1457

293. Preston FE, Rosendaal FR, Walker ID, et al. Increased fetal loss in women with heritable thrombophilia. Lancet 1996; 348: 913–916

294. Grandone E, Margaglione M, Colaizzo D, et al. Factor V Leiden is associated with repeated and recurrent unexplained fetal losses. Thromb Haemostas 1997; 77: 822–824

295. Rees MM, Rodgers GM. Homocysteinemia: association of a metabolic disorder with vascular disease and thrombosis. Thromb Res 1993; 71: 337–359

296. Arruda VR, von Zuben PM, Chiaparini LC, Annichino-Bizzacchi JM, Costa FF. The mutation Ala^{677} – Val in the methylene tetrahydrofolate reductase gene: a risk factor for arterial disease and venous thrombosis. Thromb Haemostas 1997; 77: 818 – 821

297. Mudd SH, Levy HL, Skovby F. Disorders of transulfuration. In: Scriver C, Beaudet AL, Sly WS, Valle D (eds). The metabolic basis of inherited disease. McGraw-Hill, New York, 1989: 693 – 734

298. Wall RT, Harlan JM, Harker LA, Striker GE. Homocysteine-induced endothelial cell injury in vitro: a model for the study of vascular injury. Thromb Res 1980; 18: 113 – 121

299. De Groot PG, Willems C, Boers GH, Gonsalves MD, Van Aken WG, Van Mourik JA. Endothelial cell dysfunction in homocystinuria. Eur J Clin Invest 1983; 13: 405 – 410

300. Starkebaum G, Harlan JM. Endothelial cell injury due to copper-catalyzed hydrogen peroxide generation from homocysteine. J Clin Invest 1986; 77: 1370 – 1376

301. Rodgers GM, Kane WH, Pitas RE. Formation of factor Va by atherosclerotic rabbit aorta mediates factor Xa-catalyzed prothrombin activation. J Clin Invest 1988; 81: 1911 – 1919

302. Rodgers GM, Conn MT. Homocysteine, an atherogenic stimulus, reduces protein C activation by arterial and venous endothelial cells. Blood 1990; 75: 895 – 901

303. Boers GHJ, Smals AGH, Trijbels FJM, et al. Heterozygosity for homocystinuria in premature peripheral and cerebral occlusive arterial disease. N Engl J Med 1985; 313: 709 – 715

304. Selhub J, Jacques PF, Bostom AG, et al. Association between plasma homocysteine concentrations and extracranial carotid-artery stenosis. N Engl J Med 1995; 332: 286 – 291

305. Stampfer MJ, Malinow MR, Willett WC, et al. A prospective study of plasma homocyst(e)ine and risk of myocardial infarction in US physicians. JAMA 1992; 268: 877 – 881

306. Brattström L, Tengborn L, Israelsson B, Hultberg B. Plasma homocysteine in venous thromboembolism. Haemostasis 1991; 21: 51 – 57

307. Beaumont V, Malinow MR, Sexton G, et al. Hyperhomocysteinemia, anti-estrogen antibodies and other risk factors for thrombosis in women on oral contraceptives. Atherosclerosis 1992; 94: 147 – 152

308. Bienvenu T, Ankri A, Chadefaux B, Kamoun P. Plasma homocysteine assay in the exploration of thrombosis in young subjects. Press Med 1991; 20: 985 – 988

309. Den Heijer M, Koster T, Blom HJ, et al. Hyperhomocysteinemia as a risk factor for deep-vein thrombosis. N Engl J Med 1996; 334: 759 – 762

310. Simioni P, Prandoni P, Burlina A, et al. Hyperhomocysteinemia and deep-vein thrombosis. A case control study. Thromb Haemostas 1996; 76: 883 – 886

311. Falcon CR, Cattaneo M, Panzeri D, Martinelli I, Mannucci PM. High prevalence of hyperhomocysteinemia in patients with juvenile venous thrombosis. Arterioscl Thromb 1994; 14: 1080 – 1083

312. Fermo I, Viganò D'Angelo S, et al. Prevalence of moderate hyperhomocysteinemia in patients with early-onset venous and arterial occlusive disease. Ann Intern Med 1995; 123: 747 – 753

313. Den Heijer M, Blom HJ, Gerrits WB, Rosendaal FR, Wijermans PW, Bos GM. Is hyperhomocysteinaemia a risk factor for recurrent venous thrombosis? Lancet 1995; 345: 882 – 885

314. Eichinger S, Stümpflen A, Hirschl M, et al. Hyperhomocysteinemia is a risk factor of recurrent venous thromboembolism in male patients. Thromb Haemostas 1997; Suppl.1: OC-745

315. Widimsky J. Acute pulmonary embolism and chronic thromboembolic pulmonary hypertension: is there a relationship? Eur Respir J 1991; 4: 137 – 140

316. Heit JA. An analysis of current pulmonary embolism therapy. Intern Angiol 1992; 11: 57 – 63

317. Leclerc JR. Natural history of venous thromboembolism. In Leclerc JR (ed): Venous thromboembolic disorders. Lea & Febiger, Philadelphia, 1991: 166 – 175

318. Dalen JE, Alpert JS. Natural history of pulmonary embolism. Progr Cardiovasc Dis 1975; 17: 259 – 270

319. Hall RJC, Sutton GC, Kerr IH. Long-term prognosis of treated acute massive pulmonary embolism. Br Heart J 1977; 39: 1128 – 1134

320. Urokinase Pulmonary Embolism Trial: a national cooperative study. Circulation 1973; 47 (Suppl. 2): 1 – 108

321. Paraskos JA. Late prognosis of acute pulmonary embolism. N Engl J Med 1973; 289: 55 – 58

322. Goldhaber SZ, Haire WD, Feldstein ML, et al. Alteplase versus heparin in acute pulmonary embolism: randomised trial assessing right-ventricular function and pulmonary embolism. Lancet 1993; 341: 507 – 511

323. Donnamaria V, Palla A, Petruzzelli S, Carrozzi L, Pugliesi O, Giuntini C. Early and late follow-up of pulmonary embolism. Respiration 1993; 60: 15 – 20

324. Riedel M, Stanek V, Widimsky J, Prerovsky I. Long-term follow-up of patients with pulmonary thromboembolism. Chest 1982; 81: 151 – 158

325. Tow DE, Wagner HN. Recovery of pulmonary arterial blood flow in patients with pulmonary embolism. N Engl J Med 1967; 276: 1053 – 1059

326. Yoo HS, Intenzo CM, Park CH. Unresolved major pulmonary embolism: importance of follow-up lung scan in diagnosis. Eur J Nucl Med 1986; 12: 252 – 253

327. Chait A, Summers D, Kransnow N. Observations on the fate of large pulmonary embolism. Am J Roentgenol 1967; 100: 364 – 373

328. Urokinase-Streptokinase Pulmonary Embolism Trial: phase 2 results. JAMA 1974; 229: 1606 – 1613

329. Benotti JR, Dalen JE. The national history of pulmonary embolism. Clin Chest Med 1984; 5: 403 – 410

330. Fred HL, Axelrad MA, Lewis GM, Alexander JK. Rapid resolution of pulmonary thromboembolism in man. JAMA 1966; 196: 1137 – 1142

331. Dalen JE, Banas JS Jr, Brooks HL, Evans GL, Paraskos JA, Dexter L. Resolution rate of acute pulmonary embolism in man. N Engl J Med 1969; 280: 1194 – 1199

332. Sutton GC, Hall RJC, Kerr IH. Clinical course and late prognosis of treated subacute massive, acute minor, and chronic pulmonary thromboembolism. Br Heart J 1977; 39: 1135–1142

333. Moser KM., Auger WR, Fedullo PF. Chronic major-vessel thromboembolic pulmonary hypertension. Circulation 1990; 81: 1735–1743

334. Dexter L, Smith GT. Quantitative studies of pulmonary embolism. Am J Med Sci 1964; 247: 641–648

335. Ansari A. Acute and chronic pulmonary thromboembolism: current perspectives. Part I. Glossary of terms, historic evolution and prevalence. Clin Cardiol 1986; 9: 398–402

336. Hirsh J, Lensing AWA. Natural history of minimal calf deep vein thrombosis. In: Bernstein EF (ed). Vascular diagnosis. CV Mosby, St. Louis, 1993: 779–781

337. Kakkar VV, Flank C, Howe CT, et al. Natural history of postoperative deep vein thrombosis. Lancet 1969; 2: 230–233

338. Browse NL, Thomas M. Source of non-lethal pulmonary emboli. Lancet 1974; 1: 258–259

339. Doyle DJ, Turpie AGG, Hirsh J, et al. Adjusted subcutaneous heparin or continuous intravenous heparin in patients with acute deep vein thrombosis. Ann Intern Med 1987; 107: 441–445

340. Anderson M, Willie-Jorgensen P. Late venous function after asymptomatic deep venous thrombosis. Thromb Haemostas 1989; 62: 336–340

341. Cogo A, Lensing AWA, Prandoni P, Hirsh J. Distribution of thrombosis in patients with symptomatic deep vein thrombosis. Implications for simplifying the diagnostic approach with compression ultrasound. Arch Intern Med 1993; 153: 2777–2780

342. Markel A, Manzo RA, Bergelin RO, Strandness D. Pattern and distribution of thrombi in acute venous thrombosis. Arch Surg 1992; 127: 305–309

343. Mattos MA, Melendres G, Sumner DS, et al. Prevalence and distribution of calf vein thrombosis in patients with symptomatic deep venous thrombosis: a color-flow duplex study. J Vasc Surg 1996; 24: 738–744

344. Philbrick JT, Becker DM. Calf deep venous thrombosis. A wolf in sheep's clothing? Arch Intern Med 1988; 148: 2131–2138

345. Lagerstedt CJ, Olsson CG, Fagher BO, Oqvist BW, Albrechtsson U. Need for long-term anticoagulant treatment in symptomatic calf-vein thrombosis. Lancet 1985; 2: 515–518

346. Hirsh J, Salzman EW, Marder VJ. Treatment of venous thromboembolism. In: Colman RW, Hirsh J, Marder VJ, Salzman EW (eds). Hemostasis and Thrombosis. Basic principles and clinical practice. JB Lippincott, Philadelphia, 1993: 1346–1366

347. Brandjes DPM, Heijboer H, Büller HR, de Rijk M, Jagt H, ten Cate JW: Acenocoumarol and heparin compared with acenocoumarol alone in the initial treatment of proximal-vein thrombosis. N Engl J Med 1992; 327: 1485–1489

348. Hull RD, Raskob GE, Hirsh J, et al. Continuous intravenous heparin compared with intermittent subcutaneous heparin in the initial treatment of proximal-vein thrombosis. N Engl J Med 1986; 315: 1109–1114

349. Hull RD, Raskob GE, Rosenbloom D, et al. Heparin for 5 days as compared with 10 days in the initial treatment of proximal venous thrombosis. N Engl J Med 1990; 322: 1260–1264

350. Prandoni P, Lensing AWA, Büller HR, et al. Comparison of subcutaneous low-molecular-weight heparin with intravenous standard heparin in proximal deep-vein thrombosis. Lancet 1992; 39: 441–445

351. Hull RD, Raskob GL, Pineo GF, et al. Subcutaneous low molecular-weight heparin compared with intravenous heparin in the treatment of proximal-vein thrombosis. N Engl J Med 1992; 326: 975–982

352. Koopman MMW, Prandoni P, Piovella F, et al. Treatment of venous thrombosis with intravenous unfractionated heparin administered in hospital as compared with subcutaneous low-molecular-weight heparin administered at home. N Engl J Med 1996; 334: 682–687

353. Levine M, Gent M, Hirsh J, et al. A comparison of low-molecular-weight heparin administered primarily at home with unfractionated heparin administered in the hospital for proximal deep-vein thrombosis. N Engl J Med 1996; 334: 677–681

354. Bergqvist D, Jendteg S, Johansen L, Persson U, Ödegaard K. Cost of long-term complications of deep venous thrombosis of the lower extremities: an analysis of a defined patient population in Sweden. Ann Intern Med 1997; 26: 454–457

355. Franzeck UK, Schalch I, Jager KA, Schneider E, Grimm J, Bollinger A: Prospective 12-year follow-up of clinical and hemodynamic sequelae after deep vein thrombosis in low-risk patients (Zurich Study). Circulation 1996; 93: 74–79

356. Immelman EJ, Jeffery PC. The postphlebitic syndrome. Pathophysiology, prevention and management. Clin Chest Med 1984; 5: 537–550

357. Bauer GA. Roentgenological and clinical study of the sequels of thrombosis. Acta Chir Scand 1942; 86 (suppl.74): 1–110

358. Gjores J. The incidence of venous thrombosis and its sequelae in certain districts of Sweden. Acta Chir Scand 1956; 206 (suppl.1): 1–88

359. O'Donnell FF, Browse NL, Burnand KG, Lea Thomas M. The socioeconomic effects of an ilio-femoral venous thrombosis. J Surg Res 1977; 22: 483–488

360. Strandness DE, Langlois Y, Cramer M, Randlett A, Thiele BL. Long-term sequelae of acute venous thrombosis. JAMA 1983; 250: 1289–1292

361. Widmer LK, Zemp E, Widmer MTH, et al. Late results in deep-vein thrombosis of the lower extremities. Vasa 1985; 14: 264–268

362. Lindner DJ, Edwards JM, Phinney ES, Taylor LM, Porter JM. Long-term hemodynamic and clinical sequelae of lower extremity deep-vein thrombosis. J Vasc Surg 1986; 4: 436–442

363. Heldal M, Seem E, Snadset PM, Abildgaard U. Deep-vein thrombosis: a 7-year follow-up study. J Intern Med 1993; 234: 71–75

364. Monreal M, Martorell A, Callejas JM, et al. Venographic assessment of deep-vein thrombosis and risk of developing post-thrombotic syndrome: a prospective study. J Intern Med 1993; 233: 854–859

31

365. Milne AA, Ruckley CV. The clinical course of patients following extensive deep venous thrombosis. Eur J Vasc Surg 1994; 8: 56–59

366. Saarinen J, Sisto T, laurikka J, Salenius JP, Tarkka M. Late sequelae of acute deep venous thrombosis: evaluation five and ten years after. Phlebology 1995; 10: 106–109

367. Beyth RJ, Cohen AM, Landefeld S. Long-term outcomes of deep-vein thrombosis. Arch Intern Med 1995; 155: 1031–1037

368. Brandjes DPM, Büller HR, Heijboer H, et al. Randomised trial of effect of compression stockings in patients with symptomatic proximal-vein thrombosis. Lancet 1997; 349: 759–762

Chapter II
Clinical Symptoms

II The clinical presentation of deep vein thrombosis and pulmonary thromboembolism

S. A. Renshaw, S. R. Brennan, T. W. Higenbottam

There are many occasions in clinical medicine when a single pathological process is modified by host characteristics and disease factors, which interact to determine the nature of the clinical presentation. To reach the correct diagnosis can be challenging, especially when there are few reliable diagnostic features in the history, examination or bedside investigation. A combination of high clinical suspicion, and a thoughtful analysis of all available information is required in order to steer investigations safely toward the correct diagnosis. This is particularly important for deep vein thrombosis (DVT) and pulmonary thromboembolism, which are part of one clinical entity: venous thromboembolism. Once diagnosed, the treatment of venous thromboembolism is relatively straightforward and effective (see Chapter VI.1). Unfortunately, it is often diagnosed too late, and many cases of pulmonary embolism (PE) are not diagnosed before death [1 – 3]. In one recent study, PE was not diagnosed until the post-mortem exam in 70 % of those in whom it was the fatal event [4]. Primary prevention of venous thromboembolic disease is of vast importance. Similarly, to have any impact on the mortality of this condition, the diagnosis has to be made more reliably at a time when therapeutic options are still available.

The variety of clinical presentation in venous thromboembolism is due to variations in location, size, number and chronicity of emboli, and in the patient's underlying cardiorespiratory status. Additional confounding factors exist: the presenting features are often non-specific, and other pathologies may coexist which may themselves mimic DVT or PE.

As in all clinical encounters, features of the history, examination and initial investigations need to be interpreted in light of the underlying risk. This is determined by the presence of various risk factors, which have been discussed in detail in Chapter I. For instance, it is well recognised that prolonged immobilisation (especially following surgery) and the combined oral contraceptive pill increase the risk of thrombosis. Less readily appreciated, but equally important situations are present with inherited thrombophilia, use of hormone replacement therapy, (occult) malignancy, and low cardiac output states. It is important to mention primary pulmonary hypertension at this point, as it has a unique relationship to pulmonary thromboembolic disease. The two may be difficult to distinguish clinically, and endothelial dysfunction in primary pulmonary hypertension leads to in-situ thrombosis, which can worsen the pulmonary hypertension and its prognosis (this is more fully discussed in Chapter VI.3). Primary pulmonary hypertension is considered a pro-thrombotic state by many, and anticoagulation is instituted accordingly [5].

Symptoms and signs of venous thromboembolic disease

It is helpful to group together this broad spectrum of disease into five clinical syndromes, which are listed below along with their pathological correlates (Table 1). These clinical syndromes often coexist; patients may present with combinations of features from more than one syndrome, or they may show only one isolated feature. Although the physical signs of lower limb venous thrombosis may be present in any of the chest syndromes, their presence is by no means invariable. About half of the DVT's are not apparent clinically [6].

Circulatory collapse caused by massive PE presents as shock or syncope. It is sometimes accompanied by severe breathlessness and anginal chest pain. There may be signs of acute right heart failure, with raised jugular venous pressure and a

Table 1. The clinical syndromes of venous thromboembolic disease.

Clinical syndromes	Pathological correlate
Circulatory collapse	massive pulmonary embolism
Sudden unexplained breathlessness	acute submassive pulmonary embolism
Pleuritic chest pain +/− haemoptysis	acute small pulmonary embolism; pulmonary infarction
Gradual onset exertional dyspnea	chronic pulmonary thromboembolic hypertension
Swollen, painful leg +/− any of the above	deep vein thrombosis +/− any of the above

loud pulmonary component of the second heart sound. The tachycardia and added third or fourth heart sounds may combine to produce a gallop rhythm. In contrast to cardiogenic shock, the lungs are usually clear, and there may be pulsus paradoxus. Hypotension is a predominant feature, and in the presence of prior cardiorespiratory embarrassment, cardiac arrest and death often follow. A massive embolus may follow a smaller event (or events), and other clinical syndromes may follow the break up of a massive embolus. Although the most dramatic syndrome in PE, it is seen infrequently: in a study in 155 patients with proven PE, circulatory collapse was encountered in only 5 patients (3 %) [7].

Acute breathlessness, often with tachycardia, may be the result of a submassive embolus. There may be chest pain, tachycardia, tachypnea, cyanosis, and a feeling of apprehension. Infarction is avoided as the clot is in proximal pulmonary circulation [8]. There are fewer specific clues to the diagnosis when it presents in this way. It is important to record the forced expiratory volume in one second (FEV$_1$); although a non-specific finding, a breathless patient with values in excess of 1.5l raises the suspicion of pulmonary embolus. This is particularly the case when there are no abnormal lung sounds to be heard on auscultation.

Smaller solitary emboli classically cause the clinical syndrome of pleuritic chest pain, with or without breathlessness and haemoptysis. Infarction is not invariable, and pulmonary haemorrhage and inflammation may be the cause of the symptoms described [8]. There may be dyspnea, or tachypnea, and the inflamed pleura may yield a rub on auscultation. Infarction occurs if the collateral circulation through the bronchial circulation is insufficient, or if an end-artery is occluded. This may produce haemoptysis although this is an uncommon feature, occurring in about 13 % of patients with proven emboli [9, 10]. The most common auscultatory findings are of crepitations (crackles) or reduced air entry [9], but such non-specific signs are of little diagnostic value. Pleural effusions may be

too small to be detected clinically. Pulmonary emboli, like pneumonia, may rarely present as abdominal pain, suggesting alternative diagnoses such as gall bladder disease [11].

Often a small embolus can be completely silent, or present with minimal symptoms, which may be attributed to many other pathologies. Some 40 % of patients under investigation for DVT have unsuspected pulmonary emboli demonstrated at angiography [12]. Most of these resolve without further complications, but if resolution is incomplete, then insidiously progressive exertional breathlessness and hypoxaemia can ensue. On careful questioning, there may be a history of minor chest or leg pain and paroxysmal breathlessness, although these rarely raise suspicion of PE. On occasion, proven venous thromboembolism may be the forerunner of chronic thromboembolic pulmonary hypertension. This condition is particularly difficult to diagnose, as it is often confused with airways and cardiac disease, with which it may coexist. It often remains undiagnosed until right heart failure supervenes, or until the diagnosis is established at autopsy. Again, breathlessness is inappropriately severe for the spirometric values of FEV$_1$. There are few abnormal chest signs.

Once there is right heart failure, the expected findings of a raised jugular venous pulse, right ventricular lift, and a loud pulmonary second sound may be present. When severe, there may be palpable S2, a right ventricular S3, or tricuspid regurgitation [13]. As in any cause of right-sided heart failure, there may be peripheral oedema, hepatic congestion and ascites. The finding of a high pitched flow murmur over the lung fields, due to partial occlusion of the pulmonary circulation, may further increase the likelihood of this diagnosis [14]. Once right heart failure has supervened, the prognosis is poor, but surgical pulmonary thromboendarterectomy is potentially curative (as described in Chapter VI.3).

DVT usually presents with a gradual swelling of the leg, which may be warm, discoloured and tender to touch [15, 16]. Sometimes, a red, palpable string may be seen, but this is equally frequent in superficial vein thrombosis. The most extreme form of DVT is related to cerulea alba dolens: the extreme swelling results in a compartment syndrome with arterial insufficiency leading to a painful, white discoloured leg. This form of deep vein thrombosis is a surgical emergency, and may result in loss of the limb. The average duration of symptoms, before the patient is referred for further investigation, is approximately 5 to 7 days, indicating the insidious nature of the illness [17, 18].

Many methods have been derived, and discarded for the diagnosis, such as measurement of leg circumference and increased tenderness of the calf on dorsal flexion of the foot (Homan's sign) [19]. Although only a minority of patients will have coexistent chest symptoms, PE may be shown by objective tests in 40% to 50% of patients with proven DVT of the leg veins [13, 20].

Pulmonary thromboembolic disease may, at times, present with even less specific features. In the el-derly, due to the presence of other pathologies and often borderline functional state, it can be the cause of confusion, falls, or reduced mobility. In all age groups, it can present as pyrexia, wheezing, resistant heart failure, cardiac arrhythmias, or the cause of unexplained syncope. Similarly, in bed-ridden patients DVT may go unnoticed and may be extensive due to the lack of symptoms. Once patients mobilise, the legs will show progressive oedema and may become tender. Venous thromboembolism is a great mimic of other diseases. It must be considered part of the differential diagnosis where any of the features described above are present, or when any of the bedside investigations yield suggestive results. Likewise, it has a broad differential diagnosis, which may be narrowed by eliciting the appropriate points in the history and examination, and by judicious use of investigations.

Differential diagnosis

As might well be expected with such a broad spectrum of clinical presentation, the list of differential diagnoses is broad and dependent on the clinical syndrome in question. PE is not exclusively the result of thromboembolism, and other forms of embolic material should be considered individually, as the risk factors, presentation and management are very different. In patients with long bone fractures, for example, fat embolism is a common occurrence, albeit that this is usually silent. Causes of non-thrombotic PE are shown in Table 2. It should be noted that almost all patients at risk of the conditions mentioned are also at risk of thrombotic PE, and may initially require treatment with heparin until a firm diagnosis is established.

The differential diagnosis of venous thromboembolism is listed in Table 3. Since the prognosis of undiagnosed PE is so poor, it is important to consider the diagnosis specifically when diagnosing any of the conditions listed. When there remains doubt, heparin therapy may be initiated while appropriate diagnostic tests are performed with some urgency.

Table 2. Non-thrombotic pulmonary embolism.

Type of embolism	Those at risk
Air	following large vein instrumentation, gynaecological surgery, baro trauma
Amniotic fluid	during labour
Fat	following trauma, orthopaedic surgery
Catheter	iatrogenic
Septic	any abscesses, right sided bacterial endocarditis
Injected matter	intravenous drug abusers, iatrogenic

Table 3. Differential diagnosis of venous thromboembolism.

Clinical syndrome	Differential diagnosis
Circulatory collapse	myocardial infarction, cardiogenic shock, pericardial tamponade, hypo-volaemia, sepsis, anaphylaxis, tension pneumothorax, poisoning (e. g. opiates), aortic dissection, ruptured aortic aneurysm, addisonian crisis
Sudden unexplained breathlessness	asthma, hyperventilation, cardiac ischaemia, arrhythmias, carcinoid syndrome, phaeochromocytoma, cardiomyopathy, pulmonary endema
Pleuritic chest pain	viral pleurisy, musculoskeletal chest pain, rib fracture, costochondritis, pneumonia, pericarditis, pneumothorax
Haemoptysis	bronchiectasis, bronchus carcinoma, pneumonia, nose bleed, fictitious haemoptysis
Gradual onset exertional dyspnea	asthma, congestive cardiac failure, cardiac ischaemia, primary pulmonary hypertension, chronic obstructive airways disease, interstitial lung disease, constrictive pericarditis, cardiomyopathy, valvular and congenital heart disease, pulmonary vasculitis
Swollen, painful leg	trauma, cellulitis, superficial phlebitis, muscle injury, venous reflux, ruptured Baker's cyst, haematoma, lymphangitis, inguinal abscess, contact dermatitis, arthritis, erytema nodosum

Early investigations in the diagnosis of pulmonary thromboembolic disease

The chest radiograph

Abnormalities of the chest radiograph have been described frequently in association with PE. In one series of patients with proven pulmonary emboli, over 90% had an abnormal chest X-ray [21]. However, the lack of sensitivity or specificity of the plain chest radiograph has limited its use in the diagnosis of PE. A chest radiograph is invaluable for excluding other pathologies that mimic pulmonary embolus, and it is a useful adjunct to the interpretation of lung scintigraphy. Although an unreliable tool itself [22], the chest radiograph may show abnormalities suggestive of PE. The radiograph is most commonly abnormal where there is pulmonary haemorrhage; the radiological signs corresponding to the site of pain. A normal chest radiograph in the context of dyspnea or hypoxia raises the suspicion of PE [23, 24], but the diagnosis can not be confirmed on further investigation in approximately half of these patients [9, 10]. Table 4 summarised the findings of chest radiographs in a cohort of patients who underwent pulmonary arteriography for confirmation [9].
Certain radiological features are associated with increased pulmonary artery pressure, and hence with increased severity of embolism. Prominent central pulmonary arteries and cardiomegaly are associated with the highest pulmonary arterial pressures, followed by atelectasis, pulmonary parenchymal abnormalities and pleural effusion. Patients with normal chest radiographs had the lowest pulmonary artery pressure [25].

Table 4. Radiographic signs in pulmonary embolism, and their frequency in the pulmonary embolism group in the POPU-MEfT series (without co-existing pulmonary disease) [8]

Radiological sign	Frequency (%)
Atelectasis, or pulmonary parenchymal abnormality	68*
Pleural effusion	48*
Pleural based opacity (Hampton's hump)	35*
Elevation of diaphragm	24
Decreased pulmonary vascularity	21*
Distention of proximal pulmonary vessels	15
Cardiomegaly	12
Focal oligaemia (Westermark's sign)	7
Pulmonary oedema	4**

* = significantly more common in group with pulmonary embolism

** = significantly less common in group with pulmonary embolism

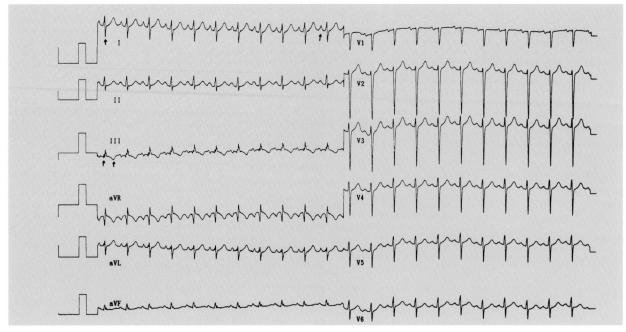

Fig. 1. Electrocardiogram showing sinus tachycardia, $S_1Q_3T_3$ and right bundle branch block in patient with massive pulmonary embolism.

The electrocardiogram

The electrocardiograph is an essential part of the assessment of any patient with chest pain, breathlessness or collapse. As well as being diagnostic of some conditions in the differential diagnosis, it gives information on underlying cardiac disease, and may itself suggest the diagnosis of PE. The most common abnormality in acute pulmonary embolism is a sinus tachycardia; other tachyarrhythmias occurring relatively rarely. Atrial fibrillation, commonly stated as a consequence of pulmonary embolism is seen in only 4 – 18 % of pulmonary emboli depending on the presence or absence of co-existing cardiac disease [10, 26]. The ECG is most commonly abnormal in massive or multiple submassive pulmonary emboli. The changes may be the classical pattern of $S_1Q_3T_3$, T-wave inversion in the right ventricular leads, right or left axis deviation, as demonstrated in Figure 1 [27, 28]. In chronic thromboembolic disease, there may be evidence of right ventricular hypertrophy [29]. In spite of all these potential findings, it should be emphasised that one study in 155 patients with proven PE showed normal ECG findings in 48 (30 %) patients [7].

Arterial blood gas analysis

Arterial blood gas analysis is an important part of the assessment of patients with suspected PE. Indeed, an isolated finding of hypoxia without any other clues may prompt the clinician to think of pul-

monary thromboembolic disease. In chronic pulmonary thromboembolism, the hypoxia may be the only finding to suggest the diagnosis. In the PIOPED cohort without coexisting disease, the arterial oxygen tension breathing room air was reduced in 74 % of the group with subsequently proven PE [9]. Hence, arterial oxygen tension is normal in 15 % to 25 % of patients with proven PE [9, 24, 25, 30 – 32] Since many patients will have coexisting disease, this figure can be expected to be higher. Patients with acute small pulmonary emboli are less likely to have abnormal blood gas analysis than any other group. Unfortunately, neither the arterial oxygen tension nor the alveolar-arterial oxygen gradient are significantly different between groups with suspected PE in whom the diagnosis was either refuted or proven, rendering the test useless for diagnostic purposes [9, 25]. Measurement of arterial carbon dioxide tension will likewise not make the diagnosis of pulmonary embolism, but in the presence of a low normal PaO_2, a low $PaCO_2$ can indicate, that oxygenation is being maintained only through increased respiratory drive. This is indicative of a pathological state, although not necessarily of pulmonary embolism. It is for this reason that oxygen saturation recording alone may give false reassurance.

D-dimer measurement

Thrombus is a dynamic metabolic structure: at the surface thrombus is undergoing lysis by the fibrinolytic system, while clot is built in other areas. The break-down of fibrin by plasmin releases split products. The split products, which contain the cross-links of the fibrin molecule, are more difficult to break up, and these fragments (so-called fragment D-dimer) are metabolised in the liver. Before this metabolic process, the concentration of plasma D-dimer may be measured by various methods. Unfortunately, D-dimer is formed in a great variety of clinical conditions, such as malignancy, infections, sepsis, pregnancy and following trauma or surgery [33, 34]. Hence, D-dimer is a non-specific test for venous thromboembolism [35–37]. Nevertheless, it has been shown that the more sensitive detection methods, such as enzyme-linked immunosorbent assays and tests, which use conjugated monoclonal antibodies, are able to detect minute amounts of D-dimer [35, 37–40]. This sensitivity is crucial, since the absence of plasma D-dimer could be regarded as proof for the absence of intravascular thrombi. However, a cost-effectiveness analysis has shown that with a decrease of sensitivity below 98% to 100%, too many thromboembolic events would go unnoticed with a resulting unacceptable increase in mortality and morbidity [41].

There has only been one management study where the measurement of plasma D-dimer has played a role in the management of PE [42]. In this study, 147 patients had non-diagnostic lung scan findings and intermediate clinical probability for PE. Of these, D-dimer was normal in 53 patients (35%), and anticoagulants were withheld. Long-term follow-up of 6 months was uneventful.

In patients with suspected DVT, 3 studies have been published or presented, which have incorporated D-dimer measurement in the management of patients [43–45]. In one study in 276 patients with initially normal impedance plethysmography findings, normal D-dimer values and low clinical probability was found in 177 patients (64%). Anticoagulants were withheld in these patients, and one patient proved to suffer a recurrent thromboembolic event during 3 months of long-term follow-up [43]. The other two studies were performed in 1128 patients with initially normal ultrasonography findings [44, 45]. A normal D-dimer result was obtained in 878 patients (78%), and these were followed-up for 3 months without anticoagulant therapy. Venous thromboembolic events occurred in 2 patients (0.2%).

Although the results of these studies are most promising, especially in DVT management, D-dimer measurement can not be advocated for use in general clinical practice. The final results of some of these studies as well as some ongoing trials need to be awaited before this approach can be deemed safe.

Clinical decision rules

The clinical diagnosis of DVT and PE is unreliable. Nevertheless, some recent studies have come to light which have addressed the value of clinical signs and symptoms in a more standardised and quantitated fashion.

In patients with suspected DVT, one clinical decision rule has been developed (Table 5) [46]. This score is easy to obtain, and was capable of indicating high, intermediate or low clinical probability for the presence of DVT. Using this score in combination with ultrasonography of the leg veins, repeat testing was still required in only 199 of 593 patients (34%) [46]. The clinical model was subsequently validated in a prospective study [47].

In patients with clinically suspected PE, three studies showed different approaches [48–50]. One study, which was based on data from the PIOPED study, developed a neural network which was able to outperform attending physicians in the assessment of pre-test probability for the presence of emboli [48]. Another study, which was based on a

Table 5. Clinical model for pre-test assessment of patients with suspected deep vein thrombosis [46, 47]

Data from history and physical examination	Score
Known malignancy	1
Immobilisation lower extremity	1
Recent bed rest (> 3 days)/major surgery (< 4 weeks)	1
Localised swelling in course of deep venous system	1
Swelling of leg	1
Swelling calf (left-right difference > 3 cm)	1
Pitting oedema	1
Collateral superficial veins (not varicosis)	1
Major chance of alternative diagnosis	−2

High risk = score ≥ 3
intermediate risk = score 1 or 2
low risk = score ≤ 0

prospective diagnostic survey in a large cohort of patients with suspected PE, derived a clinical decision rule based on physical signs, such as wheezing, cough, fever and perfusion scan defects [49]. This rule was able to adequately exclude PE in 16% of patients with non-diagnostic lung scan results. Finally, a clinical model was tested in a large cohort of patients with suspected PE [50]. The pretest probability was considered low in 734 patients (venous thromboembolism proven in 3.3%). The presence of thromboemboli increased to 27% of 402 patients with moderate pretest probability, while 75% of 99 patients with high pretest probability had the diagnosis confirmed.

To date no clinical decision rules or artificial neural network exist that have undergone management studies for the evaluation of their clinical validity in either the DVT or PE subgroups.

Prior cardiorespiratory disease should alert the clinician to a high risk situation: many cardiorespiratory diseases put the patient at risk of pulmanory thromboembolic disease; new pulmanory emboli may be interpreted as a deterioration in the underlying disease, and this group is less able to compensate for the additional insult. The result is an increased mortality in this group. The mortality of patients with prior cardiorespiratory disease and a low probability lung scan, who do not receive anticoagulation is at least 8.5%. This should be considered carefuly when making a clinical decision about anticoagulation in this group.

Other diagnostic tests

The most important diagnostic tests which are currently used for the diagnosis of DVT and PE will be discussed in subsequent chapters. Many other diagnostic tests have been advocated for use in patients with clinically suspected venous thromboembolism, such as strain gauge plethysmography [51, 52], liquid crystal thermography [53, 54] and radionuclide venography [55, 56]. However, these tests have failed to reach clinical applicability, and will not be discussed further.

References

1. Karwinski B, Svendsen E. Comparison of clinical and post-mortem diagnosis of pulmonary embolism. J Clin Pathol 1989; 42: 135–139

2. Goldhaber SZ, Hennekens CH, Evans DA, Newton EC, Godleski JJ. Factors associated with correct antemortem diagnosi of major pulmonary embolism. Am J Med 1982; 73: 822–826

3. Gross JS, Neufeld RR, Libouw LS, Gerber J, Rodstein M. Autopsy study of the elderly institutionalized patient. Review of 234 autopsies. Arch Intern Med 1988; 148: 170–176

4. Stein PD, Henry JW. Prevalence of acute pulmonary embolism among patients in a general hospital and at autopsy. Chest 1995; 108: 978–981

5. Chaouat A, Weitzenblum E, Higenbottam T. The role of thrombosis in severe pulmonary hypertension. Eur Resp J 1996; 9: 356–363

6. Landefeld CS, McGuire E, Cohen AM. Clinical findings associated with deep venous thrombosis: a basis for quantifying clinical judgement. Am J Med 1990; 88: 382–388

7. Stein PD, Henry JW. Clinical characteristics of patients with acute pulmonary embolism stratified according to their presenting syndromes. Chest 1997; 112: 974–979

8. Dalen JE, Haffajee CI, Alpert JS, Howe JP, Ockene IS, Paraskos JA. Pulmonary embolism, pulmonary haemorrhage and pulmonary infarction. N Engl J Med 1977; 296: 1431–1435

9. Stein PD, Terrin ML, Hales CA, Palevsky HI, Saltzman HA, Thompson BT, Weg JG. Clinical, laboratory, roentgenographic and electrocardiograhpic findings in patients with acute pulmonary embolism and no pre-existing cardiac or pulmonary disease. Chest 1991; 100: 598–603

10. Munganelli D, Palla A, Donnamaria V, Giuntine C. Clinical features of pulmonary embolism. Doubts and certainties. Chest 1995; 107: 25S–31S

11. Von Pohle WR. Pulmonary embolism presenting as acute abdominal pain. Respiration 1996; 63: 318–320

12. Moser KM, Fedullo PF, Littejohn JK, Crawford R. Frequent asymptomatic pulmonary embolism in patients with deep venous thrombosis. JAMA 1994; 271: 223–225

13. Moser KM, Auger WR, Fedullo PF. Chronic major vessel thromboembolic pulmonary hypertension. Circulation 1990; 81: 1735–1743

14. Auger WR, Moser KM. Pulmonary flow murmurs: a distinctive physical sign found in chronic pulmonary thromboembolic disease. Clin Research 1989; 37: 145A

15. Haeger K. Problems of acute deep venous thrombosis. I. The interpretation of signs and symptoms. Angiol 1969; 20: 219–223

16. Cranley JJ, Canos AJ, Sull WJ. The diagnosis of deep venous thrombosis. Fallibility of clinical symptoms and signs. Arch Surg 1976; 111: 34–36

17. Huisman MV, Büller HR, ten Cate JW, Vreeken J. Serial impedance plethysmography for suspected deep venous thrombosis in outpatients. The Amsterdam General Practitioner Study. N Engl J Med 1986; 314: 823–828

18. Heyboer H, Büller HR, Lensing AWA, Turpie AG, Colly LP, ten Cate JW. A randomized comparison of the clinical utility of real-time compression ultrasonography versus impedance plethysmography in the diagnosis of deep-vein thrombosis in symptomatic outpatients. N Engl J Med 1993; 329: 511–513

19. Homans J. Thrombosis of the deep veins of the lower leg, causing pulmonary embolism. N Engl J Med 1934; 211: 933–937

20. Huisman MV, Büller HR, ten Cate JW, et al. Unexpected high prevalence of silent pulmonary embolism in patients with deep venous thrombosis. Chest 1989; 95: 498–502

21. Moses DC, Silver TM, Bookstein JJ. The complementary roles of chest radiography, lung scanning, and selective pulmonary angiography in the diagnosis of pulmonary embolism. Circulation 1974; 49: 179–184

22. Greenspan RH, Ravin CE, Polansky SM, McLoud TC. Accuracy of the chest radiograph in diagnosis of pulmonary embolism. Invest Radiol 1982; 17: 539–543

23. Palla A, Petruzzelli S, Donnamaria V, Giuntini C. The role of suspicion in the diagnosis of pulmonary embolism. Chest 1995; 107 (suppl): 21–24

24. Stein PD, Alavi A, Gottschalk A, et al. Usefulness of non-invasive diagnostic tools for diagnosis of acute pulmonary embolism in patients with a normal chest radiograph. Am J Cardiol 1991; 67: 1117–1120

25. Stein PD, Athanasoulis C, Greenspan RH, Henry JW. Relation of plain chest radiographic findings to pulmonary artery pressure and arterial blood oxygen levels in patients with acute pulmonary embolism. Am J Cardiol 1992; 69: 394–396

26. Seeram N, Cheriex EC, Smeets JLRM, Gorgels AP, Wellens HJJ. Value of the 12-lead electrocardiogram at hospital admission in the diagnosis of pulmonary embolism. Am J Cardiol 1994; 78: 298–303

27. Hubloue I, Schoors D, Diltoer M, van Tussenbroek F, de Wilde P. Early electrocardiographic signs in acute massive pulmonary embolism. Eur J Emerg Med 1996; 3: 199–204

28. Ferrari E, Imbert A, Chevalier T, Mihoubi A, Morand P, Boudouy M. The ECG in pulmonary embolism – predictive value of negative T-waves in precordial leads – 80 case reports. Chest 1997; 111: 537–543

29. Fedullo PF, Moser KM. Advances in acute pulmonary embolism and chronic pulmonary hypertension. Adv Intern Med 1997; 42: 67–104

30. Bell WR, Simon TL, DeMets DL. The clinical features of submassive and massive pulmonary embolism. Am J Med 1977; 62: 355–360

31. Stein PD, Willis III PW, DeMets DL. History and physical examination in acute pulmonary embolism in patients without preexisting cardiac or pulmonary disease. Am J Cardiol 1981; 47: 218–223

32. Szucs MM Jr, Brooks HL, Grossman W, et al. Diagnostic sensitivity of laboratory findings in acute pulmonary embolism. Ann Intern Med 1971; 74: 161–166

33. Demers C, Ginsberg JS, Johnston M, Brill-Edwards P, Panju A. D-dimer and thrombin-antithrombin III complexes in patients with clinically suspected pulmonary embolism. Thromb Haemostas 1992; 67: 408–412

34. Raimondi P, Bongard O, de Moerloose P, Reber G, Waldvogel F, Bounameaux H. D-dimer plasma concentration in various clinical conditions: implications for the use of this test in the diagnostic approach of venous thromboembolism. Thromb Res 1993; 69: 125–130

35. Bounameaux H, de Moerloose P, Perrier A, Reber G. Plasma measurement of D-dimer as diagnostic aid in suspected venous thromboembolism: an overview. Thromb Haemostas 1994; 71: 1–6

36. Van Beek EJR, Van den Ende B, Berckmans RJ, et al. A comparative analysis of D-dimer assays in patients with clinically suspected pulmonary embolism. Thromb Haemostas 1993; 70: 408–413

37. Ginsberg JS, Wells PS, Brill-Edwards P, et al. Application of a novel and rapid whole blood assay for D-dimer in patients with clinically suspected pulmonary embolism. Thromb Haemostas 1995; 73: 35–38

38. Turkstra F, van Beek EJR, ten Cate JW, Büller HR. Reliable rapid blood test for the exclusion of venous thromboembolism in symptomatic outpatients. Thromb Haemostas 1996; 76: 9–11

39. Elias A, Appel I, Huc B, et al. D-dimer test and diagnosis of deep vein thrombosis: a comparative study of 7 assays. Thromb Haemostas 1996; 76: 518–522

40. De Moerloose P, Desmarais S, Bounameaux H, et al. Contribution of a new, rapid individual and quantitative automated D-dimer ELISA to exclude pulmonary embolism. Thromb Haemostas 1996; 75: 11–13

41. Van Beek EJR, Schenk BE, Michel BC, van den Ende A, van der Heide YT, Brandjes DPM, Bossuyt PMM, Büller HR. The role of plasma D-dimer concentration in the exclusion of pulmonary embolism. Br J Hematology 1996; 92: 725–732

42. Perrier A. Bounameaux H, Morabia A, et al. Diagnosis of pulmonary embolism by a decision analysis-based strategy including clinical probability, D-dimer levels, and ultrasonography: a management study. Arch Intern Med 1996; 156: 531–536

43. Ginsberg JS, Kearon C, Douketis J, et al. The use of D-dimer testing and impedance plethysmographic examination in patients with clinical indications of deep-vein thrombosis. Arch Intern Med 1997; 157: 1077–1081

44. Bernardi E, Prandoni P. Compression ultrasound and D-dimer in the management of patients with clinically suspected deep-vein thrombosis. Thromb Haemostas 1997 (suppl): 767

45. Kraayenhagen RA, Koopman MMW, Bernardi E, et al. Simplification of the diagnostic management of outpatients with symptomatic deep vein thrombosis with D-dimer measurements. Thromb Haemostas 1997 (suppl): 159

46. Wells PS, Hirsh J, Anderson DR, et al. Accuracy of clinical assessment of deep-vein thrombosis. Lancet 1995; 345: 1326–1330

47. Wells PS, Anderson DR, Bormanis J, et al. Value of assessment of pretest probability of deep-vein thrombosis in clinical management. Lancet 1997; 350: 1795–1798

48. Patil S, Henry JW, Rubenfire M, Stein PD. Neural network in the clinical diagnosis of acute pulmonary embolism. Chest 1993; 104: 1685–1689

49. Michel BC, Kuijer PMM, McDonnell J, van Beek EJR, Rutten FFH, Büller HR. The role of a decision rule in symptomatic pulmonary embolism patients with a non-high probability ventilation-perfusion scan. Thromb Haemostas 1997; 78: 794–798

50. Wells PS, Ginsberg JS, Anderson DR, Hirsh J, Turpie A, Bormanis J, et al. The use of a clinical model in a prospective management study of patients with suspected pulmonary embolism. Blood 1996; 88 (suppl): 625a

51. Barnes RW, Collicott PE, Mozersky DJ, Summer DS, Strandness DE. Noninvasive quantitation of maximum venous outflow in acute thrombophlebitis. Surgery 1972; 72: 971–979

52. Cranley JJ, Gay AY, Grass AM, Simeone FA. A plethysmographyic technique for the diagnosis of deep venous thrombosis of the lower extremities. Surg, Gyn and Obstet 1973; 136: 385–394

53. Holmgren K, Jacobsson H, Johnsson H, Lofsjogard-Nilsson E. Thermography and plethysmography, a non-invasive alternative to venography in the diagnosis of deep vein thrombosis. J Intern Med 1990; 228: 29–33

54. Bounameaux H, Khabiri E, Huber O, et al. Value of liquid crystal contact thermography and plasma level of D-dimer in screening of deep venous thrombosis following general abdominal surgery. Thromb Haemostas 1992; 67: 603–606

55. Webber MM, Pollak EW, Victery W, Cragin M, Resnick LH, Grollman JH. Thrombosis detection by radionuclide particle (MAA) entrapment: correlation with fibrinogen uptake and venography. Radiology 1974; 111: 645–650

56. LeClerc JR, Wolfson C, Arzoumanian A, Blake GP, Rosenthall L. Technetium-99m red blood cell venography in patients with clinically suspected deep vein thrombosis: a prospective study. J Nucl Med 1988; 29: 1498–1506

Chapter III
Diagnostic Procedures

natively, patients with an abnormal test should have the findings confirmed. When a new diagnostic test for venous thrombosis has complied with the requirements of each of these three phases, it can be recommended for clinical use. The recommendation should specify the patient category for which the diagnostic test has been shown to be appropriate, since the various objective tests have different diagnostic accuracies depending on the nature of the patient category under investigation (i. e., first or recurrent episode of symptomatic venous thrombosis, or asymptomatic DVT).

Methodologic considerations and analysis

We critically reviewed the articles published in the English literature that evaluated the accuracy of diagnostic methods for the diagnosis of proximal or calf-vein thrombosis in patients with a clinical suspicion of a first or recurrent suspected episode or asymptomatic high-risk patients. To minimise diagnostic suspicion bias, reports were only included for this review if the diagnostic test under consideration was independently compared with venography and the results were interpreted by observers who had no knowledge of the other outcome of the test [17]. In addition, reports needed to evaluate consecutive patients who were studied prospectively since the failure to meet this requirement can result in the exclusion of patients in certain risk categories and so produce false estimates of accuracy.

Diagnostic techniques

The presently available techniques for the objective diagnosis of DVT include invasive and non-invasive methods and biochemical assays. These techniques visualise the thrombus (contrast venography, real-time B-mode ultrasonography with or without (colour) Doppler facilities, and computed tomography or magnetic resonance imaging), measure venous outflow (impedance plethysmography or strain gauge plethysmography, and Doppler ultrasound), measure the incorporation of radiolabelled proteins in the developing thrombus (^{125}I-fibrinogen leg scanning and several other isotopic methods), or detect circulating fibrin formation or breakdown products. Of these methods, ultrasound imaging, impedance plethysmography, and Doppler ultrasonography are the most widely used methods.

Contrast venography is generally considered the reference method for the presence or absence of DVT against which all other tests should be compared.

Venography

With contrast venography, the entire deep venous system is visualised. Usually separate exposures are obtained of the calf and proximal veins. Although contrast venography is widely accepted as the gold standard for the diagnosis of DVT, several features have limited the general use of this method including its invasive nature, the technical requirements, and the difficulty of repeating the test. Also, the test may not be feasible or is inadequate for interpretation in approximately 10 to 20% of patients [18, 19].

The most reliable venographic criterion is the presence of an intraluminal filling defect that is constant in all films and is seen in at least two different projections (Fig. 1) [20]. Other less reliable criteria include: (1) non-filling of a segment of the deep venous system with abrupt termination of the column of contrast medium at a constant site below the segment and reappearance of the contrast medium at a constant site above the segment and (2) non-filling of the deep venous system above the knee, despite repeated injections of contrast material and adequate venographic technique. The likelihood that these appearances are due to venous thrombosis is increased if the abnormality is associated with the presence of abnormal collaterals.

Venography is a technique that requires experience to perform and interpret adequately. Unless care is taken to inject the dye into the dorsal foot vein, there may be non-filling of calf veins that is interpreted as being falsely abnormal for thrombosis because the vein is not filled, or as falsely normal because the filling defect produced by the thrombus is not seen. The proximal part of the femoral vein, the external iliac and common iliac veins may also be inadequately filled by ascending venography.

Contrast venography is contraindicated in patients with acute or chronic renal failure, a history of a reaction to contrast material, or an obvious local infection of the foot. If venography is required in pregnant women, it should be performed with the foetus shielded from radiation by covering the patient's abdomen and upper thighs with a lead-lined apron (see Chapter VII.2). With the use of low osmolar contrast materials, adverse reactions have become rare.

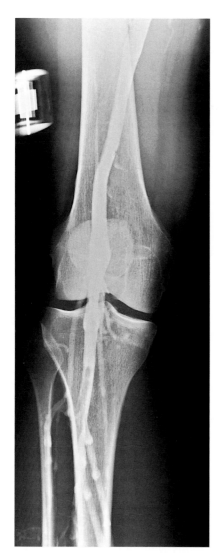

Fig. 1. Venogram demonstrating thrombus extending from the calf into the popliteal vein.

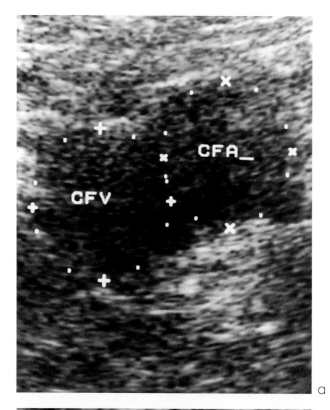

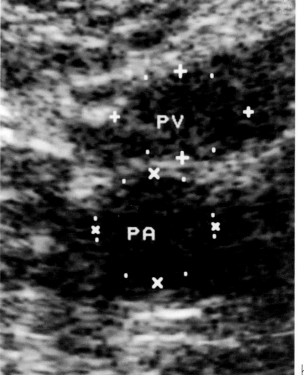

Fig. 2a, b. Ultrasound images at level of left common femoral vein (**a**) and popliteal vein (**b**) demonstrating anatomic position of deep venous system in relation to arterial system.
CFA = Common femoral artery, CFV = Common femoral vein,
PA = popliteal artery, PV = popliteal vein

Ultrasonography techniques

1) Conventional gray-scale real-time ultrasonography

Venous ultrasound imaging is performed with the patient in the supine position, with the head of the bed elevated approximately 30 degrees to ensure adequate venous filling of the legs. The ultrasound probe is placed in the groin to identify the common femoral vein, which is always medial to the common femoral artery (Fig. 2). The transducer is then moved distally to visualise the superficial femoral vein throughout its course. For examination of the popliteal vein, the patient is in the prone or the lateral decubitus position with the knees flexed to prevent spontaneous collapse of the vein. The lumen of a normal vein is free of echoes and, as opposed to arteries, veins have thin walls and are held open primarily by the low venous blood pres-

sure. Therefore, the vein lumen can be easily obliterated by a small amount of extrinsic pressure (Fig. 3).

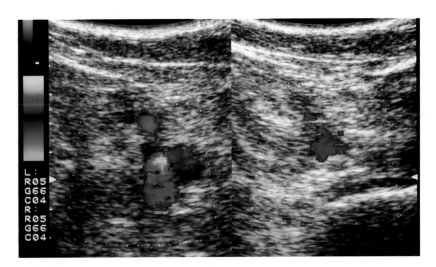

Fig. 3. Ultrasound scan at level of popliteal vein shows arterial signal (red) and disappearance of venous signal (blue) during compression.

The most accurate and simple ultrasonic criterion for diagnosing venous thrombosis is non-compressibility of the vascular lumen under gentle probe pressure (compression ultrasound) [21, 22]. Vein compressibility is considered present if no residual lumen is observed and indicates the absence of venous thrombosis. The images can be obtained in either the transverse or longitudinal plane. However, vein compressibility is best evaluated in the transverse view because it allows visualisation of both the vein and the adjacent artery (Fig. 4). With the vein imaged in the longitudinal plane, the vein may slide out of the image plane during compression with the ultrasound probe and so falsely simulate compressibility of the venous segment. The presence of echogenic bands in the vein might be helpful to diagnose venous thrombosis but they are often observed in patients in whom contrast venography proves the absence of venous thrombosis. In general, the common femoral and popliteal vein can be visualised most easily due to their superficial location. The superficial femoral vein, especially the segment that passes through the adductor canal, is localised deeper and is often more difficult to evaluate. The calf veins cannot be evaluated with conventional ultrasound techniques because they cannot be visualised adequately due to their small size and insufficient resolution of the current ultrasound device.

2) Duplex ultrasonography
Patients are examined in an identical way as with conventional compression ultrasound. In addition, blood flow characteristics may be evaluated using the pulsed Doppler capability. Blood flow in normal veins is spontaneous and phasic with respiration (Fig. 5a), can be augmented by elevating the distal lower extremity or by manual compression

distal to the ultrasound transducer, and can be interrupted by performing the Valsalva manoeuvre (Fig. 5b). When the phasic pattern is absent, flow is defined as continuous, indicating the presence of venous outflow obstruction, especially when there is no or minimal change after the Valsalva manoeuvre. Absence of spontaneous venous flow may result from complete obstruction of the vein lumen.

A major drawback of the duplex examination is the lack of objective and standardised diagnostic criteria for the Doppler assessment. Sometimes spontaneous flow cannot be detected in normal veins due to low flow in small veins and augmentation techniques will not always result in a clear venous Doppler signal. Furthermore, continuous flow with no or poor response to the Valsalva manoeuvre can be observed in patients without venous thrombosis. In patients with non-occlusive venous thrombosis the normal finding, i. e., phasic spontaneous flow interrupted by the Valsalva manoeuvre, may be observed. The assessment of the calf veins by duplex ultrasound is, as for the conventional gray-scale examination, hampered by the poor visualisation of these veins.

3) Colour-coded Doppler ultrasonography
The technique of the colour-coded Doppler ultrasonography (colour Doppler) examination is basically identical with that of compression ultrasound and duplex ultrasonography. In colour flow sonography, pulsed Doppler signals are used to produce the images. When a Doppler shift is recognised, it is assigned a colour (i. e., red or blue) according to its forward or reverse direction. Therefore, the technique of colour Doppler mapping results in a display of flowing blood as a colour overlay to the gray-scale ultrasound image which

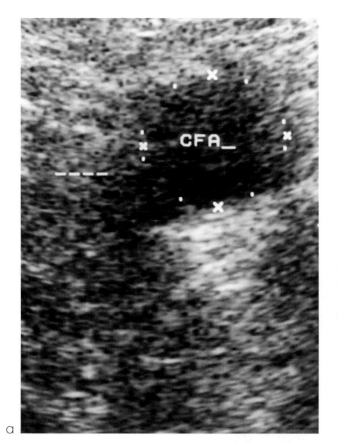

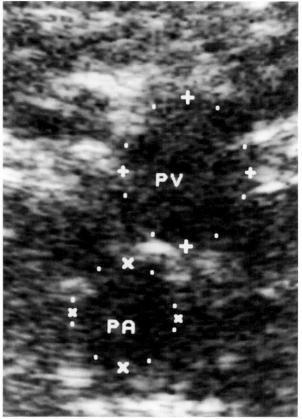

has the potential to enhance the ability to identify the veins even when they are obscured by soft tissue oedema or by excessive depth from the transducer. Colour Doppler has the potential to visualise the calf veins.

Images in the longitudinal axis are used for the assessment with colour Doppler. The interpretation of venous flow whether with colour Doppler or duplex ultrasonography is essentially the same. The criterion for an abnormal colour Doppler test is the absence of colour in a vein after augmentation or a focal intraluminal filling defect (Figs. 6a and b). As with the duplex examination, "venous flow" is Doppler wave information detected as a Doppler shift, rather than true flow measured in volume per unit of time. Therefore, Doppler detected flow may be absent in normal veins due to low flow, and augmentation does not always result in a clear colour image. The colour Doppler examination might be falsely interpreted as normal in patients with non-occlusive thrombosis due to persistent venous flow (and, therefore, normal colour coding of venous flow) around the thrombus.

Fig. 4a – c. Compression ultrasound showing (a) complete compressibility of left common femoral vein (note distortion of artery) and non-compressible popliteal vein (b). At this level was DVT (c)

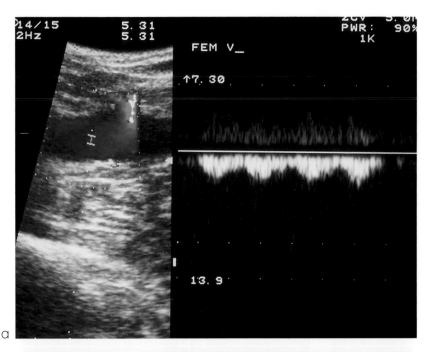

a

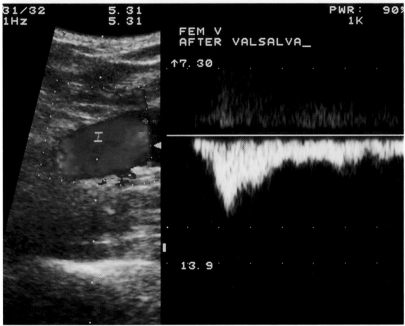

b

Fig. 5a, b. **(a)** Normal phasic venous flow pattern. **(b)** Valsalva manoeuvre stops venous flow. After cessation there is an initial increase in flow and then a return to normal phasic venous flow pattern.

Impedance plethysmography

Impedance plethysmography is performed with the patient supine and with the lower limb elevated 25° to 30°, the knee flexed 10° to 20°, and the ankle 8 cm to 15 cm higher than the knee. The cuff is inflated to a pressure of 50 cm H_2O. The test measures volume changes in the leg produced by inflation and deflation of a pneumatic thigh cuff. The volume changes in the calf are measured with the use of circumferential electrodes. The presence of proximal vein thrombosis or extensive calf vein thrombosis will result in impairment of ve-

nous outflow. Objective criteria have been defined using a discriminant line that was developed by discriminant function analysis to provide optimal separation of the impedance plethysmography test result in patients with and without proximal vein thrombosis [23]. Impedance plethysmography is relatively simple to perform, is well standardised and is an easily repeatable test which detects occlusive thrombosis in the proximal veins. The method does not distinguish between thrombotic and non-thrombotic obstruction to venous outflow. A disadvantage of impedance plethysmography is that the test is relatively insensitive to isolated calf

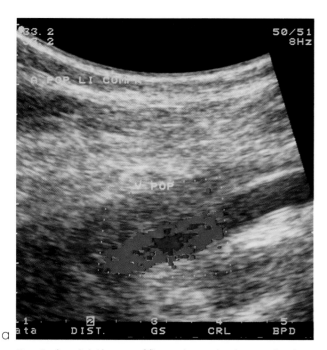
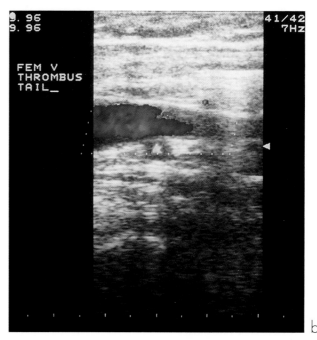

Fig. 6a, b. **(a)** Absence of flow in the popliteal vein with echogenic material suggesting DVT (during compression). **(b)** Absence of flow in the distal end of the femoral vein with return of flow more proximally. This proved a free floating thrombus tail.

vein thrombosis and non-obstructive proximal thrombi. A reliable test result can be obtained in almost all patients except in those who cannot be positioned correctly.

Doppler ultrasonography

The Doppler ultrasound examination is performed with the patient lying in bed in the semi-upright position with the hip slightly externally rotated. The common femoral vein is located by initially placing the probe over the common femoral artery, which can be easily identified, and then moving it medially until the low-pitched sound, typical of venous flow, is heard. The intensity of this low-pitched sound decreases with inspiration and increases with expiration, resulting in a phasic signal. Abdominal compression will result in interruption of venous flow in the leg and when abdominal compression is released, there is an augmented sound as blood flow in the veins suddenly increases. Manual compression of the thigh and calf produces an augmented venous sound due to sudden acceleration of venous flow. Patency of the entire superficial femoral vein can be confirmed by moving the probe distally along this vein and repeating calf and distal thigh compression. However, care must be taken not to confuse the sounds with those produced by the long saphenous vein. Augmentation of flow is also induced by sudden

release of thigh compression proximal to the probe. The probe is then placed over the posterior tibial vein, which is located adjacent to the corresponding artery behind the ankle. Augmentation of flow is produced by squeezing the foot and by suddenly releasing proximal calf compression. Doppler ultrasound is sensitive to occlusive thrombi in the popliteal and more proximal veins, but is less sensitive to non-occlusive proximal thrombi. The ultrasonic detection of isolated calf vein thrombosis is cumbersome due to slow venous flow, which is often beyond the detection limit of the Doppler equipment and the complicated anatomy of the calf veins. Obstruction to venous outflow may result in an absent venous signal, provided that the thrombus completely occludes the vein. Augmentation of the venous signal may in case of intravascular thrombus formation be diminished, high-pitched and of short duration, or absent. Manoeuvres such as deep breathing, or Valsalva's, may also result in increase of venous flow and may produce additional information regarding the patency of veins. However, venous flow may be interpreted as normal in patients with non-occlusive thrombosis, which does not cause hemodynamic changes, and in patients with collateral veins. False abnormal results may be found in patients with extrinsic venous compression, or with previous DVT, but may also be the result of inexperience of the examiner. The interpretation of Doppler ultrasound results is in part subjective and requires considerable skill and experience to perform reliably. Recordings of the signals on a strip-chart have overcome the subjective interpretation of the test [101].

^{125}I-fibrinogen leg scanning

Patients are scanned with an isotope detector probe while their legs are elevated 15° above horizontal to minimise venous pooling in the calf veins. Readings are taken over both legs and the results are expressed as a percentage of the sur-face radioactivity measured over the heart. The surface radioactivity is recorded over the femoral vein at 7 cm to 8 cm intervals, from the inguinal ligament and over the medial and posterior aspects of the popliteal fossa and calf. Venous thrombosis is suspected if there is an increase in the radioactivity of more than 20% at any point compared with the readings over the adjacent points on the limb, or with the same point on the previous day, or with the readings over the corresponding point on the opposite leg. Venous thrombosis is diagnosed if the scan remains abnormal.

Diagnosis of symptomatic DVT

Ultrasound imaging

A total of 20 ultrasound studies were selected for this analysis. In these investigations, venography was used in all patients and they included only patients with signs and symptoms of venous thrombosis of the lower extremity. Several other studies are not included in the analysis, since they did not fulfil the requirements of a systematic use of venography, a clear patient selection, or independent comparison with the reference standard [24–53]. Of the selected 20 reports, 11 evaluated compression ultrasound [54–64], 5 used duplex ultrasonography, and 4 assessed colour-coded ultrasonography.

Accuracy for proximal-vein thrombosis

a) Compression ultrasonography

Of the 11 studies evaluating compression ultrasound, 9 included symptomatic outpatients and two hospitalised patients who became symptomatic for venous thrombosis during their stay in hospital. The combined analysis of the outpatients studies demonstrated that compression ultrasound correctly identified proximal-vein thrombosis in 414 of the 430 patients, for a sensitivity of 96% (Table 2). Thrombosis was correctly excluded in 546 of the 559 patients with normal venograms, for a specificity of 98%. Therefore, the positive predictive value was 96%. Feasibility of the compression ultrasound test was consistently high in all studies. Inconclusive compression ultrasound test results occurred infrequently (less than 1% of patients). Two large studies limited the compression ultrasound evaluation to the common femoral and popliteal vein [55, 58]. Combining the data, the sensitivity and specificity for proximal-vein thrombosis was 97% and 99%, respectively: these results are fully comparable with the results of studies that evaluated the entire proximal venous system. Both compression ultrasound studies, which studied hospitalised patients who became symptomatic for venous thrombosis during hospitalisation, used correct methodology [63, 64]. In these

Table 2. Compression ultrasonography in patients with clinically suspected DVT.

Investigators	Sensitivity for Proximal DVT	Specificity
Dauzat et al. 1986 [54]	97% (89/92)	100% (45/45)
Appelman et al. 1987 [55]	92% (48/52)	97% (58/60)
Aitken, Godden 1987 [56]	94% (15/16)	100% (26/26)
Cronan et al. 1987 [57]	93% (25/27)	100% (23/23)
Lensing et al. 1989 [58]	100% (66/66)	99% (142/143)
Monreal et al. 1989 [59]	93% (40/43)	86% (18/21)
Habscheid et al. 1990 [60]	95% (57/60)	100% (91/91)
Gudmundsen et al. 1990 [61]	100% (60/60)	97% (87/90)
Chance et al. 1991 [62]	100% (14/14)	93% (56/60)
Total	96% (414/430)	98% (546/559)

patients, the combined sensitivity and specificity for proximal-vein thrombosis were 91% (135/148) and 94% (102/109), respectively. These findings in hospitalised patients appear to be comparable with the results obtained in symptomatic outpatients.

b) Duplex ultrasonography

Of the 5 selected studies evaluating the accuracy of duplex ultrasonography for the diagnosis of proximal-vein thrombosis (4 in symptomatic outpatients, 1 in hospitalised patients). The combined sensitivity for the 4 outpatients studies was 95% (98/103), whereas specificity was 93% (134/144) (Table 3) [65–68]. The positive predictive value was, therefore, 91%. In the single duplex ultrasonography study, which evaluated hospitalised patients who became symptomatic for venous thrombosis during hospitalisation, sensitivity and specificity for proximal-vein thrombosis were 97% and 98%, respectively [69].

c) Colour Doppler ultrasonography

In the 4 selected studies, colour Doppler correctly diagnosed proximal-vein thrombosis in 123 of the 127 patients, for a sensitivity of 97% (Table 4) [70–73]. The presence of proximal-vein thrombosis was correctly excluded in 207 of the 213 patients, for a specificity of 97%. The predictive value of an abnormal test result was, therefore, 96%.

Accuracy for isolated calf-vein thrombosis

Only one study correctly evaluating accuracy investigated the use of compression ultrasound in the diagnosis of isolated calf-vein thrombosis (Table 5) [60]. In this study, isolated calf-vein thrombosis was demonstrated by venography in 23 patients and compression ultrasound identified 20 of these (sensitivity, 87%). Of the duplex ultrasonography studies performed with correct methodology, the ability to detect isolated calf-vein thrombosis was addressed in one small investigation [68]. In this study, duplex ultrasonography identified 2 of the 5 patients with isolated calf-vein thrombosis (sensitivity, 40%). The sensitivity of colour Doppler ultrasonography for isolated calf-vein thrombosis was determined in 2 methodologically sound studies [70, 71]; colour Doppler correctly identified 24 of the 32 patients with isolated calf-vein thrombosis, for a sensitivity of 75%.

Table 3. Duplex ultrasonography in patients with clinically suspected DVT.

Investigators	Sensitivity for proximal DVT	Specificity
Vogel et al. 1987 [65]	95% (19/20)	100% (33/33)
O'Leary et al. 1988 [66]	92% (22/24)	96% (25/26)
Mantoni et al. 1989 [67]	97% (34/35)	97% (48/50)
Mitchell et al. 1991 [68]	96% (23/24)	80% (28/35)
Total	95% (98/103)	93% (134/144)

Table 4. Colour-coded Doppler ultrasonography in patients with clinically suspected DVT.

Investigators	Sensitivity for proximal DVT	Specificity
Baxter et al. 1990 [70]	92% (11/12)	100% (26/26)
Rose et al. 1990 [71]	92% (23/25)	100% (50/50)
Schindler et al. 1990 [72]	98% (54/55)	100% (100/100)
Mattos et al. 1992 [73]	100% (35/35)	84% (31/37)
Total	97% (123/127)	97% (207/213)

Table 5. Sensitivity for isolated calf-vein thrombosis for studies in symptomatic patients, which minimised the potential for bias.

	Sensitivity	95% Confidence Interval
Gray-scale real-time ultrasonography		
Habscheid et al. 1990 [60]	87% (20/23)	65–92%
Duplex ultrasonography		
Mitchell et al. 1991 [68]	40% (2/5)	13–93%
Colour Doppler ultrasonography		
Baxter et al. 1990 [70]	100% (2/2)	23–100%
Rose et al. 1990 [71]	73% (22/30)	54–87%
Total	75% (24/32)	56–88%

Table 6. Impedence plethysmography in patients with clinically suspected DVT.

Investigator(s)	Sensitivity	Specificity
Hull et al. 1976 [74]	93% (124/133)	97% (386/397)
Richards et al. 1976 [75]	81% (30/37)	87% (78/90)
Hull et al. 1977 [76]	98% (59/60)	95% (108/114)
Toy Schrier 1978 [77]	94% (15/16)	100% (9/9)
Hull et al. 1978 [78]	92% (155/169)	96% (305/317)
Hull et al. 1981 [79]	95% (74/78)	98% (157/160)
Peters et al. 1982 [80]	92% (36/39)	93% (115/124)
Prandoni et al. 1991 [81]	86% (44/51)	95% (134/141)
Anderson et al. 1992 [82]	66% (37/56)	–
Total	90% (574/639)	96% (1292/1352)

Table 7. Doppler ultrasonography in symptomatic patients.

Investigators	Sensitivity	Specificity
Yao et al. 1972 [92]	100% (33/33)	88% (15/17)
Holmes et al. 1973 [93]	100% (17/17)	94% (46/49)
Meadway et al. 1975 [94]	85% (29/34)	72% (55/76)
Dosick et al. 1978 [95]	96% (50/52)	93% (100/102)
Flanigan et al. 1978 [96]	65% (35/54)	96% (94/98)
Sumner Lambeth 1979 [97]	94% (34/36)	90% (35/39)
Hanel et al. 1981 [98]	92% (49/53)	91% (118/130)
Zielinsky et al. 1983 [99]	95% (20/21)	76% (117/153)
Turnbull et al. 1990 [100]	87% (13/15)	78% (33/42)
Lensing et al. 1993 [3,206]	87% (83/92)	99% (206/209)

Impedance plethysmography

Thus far, the accuracy of impedance plethysmography for the diagnosis of DVT in symptomatic patients has been evaluated in 17 studies (including one study in hospitalised patients). The inclusion of consecutive patients and independent analysis of a standardised impedance plethysmography result with venography was used in 9 studies [74–82], whereas the remaining 8 studies had a potential for bias, or did not truly evaluate accuracy [83–91]. The combined analysis of the studies using proper methodology demonstrated that impedance plethysmography detected 574 of the 639 proximal thrombi, for a sensitivity of 90% (Table 6). False positive results were obtained in 60 of the 1352 patients, for a specificity of 96%. Therefore, the predictive value of an abnormal test is 89%. The sensitivity and specificity in the single study evaluating hospitalised patients were 96% and 83%, respectively [64]. Impedance plethysmography has a very low sensitivity (approximately, 20%) for isolated calf vein thrombosis [74–82].

Doppler ultrasonography

Ten studies correctly evaluated the accuracy of Doppler ultrasound for the diagnosis of symptomatic DVT [92–102], albeit that subjective criteria for the analysis of flow sound were used, whereas the earlier Doppler ultrasound studies had methodologic weaknesses [101, 103, 104]. The pooled results of these studies demonstrated that Doppler ultrasound detected 363 of the 407 patients with venographically proven proximal-vein thrombosis, for a sensitivity of 89% (Table 7). The test result was falsely abnormal in 96 of the 915 patients without proximal-vein thrombosis, for a specificity of 90%. Consequently, the predictive value of an abnormal Doppler ultrasound test is 79%. Doppler ultrasonography is not sensitive for the detection of isolated calf vein thrombosis.

Recently, Doppler ultrasound for the diagnosis of proximal vein thrombosis was evaluated using objective criteria for normal and abnormal test results [102, 105]. A total of 155 consecutive patients with clinically suspected DVT were studied. An abnormal Doppler test was obtained in 83 of the 92 patients with proximal-vein thrombosis (sensitivity, 87%). A false abnormal Doppler test result was obtained in only 3 of the 209 patients without DVT, for a specificity of 99%.

Other methods

Various other methods, including strain gauge plethysmography [106, 107], liquid crystal (contact) thermography [108–112], light reflection rheography [113], computed tomography scanning, and magnetic resonance scanning [114–117], radionuclide venography [118–137], as well as numerous blood tests (including measurements of fibrinopeptide A [138–140], fibrin(ogen) degradation products (FDP) [141, 142], degradation products of cross-linked fibrin (D-dimer) [143–156], prothrombin fragments 1 + 2 (F1 + 2) and thrombin-antithrombin III (TAT) complexes [157–159], and Fragment E [160], have been evaluated in patients presenting with signs and symptoms of DVT. These methods are either still experimental or have not been properly evaluated in large series of consecutive patients. Therefore, at present none of these methods should be used for the diagnosis of DVT.

Diagnostic management of patients with a clinically suspected first episode of venous thrombosis

Although a normal ultrasound imaging or an impedance plethysmography result essentially excludes a diagnosis of proximal vein thrombosis, it does not exclude the presence of isolated calf vein thrombosis. A proportion of the undetected limited thrombi may extend during the ensuing days and put the patient at risk for PE [3]. In the 1980's, it was hypothesised that the use of anticoagulant therapy in symptomatic patients could be directed by results of non-invasive tests if the majority of clinically important thrombi were detected by repeated testing during a short period of time (one to two weeks). This concept was first evaluated using impedance plethysmography. In the initial impedance plethysmography study, tests were repeated five times during a period of two weeks in patients with an initial normal test result to detect proximally extending venous thrombi [161]. Patients with an abnormal test were treated, whereas patients with serial normal tests did not receive anticoagulant treatment and were followed up to evaluate the safety of this management approach. A clinically acceptable rate of thromboembolic complications occurred in patients with serial normal impedance plethysmography tests. Subsequently, several modifications of the serial non-invasive test concept have been evaluated which aimed to reduce the number of serial tests without compromising safety.

Selection and classification of clinical studies

Published and unpublished trials were identified which addressed the diagnostic management of patients with clinically suspected DVT. Studies were eligible if consecutive patients with clinically suspected DVT were included; a pre-defined and objective diagnostic strategy was used to confirm or refute the diagnosis of DVT; anticoagulant treatment was based on the results of the diagnostic strategy; and if follow-up with a duration of at least 3 months was prospectively performed to document the frequency of venous thromboembolic complications. The search included all possible diagnostic methods for DVT, including contrast venography, phleborheography, Doppler ultrasound, impedance and strain gauge plethysmography, thermography, various isotopic methods, various blood tests, computerised tomography, magnetic resonance imaging, and ultrasound imaging. We excluded studies that were duplicate reports and preliminary reports which were later presented in full. We included abstracts of interim analyses of ongoing studies. From all studies which qualified for the analysis, the frequency of venous thromboembolic complications (i. e., DVT or PE) during follow-up in patients in whom the diagnostic strategy had ruled out DVT was determined. Most diagnostic strategies with non-invasive testing consisted of a limited period in which the diagnostic tests were repeated in patients whose results remained normal. The frequency of PE during this period was also assessed. Clinically suspected venous thromboembolic complications, for which no objective testing could be performed, were considered true events. The total complication rate was defined as either a PE during the interval of serial non-invasive testing or as a PE or a DVT during 3 months of follow-up. The total complication rate was calculated using the Kaplan-Meier survival analysis and was defined as one minus the complication-free survival rate. This method takes into account the different numbers of patients at risk during the different time periods. An estimate of the exact upper 95 percent confidence limit (CL) was

Table 8. Summary of the diagnostic strategies used in patients with clinically suspected DVT.

Authors, year	Diagnostic strategy	Duration of follow-up
Venography		
Hull, 1981 [79]	venography at day 1	3 months
Impedance plethysmography		
Hull, 1985 [161]	IPG at day 1, 2, 3, 5 or 7, 10, and 14	12 months
Hull, 1985 [61]	IPG the same combined with ^{125}I-fibrinogen leg scan	12 months
Huisman, 1986 [162]	IPG at day 1,2,5, and 10	6 months
Huisman, 1989 [163]	IPG at day 1,2, and 7	6 months
Prandoni, 1991 [173]	IPG at day 1,3, and 7	6 months
Ultrasonography		
Sluzewski, 1991 [166]	ultrasound at day 1,2, and 7	3 months
Heijboer, 1993 [167]	ultrasound at day 1,2, and 8	6 months
Cogo, 1998 [174]	ultrasound at day 1, and 7	6 months
Combinations		
Kraaijenhagen, 1997 [175]	normal ultrasound and normal D-dimer: follow-up normal ultrasound and abnormal D-dimer: repeat ultrasound day 7	3 months
Bernardi, 1998 [176]	normal ultrasound and normal D-dimer: follow-up normal ultrasound and abnormal D-dimer: repeat ultrasound day 7	3 months
Wells, 1997 [177]	normal ultrasound and low clinical score: follow-up normal ultrasound and intermediate clinical score: ultrasound day 7 normal ultrasound and high clinical score: venography	3 months
Ginsberg, 1997 [178]	normal IPG and normal D-dimer and low or intermediate clinical score: follow-up normal IPG and normal D-dimer and high clinical score: ultrasound and/or venography abnormal IPG and normal D-dimer: ultrasound and/or venography normal IPG and abnormal D-dimer: ultrasound and/or venography	3 months

made using the standard deviation as calculated by the Kaplan-Meier analysis. The individual results of studies which used the same diagnostic test were pooled after testing for homogeneity using a Chi-square test. Feasibility was expressed as the mean number of extra visits to the hospital and the mean number of additional tests required per initially referred patient.

Identified trials

The search revealed a total of 19 reports [79, 161–167]. Seven reports had to be excluded from the analysis because follow-up was performed retrospectively (four studies) [165, 169–171], the results were also described in another article (one study) [79], the inception cohort exclusively consisted of pregnant women (one study)

[164], and the interim analysis results were too limited to qualify for the analysis (one study) [172]. The 12 reports which qualified for the analysis included more than 7,000 patients. In two of these reports, two diagnostic strategies were compared in a randomised design [161, 167]. The diagnostic strategies included venography, serial impedance plethysmography with and without ^{125}I-fibrinogen leg scanning, serial ultrasound imaging with and without D-dimer, serial ultrasound imaging in combination with a clinical score, and a diagnostic work up including ultrasound imaging, impedance plethysmography, D-dimer and a clinical score. The applied diagnostic strategy during the initial period and the length of follow-up are summarised in Table 8. The frequency of venous thromboembolic complications in patients with a normal test result at presentation is shown for each diagnostic strategy separately in Figure 7.

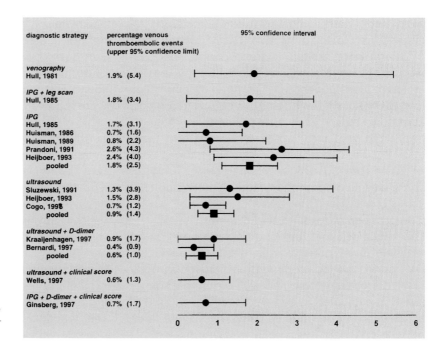

Fig. 7. Summary of diagnostic strategies in suspected DVT with respective 95% confidence intervals of venous thromboembolic events.

Diagnostic strategies

Venography

Venography was used to confirm or refute the diagnosis of DVT in a large series of consecutive patients [168]. All 160 patients with a normal venogram were not treated with anticoagulant therapy and prospectively followed up for a period of three months to document the frequency of venous thromboembolic complications. Subsequent venous thromboembolic complications occurred in three patients (1.9%; 95% upper CL: 5.4%).

Serial impedance plethysmography and ^{125}I-fibrinogen leg scanning

A single study evaluated patients with suspected DVT and a normal initial impedance plethysmography test result with serial impedance plethysmography tests and ^{125}I-fibrinogen leg scanning [161]. Impedance plethysmography was repeated 5 times during a 2-week period. In 265 (82%) of the 323 patients, the combination of both methods remained normal during serial testing and anticoagulant therapy was not initiated. All 265 patients had long-term follow-up. A single episode of PE occurred during serial testing (0.3%). Venous thromboembolic complications occurred in four patients (1.5%) during three months of follow-up (three patients had DVT and one had non-fatal PE). Therefore, the total venous thromboembolic complication rate was 1.8% (95% upper CL: 3.4%).

Serial impedance plethysmography

In five studies the usefulness of serial impedance plethysmography alone in the diagnosis of DVT in patients with clinically suspected disease was assessed [161–163, 167, 173]. Prospective follow-up was performed in all studies for a period of at least three months. The pooled results show that symptomatic PE occurred in four (0.3%) of the 1515 patients with an initial normal impedance plethysmography result during the period of serial testing, of which two were fatal. Serial impedance plethysmography remained normal in a total of 1425 patients and 1395 of these patients were available for long-term follow-up. No anticoagulant therapy was given to these patients. Venous thromboembolic complications occurred in 21 of these patients (1.5%) during the 3-month follow-up. Of these 21 patients with thromboembolic complication, 18 had DVT and 3 had PE, which was fatal in 1. The total venous thromboembolic complication rate was 1.8% (95% upper CL: 2.5%). There was no heterogeneity among these studies.

Serial compression ultrasound

Serial compression ultrasound was evaluated in three studies as a diagnostic strategy for clinically suspected DVT [166, 167, 174]. Prospective follow-up was performed in all studies for a period of at least three months. The pooled results show that PE occurred in one (0.1%) of the 1773 patients with an initial normal compression ultrasound test, during the period of serial testing; this episode was fatal. Serial compression ultrasound remained normal in a total of 1753 patients and 1738 of these patients were available for long-term follow-up. No anticoagulant therapy was initiated in these patients. During three months of follow-up, venous thromboembolic complications occurred in 15 (0.9%) of these patients; of whom 12 had deep vein thromboses and three had (nonfatal) PE. The overall venous thromboembolic complication rate was 0.9% (95% upper CL: 1.4%). There was no heterogeneity among these studies.

Compression ultrasound and D-dimer

The hypothesis that anticoagulant therapy can be withheld from patients with clinically suspected DVT and a normal compression ultrasonography result at baseline combined with a normal D-dimer test was evaluated in two studies [175, 176]. Patients with an abnormal ultrasound test were treated with anticoagulants. Patients with a normal initial ultrasound test but an abnormal D-dimer result were scheduled for repeat ultrasound testing at one week, whereas those with a normal initial ultrasound test and a normal D-dimer result were not subjected to repeat ultrasound testing but evaluated during long-term follow-up. Of the 1128 patients with an initial normal ultrasound test, only 250 (22%) had to undergo a repeat ultrasound test because of an abnormal D-dimer test. In these 250 patients, one (0.4%) PE, which was fatal, occurred during serial testing. Serial compression ultrasound remained normal in 234 patients and long-term follow-up revealed four nonfatal venous thromboembolic events. Of the 878 patients with a normal initial ultrasound and D-dimer result who had follow-up, two (0.2%) developed a nonfatal venous thromboembolic complication. The overall venous thromboembolic complication rate was 0.6% (95% upper CL: 1%); two had DVT and five had PE.

Compression ultrasonography and clinical score

In a single study a cohort of 577 patients with suspected DVT were evaluated with compression ultrasound followed by a clinical probability strategy [177]. Thus, patients were classified as high, intermediate, or low probability for DVT based on history and clinical signs and symptoms. Patients with an abnormal ultrasound test were treated with anticoagulants if they had an intermediate or high clinical probability for DVT, whereas those with a low clinical probability underwent venography. Patients with a normal ultrasound test and a high clinical probability had venography, whereas those with an intermediate clinical probability were scheduled for a repeat ultrasound at

one week. If the repeat ultrasound test remained normal, the patient was not treated and follow-up was performed. Repeat ultrasound testing was not performed in patients with a normal baseline ultrasound test and a low clinical probability; they were followed up. All patients with a normal venogram also had follow-up.
Serial testing was limited to 165 (34%) of the 491 patients with an initial normal test result, and none had PE during serial testing. Only 3 (0.6%) of the 485 patients who had follow-up developed a venous thromboembolic complication. The overall venous thromboembolic complication rate was 0.6% (95% upper CL: 1.3%).

Impedance plethysmography, D-dimer and clinical pre-test probability, combined with ultrasound and/or venography

The hypothesis that DVT can be excluded safely in patients with clinically suspected DVT and a normal baseline impedance plethysmography result in combination with a normal D-dimer test was evaluated in a cohort of 401 patients [178]. Of these, 352 had a normal initial impedance plethysmography test and the D-dimer test was abnormal in 76 (19%) of them. Most of these latter patients had confirmatory venography and DVT was identified in approximately one-third of them. Of the 276 patients with a normal D-dimer test, 177 (64%) had a low clinical score, no additional testing was done and three months of follow-up showed one (0.6%) venous thromboembolic complication. The clinical score indicated an intermediate probability in 92 (33%) patients, additional testing was done in 16 patients (and identified two patients with DVT) and a three month follow-up revealed no venous thromboembolic complications. The clinical score was high in four (1.4%) patients and venography or ultrasound was performed. In two patients a DVT was detected and they were treated with anticoagulants. One of the remaining two patients with a high clinical score developed a (contralateral) DVT during the three months of follow-up. Therefore, the total venous thromboembolic complication rate is 0.7% (95% upper CL: 1.7%).

Number of extra visits to the hospital and additional tests

The mean number of extra visits to the hospital and the mean number of additional tests required per patient is specified for each diagnostic strategy separately in Table 9. Initially, impedance plethysmography was repeated five times during a peri-

Table 9. Mean number of extra hospital visits and additional tests required per initially referred patient.

Author, year	Number of patients	Prevalence of DVT	Mean number of extra hospital visits and additional tests	Additional use of D-dimer tests (D) or clinical score (C)
Hull, 1981 [79]	160	0%*	–	–
Hull, 1985 [161]	} 992	21%	4.1	–
Hull, 1985 [161]		29%	3.9	–
Huisman, 1986 [162]	426	30%	2.1	–
Huisman, 1989 [163]	243	45%	1.3	–
Prandoni, 1991 [173]	381	18%	1.7	–
Heijboer, 1993 [167]	490	24%	1.6	–
Heijboer, 1993 [167]	491	21%	1.6	–
Sluzewski, 1991 [167]	118	37%	1.3	–
Cogo, 1998 [174]	1703	33%	0.8	–
Kraaijenhagen, 1997 [175]	552	22%	0.3	D
Bernardi, 1998 [176]	946	28%	0.1	D
Wells, 1997 [177]	577	17%	0.3**	C
Ginsberg, 1997 [178]	401	17%	0.3***Ψ	D + C

*	= by definition
**	= 15% venography
***Ψ	= at least 75% venography
Ψ	= all tests were performed on the day of referral

od of two weeks in patients with an initial normal test result, for a mean number of extra visits and additional tests of 4.1 per initially referred patient [161]. Subsequently, the number of repeat tests was reduced to three [21], and finally to two tests during a period of one week, for a mean number of extra visits and additional tests of approximately 1.5 per patient [163, 167, 173]. The reduction of the number of repeat impedance plethysmography tests was not associated with an increase in venous thromboembolic complications during the period of serial testing or long-term follow-up.

A similar phenomenon was observed for compression ultrasound. In the initial compression ultrasound studies, patients were evaluated only at the level of the common femoral vein in the groin and the popliteal vein in the mid-popliteal fossa, and two repeat tests were necessary, for a mean number of extra visits and additional tests of approximately 1.5 per initially referred patient [166, 167]. In a subsequent compression ultrasound study, the evaluation of the common femoral vein and popliteal vein in the mid-popliteal fossa was extended with an evaluation of the entire popliteal

vein until the trifurcation of the calf veins [174]. As a result of this modification, limited DVT was found in a small subset of patients with an initial normal compression ultrasound test. The improved baseline sensitivity for DVT allowed for a reduction in the number of repeat ultrasound tests from two to a single test (for a mean number of extra visits and additional tests of 0.8 per patient) without an increased risk for venous thromboembolic complications during serial testing or follow-up. The use of the D-dimer test complementary to ultrasound resulted in a further reduction in the number of additional tests needed to rule out DVT, for a mean number of extra visits and additional tests of 0.1 to 0.3 per initially referred patient [175, 176]. The ultrasound-D-dimer strategy was associated with a low number of venous thromboembolic complications.

Comparable results were obtained for the two strategies that used combinations of non-invasive tests with clinical probability scores [177]. In these studies, the mean number of additional tests per patient was also low (approximately 0.3 additional test per patient) but did include venography.

A. W. A. Lensing, R. Kraaijenhagen, E. J. R. van Beek, H. R. Büller

Summary

At present, compression ultrasound limited to the assessment of the common femoral vein and the popliteal vein down to the trifurcation of the calf veins is the test of choice in the evaluation of symptomatic patients. An abnormal compression ultrasound test justifies the initiation of anticoagulant treatment since the predictive value of an abnormal test outcome is high. Although a normal compression ultrasound result essentially excludes a diagnosis of proximal-vein thrombosis, it does not exclude the presence of isolated calf-vein thrombosis. Therefore, patients with a normal test outcome should be retested to detect the small proportion of patients (approximately 1 – 2 % of patients with an initial normal ultrasound test) with proximally extending calf-vein thrombosis. Nowadays, there appears to be no role for simple Doppler ultrasound in the diagnosis of DVT, since the subjective interpretation limits its reliability. The results of this review indicate that for the diagnosis of symptomatic DVT, duplex and colour ultrasonography do not offer any advantage over conventional compression ultrasound, since use of the former tests does not result in an increased accuracy for proximal-vein thrombosis. Duplex and colour Doppler ultrasonography have the disadvantages of being less cost-effective than compression ultrasound, since these devices are more expensive and the procedures more time-consuming.
A diagnostic algorithm for the non-invasive diagnosis of clinically suspected venous thrombosis could be as follows: compression ultrasound is performed on referral; if it is abnormal, the diagnosis of venous thrombosis is established, and the patient is treated accordingly. If the result of the initial real-time ultrasound evaluation is normal, anticoagulant therapy is withheld and the test is repeated at one week. If the ultrasound becomes abnormal during this time, a diagnosis of venous thrombosis is made, and anticoagulant therapy is commenced. If the repeat ultrasound test remains normal, the diagnosis of venous thrombosis is excluded and the patient is not treated with anticoagulant therapy. It needs to be demonstrated whether alternative strategies can be employed to limit the number of repeat tests.

DVT and PE

Although traditionally regarded as separate clinical entities, there is good evidence that DVT and PE are expressions of the one disease, namely venous thromboembolism [179 – 181]. In patients presenting with clinically suspected DVT, symptomatic PE is rarely apparent. In a prospective cohort study, the prevalence was assessed of silent PE. Perfusion ventilation lung scans were performed in 101 consecutive patients at the time of presentation to the hospital. Fifty-one percent of these patients had a high probability lung scan. In comparison, in patients referred with suspected venous thrombosis, but who on subsequent objective testing did not have venous thrombosis (n = 44), the prevalence of a high probability scan for PE was only 5 percent. The high frequency of lung scan detected silent PE has been confirmed in other series of comparable patients [182, 183].

Diagnosis of DVT in asymptomatic high risk patients

Ultrasound Imaging

A total of 15 studies (14 in orthopedic surgical patients; 1 in neurosurgical patients) reported on the accuracy of ultrasound imaging techniques for the diagnosis of asymptomatic venous thrombosis of the leg in high-risk patients. In all these studies, venography was used systematically, consecutive patients were included and the analysis was done independently. Various other studies have investigated the usefulness of ultrasound in the diagnosis of thrombosis in this patients category, but have failed to meet the criteria for the proper evaluation of a diagnostic test [35, 59, 183 – 191]. In the selected 15 reports, 8 evaluated compression ultrasound [192 – 199], 4 used duplex ultrasonography [51, 200, 201], and 3 assessed colour-coded ultrasonography [53, 73, 199].

a) Compression ultrasound
In the 8 studies using correct methodology, compression ultrasound identified 80 of the 129 legs with proximal-vein thrombosis, for a sensitivity of 62 % (Table 10). An abnormal ultrasound test was found in 21 of the 769 legs with normal venogram results, for a specificity of 97 %. The positive predictive value was 79 %.

b) Duplex ultrasonography
Four studies evaluated properly the accuracy of duplex ultrasonography for the diagnosis of proximal-vein thrombosis in asymptomatic high-risk patients (Table 11). In these studies, the sensitivity

Table 10. Compression ultrasonography in asymptomatic high-risk patients.

Investigators	Sensitivity for proximal DVT	Specificity	Positive predictive value
Borris et al. 1989 [192]	63% (15/24)	91% (29/32)	83% (15/18)
Borris et al. 1990 [193]	73% (8/11)	94% (44/47)	73% (8/11)
Ginsberg et al. 1991 [194]	52% (11/21)	99% (184/186)	89% (11/13)
Cronan et al. 1991 [195]	100% (12/12)	100% (64/64)	100% (12/12)
Agnelli et al. 1992 [196]	57% (12/21)	99% (165/166)	2% (12/13)
Tremaine et al. 1992 [197]	100% (2/2)	95% (55/58)	40% (2/5)
Jongbloets et al. 1992 [198]	38% (5/13)	96% (83/87)	56% (5/9)
Lensing et al. 1997 [199]	60% (15/25)	96% (124/129)	5% (15/20)
Total	62% (80/129)	97% (748/769)	79% (80/101)

Table 11. Duplex ultrasonography in asymptomatic high-risk patients.

Investigators	Sensitivity for proximal DVT	Specificity	Positive predictive value
Froehlich et al. 1989 [200]	100% (5/5)	97% (33/34)	83% (5/6)
Barnes et al. 1991 [201]	79% (15/19)	98% (283/289)	71% (15/21)
Woolson et al. 1991 [51]	67% (10/15)	99% (72/73)	91% (10/11)
Elliott et al. 1993 [52]	100% (4/4)	92% (85/92)	36% (4/11)
Total	79% (34/43)	97% (473/488)	69% (34/49)

Table 12. Colour Doppler ultrasonography in asymptomatic high-risk patients.

Investigators	Sensitivity for proximal DVT	Specificity	Positive predictive value
Davidson, et al. 1992 [53]	38% (8/21)	94% (225/239)	36% (8/22)
Mattos, et al. 1992 [73]	50% (5/10)	99% (179/180)	83% (5/6)
Lensing, et al. 1997 [199]	60% (15/25)	96% (124/129)	75% (15/20)
Total	50% (28/56)	96% (528/548)	58% (28/48)

was 79% (34/43), and specificity was 97% (473/488). The predictive value of an abnormal test was 69%.

c) Colour Doppler ultrasonography
The accuracy of colour Doppler ultrasonography as a screening test for proximal-vein thrombosis has thus far been investigated in 3 methodologically sound studies [48, 69, 78]; (Table 12). Colour Doppler correctly diagnosed proximal-vein thrombosis in only 28 of the 56 legs, for a sensitivity of 50%. The presence of proximal-vein thrombosis was correctly excluded in 528 of the 548 legs, for a specificity of 96%. Proximal-vein thrombosis was demonstrated by venography in only

28 of the 48 legs with an abnormal colour Doppler test result, for a positive predictive value of 58%.

Accuracy for isolated calf-vein thrombosis

Of the 8 compression ultrasound studies in which the potential for bias was minimised, four evaluated the accuracy for isolated calf-vein thrombosis [195 – 199]; (Table 13). In these studies, compression ultrasound identified 17 of the 42 isolated calf-vein thromboses, for a sensitivity of 40%. Of the four duplex ultrasonography studies, only one study evaluated the accuracy for isolated calf-vein thrombosis [52]. In this study, duplex ultrasonography identified 13 of the 23 patients with isolated calf-vein thrombosis (sensitivity 57 %). The sensitivity of colour Doppler ultrasonography for isolated calf-vein thrombosis was determined in 1 of the 3 methodologically sound studies [199]. In addition, a colour Doppler ultrasonography study that minimised the potential for bias was identified which evaluated only patients with isolated calf-vein thrombosis [202]. The combined results of these studies demonstrate that 24 of the 49 patients with isolated calf-vein thrombosis (sensitivity 49 %) were correctly diagnosed.

Table 13. Sensitivity for isolated calf-vein thrombosis for studies in asymptomatic high-risk patients which minimised the potential for bias.

	Sensitivity 95 %	Confidence Interval
Gray-scale real-time ultrasonography		
Cronan et al. 1991 [195]	0 % (0/1)	–
Tremaine et al. 1992 [197]	50 % (2/4)	12–100 %
Jongbloets et al. 1994 [198]	38 % (5/13)	8–69 %
Lensing et al. 1997 [199]	42 % (10/24)	20–63 %
Total	40 % (17/42)	24–57 %
Duplex ultrasonography		
Elliott et al. 1993 [52]	57 % (13/23)	34–79 %
Colour Doppler ultrasonography		
Rose et al. 1993 [202]	58 % (14/24)	37–80 %
Lensing et al. 1997 [199]	42 % (10/24)	20–63 %
Total	49 % (24/49)	34–64 %

Impedance plethysmography

A total of 3 studies evaluated the accuracy of IPG for the detection of asymptomatic thrombosis in postoperative patients [203–205]. All 3 studies used correct methodology. IPG detected 30 of the 134 patients with proximal-vein thrombosis, for a sensitivity of 22 %. A false abnormal result was obtained in 32 of the 1713 patients without proximal-vein thrombosis, for a specificity of 98 %. The positive predictive value was 55 % (Table 14). The addition of fibrinogen leg scanning to IPG in patients who have hip surgery improves sensitivity, but only to approximately 50 %.

Doppler ultrasonography

No studies using rigorous methodology addressed the value of Doppler ultrasound for the screening of asymptomatic DVT.

^{125}I-Fibrinogen leg scanning

The pooled analysis of studies correlating ^{125}I-fibrinogen leg scanning with contrast venography in postoperative patients who had hip surgery reported a sensitivity and specificity of leg scanning for both proximal and calf vein thrombosis of 45 % and 92 %, respectively (Table 15) [206]. Surprisingly, ^{125}I-fibrinogen leg scanning had a sensitivity for isolated calf vein thrombosis of only 55 %.

Diagnostic management of patients with asymptomatic DVT

The need for an accurate screening test for patients at high risk for asymptomatic DVT is well recognised. This patient category includes those following major orthopedic neurosurgical or abdominal-thoracic intervention as well as patients who are subjected to periods of prolonged bed rest

Table 14. Impedance plethysmography in postoperative orthopedic patients.

Investigators	Sensitivity for proximal DVT	Specificity	Positive predictive value
Paiement et al. 1988 [203]	12 % (9/73)	99 % (856/864)	53 % (9/17)
Cruickshank et al. 1989 [204]	29 % (14/49)	98 % (681/694)	58 % (18/31)
Ginsberg et al. 1991 [194]	58 % (7/12)	95 % (144/155)	50 % (7/14)
Total	22 % (30/134)	98 % (1681/1713)	55 % (34/62)

Table 15. ^{125}I-Fibrinogen leg scanning in orthopedic surgical patients.

Investigators	Sensitivity calf DVT	Sensitivity all DVT	Specificity
Harris et al. 1975 [214]	75% (6/8)	37% (7/19)	90% (53/59)
Sautter et al. 1979 [215]	59% (23/39)	58% (29/50)	70% (67/96)
Sautter et al. 1983 [216]	59% (14/24)	34% (20/50)	79% (47/59)
Paiement et al. 1988 [203]	59% (78/133)	44% (84/190)	96% (769/804)
Cruickshank et al. 1989 [204]	51% (59/116)	45% (78/175)	95% (737/776)
Faunø et al. 1990 [217]	50% (30/60)	44% (12/27)	87% (368/423)
Total	55% (210/380)	45% (230/511)	92% (2041/2217)

due to stroke or other chronic medical disorders. The ideal screening test should have a high predictive value for both ruling in and ruling out venous thrombosis, particularly of the deep calf veins. Furthermore, the test should be non-invasive, easy to perform in large numbers of patients, and cost-effective. At present, none of the available non-invasive techniques is able to satisfy these requirements.

Initially, it was believed that ^{125}I-fibrinogen leg scanning was highly accurate for the diagnosis of asymptomatic thrombosis. The more rigorously designed studies, however, have revealed its poor sensitivity for calf as well as proximal vein thrombosis. There was an initial optimism that the ultrasound imaging techniques would resolve the diagnostic problem in patients at high risk of having asymptomatic thrombosis. Unfortunately, again upon careful evaluation it was shown that none of the ultrasound devices had a sufficiently high sensitivity, even for proximal vein thrombosis. These findings are in contrast with the high clinical utility of ultrasound in the diagnosis of symptomatic venous thrombosis. This discrepancy is most likely caused by the different features of the thrombus in the two patient categories (Table 1). Therefore, at this time the only reliable technique remains contrast venography.

Diagnosis of recurrent DVT

The diagnosis of recurrent DVT still remains a difficult problem, because the clinical diagnosis of recurrent DVT is highly non-specific and because each of the objective diagnostic tests for DVT has potential limitations in this setting [8, 9]. Approximately one-third of patients with an initial episode of DVT will present during the following year with signs and symptoms suggestive of recurrent DVT. These symptoms will indeed be caused by acute recurrent DVT in approximately one out of three patients, whereas in the remaining subjects the suspected episode is due to the post-thrombotic syndrome, or a variety of other non-thrombotic disorders. Differentiation among these three causes for recurrent leg symptoms is important because anticoagulant therapy is not required in patients with either the post-thrombotic syndrome or a non-thrombotic cause for leg symptoms. Of the available diagnostic tests for venous thrombosis, venog-

raphy, impedance plethysmography alone or in combination with ^{125}I-fibrinogen leg scanning and ultrasound imaging have been evaluated for the diagnosis of recurrent DVT.

Venography

Venography is a useful test for the diagnosis of recurrent DVT if films are available of the initial thrombotic episode and repeat venography demonstrates a new constant intraluminal filling defect [8]. The use of venography as a diagnostic tool for recurrent DVT is limited if a base-line venogram is not available or if the presence of recurrent thrombosis is masked by obliteration and recanalisation of the vein as a consequence of previous disease. The latter may occur in up to 30% of patients.

Impedance plethysmography and ^{125}I-Fibrinogen leg scanning

In patients with suspected recurrent DVT, IPG can only be used if a normal previous test result is available. In prospective cohort studies it has been shown that 1 year after the initial thrombosis 95 % of the IPG tests have been normalised [9, 207]. If the IPG test has been normalised, it can be used alone or in combination with fibrinogen leg-scanning to confirm or refute the diagnosis of recurrent DVT in symptomatic patients [17, 42]. The utility of IPG in symptomatic recurrent DVT has been determined in 2 studies [8, 9]. In the first study, 270 patients were referred with clinical signs and symptoms of recurrent DVT. In 200 of these patients the IPG result was normal and subsequently leg scanning was performed. The results of leg scanning were normal in 181 patients. These patients were not treated with anticoagulants. During 3 months of follow-up, recurrent DVT was demonstrated in 3 of the 181 patients (1.7 %). In another study of patients with suspected recurrent DVT, anticoagulants were withheld safely in all 18 patients with repeated normal IPG tests.

Ultrasound imaging

The use of ultrasound imaging for the diagnosis of recurrent DVT is complicated by the high rate of patients with persistent abnormal ultrasound results. In prospective cohort studies, the compression ultrasound results became normal in only 50 % to 60 % of the patients after one year [208 – 211]. An alternative quantitative compression ultrasound method based on measuring vein diameter during maximal compressibility has recently been introduced [212, 213]. To obtain a baseline result, compression measurements were performed every 3 months after a first episode of DVT. If a patient returned with recurrent symptoms, the measurements were repeated and compared to the previous results. The hypothesis is that new thrombosis correlates with an increase in diameter. Currently, a study is ongoing to demonstrate the safety and effectiveness of this method in a large sample of patients with a suspected episode of recurrent DVT.

Diagnostic management of patients with suspected recurrent DVT

No general recommendations can be given for the diagnostic management of patients with suspected recurrent DVT since the use of all available methods is limited in this setting. Contrast venography gives indeterminate results in a substantial proportion of patients. IPG alone has not been sufficiently documented to be a safe approach, whereas the addition of ^{125}I-fibrinogen leg scanning is hampered by the limited availability of the radiofarmacon. Finally, ultrasound imaging has the potential to become the method of choice.

References

1. Bauer G. A venographic study of thromboembolism problems. Acta Chir Scand 1940; 84 (Suppl 161): 1

2. Haeger K. Problems of acute deep venous thrombosis. I. The interpretation of signs and symptoms. Angiology 1969; 20: 219

3. Lensing AWA, Hirsh J, Büller HR. Diagnosis of DVT. In: Colman RW, Hirsh J, Marder VJ, Salzman EW (eds). Hemostasis and Thrombosis. JB Lippincott Company, Philadelphia 1993: 1297–1321

4. Büller HR, Lensing AWA, Hirsh J, Ten Cate JW. Deep venous thrombosis: new noninvasive tests. Thromb Haemost 1991; 66: 133

5. Cranley JJ, Canos AJ, Sull WJ. The diagnosis of DVT. Fallibility of clinical signs and symptoms. Arch Surg 1976; 111: 34

6. O'Donnel TF, Abbott WM, Athanasoulis CA, et al. Diagnosis of DVT in the outpatient by venography. Surg Gynecol Obstet 1980; 150: 69

7. Cogo A, Lensing AWA, Prandoni P, Hirsh J. Distribution of deep vein thrombi in symptomatic patients. Arch Intern Med 1993; 153: 2777–2780

8. Hull RD, Carter C, Jay R, et al. The diagnosis of acute recurrent DVT: A diagnostic challenge. Circulation 1983; 67: 901

9. Huisman MV, Büller HR, Ten Cate JW. Utility of impedance plethysmography in the diagnosis of recurrent DVT. Arch Intern Med 1988; 148: 681

10. Consensus Conference. Prevention of Venous Thrombosis and PE. JAMA 1986; 256: 744

11. Leyvraz PF, Richard J, Bachman F, et al. Adjusted versus fixed dose subcutaneous heparin in the prevention of DVT after total hip replacement. N Engl J Med 1983; 309: 954

12. Francis CW, Marder VJ, Evarte CM, Yaukoolbodi S. Two step warfarin therapy. Prevention of postoperative venous thrombosis without excessive bleeding. JAMA 1983; 249: 374

13. Turpie AG, Levine MN, Hirsh J, et al. A randomized controlled trial of low molecular weight heparin to prevent DVT in patients undergoing elective hip surgery. N Engl J Med 1986; 315: 925

14. Hirsh J, Levine M. Prevention of venous thrombosis in patients undergoing major surgical procedures. Br J Clin Pract 1988; 65 (suppl) 43: 2

15. Levine MN, Hirsh J, Gent M, Turpie AG, Leclerc J, Powers PJ, et al. Prevention of DVT after elective hip surgery. A randomized trial comparing low molecular weight heparin with standard unfractionated heparin. Ann Intern Med 1991; 114: 545

16. Hull R, Raskob G, Pineo G, et al. A comparison of subcutaneous low-molecular-weight heparin with warfarin sodium for prophylaxis against DVT after hip or knee implantation. N Engl J Med 1993; 329: 1370

17. Sackett DL, Haynes RB, Guyatt GH, Tugwell P. The interpretation of diagnostic data. In: Sackett DL, Haynes RB, Guyatt GH, Tugwell P (eds). Clinical Epidemiology. A basic science for clinical medicine. Little, Brown and Company, Boston/Toronto 1991: 51–68

18. Lensing AWA, Prandoni P, Büller HR, et al. Lower extremity venography with iohexol: results and complications. Radiology 1990; 177: 503

19. McLachlan MSF, Thomson JG, Taylor DW, Kelly ME, Sackett DL. Observer variation in the interpretation of lower limbs venograms. Am J Radiol 1979; 132: 227

20. Lensing AWA, Büller HR, Prandoni P, et al. Contrast venography, the gold standard for the diagnosis of DVT: improvement in observer agreement. Thromb Haemost 1992; 67: 8

21. White RH, McGahan JP, Dasenbach MM, Hartling RP. Diagnosis of DVT using duplex ultrasound. Ann Intern Med 1989; 111: 297

22. Becker DM, Philbrick JT, Abbitt PL. Real-time ultrasonography for the diagnosis of lower extremity deep venous thrombosis. Arch Intern Med 1989; 149: 1731

23. Hull RD, van Aken WG, Hirsh J, et al. Impedance plethysmography using the occlusive cuff technique in the diagnosis of venous thrombosis. Circulation 1976; 53: 696

24. Langsfeld M, Hershey FB, Thorpe L, et al. Duplex B-mode imaging for the diagnosis of deep venous thrombosis. Arch Surg 1987; 122: 587

25. Rollins DL, Semrow CM, Friedell ML, Calligaro KD, Buchbinder D. Progress in the diagnosis of deep venous thrombosis. J Vasc Surg 1988; 7: 638

26. Rosner NH, Doris PE. Diagnosis of femeropopliteal venous thrombosis. Am J Roentgenol 1988; 150: 623

27. Persson AV, Jones C, Zide R, Jewell ER. Use of triplex scanner in diagnosis of deep venous thrombosis. Arch Surg 1989; 124: 593

28. Fobbe F, Koennecke HC, Bedewi M, Heidt P, Boese-Landgraf J, Wolf KJ. Diagnostik der tiefen beinvenenthrombose mit der farbkodierten duplexsonographie. Fortschr Roentgenstr 1989; 151: 569

29. Killewich LA, Bedford GR, Beach KW, Strandness DE. Diagnosis of deep venous thrombosis. Circulation 1989; 79: 810

30. Cavaye D, Kelly AT, Graham JC, Appleberg M, Briggs GM. Duplex ultrasound diagnosis of lower limb venous thrombosis. Aust N Z J Surg 1990; 60: 283

31. George JE, Berry RE. Noninvasive detection of deep venous thrombosis. Am Surg 1990; 56: 76

32. Wright DJ, Shepard AD, McPharlin M, Ernst CB. Pitfalls in lower extremity venous duplex scanning. J Vasc Surg 1990; 5: 675

33. Foley WD, Middleton WD, Lawson TL, Erickson S, Quiroz FA, Macrander S. Color Doppler ultrasound imaging of lower-extremity venous disease. Am J Roentgenol 1991; 152: 371

34. AbuRahma AF, Kennard W, Robinson PA, et al. The judicial use of venous duplex imaging and strain gauge plethysmography (single or combined) in the diagnosis of acute and chronic DVT. Surg Gynecol Obstet 1992; 174: 52

35. Mussurakis S, Papaioannou S, Voros D, Vrakatselis T. Compression ultrasonography as a reliable imaging monitor in deep venous thrombosis. Surg Gynecol Obstet 1990; 171: 233

36. Greer IA, Barry J, Mackon N, Allan PL. Diagnosis of deep venous thrombosis in pregnancy: a new role for diagnostic ultrasound. Br J Obstet Gyn 1990; 97: 53

37. Ramshorst B, Legemate DA, Verzijlbergen JF, et al. Duplex scanning in the diagnosis of acute DVT of the lower extremity. Eur J Vasc Surg 1991; 5: 255

38. Irvine AT, Thomas ML. Colour-coded duplex sonography in the diagnosis of DVT: a comparison with phlebography. Phlebography 1991; 6: 103

39. Lindqvist R. Ultrasound as a complementary diagnostic method in DVT of the leg. Acta Med Scand 1977; 201: 435

40. Montefusco-von Kleist CM, Bakal C, Sprayregen S, Rhodes BA, Veith FJ. Comparison of duplex ultrasonography and ascending contrast venography in the diagnosis of venous thrombosis. Angiology 1993; 44: 169

41. Yucel EK, Fisher JS, Egglin TK, Geller SC, Waltman AC. Isolated calf vein thrombosis: diagnosis with compression ultrasound. Radiology 1991; 179: 443

42. Effeney DJ, Friedman MD, Gooding GAW. Iliofemoral venous thrombosis: real-time ultrasound diagnosis, normal criteria, and clinical application. Radiology 1984; 150: 787

43. Raghavendra BN, Rosen RJ, Lam S, et al. Deep venous thrombosis: detection by high resolution real-time ultrasonography. Radiology 1984; 152: 789

44. Raghavendra BN, Horii SC, Hilton S, et al. Deep venous thrombosis: detection by probe compression of veins: J Ultrasound Med 1986; 5: 89

45. Fletcher JP, Kershaw LS, Barker DS, Koutts J, Varnava A. Ultrasound diagnosis of lower limb deep venous thrombosis. Med J Aust 1990; 153: 453

46. George JE, Smith MO, Berry RE. Duplex scanning for the detection of deep venous thrombosis of lower extremities in a community hospital. Curr Surg 1987; 44: 203

47. Elias A, LeCorff G, Bouvier JL, et al. Value of real-time B-mode ultrasound imaging in the diagnosis of DVT of the lower limbs. Int Angiol 1987; 6: 175

48. Comerota AJ, Katz ML, Greenwald LL, et al. Venous duplex imaging: should it replace hemodynamic tests for deep venous thrombosis? J Vasc Surg 1990; 11: 53

49. Belcaro GV, Laurora G, Cesarone MR, Errichi BM. Colour duplex scanning and phlebography in DVT. Panminerva Med 1992; 34: 1

50. Bradley MJ, Spencer PA, Elaxander L, Milner GR. Colour flow mapping in the diagnosis of calf DVT. Clin Radiol 1993; 47: 399

51. Woolson ST, Pottorf G. Venous ultrasonography in the detection of proximal vein thrombosis after total knee arthroplasty. Clin Orthop 1991; 273: 131

52. Elliott GC, Suchyta M, Rose SC, et al. Duplex ultrasonography for the detection of deep vein thrombi after total hip or knee arthroplasty. Angiology 1993; 44: 26

53. Davidson B, Elliott GC, Lensing AWA. Low accuracy of color Doppler ultrasound to detect proximal leg vein thrombosis during screening of asymptomatic high-risk patients. Ann Intern Med 1992; 117: 735

54. Dauzat MM, Laroche JP, Charras C et al: Real-time B-mode ultrasonography for better specificity in the noninvasive diagnosis of deep venous thrombosis. J Ultrasound Med 1986; 5: 625

55. Appelman PT, De Jong TE, Lampman LE, et al. Deep venous thrombosis of the leg: US findings. Radiology 1987; 163: 743

56. Aitken AGF, Godden DJ. Real-time ultrasound diagnosis of DVT: a comparison with venography. Clin Radiol 1987; 38: 309

57. Cronan JJ, Dorfman GS, Scola FH, Schepps B, Alexander J. Deep venous thrombosis: US assessment using vein compressibility. Radiology 1987; 162: 191

58. Lensing AWA, Prandoni P, Brandjes D, et al. Detection of DVT by real-time B-mode ultrasonography. N Eng J Med 1989; 320: 342

59. Monreal M, Montserrat E, Salvador R, et al. Real-time ultrasound for diagnosis of symptomatic venous thrombosis and for screening of patients at risk. Angiology 1989; 40: 527

60. Habscheid W, Hohmann M, Wilhelm T, Epping J. Real-time ultrasound in the diagnosis of acute deep venous thrombosis of the lower extremity. Angiology 1990; 41: 599

61. Gudmundsen TE, Vinje B, Pedersen T. DVT of lower extremities. Diagnosis by real time ultrasonography. Acta Radiol 1990; 31: 473

62. Chance JF, Abbitt PL, Tegtmeyer CJ, Powers RD. Real-time ultrasound for the detection of deep venous thrombosis. Ann Emerg Med 1991; 20: 494

63. Pedersen OM, Aslaksen A, Vik-Mo H, Bassoe AM. Compression ultrasonography in hospitalized patients with suspected deep venous thrombosis. Arch Intern Med 1991; 151: 2217

64. Heijboer H, Cogo A, Büller HR, et al. Detection of DVT with impedance plethysmography and real-time compression ultrasonography in hospitalized patients. Arch Intern Med 1992; 152: 1901

65. Vogel P, Laing FC, Jeffrey RB, Wing VW. Deep venous thrombosis of the lower extremity: US evaluation. Radiology 1987; 163: 747

66. O'Leary DH, Kane RA, Chase BM. A prospective study of the efficacy of B-scan sonography in the detection of deep venous thrombosis in the lower extremities. J Clin Ultrasound 1988; 16: 1

67. Mantoni M: Diagnosis of deep venous thrombosis by duplex sonography. Acta Radiol 19 889; 30: 575

68. Mitchell DC, Grasty MS, Stebbings WSL, et al. Comparison of duplex ultrasonography and venography in the diagnosis of deep venous thrombosis. Br J Surg 1991; 78: 611

69. Quintavalla R, Larini P, Miselli A, Mandrioli R, Ugolotti U, Pattacini C, Pini M. Duplex ultrasound diagnosis of symptomatic proximal DVT of lower limbs. Eur J Radiol 1992; 15: 32

70. Baxter GM, McKechnie S, Duffy P. Colour Doppler ultrasound in deep venous thrombosis: a comparison with venography. Clin Radiol 1990; 42: 32

71. Rose ST, Zwiebel WJ, Nelson BD, Priest DL, Knighton RA, Brown JW, et al. Symptomatic lower extremity deep venous thrombosis: accuracy, limitations, and role of color duplex flow imaging in diagnosis. Radiology 1990; 175: 639

72. Schindler JM, Kaiser M, Gerber A, et al. Colour coded duplex sonography in suspected DVT of the leg. Br Med J 1990; 301: 1369

73. Mattos MA, Londey GL, Leutz DW, et al. Color-flow duplex scanning for the surveillance and diagnosis of acute deep venous thrombosis. J Vasc Surg 1992; 15: 366

74. Hull RD, Van Aken WG, Hirsh J, et al. Impedance plethysmography using the occlusive cuff technique in the diagnosis of venous thrombosis. Circulation 1976; 53: 696

75. Richards KL, Armstrong DJ, Tikoff G, et al. Noninvasive diagnosis of deep venous thrombosis. Arch Intern Med 1976; 136: 1091

76. Hull RD, Hirsh J, Sackett DL, et al. Combined use of leg scanning and impedance plethysmography in suspected venous thrombosis: An alternative to venography. N Engl J Med 1977; 296: 1497

77. Toy PTC, Schrier SL. Occlusive impedance plethysmography: a non-invasive method of diagnosis of DVT. West J Med 1978; 129: 89

78. Hull RD, Taylor DW, Hirsh J, et al. Impedance plethysmography: The relationship between venous filling and sensitivity and specificity for proximal vein thrombosis. Circulation 1978; 58: 898

79. Hull RD, Hirsh J, Sackett DL, et al. Replacement of venography in suspected venous thrombosis by impedance plethysmography and ^{125}I-fibrinogen leg scanning: A less invasive approach. Ann Intern Med 1981; 94: 12

80. Peters SHA, Jonker JJC, De Boer AC, et al. Home diagnosis of deep venous thrombosis with impedance plethysmography. Thromb Haemost 1982; 48: 297

81. Prandoni P, Lensing AWA, Huisman MV, et al. A new computerized impedance plethysmograph: accuracy in the detection of proximal DVT in symptomatic outpatients. Thromb Haemost 1991; 65: 229

82. Anderson DR, Lensing AWA, Wells PS, Levine MN, Weitz JI, Hirsh J. Limitations of impedance plethysmography in the diagnosis of clinically suspected DVT. Ann Intern Med 1993; 118: 25

83. Johnston KW, Kakkar VV. Plethysmographic diagnosis of DVT. Gynecol Obstet 1974; 139: 41

84. Wheeler HB, Pearson D, O'Connell D, Mullick SC. Impedance phlebography: Technique, interpretation and results. Arch Surg 1972; 104: 164

85. Wheeler B, O'Donnel JA, Anderson F, et al. Bedside screening for venous thrombosis using occlusive impedance plethysmography. Angiology 1975; 26: 199

86. Flanigan DP, Goodreau JJ, Burnham SJ, et al. Vascular laboratory diagnosis of clinically suspected acute DVT. Lancet 1978; 2: 331

87. Cooperman M, Martin EW Jr, Satiani B, et al. Detection of deep venous thrombosis by impedance plethysmography. Am J Surg 1979; 137: 252

88. Gross WS, Burney RE. Therapeutic and economic implications of emergency department evaluation for venous thrombosis. Ann Emerg Med 1979; 8: 110

89. Wheeler HB, Anderson FA, Cardullo PA. Suspected DVT. Management by impedance plethysmography. Arch Surg 1982; 117: 1206

90. Sandler DA, Martin JF, Duncan JE, et al. Diagnosis of DVT. comparison of clinical evaluation, ultrasound, plethysmography and venoscan with X-ray venogram. Lancet 1984; i: 716

91. Comerota A, Katz ML, Grossy RJ, et al. Comparative value of noninvasive testing for diagnosis and surveillance of DVT. J Vasc Surg 1988; 7: 40

92. Yao ST, Gourmos C, Hobbs JT. Detection of proximal vein thrombosis by Doppler ultrasound flow detection. Lancet 1972; 1: 1

93. Holmes MCG. Deep venous thrombosis of the lower limbs diagnosed by ultrasound. Med J Aust 1973; 1: 427

94. Meadway J, Nicolaides AN, Walker CJ, et al. Value of Doppler ultrasound in diagnosis of clinically suspected DVT. Br Med J 1975; 4: 552

95. Dosick SM, Blakemore WS. The role of Doppler ultrasound in acute DVT. Am J Surg 1978; 136: 265

96. Flanigan DP, Goodreau JJ, Burnham SJ, et al. Vascular laboratory diagnosis of clinically suspected acute DVT. Lancet 1978; 2: 331

97. Sumner DS, Lambeth A. Reliability of Doppler ultrasound in the diagnosis of acute venous thrombosis both above and below the knee. Am J Surg 1979; 138: 205

98. Hanel KC, Abbott WM, Reidy NC, Fulchino D, Miller A, Brewster DC, Athanasoulis CA. The role of two noninvasive tests in deep venous thrombosis. Ann Surg 1981; 194: 725

99. Zielinsky A, Hull R, Carter C, Raskob G, Hirsh J. Doppler ultrasonography in patients with clinically suspected DVT. Thromb Haemost 1983; 50: 153

100. Turnbull T, Dymowski JJ, Zalut TE. A prospective study of hand-held Doppler ultrasonography by emergency physicians in the evaluation of suspected DVT. Ann Emergency Med 1990; 19: 691

101. Sigel B, Felix WR, Popky GL, Ispen J. Diagnosis of lower limb venous thrombosis by Doppler ultrasound technique. Arch Surg 1972; 104: 174

102. Evans DS. The early diagnosis of thromboembolism by ultrasound. Ann R Coll Surg Engl 1971; 49: 225

103. Strandness DE, Sumner DS. Ultrasonic velocity detector in the diagnosis of thrombophlebitis. Arch Surg 1972; 104: 180

104. Lensing AWA, Levi MM, Büller HR, et al. An objective Doppler method for the diagnosis of DVT. Ann Intern Med 1990; 113: 9

105. Cogo A, Lensing AWA, Prandoni P, et al. Comparison of real-time B-mode ultrasonography and Doppler ultrasound with contrast venography in symptomatic outpatients. Thromb Haemost 1993; 70: 404

106. Barnes RW, Collicott PE, Mozersky DJ, et al. Non-invasive quantitation of maximum venous outflow in acute thrombophlebitis. Surgery 1972; 72: 971

107. Cranley JJ, Gay AY, Grass AM, Simeone FA. A plethysmographic technique for the diagnosis of deep venous thrombosis of the lower extremities. Surg Gynecol Obstet 1973; 136: 385

108. Cooke ED, Pilcher MF. DVT: A preclinical diagnosis by thermography. Br J Surg 1974; 61: 971

109. Jensen C, Lomboldt Knudsen L, Hegedüs V. The role of contact thermography in the diagnosis of deep venous thrombosis. Europ J Radiol 1983; 3: 99

110. Sandler DA, Martin JF. Liquid crystal thermography as a screening test for DVT. Lancet 1985; i: 665

111. Holmgren K, Jacobsson H, Johnsson H, Lofsjogard-Nilsson. Thermography and plethysmography, a non-invasive alternative to venography in the diagnosis of DVT. J Int Med 1990; 228: 29

112. Bounameaux H, Khabiri E, Huber O, et al. Value of liquid crystal contact thermography and plasma level of D-dimer for screening of deep venous thrombosis following general abdominal surgery. Thromb Haemost 1992; 67: 603

113. Thomas PRS, Butler CM, Bowman J, et al. Light reflection rheography: an effective non-invasive technique for screening patients with suspected deep venous thrombosis. Br J Surg 1991; 78: 207

114. Spritzer CE, Sussman SK, Blinder RA, et al. Deep venous thrombosis evaluation with limited-flipangle, gradient-refocused MR imaging: preliminary experience. Radiology 1988; 166: 371

115. Erdman WA, Jayson HT, Redman HC, et al. Deep venous thrombosis of extremities: role of MR imaging in the diagnosis. Radiology 1990; 174: 425

116. Spritzer CE, Sostman HD, Wilkes DC, Coleman RE. Deep venous thrombosis: experience with gradient echo MR imaging in 66 patients. Radiology 1990; 177: 235

117. Evans AJ, Sostman HD, Knelson MH, et al. Detection of deep venous thrombosis; prospective comparison of MR imaging with contrast venography. Am J Roentgenol 1993; 161: 131

118. Webber MM, Bennett LR, Cragin M, Webb R Jr. Thrombophlebitis-demonstration by scintiscanning. Radiology 1969; 92: 620

119. Rosenthal L, Greyson ND. Observations on the use of ^{99m}Tc albumin macroaggregates for the detection of thrombophlebitis. Radiology 1970; 94: 413

120. Webber MM, Victery W, Cragin MD. Demonstration of thrombophlebitis and endothelial damage by scintiscanning. Radiology 1971; 100: 93

121. Webber MM, Pollack EW, Victery W, et al. Thrombosis detection by radionuclide particle (MAA) entrapment: Correlation with fibrinogen uptake and venography. Radiology 1974; 111: 645

122. Millar WT, Smith JFB. Localization of deep venous thrombosis using technetium-99m-labelled urokinase. Lancet 1974; 2: 695

123. Kempi V, Van Der Linden V, Von Scheele C. Diagnosis of DVT with ^{99m}Tc-streptokinase: A clinical comparison with phlebography. Br Med J 1974; 4: 748

124. Ryo UY, Qazi M, Srikantaswamy S, Pinsky S. Radionuclide venography: Correlation with contrast venography. J Nucl Med 1977; 18: 11

125. Knight LC, Primeau JL, Siegel BA, Welch MJ. Comparison of In-111-Labelled platelets and iodinated fibrinogen for the detection of DVT. J Nucl Med 1978; 19: 891

126. Bentley PG, Kakkar VV. Radionuclide venography for the demonstration of the proximal deep venous system. Br J Surg 1979; 66: 687

127. Beswick W, Chmiel R, Booth R, et al. Detection of deep venous thrombosis by scanning of ^{99m}technetium-labelled red-cell venous pool. Br Med J 1979; 1: 82

128. Deacon JM, Ell PJ, Anderson P, Khan O. Technetium-99m-plasmin: A new test for the detection of DVT. Br J Radiol 1980; 53: 673

129. Uphold RE, Knopp R, DosSantos PAL. Radionuclide venogaphy as an outpatient screening test for deep venous thrombosis. Ann Emerg Med 1980; 9: 613

130. Fenech A, Hussey JK, Smith FW, et al. Diagnosis of DVT using autologous indium-111-labelled platelets. Br Med J 1981; 282: 1020

131. Grimley RP, Rafiqi E, Hawker RJ, Drolc Z. Imaging of ^{111}In-labelled platelets-a new method for the diagnosis of DVT. Br J Surg 1981; 68: 714

132. Lisbona R, Stern J, Derbekyan V. ^{99m}Tc red blood cell venography in DVT of the legs: A correlation with contrast venography. Radiology 1982; 143: 771

133. Adolfsson L, Nordenfelt I, Olsson H, Torstensson I. Diagnosis of DVT with ^{99}Tc^m-plasmin. Acta Med Scand 1982; 211: 365

134. Fedullo PF, Moser KM, Moser KS, et al. Indium-111-labelled platelets: Effect of heparin on uptake by venous thrombi and relationship to the activated partial thromboplastin time. Circulation 1982; 66: 632

135. Singer I, Royal HD, Uren RF, et al. Radionuclide plethysmography and Tc-99m red blood cell venography in venous thrombosis: Comparison with contrast venography. Radiology 1984; 150: 213

136. Zorba J, Schier D, Posmituck G. Clinical value of blood pool radionuclide venography. Am J Roentgenol 1986; 146: 1051

137. Leclerc JR, Wolfson C, Arzoumanian A, et al. Technetium-99m red blood cell venography in patients with clinically suspected DVT: a prospective study. J Nucl Med 1988; 29: 1498

138. Yudelman IM, Nossel HL, Kaplan KL, Hirsh J. Plasma fibrinopeptide A levels in symptomatic venous thromboembolism. Blood 1978; 51: 1189

139. Kockum C. Radioimmunoassay of fibrinopeptide A – clinical applications. Thromb Res 1976; 8: 225

140. Yudelman IM, Nossel HL, Kaplan KL, Hirsh J. Plasma fibrinopeptide A levels in symptomatic venous thromboembolism. Blood 1978; 51: 1189–1195

141. Tibbutt DA, Chesterman CN, Allington MJ, et al. Measurement of fibrinogen-fibrin-related antigen in serum as aid to diagnosis of DVT in outpatients. Br Med J 1975; 1: 367

142. Hunt FA, Rylatt DB, Hart RA, et al. Serum crosslinked fibrin (XDP) and fibrinogen/fibrin degradation products (FDP) in disorders associated with activation of the coagulation or fibrinolytic systems. Br J Haematol 1985; 60: 715

143. Heaton DC, Billings JD, Hickton CM. Assessment of D dimer assays for the diagnosis of DVT. J Lab Clin Med 1987; 110: 588

144. Declerck PJ, Mombaerts P, Holvoet P, et al. Fibrinolytic response and fibrin fragment D-dimer levels in patients with DVT. Thromb Haemost 1987; 58: 1024

145. Ott P, Astrup L, Jensen RH, et al. Assessment of D-dimer in plasma: diagnostic value in suspected deep venous thrombosis of the leg. Acta Med Scand 1988; 224: 263

146. Bounameaux H, Schneider PA, Reber G, et al. Measurement of plasma D-dimer for diagnosis of deep venous thrombosis. Am J Clin Pathol 1989; 91: 82

147. Wilde JT, Kitchen S, Kinsey S, et al. Plasma D-dimer levels and their relationship to serum fibrinogen/fibrin degradation products in hypercoagulable states. Br J Haematol 1989; 71: 65

148. Elms MJ, Bunce IK, Bundesen PG, et al. Measurement of crosslinked fibrin degradation products – an immunoassay using monoclonal antibodies. Thromb Haemost 1983; 50: 591

149. Rowbotham BJ, Carroll P, Whitaker AN, et al. Measurement of crosslinked fibrin derivatives – use in the diagnosis of venous thrombosis. Thromb Haemost 1987; 57: 59

150. Heaton DC, Billings JD, Hickton CM. Assessment of D-dimer assays for the diagnosis of DVT. J Lab Clin Med 1987; 1110: 588

151. Ott P, Astrup L, Jensen RH, Nyeland B, Pederson B. Assessment of D-dimer in plasma: diagnostic value in suspected deep venous thrombosis of the leg. Acta Med Scand 1988; 224: 263

152. Bounameaux H, Schneider PA, Reber G, de Moerloose P, Krahenbuhl B. Measurement of plasma D-dimer for diagnosis of deep venous thrombosis. Am J Clin Pathol 1989; 91: 82

153. Speiser W, Mallek R, Koppensteiner R, et al. D-dimer and TAT measurements in patients with deep venous thrombosis: utility in diagnosis and judgement of anticoagulant treatment effectiveness. Thromb Haemost 1990; 64: 196

154. Rowbotham BJ, Carroll P, Whitaker AN, et al. Measurement of crosslinked fibrin derivatives – use in the diagnosis of venous thrombosis. Thromb Haemost 1987; 57: 59

155. Boneu B, Bes G, Pelzer H, Sié P, Boccalon H. D-dimers, thrombin-antithrombin III complexes and prothrombin fragments 1+2: diagnostic value in clinically suspected DVT. Thromb Haemost 1991; 65: 28

156. Heijboer H, Ginsberg JS, Büller HR, Lensing AWA, Colly LP, Ten Cate JW. The use of the D-dimer test in combination with non-invasive testing versus serial non-invasive testing alone for the diagnosis of DVT. Thromb Haemost 1992; 67: 510

157. Hoek JA, Nurmohamed MT, Ten Cate JW, et al. Thrombin-antithrombin III complexes in the prediction of DVT following total hip replacement. Thromb Haemost 1989; 62: 1050

158. Boneu B, Bes G, Pelzer, et al. D-dimers, thrombin antithrombin III complexes and prothrombin fragments 1 + 2: diagnostic value in clinically suspected DVT. Thromb Haemost 1991; 65: 28

159. Cogo A, Lensing AWA, Prandoni P, et al. Failure of T-AT complexes in the diagnosis of DVT in symptomatic patients. Angiology 1992; 43: 975–979

160. Zielinsky A, Hirsh J, Hull R, et al. Evaluation of radioimmunoassay for Fragment E in the diagnosis of venous thrombosis. Thromb Haemost 1979; 42: 28

161. Hull RD, Hirsh J, Carter C, et al. Diagnostic efficacy of impedance plethysmography for clinically suspected DVT: A randomized trial. Ann Intern Med 1985; 102: 21

162. Huisman MV, Büller HR, Ten Cate JW, Vreeken J. Serial impedance plethysmography for suspected deep venous thrombosis in outpatients. The Amsterdam General Practioner Study. N Engl J Med 1986; 314: 823

163. Huisman MV, Büller HR, Ten Cate JW, et al. Management of clinically suspected acute venous thrombosis in outpatients with serial impedance plethysmography in a community hospital setting. Arch Intern Med 1989; 149: 511

164. Hull RD, Raskob GE, Carter CJ, et al. Serial impedance plethysmography in pregnant patients with clinically suspected DVT. Ann Intern Med 1990; 112: 663

165. Vaccaro JP, Cronan JJ, Dorfman GS. Outcome analysis of patients with normal compression US-examinations. Radiology 1990; 175: 645

166. Sluzewski M, Koopman MMW, Schuur KH, Vroonhoven TJMV, Ruijs JHJ. Influence of negative ultrasound findings on the management of in- and outpatients with suspected DVT. Eur J Radiol 1991; 13: 174

167. Heijboer H, Büller HR, Lensing AWA, et al. A comparison of real-time compression ultrasonography with impedance plethysmography for the diagnosis of DVT in symptomatic outpatients. N Engl J Med 1993; 329: 1365

168. Hull R, Hirsh J, Sackett DL, et al. Clinical validity of a negative venogram in patients with clinically suspected venous thrombosis. Circulation 1981; 64: 622–625

169. Wheeler HB, Anderson FA Jr. Can noninvasive tests be used as the basis for treatment of DVT? In: Bernstein EF (ed). Noninvasive diagnostic techniques in vascular disease. 3rd ed. C.V. Mosby Co., St. Louis 1985: 805–818

170. Wheeler HB, Anderson FA Jr., Cardullo PA, et al. Suspected DVT. Management by impedance plethysmography. Arch Surg 1982; 117: 1206–1209

171. Jonker JJC. Computerized impedance pletysmography. Thromb Haemost 1991; 66: 743

172. Kearon C, Ginsberg JS, Douketis J, et al. Diagnosis of a first DVT in outpatients: interim analysis of a strategy based on clinical evaluation and D-dimer (SimpliRED™) results. Thromb Haemost 1997; Suppl: 588

173. Prandoni P, Lensing AWA, Buller HR, et al. Failure of computerized impedance plethysmography in the diagnostic management of patients with clinically suspected DVT. Thromb Haemost 1991; 65: 233–236

174. Cogo A, Lensing AWA, Koopman MMW, et al. Compression ultrasonography for the diagnostic management of patients with clinically suspected venous thrombosis. Br Med J 1998; 316: 17–20

175. Kraaijenhagen RA, Koopman MMW, Bernardi E, et al. Simplification of the diagnostic management of outpatients with symptomatic DVT with D-dimer measurements. Thromb Haemost 1997; Suppl.: 159

176. Bernardi E, Prandoni P., Lensing AWA, et al. D-dimer testing as an adjunct to ultrasonography in patients with clinically suspected deep vein thrombosis: prospective cohort study. BMJ 1998; 317: 1037

177. Wells PS, Anderson DR, Bormanis J, et al. Value of assessment of pretest probability of DVT in clinical management. Lancet 1997; 350: 1795–1798

178. Ginsberg JS, Kearon C, Douketis J, et al. The use of D-dimer and impedence pletysmographic examination in patients with clinical indications of DVT. Arch Intern Med 1997; 157: 1077–1081

179. Huisman MV, Buller HR, ten Cate JW, et al. Unexpected high prevalence of silent PE in patients with deep venous thrombosis. Chest 1989; 95: 498–502

180. Hull RD, Hirsh J, Carter CJ, et al. Pulmonary angiography, ventilation lung scanning, and venography for clinically suspected PE with abnormal perfusion lung scan. Ann Intern Med 1983; 98: 891–899

181. Kruit WHJ, De Boer AC, Sing AK, Van Roon F. The significance of venography in the management of patients with clinically suspected PE. J Intern Med 1991; 230: 333–339

182. Prandoni P, Lensing AWA, Buller HR, et al. Comparison of subcutaneous low molecular weight heparin with adjusted dose unfractionated heparin for the treatment of DVT. Lancet 1992; 339: 441–445

183. Nix ML, Nelson CL, Harmon BH, Ferris EF, Barnes RW. Duplex venous scanning: image vs Doppler accuracy. J Vasc Tech 1989; 13: 123

184. Barnes RW, Nix ML, Barnes CL, et al. Perioperative asymptomatic venous thrombosis: Role of duplex scanning versus venography. J Vasc Surg 1989; 9: 251

185. Flinn WR, Sandager GP, Cerullo LJ, Havey RJ, Yao JST. Duplex venous scanning for the prospective surveillance of perioperative venous thrombosis. Arch Surg 1989; 124: 901

186. Kraay MJ, Goldberg VM, Herbener TE. Vascular ultrasonography for deep venous thrombosis after total knee arthroplasty. Clin Orthop 1993; 286: 18

187. Vanninen R, Manninen H, Soimakallio S, Katila T, Suomalainen O. Asymptomatic deep venous thrombosis in the calf: accuracy and limitations of ultrasonography as a screening test after total knee arthroplasty. Br J Radiol 1993; 66: 199

188. Woolson ST, McCrory DW, Walter JF, et al. B-mode ultrasound scanning in the detection of proximal venous thrombosis after total hip replacement. J Bone Joint Surg 1990; 72: 983

189. Dorfman GS, Froehlich JA, Cronan JJ, Urbanek PJ, Herndon JH. Lower-extremity venous thrombosis in patients with acute hip fractures. Am J Roentgenol 1990; 154: 851

190. Comerota AJ, Katz ML, Greenwald LL, et al. Venous duplex imaging: should it replace haemodynamic tests for deep venous thrombosis? J Vasc Surg 1990; 11: 53

191. White RH, Goulet JA, Bray TJ, et al. DVT after fracture of the pelvis: assessment with serial duplex ultrasound screening. J Bone Joint Surg 1990; 4: 495

192. Borris LC, Christiansen HM, Lassen MR, et al. Comparison of real-time B-mode ultrasonography and bilateral ascending phlebography for detection of postoperative DVT following elective hip surgery. Thromb Haemost 1989; 61: 363

193. Borris LC, Christiansen HM, Lassen MR, et al. Real-time B-mode ultrasonography in the diagnosis of postoperative DVT in non-symptomatic high-risk patients. Eur J Vasc Surg 1990; 4: 473

194. Ginsberg JS, Caco CC, Brill-Edwards P, et al. Venous thrombosis in patients who have undergone major hip or knee surgery: Detection with compression US and impedance plethysmography. Radiology 1991; 181: 651

195. Cronan JJ, Froehlich JA, Dorfman GS. Image-directed Doppler ultrasound: a screening technique for patients at high risk to develop DVT. JCU 1991; 19: 133

196. Agnelli G, Volpato R, Radicchia S, et al. Detection of asymptomatic DVT by real-time B-mode compression ultrasound in hip surgery patients. Thromb Haemost 1992; 68: 257

197. Tremaine MD, Choroszy CJ, Gordon GH, Menking SA. Diagnosis of DVT by compression ultrasound in knee arthroplasty patients. J Arthroplasty 1992; 7: 187

198. Jongbloets LMM, Lensing AWA, Koopman MMW, Büller HR, Ten Cate JW. Limitations of compression ultrasound imaging for the detection of symptomless postoperative DVT. Lancet 1994; 343: 1142–1144

199. Lensing AWA, McGrath FP, Doris CI, et al. A comparison of compression ultrasound with color Doppler ultrasound for the diagnosis of symptomless postoperative DVT. Arch Intern Med 1997; 157: 765

200. Froehlich JA, Dorfman GS, Cronan JJ, et al. Compression ultrasonography for the detection of deep venous thrombosis in patients who have a fracture of the hip. J Bone Joint Surg 1989; 71: 249

201. Barnes CL, Nelson CL, Nix ML, et al. Duplex scanning versus venography as a screening examination in total hip arthroplasty patients. Clin Orthop 1991; 271: 180

202. Rose SC, Zwiebel WJ, Murdock LE, et al. Insensitivity of color Doppler flow imaging for detection of acute calf deep venous thrombosis in asymptomatic postoperative patients. J Vasc Intervent Radiol 1993; 4: 111

203. Paiement G, Wessinger SJ, Waltman AC, Harris WH. Surveillance of DVT in asymptomatic total hip replacement patients. Impedance plethysmography and fibrinogen scanning versus roentgenographic phlebography. Am J Surg 1988; 155: 400

204. Cruickshank MK, Levine MN, Hirsh J, et al. An evaluation of impedance plethysmography and ^{125}I-fibrinogen leg scanning in patients following hip surgery. Thromb Haemost 1989; 62: 830

205. Ginsberg JS, Caco CC, Brill-Edwards P, et al. Venous thrombosis in patients who have undergone major hip or knee surgery: Detection with compression US and impedance plethysmography. Radiology 1991; 181

206. Lensing AWA, Hirsh J. ^{125}I-fibrinogen leg scanning: reassessment of its role for the diagnosis of venous thrombosis in post-operative patients. Thromb Haemost 1993; 69: 2

207. Jay R, Hull RD, Carter C, et al. Outcome of abnormal impedance plethysmography results in patients with proximal-vein thrombosis: Frequency of return to normal. Thromb Res 1984; 36: 259

208. Murphy TP, Cronan JJ. Evolution of deep venous thrombosis: a prospective evaluation with US. Radiology 1990; 177: 543

209. Cronan JJ, Leen V. Recurrent deep venous thrombosis: Limitations of US. Radiology 1989; 170: 739

210. Heijboer H, Jongbloets LMM, Büller HR, Lensing AWA, Ten Cate JW. The clinical utility of real-time compression ultrasound in the diagnostic management of patients with recurrent venous thrombosis. Acta Radiol Scan 1992; 33: 297

211. Heijboer H, Ginsberg JS, Büller HR, Lensing AWA, Colly LP, Ten Cate JW. The use of the D-dimer test in combination with non-invasive testing versus serial non-invasive testing alone for the diagnosis of DVT. Thromb Haemost 1992; 67: 510

212. Prandoni P, Cogo A, Bernardi E, et al. A simple approach for detection of recurrent proximal vein thrombosis. Circulation 1993; 88: 1730

213. Koopman MMW, Jongbloets LMM, Lensing AWA, Büller HR, Ten Cate JW. Clinical utility of a quantitative B-mode ultrasonography method in patients with suspected recurrent DVT (DVT). Thromb Haemost 1993; 69: 623

214. Harris WH, Salzman EW, Athanasoulis C, et al. Comparison of 125I fibrinogen count scanning with phlebography of venous thrombi after elective hip surgery. N Engl J Med 1975; 292: 665–667

215. Sautter RD, Larson DE, Bhattacharyya SK, et al. The limited utility of I125 leg scanning. Arch Intern Med 1979; 139: 148–153

216. Sautter RD, Koch EL, Myers WG, et al. Aspirin-sulfinpyrazone in prophylaxis of deep venous thrombosis in total hip replacement. JAMA 1983; 250: 2649–2654

217. Faunø P, Suomalainen O, Bergquist D, et al. The use of fibrigen uptake test in screening for DVT in patients with hip fracture. Thromb Res 1990; 60: 185–190

III.2 Arm vein thrombosis

M. Monreal

Introduction

Deep venous thrombosis (DVT) of the arm was long believed to be an uncommon disorder caused by malrotation of the upper extremity especially when associated with strenuous exercise. However, with the increasingly common use of subclavian venous access, arm DVT has been recognised as being more common than previously reported. Earlier reports have suggested that it is an innocuous, self-limiting disease. As more experience has accrued, it is becoming evident that this is not correct. Arm DVT can cause superior vena cava syndrome, long-term upper-extremity disability, pulmonary embolism, and death. Furthermore, catheter-associated arm DVT can cause septic thrombophlebitis, loss of central venous access and extravasation of infusate.

The diagnosis of arm DVT is often obvious from the clinical picture. However, it is important to confirm the clinical diagnosis in order to avoid empiric anticoagulation in patients with other problems, such as hematoma, lymphedema or cellulitis. Recommended treatments have ranged from symptomatic care alone to aggressive management with anticoagulants, thrombolytic agents, and surgery.

Risk factors

There are three general etiologic categories of arm DVT: *a) external compression of the subclavian vein*, including trauma, thoracic tumours, and thrombosis related to strenuous effort; *b) hypercoagulable states*, such as malignancy, anti-phospholipid syndrome or congenital thrombophilia; and *c) catheter-induced DVT*, including thrombus related to pacemaker electrodes, central venous cannulation for parenteral nutrition or medication, and catheterisation for hemodynamic monitoring (Table 1).

a) External compression of the subclavian vein

Compression may result from anatomic abnormalities in the anterior part of the thoracic outlet, such as a hypertrophied scalene or subclavian muscle, compression between the clavicle and a cervical rib, a hypertrophic costoclavicular ligament, callus from a fractured clavicle, congenital fibromuscular bands, or the tendonous insertion of the pectoralis minor muscle [1 – 4]. Even in a normal person the thoracic outlet is a point of anatomic constriction, being narrowed even more when one is carrying heavy loads, or sleeping with the arm in an overhead position. Repetitive shoulder movements in these positions may intermittently compress the subclavian vein, and induce thrombosis.

Descriptions of arm DVT in the past have usually emphasised effort thrombosis, being more frequent in healthy young men, especially after unusual arm exertion. In 1968, Swinton et al. reported that 12 of 25 patients with arm DVT developed symptoms within 24 hours of vigorous activity [2]. Some years later, Prescott et al. found a traumatic etiology in 5 of their 12 patients, including 3 cases of effort thrombosis [5]. However, in more recent series [6 – 14] the percentage of patients with arm DVT associated to a strenuous effort or an anatomic abnormality has become less and less common (Table 1).

Table 1. Predisposing factors for arm DVT.

Authors	Year	Patients (N)	Effort	Anatomic	Cancer	Catheter
Tilney et al. [3]	1970	48	21%	10%	6%	17%
Prescott et al. [5]	1979	12	25%	17%	17%	0%
Demeter et al. [6]	1982	16	19%	25%	6%	31%
Donayre et al. [7]	1986	41	22%	2%	12%	24%
Horattas et al. [8]	1987	33	6%	6%	24%	39%
Lindblad et al. [9]	1988	120	6%	4%	11%	24%
Kerr et al. [10]	1990	85	6%	4%	31%	69%
Hill et al. [11]	1990	40	0%	not reported	22%	32%
Monreal et al. [12]	1991	30	13%	3%	33%	67%
Burihan et al. [13]	1993	52	6%	12%	23%	29%
Prandoni et al. [14]	1997	27	11%	0%	22%	30%

b) Hypercoagulable states

In addition to the above-mentioned anatomic abnormalities, co-existing hematologic abnormalities can contribute to arm DVT [14, 15]. Seven out of 120 patients in the study by Lindblad et al. were taking contraceptive pills containing estrogen [9]. In a prospective study by Prandoni et al. [14] 27 patients with arm DVT underwent testing of antithrombin, protein C and S levels, resistance to activated protein C and lupuslike anticoagulants; a thrombophilic state was identified in 4 of the 11 patients who presented with an apparently spontaneous DVT and in 2 of the 3 DVT patients who experienced this complication after strenuous effort. Thus, spontaneous or "effort" thrombosis of the upper extremity is really a syndrome associated with many diverse etiologies. To our knowledge, this is the first study in which such abnormalities have been systematically searched in a series of patients with arm DVT.

A DVT of the arm unrelated to central venous cannulation is sometimes present in patients with malignancy. A broad variety of tumour types have been found in patients with arm DVT; predominantly located in the lung and the gastrointestinal tract [6, 16, 17]. Subclavian thrombosis could result from direct invasion of the vein by the tumour, compression or distortion of the vein by the neoplasm, or a hypercoagulable state associated with malignancy or therapy.

c) Catheter-induced DVT

The incidence of arm DVT has undoubtedly risen with the increasing use of central venous catheters and these are considered today the most frequent cause of arm DVT. Excluding these cases, the incidence in the upper extremities is much lower than that in the lower limbs. In any case, the true incidence of arm DVT in patients with indwelling catheters is difficult to estimate since there are very few studies in which diagnosis of thrombosis was based on anything but clinical grounds.

Two types of catheter thrombosis occur. Hoshal et al. reported an autopsy series of 55 patients with indwelling subclavian catheters [18]. Regardless of catheter composition, circumferential fibrin sleeves had developed on the indwelling catheter in all 55 as early as 24 hours after insertion. This high prevalence of fibrin-sleeve thrombosis around catheters was confirmed by Ahmed and Payne [19], who found them in 80% of patients who had catheters; Brismar et al. [20], who found them on phlebographic studies in 42% of patients; and more recently by Stakhammar et al. [21], who found fibrin sleeves along the route of the catheter in all 16 cases investigated. Although sleeve thrombosis seldom gives rise to any signs or symptoms, parts of the thrombus may detach and cause pulmonary embolism when the catheter is removed [19, 20].

The second type of thrombosis is mural thrombosis, which can partially block or occlude the vessel lumen. In a prospective study [22], venography showed asymptomatic DVT in 15/52 (29%) cancer patients who underwent percutaneous subclavian vein catheterisation, while the incidence of

DVT was significantly lower for silicone catheters than for polyvinyl chloride catheters. Anderson et al. [23] clinically detected catheter-related DVT in 22 out of 168 cancer patients (13%) with a Hickman catheter, and at autopsy in six further patients (3.5%). The frequency of subclavian DVT varies according to the test used for DVT diagnosis: 15% when Doppler ultrasonography was used [24], or 34% when venography was performed [25]. Finally, the frequency of catheter-related DVT may also vary according to catheter tip location: Kearns et al. [26] found DVT in 60% of patients with tips in the axillosubclavian-innominate vein compared with 21% of patients with tips in the superior vena cava (p < 0.05).

In another prospective study 57 oncologic patients with short- or long-term central venous catheters and without clinical signs of arm DVT were evaluated venographically [27]. Different degrees of non-obstructive thrombosis were found in 26 patients (45%) and (clinically silent) obstructive thrombosis, was found in six patients (10.5%). A fibrin sleeve around the central venous catheter was radiologically demonstrated in 45 (78%) patients, 21 of them (46%) with a normal venogram. There was no evidence of fibrin sleeve or parietal thrombosis in only 4 patients. It is concluded that parietal thrombosis of the axillary-subclavian veins is a frequent event, even if there is no clinical evidence of flow obstruction, and that a fibrin coating is present in the majority of the central venous catheters.

Köksoy et al. prospectively assessed the risk factors that may be important in the development of catheter-related DVT [28]. Multiple lumen and single lumen polyurethane catheters were inserted into the subclavian vein in 44 consecutive patients. Two factors were found to correlate significantly with the development of central venous catheter-related DVT, namely the number of vein punctures (one vs. two punctures, p < 0.01) and the type of infusion (fluid replacement vs. total parenteral nutrition, p = 0.01). Furthermore, De Cicco et al. prospectively evaluated the role of acquired antithrombin (AT) deficiency as a risk factor for DVT in cancer patients undergoing central venous catheterisation. They compared 20 consecutive patients with reduced AT activity (<70%) requiring chemotherapy and/or total parenteral nutrition with 20 randomly selected patients with normal AT values [29]. The group with AT deficiency presented a higher degree of both parietal (p < 0.05) and overall thrombus (p < 0.02).

The introduction of central venous catheters, pacemaker leads, and dialysis catheters, is an everyday event in our time. Considering the number and frequency of all these contributing factors, the question why arm DVT occurs is less puzzling than why it does not occur more often.

Symptoms

With primary or spontaneous arm DVT, following unusually strenuous activity, symptoms generally do occur within 24 hours. Dull, aching pain in the shoulder or axilla and swelling of the arm and hand are present in the majority of patients (Fig. 1). Prior to the onset of swelling, the extremity often feels uncomfortable, heavy or achy. Depending upon the extent of the involvement, the swelling may spread from the upper arm down to and include the hand. Both swelling and pain tend to worsen with vigorous use of the arm and improve with rest and elevation. Physical examination generally shows a mild to moderate amount of non-pitting edema. Mild cyanosis of the hand and fingers and dilatation of subcutaneous collateral veins over the upper arm and chest are occasionally noted.

Catheter-related thrombosis is usually associated with even mild or no swelling. Frequently, the development of thrombosis is associated with the inability to draw blood from the catheter, even though flushing the catheter may be unimpeded. The reasons that catheter-induced DVT are clinically much more benign than spontaneous thromboses is that the thrombi develop more gradually, do involve shorter vein segments, or are non-obstructive.

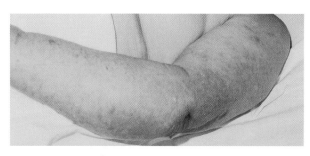

Fig. 1. Swelling of the arm, with cyanosis and subcutaneous collateral veins, in a patient with arm DVT.

Lindblad et al. [9] reviewed the case-reports of 296 patients undergoing contrast venography for a clinical suspicion of arm DVT. One-hundred and sixty five venograms (56%) did not reveal any thrombi. Edema of the arm was very frequent and often occurred in patients with a normal venogram; on the contrary, distension of the superficial veins or pain in the arm-shoulder area were more often seen in patients with arm DVT. They concluded that the clinical diagnosis is unreliable, hence objective diagnostic methods must be used to confirm or reject the diagnosis of thrombosis to correctly apply or withhold anticoagulant treatment.

Diagnostic tests

The abrupt onset of arm swelling and pain, in the absence of swelling of the contralateral upper extremity, is typical (Fig. 1). A history of unusual exertion is helpful in the diagnosis of spontaneous arm DVT, as is the awareness of recent catheterisation in the hospital setting. Inflammatory causes are less likely in case of absence of redness or warmth of the skin, and the abruptness of the swelling speaks against lymphedema. Radical mastectomy followed by radiotherapy is a notorious clinical setting in which either lymphedema or venous occlusion, or both can contribute to chronic edema. However, all these clinical manifestations are highly non-specific, and objective tests are required to confirm or reject the diagnosis.

Contrast venography remains the standard of reference for evaluating both the presence and extent of arm DVT (Figs. 2 and 3). It provides excellent spatial and contrast resolution, documents the presence of collaterals, and determines whether the obstruction is total or partial, but its use in certain patients with arm DVT may be problematic. Venography is an invasive procedure that usually must be performed in the radiology department.

The examination may be uncomfortable for the patient, venous catheterisation may be difficult because of severe arm swelling, and the contrast material itself may contribute to thrombus formation.

Ultrasound (US) evaluation overcomes these difficulties. Over the past decade, real-time B-mode US, duplex US, and colour Doppler US imaging have been used for the diagnosis of arm DVT [30–34]. Real-time US is reliable, non-invasive, repeatable, safe, and low in cost. Examinations can be performed at bedside in critically ill patients, no venous access is required, and it can be used regardless of renal function. There is a high degree of patient acceptance, and serial examinations are easy to perform. The established criteria for the sonographic diagnosis of lower limb DVT are identification of the thrombus as an intraluminal echogenic mass (Fig. 4), absence of response of the involved veins to respiratory manoeuvres and non-compressibility of the veins on increased pressure exerted with the transducer probe. The same criteria are valid in the diagnosis of arm DVT.

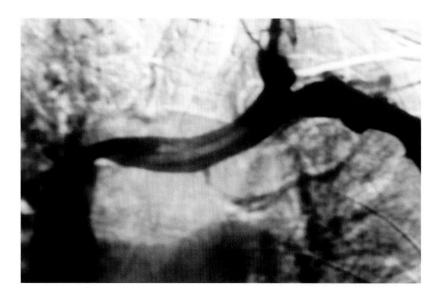

Fig. 2. Venography: Mural subclavian thrombosis in a patient with a central venous line.

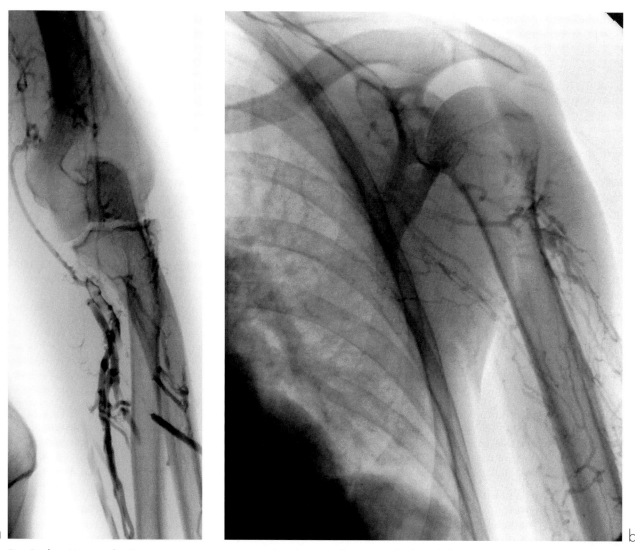

Fig. 3a, b. Venography. Extensive acute upper extremity thrombosis involving antecubital to subclavian vein segment in patient with axillary malignant lymphadenopathy **(a)**. Early collateral vessels present in the upper arm **(b)**.

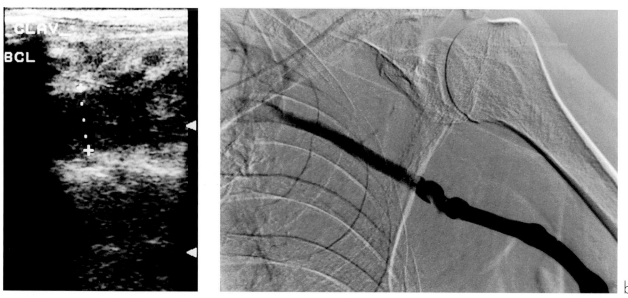

Fig. 4a, b. Sonogram **(a)** showing echogenic material in non-compressible subclavian vein. Note clavicle shadowing. The corresponding venogram **(b)** shows filling defect in subclavian vein before confluence with jugular vein.
CLAV = Clavicle, BCL = Acoustic shadow of clavicle

Doppler examinations can improve the diagnostic accuracy of high-resolution B-scanning. As venous Doppler signals increase with inspiration and decrease with expiration, Doppler is especially useful when respiratory manoeuvres are impractical [31]. Prandoni et al. compared real-time compression US, colour flow Doppler imaging, and Doppler US in a series of 58 consecutive patients with signs and symptoms of arm DVT [14]. All three non-invasive tests were performed prior to venography. Twenty-seven out of these patients had venographically proven DVT, and the accuracy of compression US (95%) was significantly higher than that of Doppler US (79%). The accuracy of colour flow Doppler imaging was slightly higher (97%), but since this test is far more expensive and time-consuming, the authors consider that real-time compression US should be considered as

the first choice alternative to contrast venography for the diagnosis of arm DVT.

Other non-invasive diagnostic techniques have also received attention. Magnetic resonance imaging is very specific in its ability to image subclavian vein thrombi, but its sensitivity is too low to be a reliable screening method [35]. Impedance plethysmography has not been sufficiently investigated to allow statements of its sensitivity and specificity for this anatomic location [25, 36]. Therefore, real-time US should be considered as the primary non-invasive test in patients with suspected arm DVT; if US establishes the diagnosis of subclavian thrombosis, further invasive diagnostic procedures can be omitted; in the case of normal findings, venography may be necessary if the clinical suspicion remains high.

Arm vein thrombosis and pulmonary embolism

The significance of arm DVT has received considerably less attention in comparison to femoral vein thrombosis, likely due to the erroneous belief that subsequent pulmonary embolism (PE) is rare. Accordingly, in the past several authors have questioned the need for anticoagulant therapy in such patients. However, recent prospective studies using sensitive methods for detecting PE have demonstrated that the prevalence of both symptomatic and asymptomatic PE in patients with arm DVT is high, and it is close to that observed in cohorts of patients with lower-extremity DVT (Table 2). In fact, in a study comprising all autopsies in a single hospital over a period of 30 years thrombi were detected in the veins of the upper extremity in 19 of 154 cases with fatal pulmonary embolism, and in the superior caval vein in eight [37].

In a review of the literature we found 16 cases of PE in 237 patients (6.7%) with arm DVT [12]. In all these studies the diagnosis of PE was based on clinical criteria only. However, now it is well established that PE most often may occur without clinical symptoms [38, 39]. Accordingly, we prospectively evaluated the prevalence of PE in a series of 30 consecutive patients with confirmed DVT of the upper extremity [12]. Ten patients had arm DVT arising spontaneously or following strenuous exertion, and 20 patients had a catheter-induced DVT. Ventilation-perfusion lung scans were routinely performed at the time of hospital admission in all but one patient (this patient was critically ill, and he died 4 days after DVT diagnosis because of mas-

sive PE despite adequate heparin therapy). Lung scan findings were normal in 9/10 patients with primary DVT, and they were indeterminate in the remaining patient. By contrast, perfusion defects with a high likelihood of PE were observed in 4 of 19 patients (21%) with catheter-related DVT. We concluded that PE is not a rare complication in arm DVT, and that patients with catheter-related DVT appeared to be at a higher risk. In another prospective study, Prandoni et al. found PE confirmed by ventilation-perfusion lung scans in 8 of 27 patients (30%) with arm DVT [14]. Lindblad et al. also found PE to be far more common in patients with catheter-related thrombosis [9]: they reviewed the case records of 120 patients with arm DVT, and none of the 73 patients with primary DVT had PE symptoms, as compared to 5/47 patients with secondary DVT (catheter-related, malignancy). Three patients had a fatal (6.4%) and one contributory PE verified at autopsy. The remaining patient had a clinically and scintigraphically confirmed PE. In a similar study by Kerr et al. [10] 5 out of 61 patients with arm DVT had PE, and 2 of these patients died; all 5 patients had a catheter-related DVT.

Searching of the frequency of thromboembolic complications in patients with central venous lines, Dollery et al. prospectively studied clinical events, lung perfusion scans, and echocardiographic screens in 34 children and adolescents with gut failure who received cyclical parenteral nutrition for 2 months to 9 years [40]. Sixteen thrombotic

Table 2. Frequency of pulmonary embolism (PE) in patients with arm DVT.

Authors	Year	Design of the study	Patients (N)	Patients with PE
Swinton et al. [2]	1968	Retrospective	23	1 (4%)
Tilney et al. [3]	1970	Retrospective	48	0
Prescott et al. [5]	1979	Prospective	12	1 (8%)
Demeter et al. [6]	1981	Retrospective	16	0
Donayre et al. [7]	1986	Retrospective	41	5 (12%)
Horattas et al. [8]	1988	Retrospective	33	4 (12%)
Lindblad et al. [9]	1988	Retrospective	120	4 (3%)
Monreal et al. [12]	1991	Prospective	30	5 (17%)
Burihan et al. [13]	1993	Retrospective	52	2 (4%)
Dollery et al. [35]	1994	Prospective	34	10 (29%)
Monreal et al. [15]	1994	Prospective	86	13 (15%)
Prandoni et al. [14]	1997	Prospective	27	8 (36%)

events (10 PE, 5 right atrial thrombi, and 1 superior vena cava obstruction) occurred in 12 patients. Eight of these patients had symptoms attributable to their thromboembolic disease; the other 4 had asymptomatic echocardiographic or perfusion-scan abnormalities. Four patients died, and in 2 cases PE was diagnosed at necropsy.

In a further study we validated our initial findings in a larger series of patients with catheter-related arm DVT; moreover, we attempted to identify clinical variables that would increase the likelihood of developing PE [15]. Eighty-six consecutive patients with central vein catheter-related DVT of the upper extremity underwent ventilation-perfusion lung scan within 24 hours of DVT diagnosis, whether PE symptoms were present or not. Thirteen patients (15%) were considered to have PE. Two out of these 13 patients subsequently died because of recurrent, massive embolism despite adequate heparin therapy. No differences were found between groups (PE versus normal scan) according to age, sex, underlying diseases, type of drugs administered through the catheter or the duration of cannulation. However, PE was more commonly found in patients with polyvinyl chloride or polyethylene catheters (10/38, 26%). These complications have been considerably reduced (3/41, 7%) due to the introduction of new catheter materials, i. e. polyurethane or silicone.

Treatment

In 1960, the standard treatment of arm DVT included sympathic ganglion blocks, anticoagulation with heparin and coumarins, application of heat, and elevation of the extremity [41]. In this series, 75% of patients reported chronic pain, edema, and limitation of movement at follow-up. In 1968, Swinton et al. [2] treated patients with bed rest, heparinisation, and ganglion blocks; only 11 of the 23 patients received full anticoagulant therapy. In 1966, thrombectomy was proposed as the method of choice to prevent the long-term sequelae of post-phlebitic syndrome [42], but thrombectomy has been refuted as the first line of treatment for effort thrombosis by others [6]. These authors reported a lower incidence of chronic post-thrombotic symptoms than previously reported and they recommended thrombectomy only for patients with chronic and disabling symptoms. More recently thrombolytic agents have been used to treat arm DVT. However, when overall considered, among the 17 articles reviewed by Becker et al. [43], 14 failed to describe the intensity and duration of this treatment. In general, many different regimens were used, and neither patients nor physicians were blinded to the therapy when the response to treatment was evaluated.

Presently, most patients receive anticoagulation according to current guidelines for lower-extremity

DVT [44]. The goal of this regimen is to halt the propagation of thrombi and to preserve collateral vein patency. In our series of 86 patients with catheter-related arm DVT all patients received intermittent intravenous heparin therapy, the dose being adjusted to maintain the aPTT at 1.5–2.0 times the pre-treatment value [15]. No patients experienced any bleeding complications, but 2 patients with PE signs on baseline lung scan suddenly died during the 8-day period, and necropsic studies demonstrated the presence of massive, recurrent PE as the cause of death in both patients. Furthermore, one additional patient with baseline evidence of asymptomatic PE developed chest pain 5 days after heparin was started and the repeat lung scan showed new perfusion defects. By contrast, in the study by Prandoni et al. none of the 27 patients receiving intravenous heparin and oral anticoagulants developed recurrent VTE during the 3-month period of therapy [14].

The role of thrombolytic agents in arm DVT remains controversial. AbuRahma et al. retrospectively compared the efficacy of thrombolysis vs heparin therapy in a small series of 10 consecutive patients with effort arm DVT [45]. Three out of 4 patients receiving thrombolytic therapy had complete resolution, and one patient had partial resolution of the symptoms and of the thrombus confirmed by repeat venogram. Three out of 6 patients receiving heparin had no resolution, one patient had complete resolution of the symptoms and of the thrombus, and two patients had only partial resolution of symptoms but no resolution of thrombus. By contrast, in the study by Lindblad et al. none of the 5 patients receiving thrombolysis showed recanalisation at repeat venogram [9]. In the review article by Becker et al. [43], 28/52 patients (54%) who had post-streptokinase venograms had the obstructing thrombus completely lysed, and 21 (40%) had partial relief of the obstruction. However, all three patients with arm DVT who were reported to have had PE while on any therapy were receiving streptokinase [46–48].

Due to the low incidence rate of arm DVT, only a few have prospectively assessed the efficacy and safety of either anticoagulant or thrombolytic therapy in patients with arm DVT. A recent study compared the early and late results of lytic versus anticoagulant therapy in 19 consecutive patients with arm DVT. Two of 9 patients (22%) receiving heparin and 8 of 10 patients (80%) receiving thrombolysis had total venous recanalisation and symptom resolution (p < 0.02) [49].

The role of surgery for arm DVT has not been well established. Except for thrombectomy, surgical procedures were selected to correct anatomic abnormalities identified by venography, the most common interventions being rib or clavicle resection to relieve subclavian vein compression [43, 50]. A recent study reported 65 patients with effort arm DVT who received direct lytic (urokinase) therapy followed by surgery. An anterior subclavicular approach was used to remove the first rib, subclavius, and anterior scalene muscles to have safe access to the vein [51]. In acute cases (8 patients only) decompression of the vein at the thoracic outlet was effective in all cases. Vein patch angioplasty was needed in recurrent, subacute, and chronic cases. This procedure was 100% effective if stenosis was less than 2 cm long. The authors recommend that effort DVT of the subclavian vein should be treated acutely with thrombolytic agents followed by surgery.

In a recent consensus conference, 15 multiple-choice questions concerning various options in the management of primary (no catheter-related) arm DVT were discussed by a panel of experts [52]. The large majority agreed upon early clot removal for active, healthy patients by catheter-directed thrombolysis as initial therapy. Further therapy should be based on venographic findings: surgical relief of demonstrated thoracic outlet compression or conservative therapy if post-lysis venogram showed either no extrinsic compression or short residual occlusion.

In summary, a review of published studies comparing thrombolytic therapy to anticoagulation alone indicates that substantial venographic improvement occurs more commonly in patients receiving thrombolysis (Figs. 5a and b). However, bleeding complications are also more frequent, and the long-term benefits of thrombolytic therapy in preventing chronic venous insufficiency are to be demonstrated. For the present, most patients should receive anticoagulation according to current guidelines for lower-extremity DVT [44]. Alternatively, some authors consider that, since patients with effort arm DVT are usually young and most of them continue to have upper extremity edema or pain, aggressive attempts to re-establish normal venous return through the subclavian vein should be warranted [47]. In this case, thrombolytic therapy could be indicated, and perhaps even surgery. On the other hand, in patients with catheter-related arm DVT it could be prudent to treat the patient by removing the catheter and with anticoagulant therapy.

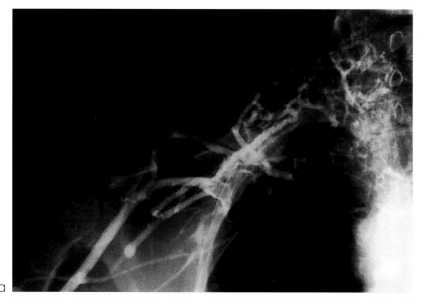
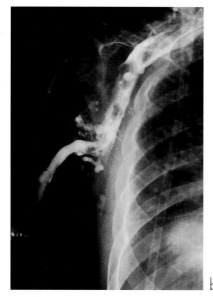

a   b

Fig. 5a, b. Venography: Axillo-subclavian DVT, **(a)** before and **(b)** after thrombolytic therapy.

Prophylaxis

Today many patients with cancer have indwelling long-term central venous catheters. Benefits from this approach include increased ease of administration of either chemotherapy or drugs, and increased ease of blood sampling for clinical laboratory tests. However, as previously reported, these patients are prone to a number of complications, including subclavian DVT. Trying to avoid this problem, Bern et al. [53] conducted a study in which 121 cancer patients with chronic indwelling central venous catheters were prospectively and randomly assigned to receive or not to receive 1 mg of warfarin, beginning 3 days before catheter insertion and continuing for 90 days. Of 42 patients completing the study while receiving warfarin, 4 had venogram-confirmed DVT. Of 40 patients completing the study while not receiving warfarin, 15 had DVT (p < 0.001). Since then, the American College of Chest Physicians [54] advocated prophylactic anticoagulation for patients with indwelling catheters. However, warfarin is reluctantly given in most cancer patients. In fact, patients taking drugs that suppress platelet function were not included in the study by Bern et al.

Furthermore, warfarin had to be discontinued in 10% of patients in whom the prothrombin time exceeded 15.0 seconds. Accordingly, we decided to investigate the effectiveness of fixed doses of a low-molecular-weight heparin in this setting. In an open, prospective study, patients with cancer who underwent placement of a Port-a-Cath subclavian venous catheter were randomised to receive or not 2,500 IU of Fragmin® once daily for 90 days [55]. Venography was routinely performed 90 days after catheter insertion, or sooner if DVT symptoms had appeared. On the recommendation of the Ethics Committee, patient recruitment was terminated earlier than planned: DVT developed in 1/16 patients (6%) taking Fragmin® and 8/13 patients (62%) without prophylaxis. Accordingly, the Ethics Committee decided to recommend prophylaxis with low-molecular-weight heparin to all cancer patients with central venous catheters, at least during the first 3 months. It has to be demonstrated if Fragmin® may be superior to warfarin, but some kind of prophylaxis seems to be mandatory.

Sequelae and long-term outcome

The acute symptoms of arm thrombosis usually regress rapidly regardless of therapy, and the affected extremity is often normal upon discharge from the hospital in most patients. However, with return to routine activity many patients experience recurrence of discomfort of varying intensity. Symptoms include aching and fullness accentuated by dependency or by extremes in the weather, repetitive motion often elicits cramping and fatigue of muscles of the forearm. Such symptoms usually resolve with the arm at rest for several minutes.

A number of studies have addressed the frequency of the post-thrombotic syndrome after arm DVT. Early reports implied that most patients had residual symptoms for years: as many as 74–91% of patients with arm DVT experienced late sequelae [2, 3]. However, more recent studies suggest that most patients suffer minimal, if any, sequelae. None of the 120 patients in one series were reported to have to change occupation due to disability of the arm [9]; moderate pain restricting daily activity in some way was found in five patients (4%) and mild discomfort with occasional swelling of the arm was noted in 26 patients (22%). Prandoni et al. [14] found late post-thrombotic sequelae two years after discharge in 4 of 27 patients (18%); these sequelae were severe in one patient and moderate in the remaining three.

The etiologic factor causing the subclavian DVT may explain the discrepant outcomes of these studies. Those patients with an anatomic basis for arm DVT will continue with recurrences and propagation of the thrombus and with occlusion of collaterals. The end result is venous hypertension, edema, and pain. Those patients who did not have an anatomic cause but instead had a catheter or transient hypercoagulable state will have resolution of the immediate problem and avoid sequelae or recurrences.

References

1. Coon WW, Willis PW. Thrombosis of axillary and subclavian veins. Arch Surg 1966; 94: 657–663.

2. Swinton NW, Edgett JW, Hall RJH. Primary subclavian-axillary vein thrombosis. Circulation 1968; XXXVIII: 737–745.

3. Tilney NL, Griffiths HJG, Edwards EA. Natural history of major venous thrombosis of the upper extremity. Arch Surg 1970; 101: 792–796.

4. Molina JE. Surgery for effort thrombosis of the subclavian vein. J Thorac Cardiovasc Surg 1992; 2: 341–346.

5. Prescott SM, Tikoff G. Deep venous thrombosis of the upper extremity: a reappraisal. Circulation 1979; 59: 350–355.

6. Demeter SL, Pritchard JS, Piedad OH, Cordasco EM, Taherj S. Upper extremity thrombosis: etiology and prognosis. Angiology 1982; November: 743–755.

7. Donayre CE, White GH, Mehringer SM, Wilson SE. Pathogenesis determines late morbidity of axillosubclavian vein thrombosis. Am J Surg 1986; 152: 179–184.

8. Horattas MC, Wright DJ, Fenton AH, Evans DM, Oddi MA, Kamienski RW, Shields EF. Changing concepts of deep venous thrombosis of the upper extremity – Report of a series and review of the literature. Surgery 1988; 104: 561–567.

9. Lindblad B, Tengborn L, Bergqvist D. Deep vein thrombosis of the axillary-subclavian veins: epidemiologic data, effects of different types of treatment and late sequelae. Eur J Vasc Surg 1988; 2: 161–165.

10. Kerr TM, Lutter KS, Moeller DM, Hasselfeld KA, Roedersheimer LR, McKenna PJ, Spirtoff K, Sampson MG, Cranley JJ. Upper extremity venous thrombosis diagnosed by duplex scanning. Am J Surg 1990; 160: 202–206.

11. Hill SL, Berry RE. Subclavian vein thrombosis: a continuing challenge. Surgery 1990; 108: 1–9.

12. Monreal M, Lafoz E, Ruiz J, Valls R, Alastrue A. Upper-extremity deep venous thrombosis and pulmonary embolism. A prospective study. Chest 1991; 9: 280–283.

13. Burihan E, Poli de Figueiredo LF, Francisco J, Miranda F. Upper-extremity deep venous thrombosis: analysis of 52 cases. Cardiovasc Surg 1993; 1: 19–22.

14. Prandoni P, Polistena P, Bernardi E, Cogo A, Casara D, Verlato F, Angelini F, Simioni P, Signorini GP, Benedetti L, Girolami A. Upper-extremity deep vein thrombosis. Risk factors, diagnosis, and complications. Arch Intern Med 1997; 57: 57–62.

15. Haire WD. Arm vein thrombosis. Clinics in Chest Medicine 1995; 16: 341–351.

16. Monreal M, Raventós A, Lerma R, Ruíz J, Lafoz E, Alastrué A, Llamazares JF. Pulmonary embolism in patients with upper extremity DVT associated to venous central lines. A prospective study. Thromb Haemost 1994; 72: 548–550.

17. Hung SSJ. Deep vein thrombosis of the arm associated with malignancy. Cancer 1989; 64: 531–535.

18. Hoshal VL Jr, Ause RG, Hoskins PA. Fibrin formation on indwelling subclavian central venous catheters. Arch Surg 1971; 102: 353–358.

19. Ahmed N, Payne RF. Thrombosis after central venous cannulation. Med J Aust 1976; 1: 217–220.

20. Brismar B, Hardstedt C, Jacobson S. Diagnosis of thrombosis by catheter phlebography after prolonged central venous catheterization. Ann Surg 1981; 194: 779–783.

21. Starkhammar H, Bengtsson M, Morales O. Fibrin sleeve formation after long term brachial catheterisation with an implantable port device. A prospective venographic study. Eur J Surg 1992; 158: 481–484.

22. Bozzetti F, Scarpa D, Terno G, Scotti A, Ammatuna M, Bonalumi MG, Ceglia E. Subclavian venous thrombosis due to indwelling catheters: A prospective study on 52 patients. JPEN 1983; 7: 560–562.

23. Anderson AJ, Krasnow SH, Boyer MW, Cutler DJ, Jones BD, Citron ML, Ortega LG, Cohen MH. Thrombosis: the major Hickman catheter complication in patients with solid tumor. Chest 1989; 95: 71–75.

24. Pucheu A, Leduc B, Sillet-Bach I, Payen C, Pucheu ME. Thromboses veineuses profondes sur dispositifs de perfusion implantables. Étude prospective de 72 patients par échotomographie-doppler des veines du cou (jugulaire, sous-clavière et tronc brachio-céphalique veineux). Bull Cancer 1993; 80: 680–688.

25. Horne MDK, Mayo DJ, Alexander HR, Stelnhaus EP, Chang RC, Whitman E, Gralnick HR. Upper extremity impedance plethysmography in patients with venous access devices. Thromb Haemost 1994; 72: 540–542.

26. Kearns PJ, Coleman S, Wehner JH. Complications of long-arm catheters: a randomized trial of central vs peripheral tip location. J Parenter Enteral Nutr 1996; 20: 20–24.

27. Balestreri L, De Cicco M, Matovic M, Coran F, Morassut S. Central venous catheter-related thrombosis in clinical asymptomatic oncologic patients: a phlebographic study. Eur J Radiol 1995; 2: 108–111.

28. Köksoy C, Kuzu A, Erden I, Akkaya A. The risk factors in central venous catheter-related thrombosis. Aust N Z J Surg 1995; 65: 796–798.

29. De Cicco M, Matovic M, Balestreri L, De Angelis V, Fracasso A, Morassut S, Coran F, Barbare R, Buonadonna A, Testa V. Antithrombin III deficiency as a risk factor for catheter-related central vein thrombosis in cancer patients. Thromb Res 1995; 78: 127–137.

30. Falk RL, Smith DF. Thrombosis of upper extremity thoracic inlet veins: Diagnosis with duplex doppler sonography. AJR 1987; 149: 677–682.

31. Gaitini D, Kaftori JK, Pery M, Engel A. High-resolution real-time ultrasonography. Diagnosis and follow-up of jugular and subclavian vein thrombosis. J Ultrasound Med 1988; 7: 621–627.

32. Knudson GJ, Wiedmeyer DA, Erickson SJ, Foley WD, Lawson TL, Mewissen MW, Lipchik EO. Color doppler sonographic imaging in the assessment of upper-extremity deep venous thrombosis. AJR 1990; 154: 399–403.

33. Haire WD, Lynch TG, Lieberman RP, Lund GB, Edney JA. Utility of duplex ultrasound in the diagnosis of asymptomatic catheter-induced subclavian vein thrombosis. J Ultrasound Med 1991; 10: 493–496.

34. Köksoy C, Kuzu A, Kutlay J, Erden I, Ozcan H, Ergîn K. The diagnostic value of colour Doppler ultrasound in central venous catheter related thrombosis. Clin Radiol 1995; 50: 687–689.

35. Haire WD, Lynch TG, Lund GB, Lieberman RP, Edney JA. Limitations of magnetic resonance imaging and ultrasound-directed (duplex) scanning in the diagnosis of subclavian vein thrombosis. J Vasc Surg 1991; 13: 391–397.

36. Zufferey P, Pararas C, Monti M, Depairon M. Assessment of acute and old deep venous thrombosis in upper extremity by venous strain gauge plethysmography. Vasa 1992; 21: 263–267.

37. Lindblad B, Sternby NH, Bergqvist D. Incidence of venous thromboembolism verified by necropsy over 30 years. Br Med J 1991; 302: 709–711.

38. Huisman MV, Büller HR, ten Cate JW, Van Royen EA, Vreeken J, Kersten MJ, Bakx R. Unexpected high prevalence of silent pulmonary embolism in patients with deep venous thrombosis. Chest 1989; 95: 498–502.

39. Monreal M, Rey-Joly C, Ruíz J, Salvador R, Lafoz E, Viver E. Asymptomatic pulmonary embolism in patients with deep vein thrombosis: is it useful to take lung scan to rule out this condition? J Cardiovasc Surg 1989; 30: 104–107.

40. Dollery CM, Sullivan ID, Bauraind O, Bull C, Milla PJ. Thrombosis and embolism in long-term central venous access for parenteral nutrition. Lancet 1994; 344: 1043–1045.

41. Crowell DL. Effort thrombosis of the subclavian and axillary vein: review of the literature and case-report with two-year follow-up with venography. Ann Intern Med 1960; 52: 1337–1343.

42. Drapanas T, Curran WL. Thrombectomy in the treatment of "effort" thrombosis of the axillary and subclavian veins. J Trauma 1966; 6: 107–119.

43. Becker DM, Philbrick JT, Walker FB. Axillary and subclavian venous thrombosis. Prognosis and treatment. Arch Intern Med 1991; 151: 1934–1943.

44. Hyers TM, Hull RD, Weg JG. Antithrombotic therapy for venous thromboembolic disease. Chest 1995; 108 (suppl): 335S–351S.

45. AbuRahma AF, Sadler D, Stuart P, Khan MZ, Boland JP. Conventional versus thrombolytic therapy in spontaneous (effort) axillary-subclavian vein thrombosis. Am J Surg 1991; 161: 459–465.

46. Rubenstein M, Creger WP. Successful streptokinase therapy for catheter-induced subclavian vein thrombosis. Arch Intern Med 1980; 140: 1370–1371.

47. Druy EM, Trout HH III, Giordano JM, Hix WR. Lytic therapy in the treatment of axillary and subclavian vein thrombosis. J Vasc Surg 1985; 2: 821–827.

48. Jones JC, Balkcom IL, Worman RK. Pulmonary embolus after treatment for subclavian-axillary vein thrombosis. Postgrad Med 1987; 82: 244–249.

49. AbuRahma AF, Short YS, White JF, Boland JP. Treatment alternatives for axillary-subclavian vein thrombosis: long-term follow-up. Cardiovasc Surg 1996; 4: 783–787.

50. Daskalakis E, Bauhoutsos J. Subclavian and axillary vein compression of musculoskeletal origin. Br J Surg 1980; 67: 573–576.

51. Molina JE. Need for emergency treatment in subclavian vein effort thrombosis. J Am Coll Surg 1995; 181: 414–420.

52. Rutherford RB, Hurlbert SN. Primary subclavian-axillary vein thrombosis: consensus and commentary. Cardiovasc Surg 1996; 4: 420–423.

53. Bern MM, Lokich JJ, Wallach SR, Bothe A, Benotti PN, Arkin CF, Greco FA, Huberman M, Moore C. Very low doses of warfarin can prevent thrombosis in central venous catheters. A randomized prospective trial. Ann Intern Med 1990; 112: 423–428.

54. Clagett GP, Anderson FA, Levine MN, Salzman EW, Wheeler HB. Prevention of venous thromboembolism. Chest 1992; 102 (suppl): 391S–407S.

55. Monreal M, Alastrué A, Rull M, Mira X, Muxart J, Rosell R, Abad A. Upper extremity deep venous thrombosis in cancer patients with venous access devices. Prophylaxis with a low molecular weight heparin (Fragmin). Thromb Haemost 1994; 75: 251–253.

Chapter IV
Imaging Procedures

IV.1 The role and value of ventilation perfusion imaging in pulmonary embolism

H. W. Gray, J. B. Neilly

Introduction

While increasing knowledge of the pathogenesis of venous thromboembolism expands our role in prophylaxis, the diagnosis of pulmonary embolism (PE) remains problematical and as such, continues to challenge the skills and commitment of both physician and diagnostic imager.

The most important clinical application of radiopharmaceuticals to the study of lung pathophysiology is in the evaluation of the patient with suspected PE. Abnormalities of perfusion and ventilation are common to all lung conditions. Over the last 25 years, much of the focussed research effort has been oriented towards correct categorisation of ventilation perfusion (VQ) scans to provide improved overall accuracy of reporting. More recently, the application of Bayes' theorem as a tool for the diagnostic imager has improved our understanding of the strengths and weaknesses of VQ scintigraphy and has provided evidence on which to base a coherent reporting policy. Improved technology has provided Magnetic Resonance Imaging and Spiral Computed Tomography. These new modalities and other advances challenge our understanding of the role of VQ imaging in PE diagnosis and mandate a reassessment of our own diagnostic strategies.

This chapter will discuss the principles and practice of VQ imaging including radiopharmaceuticals, instrumentation and imaging techniques. The uncertainties relating to PE diagnosis with VQ imaging will be explored, the difficulties in scan interpretation outlined and the formulation of a post-test diagnosis discussed. Finally, an overall strategy for PE diagnosis using VQ imaging, B-mode or Doppler ultrasonography, D-dimer measurement and conventional or spiral CT pulmonary angiography will be outlined.

Pulmonary Circulation

Functional structure

The pulmonary circulation possesses certain distinctive properties, which differentiates it from other vascular beds. It accommodates the entire circulating blood volume (6 l/m) and provides a vast surface area for gas exchange at low pressure. Venous blood is transported to the gas exchanging areas via the mixing chambers of the right atrium and ventricles entering the main pulmonary artery through the pulmonary valve. Blood is diverted to each lung via the right and left pulmonary arteries entering the lung at the hilum and spreading axially in the direction of the lung periphery. The arteries divide sequentially into lobar and segmental branches following the route of their bronchial divisions forming bronchopulmonary segments. Successive divisions numbering 17 result in a prodigious number of vessels numbering roughly 200 to 300 million [1]. The internal diameter of the pulmonary vessels diminishes from 1.86 cm in the main pulmonary artery to 8.3 μm in the alveolar capillaries. In children the number of vessels is reckoned to be 10% and 33% of the adult number in those aged less than 1 year and 3 years respectively. The extra-alveolar vessels are protected from the influence of alveolar pressures by the presence of a supporting sheath, but are influenced by changes in lung volume during the normal breathing cycle. Regional blood flow in the normal human lung has a non-uniform distribution [2]. It is subject to gravity so that perfusion per unit volume is less at the lung apex than at the lung base in the upright position. Not all of the lung circulation is actively perfused at any one time. Increasing pulmonary blood flow and/or left atrial pressure leads to the recruitment of blood vessels which are normally closed. The pulmonary vessels also display the phenomenon of hypoxic vasoconstriction. When alveolar pO_2 falls below 70 mmHg, regional perfusion diminishes to prevent physiological shunt. The pulmonary circulation may be affected by a wide range of disease processes including primary disorders of the heart, pulmonary vasculature and lung parenchyma. The clinical features of pulmonary thromboembolism are due to obstruction of pulmonary arteries [3], principally the lobar or segmental branches. Rarely, pulmonary thromboembolism affects the lung microcirculation where its effects are mediated by reflex pulmonary arterial vasoconstriction. Occasionally, thrombus occupies the central circulation (the so-called saddle embolus) without causing complete obstruction to blood flow.

Principles of perfusion imaging

The unique properties of the pulmonary circulation have been utilised to image regional pulmonary perfusion. The latter can be measured by particle infusion and regional particle deposition is proportional to the quantity of tracer injected and the blood flow to the region if certain conditions are met [4]. These conditions include the uniform distribution and trapping of all infused particles within the lung vasculature, and a residence time long enough to afford detection by external means. The particles must therefore be capable of detection and should not be subject to immediate metabolism. The outworking of this principle was demonstrated in an experimental model of PE using radiolabelled inert ceramic microspheres [5]. However, the application of this technology to humans awaited the development of biodegradable particles of suitable size and capable of accepting a radiolabel. The breakthrough came from research into small particle for the study of phagocytosis. Halpern described a method for the production of albumin particles in 1956 [6], which were noted to entrap in the lung circulation. The method was adapted by Taplin and colleagues [7] to produce particles of macroaggregated albumin (MAA) which could be radiolabelled. Following rigorous safety checks with particular emphasis on potential pulmonary and cerebral toxicity, the first human studies using radio-labelled MAA were reported in 1964 [4, 7]. The resultant images successfully predicted lobar and segmental perfusion abnormalities in both experimental and actual PE [4].

Safety

The safety record of perfusion studies since their introduction more than 30 years ago has been outstanding. However, a number of deaths occurred immediately following the administration of MAA in several patients with severe pulmonary arterial hypertension of varying aetiology [8–11]. These studies employed up to 11 mg of albumin and 5 million particles and prompted the debate as to the optimal albumin dose and number of particles employed in perfusion studies. Assuming that particles are perfect spheres and of uniform distribution, Harding reasoned that 1 mg of albumin given as microspheres of size 0.15 µm and 60 µm would occupy only 0.14% and 0.31% of the available pulmonary capillaries respectively [12]. Studies in experimental animals showed that a doubling of pulmonary artery pressure required doses of albumin 2,000 times that normally used in human studies when the particle size was 15.8 µm [13]. This margin of safety reduced to 25 when the particle size employed was increased to 90.7 µm. The infusion of up to 250,000 microspheres directly into the pulmonary circulation in humans produced no change in systemic or pulmonary pressures [14]. On the other hand, there were concerns that the use of low numbers of particles would produce perfusion artefacts. Heck showed that the minimum number of particles required to avoid particle non-uniformity is 60,000 [15]. Non-uniform spatial distribution of particles is observed when the number of particles falls to less than 30,000 resulting in patchy perfusion abnormalities at the lung peripheries. Increasing the number of particles above 200,000 had little effect on image quality [16]. On the basis of these data, most agree that the ideal number of particles for injection lies between 100,000 to 200,000 per study and that the ideal particle size is in the region of 10–40 µm [17]. In patients with pulmonary hypertension, the number of particles should be reduced to about 60,000. For children the number of particles needs to be reduced to 10,000 to 20,000 for those under 1 year and to 30,000 to 50,000 for those under 3 years [18]. Adverse effects may also arise as a result of reaction to the introduction of foreign protein or ferrous ions to the circulation. The frequency of such side-effects is low. Between 1967 to 1992, in the United Kingdom, a total of 32 adverse reactions were reported [17]. The majority of these were allergic in nature. Initial concerns about cerebral toxicity of radio-labelled aggregates of albumin proved unfounded [19]. Direct injections of radio-labelled MAA into the carotid and vertebral arteries in humans were uncomplicated by any neurological sequelae [20]. Indeed, ^{99m}Tc-MAA has been used to assess right-to-left intra-cardiac shunts in both children [21] and adults [22] although the dose of albumin should be limited to 0.2 mg albumin and 100,000 particles respectively.

Kit formulations

MAA is produced [23] by heating human serum albumin to 80–90°C in the presence of stannous ions at pH 5–6 for 30 minutes. After washing with saline the suspension is freeze-dried giving a shelf life of up to one year. The albumin particles so derived are polygonal with a range of particle sizes and shapes [24]. The heterogeneity of MAA shape led to the development of microspheres of human albumin (MSA) which are spherical and of uniform size [25]. MSA is prepared by agitating human serum albumin in vegetable oil, sieving to the desired particle size and impregnating with tin as the reducing agent. MAA is available in kit form although MSA is no longer commercially available. Kit specifications differ according to the manufacturer and may create difficulties with administration of the appropriate number of particles. Typically, MAA kits contain 1 to 2 mg of albumin but particle numbers are widely disparate, ranging from 1 to 15 million particles per vial [26]. Particle size in different kits is more uniform ranging between 7 and 70 μm (mean 17–32 μm). Few kits contain particles smaller than 10 μm and none contained particles larger than 150 μm [27]. Kits are re-constituted by the addition of sodium ^{99m}Tc-pertechnetate and the dosing instructions vary widely between manufacturers. The maximum recommended activity of ^{99m}Tc pertechnetate ranges from 1.48 to 3.70 GBq depending on the kit used and this affects substantially the number of particles infused for standard activity of ^{99m}Tc-MAA (about 100 MBq) injected depending on whether the dose is reconstituted for immediate or delayed use [26]. These disparities have led to calls for standardisation in kit formulations.

Administration and kinetics

Following reconstitution with ^{99m}Tc-pertechnetate, the solution has a maximum shelf life of 8 hours and should be stored at temperatures of 2–8°C

[28]. Quality control is necessary to determine radiochemical purity and particle size. Radiochemical purity as measured by the supernatant activity may vary from 0.5% to 16% [29]. Particles tend to settle on standing and should be shaken gently before use. The use of plastic giving sets should be avoided because of particle adherence. Withdrawal of blood into the syringe should be avoided, as this will cause aggregation of particles and perfusion artefacts. The solution should be given by slow intravenous bolus injection over 30 seconds while the patient breathes at normal tidal volumes. This will ensure that the particles are infused over several respiratory cycles and facilitate uniform distribution within the pulmonary circulation. Although particle dispersion is inhomogeneous as measured by autoradiography [30], particle distribution within the pulmonary circulation appears uniform at the macroscopic level. Controversy remains as to the correct patient posture at the time of the injection of the radio-labelled albumin. However, gravity-dependent perfusion gradients are unavoidable. With the patient in the upright posture the distribution of particles is predominantly caudal with relative apical hypoperfusion while in the supine position there is dorsal pre-dominance with relative sparing of the anterior aspects of the lungs. The implication is that the perfusion and ventilation scans should be acquired in the same posture. Following administration, the albumin particles are eliminated from the lungs by mechanical dispersion and by dissociation of the ^{99m}Tc-MAA linkage. There is bi-modal elimination with effective half-lives of 0.88 and 4.56 hours [31]. The short half-life component reflects the release of large amounts of unbound ^{99m}Tc within 1 hour of injection and the longer component reflects mechanical dispersion of the more tightly bound radio-labelled albumin.

Radiation absorbed dose

The radiation absorbed dose (effective dose equivalent) following a standard ^{99m}Tc perfusion scan is estimated to be 0.013 mSv/MBq (0.047 rem/mCi) [28]. As might be expected, the lungs receive the highest dose of absorbed radiation estimated to be 0.067 mGy/MBq (0.25 rad/mCi). Up to 10% of capillaries contain more than one particle and the heterogeneous dispersion of albumin particles within the pulmonary circulation at a microscopic level means that the dose of radiation received by individual endothelial cells varies widely (30). Perfusion imaging using ^{99m}Tc-labelled aggregates of human albumin is not contra-indicated in pregnancy. The dose to the uterus is 0.0023 mGy/MBq (0.0085 rad/mCi) and the risk to the mother and foetus of undiagnosed and untreated PE is reckoned to be substantially greater than the negligible risk to the foetus from the radiation exposure [32]. However, most authorities recommend a 50% reduction in the dose of administered ^{99m}Tc-MAA. Breast feeding should be interrupted for only 24 hours following the administration of a standard dose of ^{99m}Tc-MAA [33, 34].

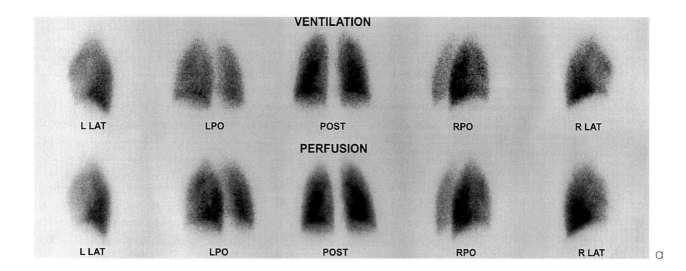

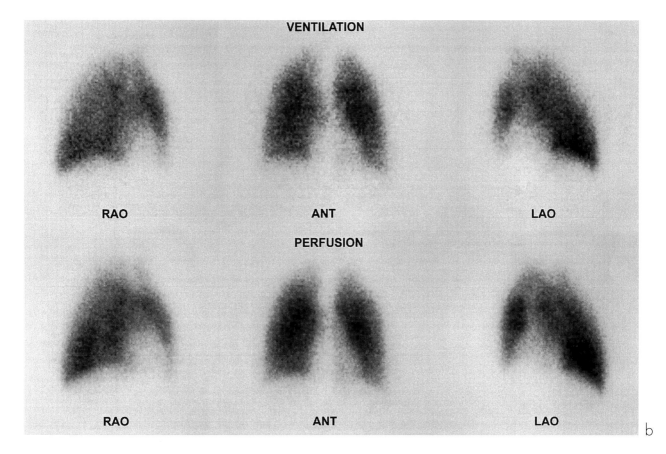

Fig. 1a, b. Normal 8-view Technegas ventilation (upper) and MAA perfusion (lower) scan performed sequentially (**a**: posterior, **b**: anterior). Count rate of perfusion was at least 5 times that of ventilation images. Normal areas of decreased activity are seen in the region of the mediastinum, hila and heart. Mild photon attenuation can also be seen normally due to overlying bone and soft tissue such as the scapulae and the patient's arms.

Imaging

Since its introduction, perfusion imaging has been performed routinely using multiple view planar imaging. Images are acquired via low-energy, all purpose collimator interfaced to a large field-of-view gamma camera centred on a 140 keV peak with a 20% window. Images are acquired for 200,000 to 1,000,000 counts in six projections: anterior; posterior; left and right posterior obliques; and left and right lateral projections. Some departments use anterior oblique projections rather than lateral views. The clarity of the perfusion images are excellent and the method has proved to be robust. In the normal study the lung margins are concave and uninterrupted, reflecting the diaphragm, chest wall and lung apical contours (Fig. 1). On the anterior and posterior projections, the medial borders are indented by the hilar structures and the heart, and the vertebral column respectively. The hilar structures are observed centrally on the oblique and lateral views and the cardiac impression is seen anteriorly on the left oblique and lateral projections. Pulmonary emboli characteristically appear as segmental, pleural-based perfusion defects and are reliably detected by perfusion scintigraphy. However, the size of the perfusion defects may be underestimated by planar perfusion scintigraphy [35]. Single photon emission tomography (SPET) [36, 37] and three-dimensional surface-shaded SPET [38] following ^{99m}Tc-MAA infusion improves the detection of segmental perfusion defects and specificity in patients with suspected PE. Tomographic images require attenuation correction to avoid gravity-dependent and gravity-independent density gradients [39]. However, tomographic imaging has not yet gained widespread acceptance for perfusion imaging, possibly because of long data acquisition and processing times and the lack of formally established criteria for the evaluation of perfusion defects. The development of multi-headed, high-resolution gamma cameras and powerful computers capable of fast processing may change this.

Timing

The timing of perfusion scans both in relation to the ventilation scan and in relation to the onset of symptoms is important and has been reviewed by Coakley [40]. Resolution of thrombus within the pulmonary circulation may take place by mechanical dispersion or by activation of thrombolysis. These changes may take place over the course of several hours or be delayed for weeks or months. In some cases, the perfusion defects may remain permanently. The implications are that the perfusion scan should be performed preferably within 24 hours of the onset of symptoms and if delayed beyond this, the scan reported should be issued with a reservation attached. If a ventilation scan is required, it should be performed at the same time as the perfusion scan and certainly within 24 hours.

Pulmonary ventilation

The need for concurrent ventilation imaging became clear early in the evolution of perfusion imaging because of the poor specificity of perfusion scans for the diagnosis of PE. A review of the basic principles of ventilation is presented followed by a description of the various radio-labelled compounds used to image regional ventilation.

Functional anatomy

Gas is transported to the alveoli by a system of airways that branch by irregular dichotomy with resultant airways of decreasing calibre and length. The number of airways increases from 1 at the level of the trachea to approximately 131,000 at the level of the terminal bronchioles and decrease in internal diameter to about 0.4 mm at the level of the respiratory and alveolar ducts. The airways proximal to the terminal bronchiole are lined by ciliated epithelium and take no part in gas transfer. The respiratory tract constitutes a natural barrier to the potentially damaging effects of inhaled aerosols. The barrier is facilitated by the muco-ciliary escalator, and the rapid and irregular branching pattern of the conducting airways, which results in a vast increase in airways cross-sectional area. The velocity of airflow decreases markedly as the cross-sectional area of the airways increases. Beyond the conducting airways is the respiratory zone, which comprise respiratory bronchioles, alveolar ducts and alveolar sacs. The volume of the conducting airways is 150 ml whereas the volume of gas within the lungs at functional residual capacity (FRC) is 2.3 litres. In the conducting airways, movement of gas takes place by mass action whereas in the respiratory zones gas moves by simple diffusion. Fully developed laminar flow probably only occurs in the small airways where the Reynold's numbers are very low (approximately 1 in terminal bronchioles). In most of the bronchial tree, flow is transitional with eddies at branch points. Turbulent flow is present in the trachea only during exercise. Not all lung regions are equally ventilated. Even in the normal lung, the distribution of ventilation is influenced by a number of factors including gravity and the rate

and depth of breathing. Transpulmonary pressures are greater at the lung apices. Alveoli at the lung apices are therefore more distended at FRC and ventilation per unit lung volume is therefore greater at the lung bases. Topographical differences are greatly exaggerated in diseased states as a result of airways narrowing and diminished compliance of individual lung units.

Radiopharmaceuticals

Agents used to image regional ventilation include radioactive forms of xenon and krypton as well as ^{99m}Tc-labelled aerosol formulations. The fact that numerous compounds are used in clinical practice indicates that none is ideal for ventilation imaging. The strengths and weaknesses of the various radiopharmaceuticals used for ventilation imaging are reviewed in turn.

Xenon

Radioactive xenon was introduced by Knipping [41] for lung function assessment in 1955 and came into routine clinical use for ventilation imaging around 1970. For many years it was the benchmark for studies of regional ventilation and formed the basis of ventilation assessment in the PIOPED study [42]. There are two forms of radioactive xenon, which are in current use. Xenon-133 (^{133}Xe) decays by beta emission with a half-life of 5.3 days, and produces 81-keV photons at 37% abundance. Xenon-127 (^{127}Xe) decays by electron capture with a half-life of 36.3 days. The principal gamma emissions are 172 keV (25%), 203 keV (68%), and 375 keV (18%). Despite its suboptimal photon energy, ^{133}Xe has generally been preferred to ^{127}Xe because it is widely available and inexpensive. ^{127}Xe, by contrast, is cyclotron-produced, is expensive and is of limited availability.

As a true gas, inhaled xenon is distributed uniformly throughout the lungs permitting the acquisition of images corresponding with different phases of ventilation. Two principal methods of ventilation imaging using xenon have been advocated: single breath [43] and multi-breath steady-state [44] methods. Both methods require substantial patient co-operation and it is necessary to familiarise the patient with the breathing routine. In the single-breath method the patient is positioned before the gamma camera in the posterior projection. Noseclips are applied and a facemask is ad-

justed to produce an air-tight seal. Between 370–740 MBq of ^{133}Xe is injected into the patient's face mask while breathing at FRC. The patient inhales to total lung capacity (TLC) followed by a breath-hold until sufficient counts (25,000 to 75,000) have been acquired. The distribution of radioactivity in this image reflects regional ventilation in the posterior projection with well ventilated areas demonstrating uniform activity and poorly ventilated areas reflecting absent or reduced regional ventilation. A significant proportion of patients are unable to comply with the manoeuvre [44].

The multi-breath steady state method consists of three distinct phases: wash-in, equilibrium, and wash-out. The patient is positioned as for the single breath method and breathes naturally through a closed 3 litre circuit containing a spirometer and a CO_2 absorber. 120 MBq ^{133}Xe is introduced into the spirometer circuit. The patient breathes at normal tidal volumes for up to 5 minutes during which oxygen is continuously replaced. The 3–5 minute wash-in is generally sufficient to allow adequate mixing of xenon with alveolar gas although many patients with uneven ventilation and long time constants due to chronic obstructive pulmonary disease will fail to reach equilibration during this phase [45]. During the wash-in and equilibration phases, single or multiple images may be acquired. These images may demonstrate in-filling of ventilation as mixing occurs. The activity on the equilibrium image reflects regional lung volume rather than ventilation [46]. The equilibrium image rarely demonstrates abnormalities not observed by the single breath or wash-out images. The wash-out phase of the study is performed by letting the patient breathe room-air and exhale the xenon gas while serial images are obtained at 30–60 second intervals for up to 6 minutes. In healthy individuals, wash-out is uniform and is complete within 3 minutes (Fig. 2). Areas of slow wash-out indicate the presence of airways obstruction (Fig. 3). Right and left posterior oblique wash-out

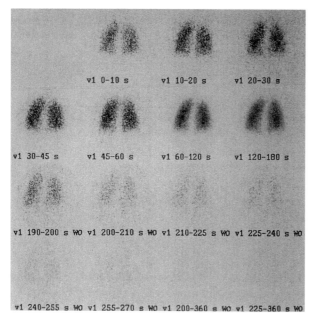

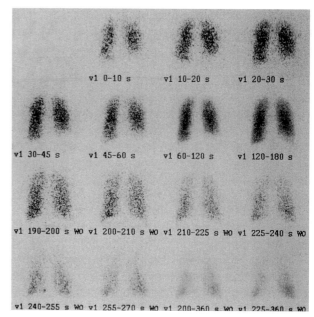

Fig. 2. Normal posterior Xenon-133 ventilation images. The first six images comprise the wash-in period from 0 to 120 seconds. The 120-180 second view represents the equilibration image. From 190 seconds, the washout phase commences. The lung uptake is symmetrical in the wash-in images followed by a symmetrical washout that is completed by 240 seconds.

Fig. 3. Abnormal posterior Xenon-133 ventilation images. The first six images comprise the wash-in period from 0 – 120 seconds and show reduced wash-in at the right base. The 120 – 180 second equilibration view shows that some ventilation has occurred at the right base. From 190 seconds, the washout phase shows persistent Xenon retention at both bases but particularly the right, a finding consistent with focal obstructive airways disease.

views may be obtained during the fourth and fifth minutes of wash-out to improve localisation of xenon retention.

Ventilation studies which rely on the single-breath manoeuvre are less sensitive to milder degrees of localised airways obstruction and have a reduced specificity compared to the multi-breath method [47]. Abnormalities identified on the delayed wash-out images are useful in detecting those ventilation abnormalities associated with non-segmental perfusion defects [48]. The wash-out phase is the most sensitive portion of the study being nearly twice as sensitive as the chest radiograph and at least comparable in sensitivity to pulmonary function testing [49]. The low photon energy of ^{133}Xe dictates the timing of the ventilation scans in relation to the perfusion scan. Compton scatter of ^{99m}Tc photons appear in the ^{133}Xe energy window and significantly degrade the ventilation images [50]. The higher energy ^{127}Xe does allow pre-ventilation perfusion scans, thus permitting the ventilation studies to be tailored to the perfusion findings or avoided altogether if the perfusion study is normal. The low photon energy of ^{133}Xe means that the absorbed dose of radiation from a ventilation study is relatively low. Doses of 220, 28 and 25 mrad to the lungs, whole body and gonads have been calculated for a 740 MBq inhaled dose [51]. The trachea bears the main burden of

radiation exposure, which takes place largely during the first 2 minutes of the study [52].

Because of the long physical half-life of radioactive xenon, radiation safety and tracer disposal must be carefully considered. Exhaled gas from the patient must be passed through a charcoal trapping mechanism or vented into the atmosphere. Escape of gas takes place through tubing connections or from accidental release round the mouthpiece. Because xenon is a heavy gas, it will descend to floor level and diffuses rapidly. The escape of xenon and its long half-life limits the number of xenon studies, which can be performed each year in a department. The use of ^{127}Xe requires more intensive disposal measures than for ^{133}Xe.

Krypton-81m

Krypton-81m (^{81m}Kr) is a radioactive inert gas, which decays to ^{81}Kr by isomeric transition with a half-life of 13 seconds. It emits 190 keV gamma rays (65 %) and 176 and 188 keV internal conversion electrons (35 %). Its parent, 81 rubidium, is cyclotron-produced and decays by electron capture (87 %) and positron emission (13 %) with a half-life of 4.7 hours.

The technique for the administration of krypton in ventilation imaging was first described in 1977

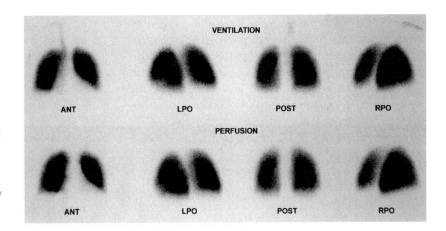

Fig. 4. Normal 4-view Krypton-81m ventilation (lower) and MAA perfusion (upper) scan. The sequential acquisition of ventilation followed by perfusion images without patient movement provides excellent correspondence between the projections of ventilation and perfusion (Courtesy of Dr. Andrew J. Hilson, Royal Free Hospital, London, United Kingdom).

[53] and rubidium generators became commercially available in 1980. [81m]Kr is eluted continuously from the rubidium source using oxygen at a flow rate of 3 litres per minute. The gas is temporarily held in a reservoir to which the patient is connected via a one-way valve and face mask. The patient breathes at normal tidal volumes while images are acquired using a high resolution, low-energy parallel-hole collimator. Images containing 100,000 to 400,000 counts each are acquired on a 128×128 matrix in multiple projections while the patient breathes the gas mixed with oxygen at flow rates of 3 litres per minute. The exhaled gases are vented via a one-way valve away from the camera head. The use of an electronic fan ensures that stray gas is blown away from the camera head.

[81m]Kr has numerous advantages over radioactive xenon for ventilation imaging [54]. The 190 keV photopeak produces superior quality images with improved spatial resolution due to increased scatter rejection, higher tissue penetration, and greater energy transfer to the sodium-iodide crystal. Because the gamma energy of [81m]Kr is higher than that of ^{99m}Tc, ventilation images may be obtained concurrently with or immediately following the perfusion scan. Simultaneous acquisition allows precise superimposition of the ventilation and perfusion images in multiple projections and reduces imaging times. Post-perfusion ventilation scans may be omitted if the perfusion scan is normal. The ultra-short half-life obviates the need for disposal precautions and reduces the hazard of airborne contamination of nuclear medicine personnel and the environment. It also means that krypton images are free of background uptake from the thoracic blood pool. Krypton ventilation imaging is technically easy to perform, is well tolerated by the patients, and is applicable to children and patients who are mechanically ventilated.

Although krypton is regarded by many as the gold standard for ventilation imaging, there are some drawbacks to its use for ventilation imaging in PE diagnosis. The generators are expensive, last only one day, and are not available on weekends or holidays. Availability is dependent on proximity to a cyclotron. The high tissue penetration results in loss of the normal anatomical landmarks witnessed on the perfusion images. Care must be exercised not to mistake the anatomical landmarks as perfusion defects. Care must also be taken when using simultaneous acquisition protocols. Two energy windows are switched back and forth during the ventilation and perfusion acquisition so there is the possibility of cross talk between technetium and krypton energy windows. As many as 40% of photons in the technetium window may be derived from krypton. This effect is particularly noticeable in older camera systems and where generator activities are greater than 300 MBq [55].

The krypton images reflect a balance between regional ventilation and radioactive decay and are comparable to the radioactive xenon single-breath images (Fig. 4). Areas of decreased ventilation appear as defects on the krypton images. [81m]Kr compliments the perfusion study better than xenon in patients with PE [56] although its short half-life precludes equilibrium and wash-out studies and ^{133}Xe has been shown to be more sensitive at detecting abnormalities of regional ventilation in patients with obstructive or parenchymal lung disease [56].

Aerosols

Aerosols are suspensions of fine particles which are small enough to remain airborne for a period of time. The aerodynamic properties of aerosols govern their interactions with matter and are determined by the size, shape and density of their constituent particles. These properties are difficult to predict but may be measured and expressed as an aerodynamic equivalent diameter. The mass median aerodynamic diameter (MMAD) describes the median diameter of particles above and below which 50 % of the mass of solute is contained. The dispersion of particles is described by geometric standard deviation (monodisperse particles have a value of < 1.2).

Aerosol particles may be removed from inhaled air by inertial and gravitational forces. Impaction occurs due to changes in airflow direction at high speed, such as at the bifurcation of large airways. Interception occurs when the aerosol makes contact by chance with the bronchial wall. Sedimentation of airway particles is the result of settlement due to gravity and occurs in the smaller airways and alveolar spaces. Diffusion describes the natural entropic tendency of particles to drift randomly within the suspended medium resulting in chance contact with the respiratory membranes. The chances of aerosol deposition are enhanced by hygroscopic growth and coalescence of particles and by electrostatic forces [57]. The size of aerosol particles critically affects their deposition in the respiratory tract. Large particles (above 5 μm MMAD) are removed by impaction in the upper respiratory tract (nasopharynx, oropharynx, trachea and larger bronchi). Particles in the size range 1 – 5 μm are deposited in the lower respiratory tract whereas ultrafine particles (less than 1 μm MMAD) exhibit virtually no tracheobronchial deposition and penetrate to the alveolar compartment [58], although only a small fraction of the particles are retained (< 16 %). For these reasons, submicronic particles are regarded as optimal for assessing regional ventilation. The deposition of aerosols is influenced by the rate and pattern of breathing. Deposition is enhanced by slower tidal breathing and by breath-holding [59]. The pattern of aerosol deposition is influenced by airways obstruction and cough [60].

While the use of radiolabelled aerosols was advocated from 1965 [61, 62], the introduction of aerosols for ventilation imaging was delayed until development in nebuliser technology in the early 1980's [63]. Both jet and ultrasound nebuliser systems are used in clinical practice although for regional ventilation imaging the jet nebuliser is more frequently used. The jet nebuliser is based on the Bernouilli principle. Gas is passed under pressure through a small hole known as a Venturi and the resultant fall in pressure produces atomisation of the liquid in the feeding tube. Larger particles are removed by baffles placed in the path of the jet. The design and geometry of the jet nebuliser influ-

ences the characteristics of the particles produced. Driven by compressed air or oxygen at standard flow rates of 8 litres/minute, commercially available jet nebulisers reliably produce aerosols with 95 % of the particles less than 1 μm in diameter.

With the introduction of reliable, inexpensive and disposable jet nebulisers, the popularity for regional ventilation studies grew and by the late 1980's in the United Kingdom, almost 60 % of such studies were carried out using radiolabelled aerosols [64].

Various solutes have been employed including sulphur colloid, diethylene triaminepentaacetate (DTPA) and human serum albumin [65] with ^{99m}Tc-DTPA the most frequently used [64]. Ventilation studies using aerosols of ^{99m}Tc-DTPA are normally carried out in a separate room within Nuclear Medicine departments, preferably fitted with negative pressure or other venting facilities. The nebuliser unit is housed in a lead-lined container and charged with 5 milligrams of sodium-DTPA labelled with between 740 to 1110 MBq of ^{99m}Tc in 2 ml of saline. The patient is fitted with a nose clip and is connected to the nebuliser unit via a plastic tube and mouthpiece. The gas supply is turned on and the patient is told to breathe at normal tidal breathing for 3 minutes. If the patient has difficulty, the procedure can be interrupted and then continued for the required time of 3 minutes. The efficiency of the system is low and less than 1 % of the aerosol is retained by the lung. The exhaled aerosol is trapped in a bacteriologic filter. Images are acquired in multiple projections with a large field-of-view gamma camera fitted with a high-resolution, low-energy collimator. Images of 50,000 to 100,000 counts can be acquired in about 100 seconds. ^{99m}Tc-DTPA aerosol studies are technically simple to perform and can be performed in children and by use of appropriate adapters in intubated patients. Following an aerosol ventilation study, breast feeding need not be interrupted for more than 4 hours after the test [66].

The quality of the images obtained with ^{99m}Tc-DTPA aerosol is good [63] and reliably demonstrate areas of regional hypoventilation [65]. Sequential imaging using radiogas and radioaerosol studies in patients with suspected PE [63] showed good agreement in the majority of cases (86 % with xenon and 80 % with krypton-81). Central deposition of the aerosol may confound interpretation of the study and is particularly problematic in patients with severe major airways narrowing. In one study, 6 % of the ventilation studies could not be interpreted [63]. One other disadvantage of radio-labelled aerosols is that there is airborne radioactive contamination which increases with the degree of breathing difficulty. Surface contamination has been shown to exceed maximal permitted levels and the use of protective clothing has been advocated for nuclear medicine personnel [67].

One issue which has not been satisfactorily resolved is whether nebuliser circuits should be for single or multiple use. Ventilation scans using radio-labelled aerosol are inexpensive and the cost largely relates to the policy of single versus re-use of nebuliser circuits. In determining policy of re-use of nebuliser circuits, the risks of the additional radiation hazard compared with the risk of transfer of infection must be balanced [68]. Re-use of nebuliser circuits is widely practised, but has been called into question [68].

Technegas

A new radiopharmaceutical for ventilation scintigraphy was reported by Burch and colleagues in 1986 [69]. This radiopharmaceutical, called 'Technegas', is an ultrafine dispersion of ^{99m}Tc-labelled carbon particles produced in a Technegas generator. The generator is a compact, commercially available microprocessor-controlled unit which consists of a lead-shielded 7 litre chamber above two electrodes between which a graphite crucible is inserted via a drawer in front of the device. Technegas is produced by first wetting the crucible with alcohol followed by the placement of 250–400 MBq of ^{99m}Tc-sodium-pertechnetate in a volume of 0.1 ml saline. Closing the drawer initiates a simmer for 6 minutes during which the liquid within the crucible evaporates. When ready to perform the ventilation study, the crucible is heated to 2,500 °C in an atmosphere of 100 % argon. Once generated, the Technegas can be used for up to 10 minutes. The Technegas particles have a structure similar to the Buckminsterfullerine molecule in which ^{99m}Tc atoms are trapped [70]. The actual size of Technegas particles is not firmly established although a figure of less than 200 nm is generally accepted [71]. From these measurements it has been estimated that approximately 20 % of the inhaled Technegas will deposit in the alveolar compartments with only 5 % in the upper airways.

The inhalation of Technegas requires patient co-operation: lung deposition of Technegas is enhanced by slow-inhalation and by breath-holding [72]. The patient is positioned in front of the gamma camera as for a posterior lung view and fitted with noseclips and a disposable delivery set consisting of a mouthpiece, a filter, two one-way valve and a 1 metre length of tubing which is attached to the generator outlet port. By depressing or releasing the plunger on top of the generator unit, the operator determines whether the patient breathes Technegas or room air respectively. When ready, the patient is asked to take a long, slow, deep inhalation of Technegas from FRC to TLC and then to hold their breath for 5 seconds before expiration and a return to breathing room air. The count rate is monitored during inhalation and the manoeuvre repeated as necessary until a count rate of 1,600 counts/second is reached. This results in a deposited activity of 20 MBq and a ventilation:perfusion ratio of 1 : 5 (assuming 100 MBq of ^{99m}Tc-MAA is administered for the perfusion study). On average patients require 4 breaths (range 1 – 12) to achieve the desired count rate. A minority of patients cannot achieve sufficient counts and acquisition times have to be extended. On occasions, the patient may exceed the target count rate in which case the dose of ^{99m}Tc-MAA will have to be increased or the perfusion study delayed.

The resultant images are of excellent technical quality and permit planar images in multiple projections (Fig. 1). As with radioaerosol studies, Technegas images may contain areas of excess particle deposition in the proximal airways. These 'hot spots' are more commonly seen in chronic obstructive airways disease and their presence correlates with the degree of lung function abnormality [73]. Comparisons of Technegas with ^{133}Xe [74] and ^{81m}Kr [75] have shown a high degree of concordance in patients with suspected PE although concern has been expressed that Technegas may lead to false-positive diagnoses of PE [76].

Inhalation of Technegas (Argon) is associated with transient falls in oxygen saturation [77] and monitoring of pulse oximetry with pre-scan administration of supplemental oxygen is recommended for patients known to have significant cardiorespiratory disease. Despite these falls, in practice there have been no published reports of serious adverse reactions following Technegas administration since its introduction in 1986. While the short-term safety is known, the long-term effects of inhaling fine carbon particles beyond the mucociliary escalator remains to be established. The fate of inhaled carbon particles is at present unknown. However, the total mass of graphite inhaled into the lungs during a Technegas ventilation study is 50 µg which is considerably less than is normally inhaled from the urban air over several hours [78].

Uncertainty in pulmonary embolism diagnosis

L. B. Lusted has quoted [79] Sir George W. Pickering as writing "Diagnosis is a matter of probability, as those of us who follow the fate of our patients into the post-mortem room know only too well. Prognosis is a matter of probability and, in judging treatment, we have to base our judgement on knowledge of probabilities". Many physicians struggle with the use of any concept of probability in clinical medicine because of the statistical connotation with a population frequency and the need to apply this relative population frequency to a single patient. Some feel that probabilities are guesses and not real numbers while others feel that not only does decision analysis take the art out of clinical medicine but that reducing the patient's problem to numbers somehow dehumanises patient care [80].

A mathematical representation of uncertainty is not the only stumbling block for physicians in the area of medical decision making. The requirement for accurate clinical information to enable test interpretation is another area of intense debate. Yet the facts speak for themselves. Provided only with thyroid function tests revealing a total thyroxine of 170 mmol/l (range 55–144) and a TSH of < 0.2 mmol/l (range 0.35–5), most physicians would include both hyperthyroidism and thyroxine replacement in their differential diagnosis. However, the clinical history that the patient was euthyroid on thyroxine following post-^{131}I hypothyroidism permits accurate interpretation of the thyroid function tests. Again, provided only with a set of normal electrolytes including a serum urea of 7 mmol (range 2.5–8) and creatinine of 118 micromol/litre (range 40–130), most physicians would note that the urea and creatinine are at the upper end of normal. If the patient had been 75 years old, the result would have been truly normal. On the other hand, in a 23 year old woman with a history of type 1 diabetes mellitus, it indicates the presence of mild renal failure since in that age group, 99 % of healthy subjects have a serum urea of <6.5 mmol and a serum creatinine of < 105 micromol/litre.

It is now recognised that tests, whether biochemical, pathological or imaging related, can only properly be interpreted for a particular disease given a complete knowledge of the pre-test probability of that disease. Further, parameters of test efficiency such as sensitivity and specificity for various diseases are also essential ingredients of test interpretation.

In summary, the interpretation of a VQ scan or any new information on a patient depends upon what one believes about the patient beforehand.

Which Test?

There is a hierarchy of tests for PE which increase in specificity from chest X-ray, blood gases, D-dimer measurement and heart echocardiography, through VQ imaging to spiral computed tomography (CTPA), MR angiography and finally to pulmonary angiography. It is appropriate in this text to consider the characteristics of VQ imaging and pulmonary angiography as they are used for PE diagnosis.

In an ideal world, a test for PE would provide a binary answer for the clinician, PE or no PE. In the real world, test results carry with them varying degrees of uncertainty. Not only do we find true positive (TP) results in patients with disease but also false positive (FP) results in those without disease. Unfortunately, as we increase the TP rate of diagnosis, the FP rate also increases. Similarly, we find true negative (TN) results in those without disease and false negative (FN) results in those with disease. Again, as we increase the number of TN cases, the FN rate also increases. The sensitivity or true positive rate is the proportion of people with PE who have a positive test result (i. e. a high probability or HP scan). The specificity or true negative rate is the proportion of people free of PE who have a negative test result (i. e. a normal, very low probability (VLP) or low probability (LP) scan). These two indices of VQ scan performance (i. e. sensitivity and specificity) give us insight into the characteristics of the ideal test for PE.

Myocardial infarction and primary hypothyroidism are serious diseases if undiagnosed but have safe and effective treatments, aspirin and thyroxine. Not wishing to miss a case, the physician employs a highly sensitive test to detect all patients with the disease. Patients without the disease have false positive results and are therefore included in the trawl. These falsely positive cases will be treated but this disadvantage is acceptable given the simple nature of the treatment. The overriding priority for a serious disease is accurate diagnosis and treatment of all patients with the disease.

A prolactinoma is a simple pituitary tumour. It is not a serious disease but requires an invasive and potentially hazardous treatment (pituitary microsurgery). The physician wants to be absolutely sure of his diagnosis before advising surgery. He will therefore employ a highly specific test to eliminate all possible false positive results. He will be unconcerned that borderline cases are undiagnosed by this strategy because the overriding priority is to operate only on patients with the disease.

Unfortunately, PE is a serious condition with a relatively dangerous long-term treatment. The attending physician requires a sensitive test which will easily pick up the majority of patients with PE. However, the test must also be specific enough to ensure that as few normal patients as possible have false positive results and are therefore given long term anticoagulants. Only the 'gold standard' test, pulmonary angiography has been shown to approach this goal in sensitivity and specificity but the test is expensive of time and manpower and carries a finite risk. Spiral CT is less invasive and the relative sensitivity and specificity may well approach pulmonary angiography but again the test is resource weighted. While test characteristics such as sensitivity and specificity will remain crucial factors in the selection of any test, cost-effectiveness is playing an increasingly dominant role.

VQ imaging is widely used as a primary screening test for PE. PIOPED [42] revealed a HP scan sensitivity of 46% and a false positive rate of 13%. If both the HP and intermediate categories were considered a positive result, the sensitivity for PE would reach 83% but the false positive rate would rise to 48%. The hazards of long-term anticoagulation make the treatment of so many patients without PE unacceptable. For diagnosis of PE with VQ scanning therefore, the HP scan with its reduced sensitivity must be accepted as the only positive test result and a strategy agreed for optimum detection of the remaining PE patients using other non-invasive tests such as D-dimer or ultrasound examination of the legs. For some patients, the more invasive tests with greater sensitivity and specificity will be necessary.

In PIOPED, the specificity of the normal and low probability lung scans were 100% and 86% respectively. Clearly, 14% of cases with a low probability scan had PE although most of these were in the medium and high clinical pre-test groups. This false negative rate is unacceptable to clinicians [81–83] who are mindful of the dangers of untreated PE. It is clear that acceptance of VQ imaging for PE exclusion will be achieved only if the specificity of the 'negative result' categories is below 10% which is about the level of uncertainty of a negative pulmonary angiogram [42]. This < 10% standard can only be achieved if consid-

erable numbers of PIOPED's low probability VQ scan criteria are re-graded as non-diagnostic [84]. The patients in those categories with extra risk of PE would require a different more specific test.

Pre-test probability and intuition

Intuition is a matter of opinion about a set of symptoms or a test result on a single patient which enables the estimation of the probability of disease [85]. The physician is exposed to two principal factors which influence the development of intuition, namely personal experience and the published literature.

Using personal experience, a physician recalls patients with similar characteristics to the patient in question and attempts to recall how many had the disease. In cognitive terms, this is difficult and it may simply end up as informed guesswork. The cognitive principles or processes for estimating the probability of disease from any combination of symptoms, signs or test results are called 'heuristics' [86]. Using the 'representativeness heuristic', a clinician believes that the patient has the disease if he/she looks like a typical case, or the test result looks typical. This representativeness heuristic can be misleading because it can lead the physician into ignoring the overall prevalence of PE (pre-test probability) in the population from which the patient is drawn. Thus, a previously well patient at home who develops sudden dyspnea, hypoxia and tachypnea might well be thought to have developed PE. In reality, PE is quite unlikely. Sudden dyspnoea and hypoxia are known to be poor predictors of PE even in hospital populations [87] but the physician can still be led to overestimate the clinical likelihood of the disease. This judgmental error will usually occur only if the physician is young, his understanding of PE is incomplete or his personal experience is atypical and based on hospital cases.

Using 'availability heuristics' a clinician assesses the probability of disease by the ease with which similar events are remembered. An easily remembered event is thought to have a higher probability than one which is difficult to recall. Since recent cases are to the forefront, even though they may be atypical, this heuristic too can be misleading.

Despite an erroneous starting point, clinicians using representativeness or availability heuristics may correct the initial probability estimate of disease (the anchor) to take account of unusual features or various test results for the patient. This 'anchoring and adjustment heuristic' is crucial since it permits revision of initial probabilities on the basis of new information such as a lung scan or Doppler venogram result. Bayes' theorem permits a quantitative combination of evidence in this way but reasonably accurate quantitative data is required to make the task worthwhile.

Medical literature provides reports of PE prevalence in different clinical populations [42, 88]. The clinician can use these, and his own research, as a starting point which will then be modified to take into account other clinical findings or new test results. Regrettably, most published series have shortcomings. While the reports highlight the prevalence of a symptom, sign or test result in patients with a particular disease thereby providing the probability of the finding, there is usually no report of its prevalence in patients without the disease. Neither do most series report upon the prevalence of various other disorders in patients with the same clinical finding or test result. Before performing the test for PE, the 'anchor point' for estimating the pre-test likelihood of disease is the estimate of prevalence of PE in that population of new patients. Most studies of the clinical presentation of PE will report only on the prevalence of a feature, say chest pain, in PE and not on the frequency of PE given that symptom. This frequently can only be guessed at from the literature because 'gold standard tests' are rarely done in patients with scant evidence of disease. In fact, the estimation of PE prevalence in your local population can be learned only by clinical experience and by auditing previous cases.

Mathematical representation of uncertainty

A physician's language usually indicates the level of uncertainty which he is experiencing. A disease 'may' be present, is 'possibly' present, is 'likely' to be present, or there is varying degrees of 'probability' of disease. Unfortunately, words cloud the clear expression of degrees of uncertainty [89] because they fail to describe precisely how to adjust a belief in the possibility of a particular diagnosis [85]. It is also clear from clinical experience and published accounts [90] that not only do different physicians choose different words to represent the same judgement on the likelihood of a diagnosis but they also may use the same words to express different judgements.

The use of an estimate of probability eliminates ambiguity in the communication of uncertainty. Probability (P) is a number that expresses an opinion about the likelihood of an event. The extreme values of P are 1, the probability of an event that is certain to occur and 0, the probability of an event that is certain never to occur. Clearly, the probability that an event will occur plus the probability that the event will not occur will always add up to 1.

Uncertainty can also be expressed as odds. Odds are equivalent to probability and are provided by two numbers which express the judgement in PE diagnosis that 'for every time PE is present, how often is it not present'. The odds format is the ratio of the likelihood of PE occurring against the likelihood of PE not occurring. For example, odds of 9 : 1 for PE indicate that for every nine occasions when PE occurs, there is one occasion when it is absent. Odds and probability are closely related. If the probability of PE being present is P, then the probability of PE being absent is $(1-P)$. Hence

$$Odds = P/(1-P)$$

which may be rearranged to convert odds back to probability

$$P = Odds/(1 + Odds)$$

Communication between physicians will be more accurate if the traditional descriptive report using its potentially ambiguous terminology is supplemented by an expression of probability [90–92] or odds. This policy should improve the flow of information and opinion from scan reviewer to attending physician.

Post-test probability

The post-test probability of PE is the probability/likelihood/risk of PE after learning the result of the VQ scan. It is important to note that it depends not only upon the pre-test estimate of probability of PE based on clinical data but also the sensitivity and specificity of the test [93] and can be calculated by several equivalent methods [94, 95] including Bayes' theorem.

Table 1 represents data from PIOPED modified to highlight the normal and very low categories and to increase the specificity of the low probability category [84]. The probability of PE in the whole population P(PE) is $252/887 = 0.28$. The probability of a high probability (HP) scan in the whole population is P(HP) is $118/887 = 0.13$. This is also an unconditional probability. If a HP scan is found, the probability that the patient has PE is $103/118 = 0.87$. This is a conditional probability and is written P(PE / HP), the probability of PE given that the scan is HP. In the notation, the upstroke ' I ' denotes 'given'. The inverse to P(PE / HP) is P(HP / PE), the probability of a HP scan given the presence of PE. In this case, HP is regarded as the diagnosis. From Table 1, P(HP / PE) = $103/252 = 0.41$.

Bayes' theorem permits the calculation of the posterior probability of PE following an HP scan {P(PE / HP)} by employing the two unconditional probabilities P(PE) and P(HP) and the conditional probability P(HP / PE).

The theorem states that the probability of PE given the HP scan result equals the probability of the HP scan result from patients with PE divided by the total probability of the HP scan result in the population.

Written:

P(PE / HP) = P(HP / PE) x P(PE) / P(HP)

Inserting values from Table 1

P(PE / HP) = 0.41 X 0.28 / 0.13 = 0.87 which is correct

Bayes' theorem may be expressed in a form using odds in which the post-test odds can be calculated more simply. The pre-test probability must be converted to pre-test odds before use. The discriminating power of VQ scanning to distinguish PE from no PE is expressed by the Likelihood Ratio (LR). The Likelihood Ratio is a measure of how much each category of VQ scan alters the probability of disease.

The Likelihood Ratio for a positive test LR(+) is given by:

$$LR(+) = \frac{\text{Probability of a positive result in pts with PE}}{\text{Probability of a positive result in pts without PE.}}$$

The Likelihood Ratio for a negative test LR(–) is given by:

$$LR((-) = \frac{\text{Probability of a negative result in pts without PE}}{\text{Probability of a negative result in pts with PE}}$$

The calculation of the LR's for each category of lung scan is shown in Table 1. The 'normal' category excludes PE virtually completely and so the LR is zero. A test result with a LR greater than 1.0 raises the probability of disease and is referred to as a positive result. A test result with an LR of less than 1.0 lowers the probability of disease and is called a negative result.

The odds form of Bayes' theorem is:

Post-test odds after test = Pre-test clinical odds x LR of test result

In the previous example, the pre-test probability of PE was 0.28. This gives pre-test odds of 0.28 / 1 – 0.28 = 0.39 or more correctly, 0.39 : 1.

The LR of a HP scan is 17 and so the post-test odds of PE after a HP scan are

Post-test odds = 0.39 X 17 = 6.63

Odds of 6.63 : 1 for PE are equivalent to a probability of 6.63/7.63 = 0.87 as calculated before by the other method.

Bayes' theorem is crucial for interpretation of a VQ result because it defines absolutely the relationship between the pre-test probability of PE (what is known of the clinical likelihood), each lung scan category and the post-test probability (how the pre-test probability changed with the new evidence from the test). Consequently, a test result cannot be properly interpreted unless there is knowledge about the patient before the test was performed.

Figure 5 shows the conditional probability curves for high (HP), intermediate, low (LP) and very low probability (VLP) scan categories obtained from the modified PIOPED data [84]. Each curve has been determined using Bayes' theorem to calculate the post-test probability for each value of pre-test probability and incorporating the appropriate

Table 1. Calculation of likelihood ratios for lung scan categories from realigned PIOPED data [84].

		Pulmonary Embolism				
		Present		Absent		
		Number	Proportion	Number	Proportion	L Ratio
Lung	HP	103	103/252 = 0.41	15	15/635 = 0.024	0.41/.024 = 17
Scan	Indet	125	125/252 = 0.496	307	307/635 = 0.48	0.496/.48 = 1.0
Result	LP	19	19/252 = 0.075	190	190/635 = 0.3	0.075/0.3 = 0.25
	Very LP	5	5/252 = 0.02	102	102/635 = 0.16	0.02/0.16 = 0.125
	Normal	0	0	21	21/635 = 0.033	0
		252		635		

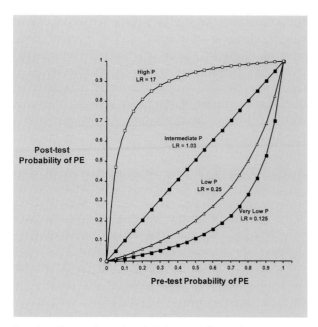

Fig. 5. The conditional probability graph for PE diagnosis is constructed using the likelihood ratios (LR) calculated from the realigned PIOPED data in Table 1. The graph combines the clinical pre-test probability of PE and the VQ categories into post-test probabilities of PE.

LR's for each scan category. It can be seen that after a HP result (+ve), the post-test probability of PE increases rapidly as the pre-test probability increases, most uncertainty occurring at the low clinical pre-test likelihood. Conversely, the post-test probability of PE for the very low and low probability scans falls rapidly as the pre-test probability falls. Sox [85] said that 'the interpretation of new information depends upon what was already known about the patient'. PIOPED confirmed this by finding the frequency of PE in a HP scan with a low pre-test clinical probability to be 56%. Such

patients without acute PE usually had unresolved changes from previous PE. When either PE or no PE is nearly certain prior to VQ scanning, a confirmatory scan has little real effect on the post-test probability of disease. A quite discordant result, however, alerts the physician to embark on further more specific testing. Only a normal scan excludes PE at any pre-test clinical likelihood.

The post-test probability from the indeterminate scan (non-diagnostic) also depends upon the pre-test probability but these two probabilities, pre and post-test, are approximately equal creating a 45° line. This line of identity represents a VQ result which does not change the probability of PE at all for the clinician.

The post-test probability for the LP and VLP decrease as the pre-test probability. The vertical distance upward from these curves to the 45° line represents the degree of change occurring from the pre- to the post-test probability after the scan result. The change is potentially maximal around a medium pre-test clinical probability (P = 0.3) where the physicians are most uncertain. It can be seen that a LP scan (LR = 0.25) easily provides a clinically acceptable low frequency of PE (2–3%) at a low clinical pre-test probability (P = 0.1) but fails to provide it (10%) at a medium pre-test (P = 0.3). The very low probability scan with a lower LR is required for PE exclusion (5%) when the clinical pre-test is medium.

In summary, a high or low probability scan result in itself is unhelpful since each category represents wide overlapping ranges of PE probability depending upon the pre-test clinical probability. Combining each scan result with the pre-test clinical probability provides a more accurate and more closely defined post-test probability of PE.

Development of categorical criteria for PE diagnosis

Early in the development of pulmonary nuclear medicine, the urokinase PE trial (UPET) [96] established the high sensitivity of perfusion ('Q' for the German 'quellen'– to flow) imaging for PE and, more importantly, the non-specificity of the abnormal perfusion scan. The study also demonstrated the uncertainties in clinical diagnosis of PE, highlighting the need for an accurate objective test. Ventilation imaging (V) was introduced [97] to improve the specificity of perfusion imaging and thereafter VQ scanning became widely adopted as the primary screening test for PE.

McNeil et al. [43, 98, 99] reported the first studies correlating VQ imaging with pulmonary angiography (PA). In a small series, they developed a basic strategy for VQ scan interpretation and introduced the concept of decision analysis. Likelihood ratios for lung scan categories were combined with the clinical presentation to provide the post-test probabilities of PE. These workers confirmed the usefulness of ventilation imaging, but their own post-perfusion ventilation technique with Xenon-133 was never widely accepted.

The Biello Criteria

In the 1970's, developments in pulmonary angiography lead to improvements in the sensitivity of this technique. In 1979, the Washington University group published their criteria for VQ analysis [100] based on a retrospective analysis of 146 highly selected patients who underwent VQ scanning, chest radiography and pulmonary angiography for suspected PE. This important work was to become a working standard for clinical VQ analysis and the criteria were called after the late Daniel Biello (see Table 2).

All 146 patients had abnormal Q scans and of these, 53 had PE (36%) by pulmonary angiography. The group found no evidence of PE in either matched (1 case) or mismatched small subsegmental defects (19 cases). Among 26 patients with matched VQ abnormalities (CXR normal), PE was present in 1 of 21 (5%) with focal matching and in 1 of 5 (20%) with severe diffuse parenchymal lung disease. One patient out of 3 with a single mismatched moderate defect (33%) had PE. In 26 patients with at least 2 moderate mismatched defects or one large mismatch, 25 (92%) had PE. Seventy-two patients had perfusion and radiographic abnormalities confined to the same regions. In 13 patients, the perfusion defect was substantially smaller than the X-ray abnormality and PE was found in 1 case (8%). In 15 patients, the perfusion defects were substantially larger than the X-ray abnormality and PE was found in 13 cases (87%). In 44 patients, the perfusion defects were equal in size to the X-ray abnormality and PE was found in 12 cases (27%).

The Biello criteria were widely used for correlation of pulmonary angiography and VQ imaging in the many retrospective series which followed [101–106]. The clinical value of VQ imaging using these criteria was confirmed and improved upon. For example, the criterion for high probability was modified to 2 or more moderate or large mismatches, the criterion for intermediate to require the extent of COPD to be greater or equal to 50% of lung zones, and the criterion for focal matches to be limited to less than or equal to 50% of the lung zones. Formal evaluation of the scheme with improvements showed better interobserver consistency and a 30% reduction in the number of intermediate studies [101]. However, such attempts to reduce the number of intermediate studies [107], particularly when the chest radiograph was abnormal, was viewed with suspicion by internists since potentially it had the effect of reducing the specificity of the low probability scan category [82].

The McMaster study

The first major prospective study of VQ imaging compared to PA was provided by the McMaster group in Canada [108–110]. They performed a great service to the nuclear medicine community by redirecting attention to the source of the venous thromboembolism in the legs and the importance of venous thrombus detection in the diagnosis and treatment of PE. Unsurprisingly, they found PE in 86% of cases with a high probability lung scan. Surprisingly, they claimed that at least 25% of cases with matched abnormalities or small subsegmental abnormalities had PE. Needless to say, this work has been the subject of debate for many years. Several factors probably account for the

---

Table 2. The Biello criteria for VQ scan analysis [100].

High probability
One or more large, or two or more moderate sized VQ mismatches with no corresponding radiographic abnormalities
Perfusion defects substantially larger than radiographic abnormalities

Intermediate probability
Diffuse, severe airway obstruction
Matched perfusion defects and radiographic abnormalities (Q = CXR)
Single moderate VQ mismatch without corresponding radiographic abnormality

Low probability
Small VQ mismatches
Focal VQ matches with no corresponding radiographic abnormalities
Perfusion defects substantially smaller than corresponding radiographic abnormalities

Normal
Normal perfusion

major differences from the previous work. Firstly, it is suspected that the patients were more highly selected than was thought by the authors. Not only did they all have plethysmography before entering the trial but the overall post-test prevalence of PE of 50% is much higher than one would find even in a tertiary referral hospital [111, 88]. For the outside observer, their unique method of categorical analysis of scans which did not follow Biello lines made comparison with other studies difficult. The emergence of the PIOPED data from the second and larger multicentre trial [42] did not confirm the McMaster group's finding in the low probability scan category and therefore their approach has not been widely used up-till-now as a basis for nuclear medicine practice.

The PIOPED Study

The controversy surrounding the clinical value of VQ imaging was addressed boldly by the National Heart, Lung and Blood Institute at the National Institutes of Health. At breathtaking financial cost, they sponsored the most ambitious and best designed multicentre trial of VQ imaging compared to pulmonary angiography in the diagnosis of PE. Known as the Prospective Investigation of Pulmonary Embolism Diagnosis (PIOPED), the goal was a prospective analysis of both VQ scanning and pulmonary angiography using state-of-the-art equipment [42]. Incorporation of follow-up data from some cases with minor VQ abnormalities who did not proceed to angiography permitted the investigators to reduce the clear selection bias towards disease which had also been prevalent within previous retrospective series. The objective reference categories for VQ scan analysis were selected as a 'best-guess' and were different in some respects from the Biello approach. For instance, a PIOPED high probability scan required two mismatched segmental equivalents [112] compared to Biello. Unfortunately, PIOPED's low probability category included a single moderate mismatch. This was really the only categorical error. The Investigators included a very low probability category of less than 3 small subsegments (< 25% segment) but did not exploit this category in the final analysis. They proposed instead a near normal/normal category for cases where disagreement between the central readers occurred as to a low, very low or normal scan.

With hindsight, the study was deficient in only two areas. Firstly, a more objective approach to the diagnosis of venous thrombosis would have permitted a more accurate and realistic pre-test clinical assessment. Secondly, xenon-133 ventilation technology, though state-of-the-art at the time, did reduce the resolution of ventilation abnormality detection and limited the total number of abnormalities seen.

PIOPED relied upon independent interpretation of the VQ and pulmonary angiography studies by two blinded central readers. A third reader was brought in upon disagreement. Agreement for VQ interpretation was 90% for high probability and normal/near normal scans but only 70 to 75% between intermediate and low probability. This was clearly a great disappointment given the experience, training and motivation of the team of investigators. Agreement with pulmonary angiography was better with 92% agreement for PE but only 83–89% for no-PE or PE uncertain. Surprisingly, the exclusion of PE by the gold standard had a degree of uncertainty in 11–17% of cases.

In many respects, the results of PIOPED validated and upgraded the underlying principles proposed by Biello and the authors of the retrospective series and countered the more pessimistic predictions of the McMaster group. The PIOPED population was selected in the sense that far fewer patients with normal, near-normal and low probability scans proceeded as planned to pulmonary angiography compared with indeterminate and high probability scans. The 33% prevalence of PE in the whole population was almost certainly higher than one might find in contemporary clinical practice but not grossly so. The prevalence of PE in those with high probability scans was 88%, for intermediate scans 33%, for low probability scans 16% and for near normal scans 4% when the results of the patients followed up for a year were taken into account. The sensitivity of the high probability scan for PE was only 41% with most of the remaining PE patients having an indeterminate scan. Table 6 of the original paper displayed the clinicians assessment of the pre-test probability of PE compared to the results of VQ scanning and PE status as determined by pulmonary angiography or by follow-up. This data confirmed that when the clinical and scan probabilities were in agreement, the diagnostic accuracy was high. A low/low or high/high accuracy was 96–98% and 96% respectively. No patient with a normal scan had PE. Accuracy was poorer when either the clinical or the scan probabilities were intermediate and most patients in the series were in this group. Three years later, the investigators published an analysis of the performance of the initial categorical selection and proffered corrections [113]. A single moderate mismatched VQ abnormality, originally low probability, was confirmed to be intermediate

Table 3. The revised PIOPED criteria for VQ scan analysis [91].

High probability (≥ 80 %)

At least 2 large mismatched segmental perfusion defects or the arithmetic equivalent in moderate or large and moderate defects

Intermediate probability (20 – 79 %)

One moderate to 2 large mismatched segmental perfusion defects or the arithmetic equivalent in moderate or large and moderate defects: one matched VQ defect with a clear chest X-ray: difficult to categorise as low or high, or not described as low or high

Low probability (≤ 19 %)

Non-segmental perfusion defects (e.g., cardiomegaly, enlarged aorta, enlarged hila, elevated diaphragm); any perfusion defect with a substantially larger abnormality at chest X-ray; Perfusion defects matched by ventilation abnormality provided that there are (a) normal chest X-ray and (b) some areas of normal perfusion in the lungs; any number of small perfusion defects with a normal chest X-ray.

Normal

No perfusion defects, perfusion outlines exactly the shape of the lungs seen on the chest radiograph (hilar and aortic impressions may be seen and the chest radiograph and/or ventilation scan may be abnormal)

with a PE prevalence of 36 % (10/28 cases). A single matched VQ abnormality was considered on balance more likely to represent an intermediate probability with a PE prevalence of 24 % (5/21 cases). Multiple large matching defects had a PE prevalence of 15 % (6/39 cases). A two segment mismatch was possibly not the ideal threshold for the high probability category (71 % PE) but two and one half segmental mismatch was much better (100 % PE). The revised categorical criteria adopted from this second analysis (Table 3) were tested and found to be more accurate than the original criteria [91].

One of the more interesting findings of the original PIOPED study was that investigators reported scans more accurately using their own experience (their 'gestalt' reading) than they did using the formal categories outlined in PIOPED. This was true for both the original [113] and the corrected criteria [91] confirming that art is as important as science in VQ lung scan reporting. Experienced readers appear to make more accurate judgements overall so it is possible that further attempts at honing the categorical analysis will not improve the overall accuracy.

Unofficial PIOPED publications and PISA-PED

Since publication of the original official PIOPED data, the individual Investigation Centres where data was collected have each separately and unofficially published further articles on PE diagnosis using some of the PIOPED data. These contributions present a sometimes bewildering mathematical analysis of the centre's own results which in some respects has muddied rather than cleared the waters of uncertainty surrounding the topic. A

table of these studies is provided (Table 4) along with the main conclusion of each paper. Certain findings have been instantly applicable to everyday practice. For example, the counting of mismatched vascular defects was as effective as counting segmental equivalents [122] for PE diagnosis. The use of neural networks was shown to be of value for inexperienced physicians. Caution is required with other conclusions, however, and great care should be exercised before incorporating them into local practice. For instance, none of the papers used matching clinical data to clarify the results of their categorical analysis. There is marginal clinical value only in knowing that 20 out of 60 cases with a certain scan category had PE unless knowledge of the clinical presentation of each case was also given. If a majority of cases came from a high clinical pre-test group, Bayesian principles and experience tell us that cases with a lower clinical probability will show a lower prevalence of PE. It is impossible to incorporate this type of data into routine clinical practice without the corresponding clinical signal.

Again, most unofficial PIOPED papers reported from a combination of two populations. To the original PIOPED cases called the 'PIOPED angiographic pursuit group' (PAP) was added the 'attending physicians angiography decision group' (APAD). This latter group was highly selected by the attending physicians own decisions to proceed with pulmonary angiography. Clearly, such a combined study population will be biased toward PE, increasing the sensitivity of the high probability scan and decreasing the specificity of the low probability scan. The patient populations have been made to resemble the many retrospective series in the literature where the decision for pulmonary angiography was made by the attending physicians.

Table 4. A synopsis for unofficial publications from the clinical teams, which made up the 'PIOPED investigators'.

Unofficial PIOPED Publications

Author	Ref	Main Conclusion
Stein et al 1991	87	Clinical features assist in identifying patients at risk of PE
Stein et al 1991	114	Clinical evaluation helps select patients for further tests for PE
Stein et al 1991	115	Pre-existing cardiac or pulmonary disease does not impair diagnostic utility of VQ imaging
Sostman et al 1992	116	Stripe sign uncommon but associated with PE in 7% of cases
Quinn et al 1992	117	Men <50 have higher PE frequency than women. Women on 'pill' needed PA to diagnose
Stein et al 1992	118	The risks of PA were sufficiently low to justify its use in the appropriate clinical setting
Stein et al 1992	119	Perfusion studies alone are reliable if the interpretation is high, low or near normal/normal
Lesser et al 1992	120	Value of VQ scans in COPD is reduced because of higher prevalence of indeterminate scans
Stein et al 1993	121	Patients without prior cardiopulmonary disease require fewer mismatched segmental equivalents than those with
Stein et al 1993	122	Mismatched vascular defects were just as accurate as seg equivalent defects for PE diagnosis
Worsley et al 1993	123	Chest X-rays exclude diagnoses that mimic PE and aid interpretation of VQ scan
Worsley et al 1993	124	PE prevalence in triple match was upper (11%), middle (12%) and lower zones (33%)
Stein et al 1993	125	Mismatched vasc defects easier to interpret than seg equivalents. Evaluation more objective
Patil et al 1993	126	Neural networks predicted PE with an accuracy comparable to experienced clinicians
Worsley et al 1993	127	Overview of PE diagnosis as seen from PIOPED
Worsley et al 1994	128	Patients with a medium clinical likelihood are more likely to have false neg VQ scans
Worsley & Alavi 1995	129	PIOPED results reinforce role of VQ scans in diagnostic evaluation of patients with suspected PE
Tourassi et al 1995	130	Artificial neural network detects or excludes PE with accuracy of an experienced physician
Stein et al 1995	131	Mild untreated PE carries a lower immediate mortality and lower mortality from recurrent PE
Stein et al 1995	132	Calf asymmetry of 1 cm or more did not distinguish patients with and without PE
Stein et al 1995	133	A non-invasive strategy including VQ scans and leg tests permits diagnosis in 71% suspects
Henry et al 1995	134	PE is infrequent with normal pulmonary angiogram but more common than in general cases
Henry et al 1996	135	Near-normal VQ scan cases had pulmonary angiography when diagnosis appeared possible
Stein et al 1996	136	Provides criteria appropriate for a very low probability (less than 10% PPV) VQ scan
Gottschalk et al 96	137	PE can be present in the normal lung where the contralateral lung has a non-high abnormality
Henry et al 1996	138	VQ scans and clinical assessment retain diagnostic value in critically ill patients
Worsley et al 1996	139	Abnormal CXR or history of PE or cardiopulmonary disease did not affect value of VQ scans
Stein et al 1996	140	Blood gases are of insufficient discriminant value to permit exclusion of PE
Gottschalk et al 96	141	Patients without prior cardiopulmonary disease require fewer VQ abnormalities for acute PE
Gottschalk et al 96	142	A triple match with PE is more likely to be in the lower zone
Stein et al 1996	143	Q scans with <3 small subsegs have 1–3% PE while those with >3 have a PPV of 11–17%
Stein et al 1996	144	Criteria appropriate for the very low probability scan (<10%) identified

Lastly, there was an implicit assumption in some unofficial PIOPED papers that a VQ abnormality caused by PE would always be related to a visible thrombus in the corresponding segmental or subsegmental pulmonary artery. This reasoning is questionable. Emboli can move peripherally and simply be unseen at angiography and some thrombus may not cause any perfusion abnormality at all [145]. The authors also reason that the evaluation of 'single lungs' rather than 'patients' is acceptable to provide sufficient numbers of cases for analysis. This means that a matched VQ defect of one lung with a thrombus in the feeding PA would be a false negative finding. If the other lung showed a mismatched VQ lesion without associated thrombus, that finding would be considered false positive. Each lung would be a unique datum point unrelated to the paired lung even when the diagnosis had been categorically established from that other lung. A more universally accepted assumption would be that the patient with PE had a matched lesion from recent visible thrombus and a mismatched one from previous clot which had become invisible after breaking up and moving peripherally. Overall therefore, the results from the unofficial PIOPED papers, though interesting, tell only part of the story and may just not be accurate enough for general use in VQ imaging.

PISA-PED, the Prospective Investigative Study of Acute Pulmonary Embolism Diagnosis [146] was the most recent large prospective study. A total of 890 consecutive cases were evaluated prospectively, 390 of them having PE, a prevalence of 39%. The investigators used perfusion imaging only without ventilation and reported predictive values of PE+ and PE- scans ranging from 87–94% and 80–87%, respectively. One of the PISA-PED investigators examined the 723 perfusion lung scans from the PIOPED study and was able to predict disease in 197 (80%) of 246 cases with PE and exclude disease in 397 (83%) of 477 cases without embolism. While these results are commendable, it remains to be seen whether this approach could be more accurate or cost-effective than the standard VQ technique.

Principles of ventilation perfusion scintigraphy interpretation

General principles

Consistent and accurate interpretation of VQ scans is a challenging cognitive task involving integration of a perfusion and ventilation signal with the chest X-ray [147]. Further integration of the scan result with the pre-test clinical probability of PE provides the final post-test diagnosis. Scan interpretation itself has been successfully refined over the last 25 years, initially with good retrospective analyses of VQ appearances compared to pulmonary angiography [148] and more recently with prospective studies [108, 109, 42]. Though well planned and executed, the prospective series do have limitations. Firstly, the invasiveness, morbidity and resource implications of pulmonary angiography [149] have resulted in fewer patients with minor disease or minimal scan findings being enrolled in the studies. This has resulted in skewing of their study populations towards PE compared with the usual mix of patients referred to nuclear medicine with suspected PE [88]. Secondly, the sensitivity of pulmonary angiography for PE may extend only to second order pulmonary arteries with the smaller more peripheral emboli never being called [108, 150, 151]. Finally, the general use of Xenon-133 for assessment of ventilation has reduced the number of mismatched defects which can be delineated particularly those positioned anteriorly and those which are small. Most nuclear medicine practitioners with experience in VQ imaging, however, recognise several principles of lung scan interpretation which transcend these difficulties and the different philosophies of VQ scan interpretation.

The first principle states that a normal lung scan excludes PE for clinical purposes no matter the clinical presentation. The retrospective study of Kipper (68 cases) [152] and prospective studies of Hull (315 cases [153] and 515 cases [154]) confirmed after follow up, that patients with a normal perfusion lung scan were at no significant risk of PE. They each concluded that the diagnostic work up for suspected PE need not extend beyond a multiple view, normal perfusion lung scan and that anticoagulants can be safely withheld except in the presence of venous thrombosis. In PIOPED [42], there were 3 patients only with a normal lung scan and each had negative pulmonary angiography.

Sostman et al. [155] emphasise the need for a 'normal' diagnosis to be reserved for unequivocally normal perfusion studies because (a) animal experiments have shown that the technique is not perfectly sensitive and (b) because of the great weight placed on a normal interpretation in the clinical management of patients. After a truly normal perfusion lung scan (Fig. 1), the search for PE should stop and attention focussed on other clinical possibilities.

There is, however, a remote risk of a normal lung scan in the presence of a large, single, non-occluding saddle embolus of the main pulmonary artery [156]. For this reason, a normal lung scan in the presence of shock or acute cardiorespiratory failure should be immediately followed by pulmonary angiography or spiral CT angiography. Lung scintigraphy is not indicated in shock.

The second principle states that *PE can be present with any lung perfusion abnormality(ies) but the risk of PE will depend in part upon the pattern of abnormality.* For example, the smaller the perfusion abnormality (ies), the more matched they are to abnormal ventilation and the less numerous, the less the risk of PE. Conversely, the larger the perfusion abnormality (ies), the more mismatched to ventilation and the more numerous, the greater the risk of PE [100, 102, 157, 158].

Pattern Analysis: The diagnosis of PE requires the presence of perfusion defects. Convention dictates that perfusion defects are described in terms of size, profile and number.

Size: Most schemes for interpretation [42, 100] estimate substantial defects as segmental or large (i. e. > 75 % segment) (Fig. 6) and less substantial as moderate subsegmental (i. e. between 25 to 75 % segment) (Fig. 7). It is with these groups of abnormalities that PE is most likely to be associated. Smaller subsegmental (< 25 % segment) (Fig. 8) and non-segmental defects are usually not associated with PE. Defects larger than a segment are considered multi-segmental (Fig. 6) while non-segmental defects relate to abnormal anatomy impinging upon the lung such as the presence of cardiomegaly, prominent hilar areas or an elevated hemi-diaphragm.

Knowledge of segmental anatomy (Fig. 9) will be essential [159] if PE diagnosis follows the hypothesis of 'segmental equivalents' where it is assumed that a moderate sized defect is of lesser significance than a large one [160]. But classification by defect size is difficult and requires skill and judgement. Some workers normalise defect size to the equivalent normal segmental configuration so that the significance of a defect size depends upon its position [147]. A segmental defect of an upper lobe would have to be almost twice the size of defects of the lower lobe to be significant. Others [155] use an idealised segmental size and apply this template for the evaluation of defects in any location. A note of caution was sounded by Morrell [161] when he reported upon the difficulties experienced by most observers in estimating defect size. In fact, the size of most defects was usually considerably underestimated. Reasons suggested were a lack of appreciation of the appearances of pure segmental defects and a range of size differences between individual segments in the lung which may be up to three-fold. The most frequently underestimated defects were the ante-

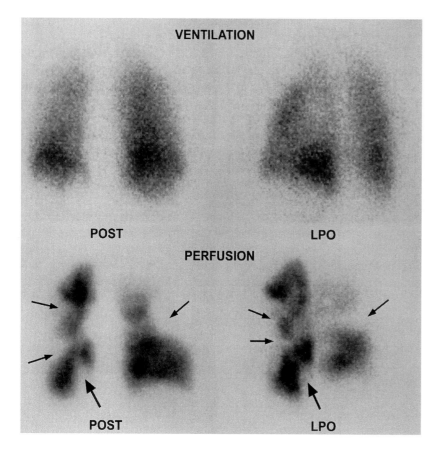

Fig. 6. Posterior and left posterior oblique perfusion (lower) and Technegas (upper) scans. This is a classical high probability scan with segmental (thick arrow) and multi-segmental (thin arrows) mismatched perfusion defects. The chest X-ray was normal but the clinical history of proximal deep vein thrombosis and sudden dyspnea was highly predictive for PE.

rior and lateral basal segments of both lower lobes (Fig. 7), the medial segment of the right middle lobe and the posterior apical segment of the right upper lobe. In light of these findings, they argued against empirical scoring criteria based on segmental size. They judged that any defect that was pleural based and triangular or concave in shape and in the anatomical distribution of a lung segment should be considered 'segmental' in nature. There is now good evidence that the total number of mismatched pulmonary vascular defects (Fig. 10), whether large or moderate, provide as accurate an assessment of PE risk as the number of mismatched segmental equivalents [125]. This is likely to make the evaluation for PE more simple, objective and reproducible.

Number: PE is usually characterised by a multiplicity of bilateral perfusion defects [162, 163]. However, it is known that the number of perfusion defects underestimates the clot burden within the pulmonary circulation [162]. In a dog model, Alderson [162] revealed that thrombi can remain unseen to perfusion imaging if they fail to obstruct the pulmonary artery. Because of this, the PIOPED investigators considered a partially perfused defect as representative of a real defect in light of this evidence [155]. Reverse mismatching where per-

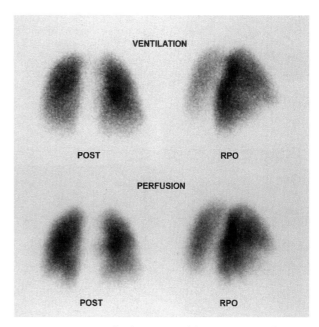

Fig. 7. Posterior and right posterior oblique 81mKr ventilation (upper) and MA perfusion (lower) scans showing multiple moderately-sized mismatched perfusion abnormalities of between 25–75% of a segment. PE was found at pulmonary angiography confirming the importance of small mismatches of the lower lobes. The chest X-ray was normal (Courtesy of Dr. Andrew J. Hilson, Royal Free Hospital, London, United Kingdom).

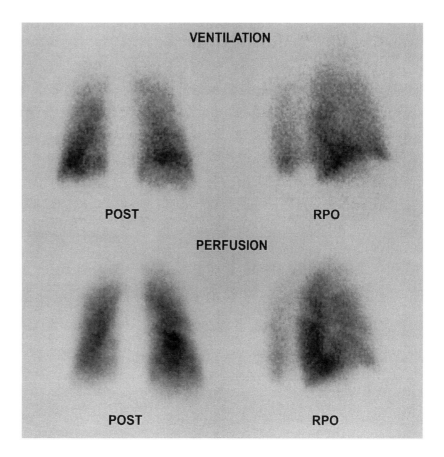

Fig. 8. Posterior and right posterior oblique perfusion (lower) and Technegas (upper) scans showing small peripheral matched perfusion abnormalities of the upper and mid-zones. The chest X-ray was normal and the pattern represents a very low probability of PE.

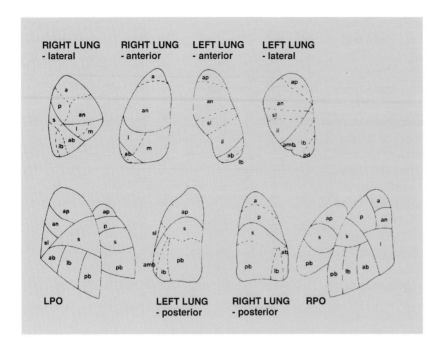

RIGHT LUNG - lateral **RIGHT LUNG** - anterior **LEFT LUNG** - anterior **LEFT LUNG** - lateral

LPO **LEFT LUNG** - posterior **RIGHT LUNG** - posterior RPO

Fig. 9. Anatomic lung segment reference chart, which should be routinely used in assessment of lung scintigraphy.

fusion is decreased less than ventilation is, however, less likely to be due to PE or infarction [164]. The PIOPED data confirmed that as the cumulative total of large and moderate sized mismatched perfusion defects increased, so the specificity of lung imaging for PE diagnosis increased significantly (Fig. 10) [125]. The positive predictive value for PE diagnosis increased from 80% for one, 89% for two, 91% for three and 92% for more than five mismatched defects.

Configuration: In the absence of pulmonary infarction, pulmonary emboli create rather typical perfusion defects which appear cut-out and always include the pleural surface. They often appear wedge shaped, are wider at the pleural surface and are truly pleural based (Fig. 11). Other defects which cross segmental boundaries are less likely to be caused by PE but there are exceptions. For example, the 'stripe sign' (Fig. 12) where perfusion defects are separated from the pleural surface by a band or stripe of perfused lung are said to be unlikely in PE [116, 165]. However, since 11 out of 50 patients with a stripe sign in that series did have PE (22%) and since the stripe sign has been reported during resolution of PE [166], there remains a question mark over its validity for PE exclusion in practice.

Ventilation: Multiple mismatched perfusion defects, with perfusion loss in areas normally ventilated, represents the classical lung scan presentation of PE [43]. Ventilation perfusion match with a normal chest radiograph were thought to be specific for parenchymal lung disease but recent prospective studies [110, 167] have clearly shown that PE can on occasion be associated with a matching of ventilation with perfusion. Initial studies had suggested that abnormalities of ventilation induced by PE were of short duration [168], but current understanding is that bronchoconstriction can be more sustained for hours or days rather than minutes or hours [169]. Wedge shaped abnormalities of perfusion cannot now be assumed to be non-embolic just because they are matched to an abnormality of ventilation (Fig. 13). In pulmonary infarction, on the other hand, as in other

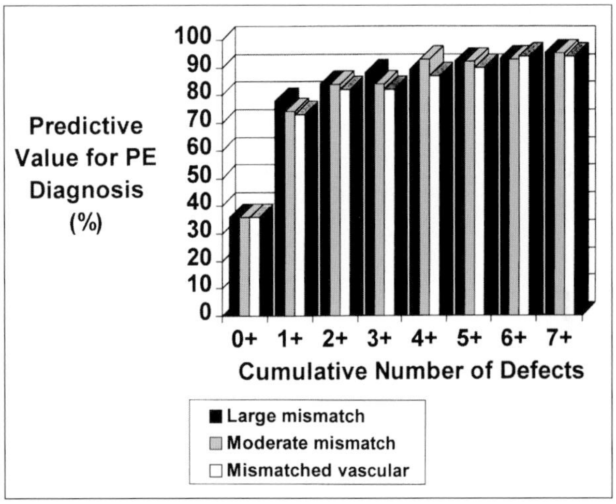

Fig. 10. Cumulative number of mismatched moderate or large-sized and vascular perfusion defects compared with the positive predictive value for PE diagnosis [125].

Predictive Value for PE Diagnosis (%)

Cumulative Number of Defects

■ Large mismatch
▨ Moderate mismatch
□ Mismatched vascular

lung pathology, the abnormality of ventilation occurs secondary to consolidation and/or pleural fluid. The combination of matched and mismatched perfusion defects (Fig. 14) is unusual and provides no clues as to the presence or absence of PE.

The third principle states that *a good quality erect and contemporaneous chest radiograph is essential for accurate VQ scan interpretation*. The only exception to this principle occurs when the perfusion scan is completely normal. The chest radio-

graph is usually the first imaging modality employed when there is a suspicion of PE. While the test is usually abnormal in some respects in PE, the prevalence of abnormalities is not significantly different from that in patients without PE (170). The chest radiograph is therefore of little value on its own for diagnosis. Indeed, it can be normal in between 20–30% of patients with PE [171]. However, the chest radiograph is important for VQ scan interpretation in two ways. Firstly, it provides a clearer understanding of the significance of

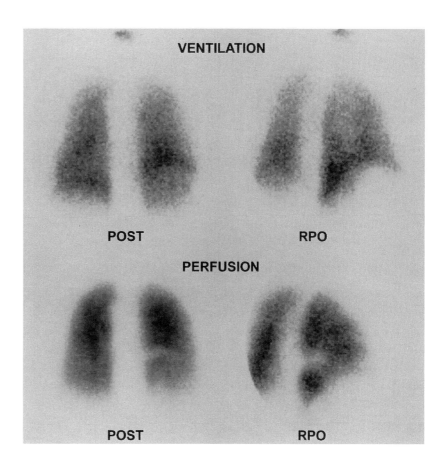

Fig. 11. Posterior and right posterior oblique perfusion (lower) and Technegas (upper) scans. The classical mismatched defect of the superior segment of the right lower lobe is wedge-shaped and wider at the pleural surface indicating that it is pleural based.

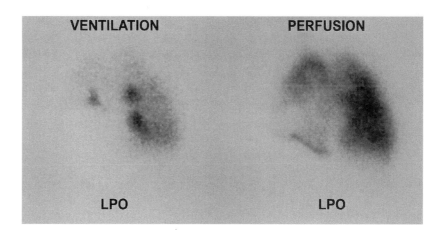

Fig. 12. Left posterior oblique perfusion (right) and Technegas (left) scans. The chest X-ray shows opacification of the middle and lower left lung zones matching the perfusion and ventilation defects (triple match). Perfusion of the lower pleural surface revealed the presence of a 'stripe sign'.

matching abnormalities of ventilation and perfusion. If atelectasis, parenchymal opacification, or blunting of the costophrenic angle caused by a small pleural effusion are present, then the triple match of V, Q and CXR prevent a useful interpretation for PE diagnosis (Fig. 15). Infarction and infection cannot be differentiated by VQ scintigraphy [148]. Interestingly, it has been shown that parenchymal opacification in the upper and mid-zones have a lower positive predictive value for the presence of PE compared with the lower zones [124]. Other even less common findings which include oligaemia, pleural based areas of increased opacity and elevated hemi-diaphragm, have no diagnostic value whatever. Secondly, the chest radiograph clarifies other lung pathology such as cancer, pneumothorax, pleural thickening and fractured ribs which can all influence VQ scan interpretation.

In many ways, interpretation of VQ scans is best approached by first examining the chest radiograph to make an assessment of possible areas of perfusion abnormality. Cardiomegaly can produce abnormalities of the left lower lobe. Prominent mediastinal structures such as a tortuous aorta or lymphadenopathy can also change the pos-

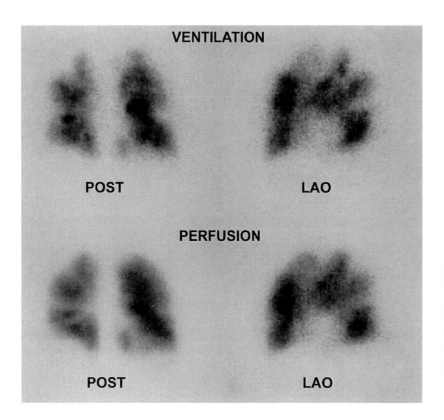

Fig. 13. Posterior and left anterior oblique perfusion (lower) and Technegas (upper) scans. The chest X-ray was normal. There are multiple matched abnormalities of both lungs indicating low probability. However, the perfusion abnormalities are segmental or vascular in character (wedge shaped and pleural based) and despite the matching, constitute a potential false negative VQ study harbouring PE. The patient was post-operative and a DVT was found on Doppler ultrasound.

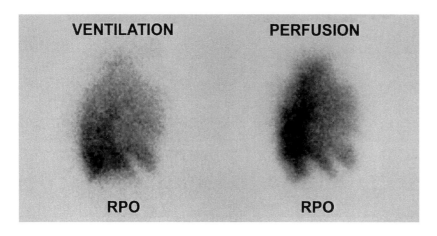

Fig. 14. Right lateral perfusion (right) and Technegas (left) scans. Two moderate segmental abnormalities are seen, one matched and the other mismatched. The chest X-ray was normal. This indicates an intermediate probability of PE.

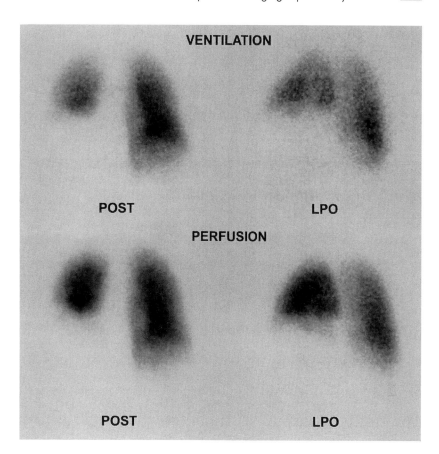

Fig. 15. Posterior and left posterior oblique perfusion (lower) and Technegas (upper) scans. Chest X-ray showed left lower specification. The classical triple match of ventilation, perfusion and X-ray opacification indicates an intermediate probability of PE.

terior views of particularly the left lobe. The position of the diaphragm can be problematical at times because of the suggestion of perfusion defects which often occur and because it is often unclear whether the diaphragm elevation is acute or chronic [160]. Since the chest radiograph appearances can change within hours of either infarction or infection it should be obtained at the same time as the VQ scan or within a couple of hours. Portable X-rays are often quite unsuitable since they can obscure areas of parenchymal opacification and thereby lead to errors in interpretation.

The fourth principle states that *the pre-test clinical probability of PE, that is the PE risk as determined by the clinical presentation, is itself an independent risk factor for PE along with the lung scan result.* Bayes' theorem defines the relationship between the pre-test clinical probability, the lung scan result and the post-test probability of PE (see above). Combining the lung scan result and pretest clinical probability provides a much more closely defined post-test probability of PE than either of these variables taken singly. This principle is only annulled by the presence of a completely normal perfusion scan because here, PE has been shown to be excluded for clinical purposes whatever the history.

The fifth principle states that *the VQ scan and chest radiograph should, whenever possible, be interpreted before becoming appraised of the clinical details of the patients presentation.* This is important because interpretation of VQ studies can be biased by prior knowledge of the clinical presentation [172]. For example, knowing the presence of several risk factors or DVT might bias the interpretation of the scan to a higher level (i. e. from low to intermediate or from intermediate to high). Conversely, the absence of risk factors might bias the interpretation to a lower level (i. e. from intermediate to low probability). A bias may be small but will inevitably lead to inaccuracy in estimation of the post-test probability of PE.

Pitfalls in ventilation perfusion imaging

Many disease processes affect the pulmonary vasculature in preference to the airways and can result in multiple VQ mismatches with the appearance of acute PE. Such false positivity or deception is thankfully uncommon and can usually be suspected from the clinical history or chest X-ray. The majority of false positive studies are likely to follow previous unresolved PE [42]. The pre-test clinical probability is usually medium with a history of previous PE only as pointer. On this basis, a strong case can be made for a routine base-line VQ scan 3 months following an attack of acute PE to document unresolved perfusion defects if required for future reference [173]. A second relatively frequent cause of perfusion mismatches is hilar or mediastinal involvement from a bronchogenic carcinoma. These mismatches are usually large and involve one lung only in our experience. The chest X-ray will often provide clues to the diagnosis. Intravenous drug abuse is the third increas-

ingly common reason for, in this case, multiple mismatches which lead to a mottled perfusion image. These features probably result from either vasculitis or non-thrombotic embolism. More rare conditions targeting pulmonary vasculature rather than airways include mediastinal fibrosis, congenital or neoplastic pulmonary vascular abnormalities or vasculitis, post-radiation fibrosis, other non-thrombotic emboli (air, fat, tumour), and patients with mitral valve disease [174, 175].

Integration of lung scan findings with clinical data

Contemporary lung scan interpretation

Interpretive algorithms for categorising VQ lung scans assist in training, in communication and are important for the production of guidelines. The lung scan category, however, represents only half of the information required to produce a post-test report, the pre-test clinical probability of PE being an equal co-variable in the assessment of PE risk. The graph of conditional probability adapted from PIOPED data [84] and relating pre- and post-test probabilities of PE with the lung scan category (Fig. 5), clearly reveals how the terms high and low probability relating to scans have been misunderstood and misinterpreted with occasional detriment to patients [81, 83]. For example, two mod-

erate matched perfusion defects with a clear chest X-ray and a low pre-test clinical probability indicates a low post-test probability of PE of 4%. The same scan features in a patient with a DVT (i. e. high clinical pre-test probability) indicate a much higher PE risk at 35%. While the low probability scan interpretation is correct in both instances, it is the addition of clinical information which puts the perceived PE risk in context. The graph illustrates how low and very-low probability scans reduce a presenting clinical probability of PE (indicated by the line of indentity) to provide a lower post-test probability of PE. When the clinical pre-test probability of PE is low (i. e. 10%), a low probability scan reduces that risk to 4% post-test while a very-low probability scan reduces it to 2%. When the

Table 5. In-house criteria for VQ scan analysis (neo-classical) which provide for a higher specificity in VQ imaging. These criteria have not been tested against pulmonary angiography at the present time.

Neo-classical criteria for VQ scan interpretation

High probability

2 moderate/large mismatched perfusion defects. Prior cardiopulmonary disease probably requires more abnormalities (i. e. ≥4). Triple match one lung with ≥1 mismatch the other lung.

Intermediate probability

Difficult to categorise or not described as very-low, low or high including all cases with a chest X-ray opacity, pleural fluid or collapse. Single moderate VQ match or mismatch without corresponding radiographic abnormality.

Low probability

Large or moderate focal VQ matches involving no more than 50% of the combined lung fields with no corresponding radiographic abnormalities.
Small VQ mismatches with a normal chest X-ray.

Very-low probability

Small VQ matches with a normal chest X-ray.
Non-segmental perfusion defects including cardiomegaly, enlarged hila or aorta.

Normal

No perfusion defects.

Large defects are > 75% segment, moderate defects 25–75% segment and small defects < 25% segment.

Table 6.   Start with the perfusion scan and move to the questions which are oblong in shape. Continue to the next questions until you finally reach a rectangle that provides the scan probability for PE. The asterisk represents a scan probability that has not been determined by prospective studies.

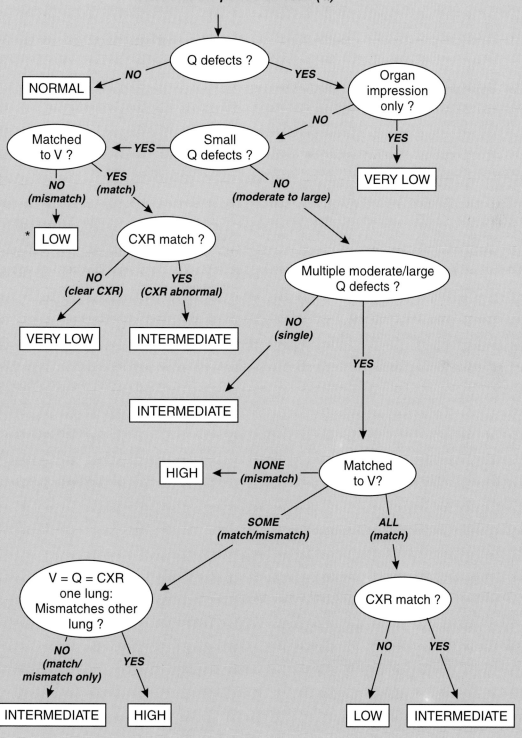

VQ SCAN INTERPRETATION:
AN ADVANCED ALGORITHM

Start with the perfusion scan (Q)

clinical pre-test is medium (i. e. 30%), a low probability scan reduces the risk to 10% and a very-low probability to 5–8% post-test. When the pre-test clinical is high (i. e. 70%), a low probability scan reduces the risk to 35% and a very low to 20% post-test. The actual risk of PE after a low probability scan may not be low at all because the risk clearly varies between 4% and 35%. It really is a 'lower-than-clinical' probability scan. The same reasoning applies to high probability which is a 'higher-than-clinical' scan.

With this important proviso about terminology in lung scanning, how then should we interpret the V, Q and chest X-ray signals from VQ imaging. A 'classical' approach would be to use the updated categorical analysis of PIOPED (Table 3). It is fair to say that this approach is finding less favour with internists and respiratory specialists [81, 82, 175, 176]. In clinical circles, the 'classical' low probability scan is becoming increasingly rejected as a stand-alone test because the category has been shown to conceal PE in a small but worrying number of cases [84, 177]. Regrettably, the official PIOPED investigators accelerated this disillusionment by erroneously categorising the single mismatched perfusion defect as low probability rather than intermediate and by accepting up to a 19% prevalence of PE for their low probability category. Clinicians who reject the low probability scan favour a *'reversionary'* approach which accepts the validity of a normal and a high probability scan, but amalgamates both the low and intermediate probability scans into a non-diagnostic [81, 82, 176] or non-high [175] grouping. This approach results in the majority of cases requiring post-test investigation. It is unsurprising therefore that a few institutions have eliminated VQ scanning and have proceeded directly to Spiral CT (CTPA) as their primary test for PE [178]. It is likely that this latter approach will eventually be shown to be wasteful of resources compared with the established cost-effectiveness of VQ imaging in the overall diagnostic algorithm [133, 179, 180]. We favour the 'neo-classical' approach to VQ scan analysis which recognises the credibility gap for the low probability scan when the pre-test clinical presentation is medium (i. e. one or more risk actors for DVT) and which therefore uses the very-low probability scan to exclude PE for clinical purposes in this important clinical group. Our current criteria for categorical analysis of those cases with suspected PE are listed in Table 5.

The pathways to scan categorisation can also be represented by an algorithm (Table 6). Doubts surround the validity of many unofficial PIOPED publications which were unsupported by clinical information and contained low numbers of cases. Therefore, many issues remain within the art and science of VQ scan interpretation. One issue for which as yet there is no reliable data, relates to the significance of the small perfusion defect. The total PE prevalence in this group is thought to be around 2.5% [128]. In PIOPED, the ventilation status of these defects was undefined because of the low intrinsic resolution of Xenon-133 imaging. Some of these defects may well have been mismatched and therefore, more likely to harbour PE than the equivalent matched variety [84]. With modern ventilation technology, such small mismatched defects are more readily identified. Until information is available, small mismatched defects will have a higher categorical risk than small matched ones in our criteria.

Formation of the post-test diagnosis

The relevance of Bayes' theorem for development of a post-test diagnosis after VQ imaging has been shown elegantly by both PIOPED [42] and PISA-PED [146]. In both reports, a combination of clinical and VQ data was shown to be more accurate than either of these co-variables alone. Modification of the PIOPED data [84] permits a reasonable match to our neo-classical criteria for lung scan reporting and provides for a more specific low probability lung scan result. A post-test diagnosis can then be provided for each clinical presentation and scan category combination dependent upon the PIOPED data. This information is illustrated in Tables 7, 8 and 9. No further investigation is required when a patient presents with a low pre-test clinical probability and a normal, very low or low probability scan since the risk of PE is extremely small. If risk factors are noted in the clinical history (i. e. medium pre-test clinical probability), a normal scan eliminates PE, a very-low probability

Table 7. Diagnosis of venous thromboembolism: *Low* pre-test clinical probability.

Scan Category	PE Risk: VQ and Clinical	Post-test Result
Normal	0%	PE excluded
Very-low Probability	2%	PE very unlikely
Low Probability	3%	PE very unlikely
Intermediate	14%	Working diagnosis no PE
High Probability	60%	Diagnosis uncertain

Table 8. Diagnosis of venous thromboembolism: *Medium* pre-test clinical probability.

Scan Category	PE Risk: VQ and Clinical	Post-test Result
Normal	0%	PE excluded
Very-low Probability	5–8%	PE unlikely
Low Probability	10%	Working diagnosis no PE
Intermediate	28%	Diagnosis uncertain
High Probability	88%	PE likely

scan makes it unlikely, while a high probability scan is almost diagnostic of PE. In cases with many risk factors or a DVT (high pre-test clinical probability), a normal VQ scan excludes PE for clinical purposes and a high probability scan is diagnostic. Most other clinical and VQ scan combinations are non-diagnostic to varying degrees and require further investigation. The exact percentage of diagnostic VQ scans will vary, rising with a lowering of total PE prevalence and falling as the PE risk in the population increases. This analysis is broadly in agreement with the recommendations of the PIOPED and McMaster combined study groups [133, 180] and awaits testing in a prospective trial.

Communication of the PE risk to the attending physicians can be difficult [90] given the jargon which is often employed [181], and it is possible that the addition of a numerical estimate of risk along with the verbal report will clarify that risk for clinicians [91, 177]. Provision of the conditional probability curve itself with the individual patients co-ordinates clearly marked thereon may be worthwhile but has not been tested. Our policy is, with others [91, 177], to verbally communicate the post-test diagnosis on completion of the VQ

scan providing both a verbal assessment and a percentage risk of PE. A discussion may then permit the nuclear medicine practitioner to clarify for the clinician the impact of the post-test result on the diagnostic strategy. This impact may be elimination of PE, its confirmation, or clarification of the degree of residual uncertainty. In the latter case, a cost-effective follow-on strategy is required.

Diagnostic strategies

Combining the clinical presentation and scan diagnosis in the original PIOPED identified certain subgroups where the predictive value for diagnosis was over 85% for a positive scan and over 90% for a negative one. The group in which Bayesian analysis provided an adequate diagnosis comprised 302 of 887 patients (34%). But the PIOPED population was unique. It was selected towards disease and contained fewer patients in the low clinical and scan groups than would be expected in a group of cases without pulmonary angiographic diagnosis. Our own department would normally expect diagnostic categories of scan plus clinical to comprise up to 45–50% of the total lung scans. Clearly, a significant number of patients require further investigation after VQ imaging.

Pulmonary angiography is the gold standard for PE diagnosis but has never been fully exploited because of resource implications. Recent pioneering work of Wheeler [182] and the McMaster group [108, 109, 153] have highlighted the importance of the search for deep vein thrombus (DVT) after a non-diagnostic VQ scan. The concept has been introduced that it is sufficient to identify and treat DVT as an alternative to proving the presence of PE in these patients since the treatment of DVT and PE is identical. The potential in this strategy is the reduction in the number of pulmonary angiograms by 50% [180]. Hull has shown that 50% of cases with PE are shown to have a DVT by non-invasive leg tests and that serial negative leg tests exclude a significant risk of PE [153]. It has also been shown that anticoagulants can be safely withheld if serial leg tests are negative [153, 184]. The risk of recurrent PE in untreated patients with PE and adequate cardiorespiratory reserve (CRR) if they have negative serial leg tests is minor (2%) [184]. Apparently, only 3% of patients with PE and a single negative leg test become positive on serial testing. Leg testing with B-mode or Doppler ultrasound or impedance plethysmography has therefore been proposed as a safe and attractive adjunct to the non-diagnostic lung scan, picking out those with clear cut proximal DVT for treatment thereby

Table 9. Diagnosis of venous thromboembolism: *High* pre-test clinical probability.

Scan Category	PE Risk: VQ and Clinical	Post-test Result
Normal	0%	PE excluded
Very-low probability	20%	Diagnosis uncertain
Low probability	40%	Diagnosis uncertain
Intermediate	70%	Working diagnosis PE
High probability	95%	Diagnosis Tic of PE

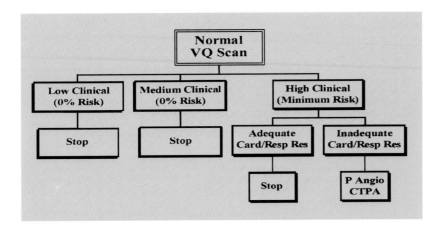

Fig. 16. This flow chart shows a diagnostic algorithm for the Normal VQ scan across the profile of clinical PE risk.

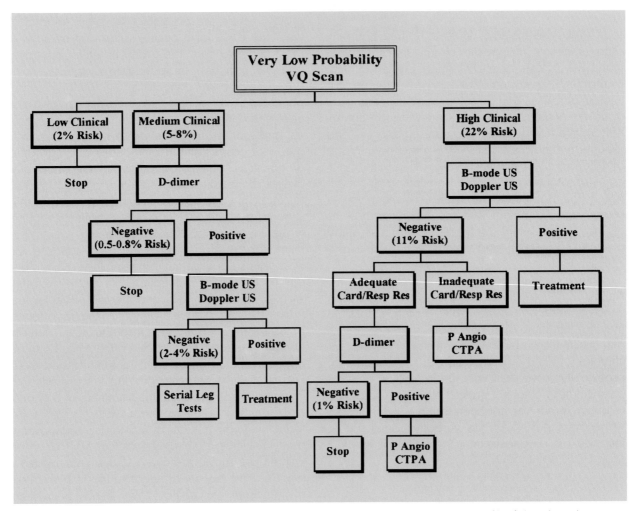

Fig. 17. This flow chart shows a diagnostic algorithm for the Very Low Probability VQ scan across the profile of clinical PE risk.

reducing the need for pulmonary angiography. It is likely that leg tests will be of greatest value in those patients with an increased risk of PE but it must be remembered that 30–50% of them will have negative leg tests despite the presence of PE [108, 185].

Spiral CT angiography (CTPA) is currently showing great promise as a less invasive alternative to pul-monary angiography. Advantages include the delineation of central pulmonary thrombus, pulmonary infarction and other non-PE causes for the patient's symptoms. It is not a complete solution to the problem of PE detection because of failure to detect subsegmental disease [186] which potentially may herald further embolic events. CTPA does, however, appear to provide a robust alternative to

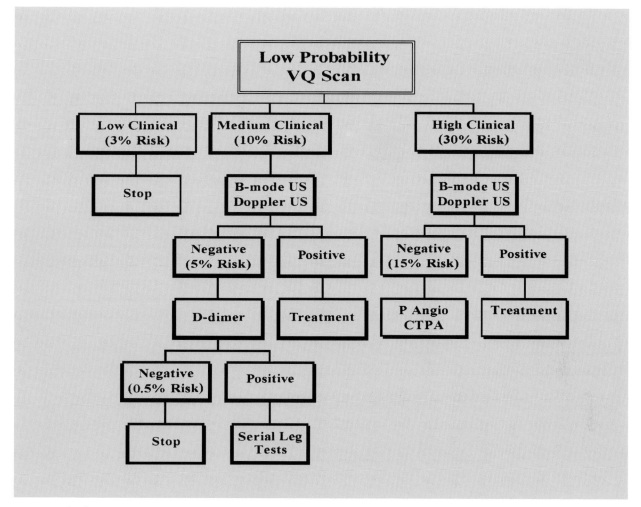

Fig. 18. This flow chart shows a diagnostic algorithm for the Low Probability scan across the profile of clinical PE risk.

pulmonary angiography for those patients with a medium risk of PE or those with inadequate cardiorespiratory reserve.

Measurement of plasma D-dimer, a specific degradation product of cross-linked fibrin, has been shown to be highly sensitive but poorly specific for the presence of intravascular thrombus. The test appears to have most value in excluding DVT and PE and initial trials have been promising [187, 188]. More widespread clinical application will be possible with the development of a rapid single-test and quantitative D-dimer assays. Initial investigation has shown a negative predictive value of a plasma D-dimer level of <500ng/ml for acute PE of 91% [189]. Given its poor specificity, the test will be of greatest value following VQ scanning in those cases with a lower prevalence of PE.

The constant drive for cost-effectiveness in our strategies for PE diagnosis will ensure that VQ imaging remains the pivotal screening test for PE [179] despite the suggestions that B-mode US [178],

D-dimer [187], or CTPA [178] are possible contenders. The PIOPED and McMaster investigators have summarised the available data and provided us with a management algorithm which can be adapted to local circumstances [190]. Our own policy (Figs. 16–20) is to advise leg tests following VQ scans when the PE risk remains medium, to perform D-dimer for those with a residual low probability, and CTPA for those with a medium to high probability of PE or when the cardiorespiratory reserve (CRR) is impaired. The following recommendations represent our current understanding of the most cost-effective strategy for PE diagnosis [191] and uses modified PIOPED data [84].

The normal VQ scan (Fig. 16). If the perfusion lung scan is completely normal, the clinical presentation is irrelevant. PE is excluded for clinical purposes and anticoagulants rendered unnecessary.

The very low probability scan (Fig. 17). If the VQ scan shows minor abnormalities and the clinical presentation is low (i. e. no risk factors), the risk of

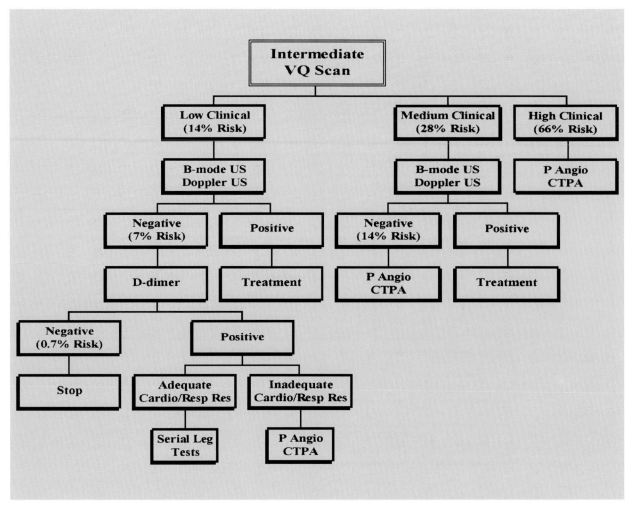

Fig. 19. This flow chart shows a diagnostic algorithm for the Intermediate Probability scan across the profile of clinical PE risk.

acute PE is 2%. No further investigation or treatment would be required. If the clinical presentation is medium (i. e. risk factors present), there is a 5–8% risk of PE. A negative D-dimer would eliminate the PE risk while a positive test should be followed by a leg study. If the leg test results are negative, there is a 2–4% PE risk. No treatment is indicated and serial leg tests are optional. If positive, treatment is recommended. With a high clinical presentation without a DVT (several risk factors), there is a 22% risk of PE. Leg tests will pick up 50% of those with PE. Those with negative leg tests (11% risk) require CTPA if there is inadequate CCR or D-dimer if CRR is adequate. A positive D-dimer may well warrant CTPA.

The low probability scan (Fig. 18). If the clinical assessment is low in a patient with a low probability scan, the PE risk is 3%. No further investigation or treatment would normally be necessary. With a medium clinical risk, the PE prevalence is 10%. A negative D-dimer would reduce the PE risk to 1%

while a positive test should be followed by a leg study. Leg tests would pick out half of those with PE while those with negative tests (5% PE risk) should have serial leg tests. If the clinical assessment is high without a DVT, leg tests are appropriate. Treatment is required if these are positive. If negative (15% risk), CTPA is probably necessary.

The intermediate scan (Fig. 19). The PE risk is 14% if the clinical assessment is low, 28% if it is medium and 66% if it is high. We suggest that patients in the low and medium clinical risk groups should proceed to a leg test and if positive, treatment instituted. If leg tests are negative, the strategy depends upon the level of risk. Following a low initial clinical presentation, the PE risk is low (i.e. 7%) and a D-dimer investigation will eliminate those with negligible risk. Cases with a positive D-dimer should probably proceed to serial leg tests or CTPA dependent upon the CRR. Cases with a high clinical likelihood without proven DVT could either proceed to leg testing as for the med-

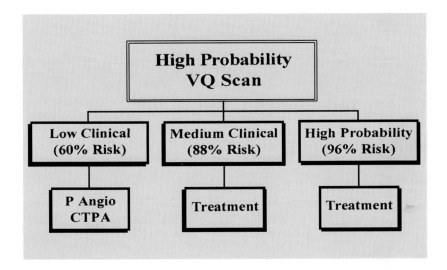

Fig. 20. This flow chart shows a diagnostic algorithm for the High Probability scan across the profile of clinical PE risk.

ium clinical group or to CTPA for definitive diagnosis. If CTPA was negative, leg testing might be prudent.

The high probability scan (Fig. 20). The high probability scan with a medium or high clinical risk indicates an 88 % or 96 % PE risk respectively. Treatment is recommended in both situations. If the clinical risk is low with no risk factors, then the high probability scan is a surprise and should be followed by pulmonary angiography or CTPA.

Conclusion/Summary

Confirmation of the relevance of Bayes' theorem to the practice of VQ scintigraphy has permitted an advance in our understanding of the analysis and reliability of lung scan categories. This improvement in the credentials of VQ scintigraphy is contingent upon our knowledge of the PE prevalence within our own patient population which may differ from the published literature. It is clear that the classical low probability scan excludes PE reliably at the lower end of the clinical pre-test probability spectrum and unreliably at the higher end. Conversely, the greater specificity of the very low probability scan in excluding PE is valuable in both low (i.e. no risk factors) and medium (i.e. risk factors) clinical pre-test presentations. Concordance between clinical and scintigraphic findings in either a low or high category is virtually diagnostic of no PE or PE respectively. A diagnostic strategy is required after scintigraphy for cases with a residual PE risk of between 10 and 80 % and the proportion of these cases will rise with increasing prevalence of PE. This strategy will be tailored to individual departments and will profitably include D-dimer measurement to exclude PE when the prevalence is low, B-mode or Doppler ultrasound for detection of DVT when the prevalence is high and pulmonary angiography or spiral CT angiography where the diagnosis remains unclear or where impaired cardiorespiratory reserve is detected.

VQ scintigraphy remains the primary non-invasive modality for the evaluation of patients with suspected PE particularly where there is a low clinical pre-test probability but also in cases with risk factors (i.e. medium risk) and a clear chest X-ray. Being realistic, it is unlikely that even pulmonary angiography could resolve all our questions about the meaning of VQ scan categories because of its intrinsic inadequacy in the peripheral lung. The best we can hope for eventually is a broad understanding of risks inherent in each scan category across the clinical spectrum. This will be achieved with an up-to-date data set comprising contemporaneous clinical, VQ scan and chest X-ray, leg studies, D-dimer and increasingly spiral CT angiography information across the whole spectrum of clinical presentations. Such information would permit the construction of accurate conditional probability curves relating lung scan results to both pre and post-test clinical probabilities of PE. Until then, we may still have to rely on our own gestalt estimations of PE risk which are so dependent upon experience.

References

1. Weibel ER. Morphometry of the human lung. Springer Verlag, Berlin, 1963

2. West JB, Dollery CT, Naimark A. Distribution of blood flow in isolated lung: relation to vascular and alveolar pressures. J Appl Physiol 1964; 19: 713–724

3. Sabiston DC, Durham NC, Wagner Jr HN. The pathophysiology of pulmonary embolism: relationships to accurate diagnosis and choice of therapy. J Thoracic & Cardiovasc Surg 1965; 50: 339–356

4. Wagner HN Jr, Sabiston DC, McAfee JG, Tow D, Stern HS. Diagnosis of massive pulmonary embolism in man by radioisotope scanning. N Engl J Med 1964; 271: 377–384

5. Haynie TP, Calhoon JH, Nasjleti CE, Nofal MM, Beierwalters WH. Visualisation of pulmonary artery occlusion by photoscanning. JAMA 1963; 185: 306–308

6. Halpern BN, Biozzi G, Benacerraf B, Stiffel C, Hillemand B. Cinétique de la phagocytose d'une sérum albumine-humaine spécialement traitée et radiomarquée et son application à l'étude de la circulation hépatique chez l'homme. Compte rend Soc de Biol 1956; 150: 1307–1311

7. Taplin GV, Johnson DE, Dore EK, Kaplan HS. Lung photoscans with macroaggregates of human serum radioalbumin. Health Phys 1964; 10: 1219–1227

8. Dworkin HJ, Smith JR, Bull FE. Reaction after administration of macroaggregated albumin (MAA) for a lung scan. N Engl J Med 1966; 275: 376

9. Vincent WR, Goldberg SJ, Desilets D. Fatality immediately following rapid infusion of macroaggrgates of 99Tc albumin (MAA) for lung scan. Radiology 1968; 91: 1181–1184

10. Williams JO. Death following injection of lung scanning agent in a case of pulmonary hypertension. Br J Radiol 1974; 47: 61–63

11. Child JS, Wolfe JD, Tashkin D, Nakano F. Fatal lung scan in a case of pulmonary hypertension due to obliterative pulmonary vascular disease. Chest 1975; 67: 308–310

12. Harding LK, Horsfield K, Singhal SS, Cumming G. The proportion of lung vessels blocked by albumin microspheres. J Nucl Med 1973; 14: 579–581

13. Allen DR, Ferens JM, Cheney FW, Nelp WB. Critical evaluation of acute cardiopulmonary toxicity of microspheres. J Nucl Med 1987; 19: 1204–1208

14. Burdine JA, Ryder LA, Sonnemaker RE, DePuey G, Calderon M. ^{99m}Tc human albumin microspheres (HAM) for lung imaging. J Nucl Med 1971; 12: 127–130

15. Heck LL, Duley JW. Statistical considerations in lung imaging with ^{99m}Tc albumin particles. Radiology 1974; 113: 675–679

16. Dworkin HJ, Gutkowski RF, Porter W, Potter M. Effect of particle number on lung perfusion images: Concise communication. J Nucl Med; 1977; 18: 260–262

17. Barrington SF, O'Docherty MJ. Is perfusion lung scanning hazardous in pulmonary hypertension? Nucl Med Comm 1995; 16: 125–127

18. Heyman S. Toxicity and safety factors associated with lung perfusion studies with radiolabelled particles. J Nucl Med 1979; 20: 1098–1099

19. Bolster AA, Murray T, Hilditch TE. Contra-indications in the administration of ^{99m}Tc-labelled macroaggregates of albumin-any basis? Nucl Med Comm 1994; 15: 188–191

20. Rosenthall L. Human brain scanning with radio-iodinated macroaggregates of human serum albumin. Radiology 1965; 85: 110–114

21. Gates GF, Orme HW, Dore EK. Cardiac shunt assessment in children with macroaggregated albumin technetium-99m. Radiology 1974; 112: 649–653

22. Dogan AS, Rezai K, Kirchner PT, Stuhlmuller JE. A scintigraphic sign for detection of right-to left shunts. J Nucl Med 1993; 34: 1607–1611

23. Subramanian G, Arnold RW, Thomas FD, McAfee JG. Evaluation of an instant ^{99m}Tc-labeled lung scanning agent. J Nucl Med 1972; 13: 790

24. McAfee JG, Subramanian G. Radioactive agents for imaging. In: Freeman LM (ed). Freeman and Johnson's Clinical Radionuclide Imaging. Third edition. Grune & Stratton, Orlando 1984: 121–125

25. Zolle I, Rhodes BA, Wagner HN Jr. Properties and uses of radioactive albumin microspheres. J Nucl Med 1968; 9: 363

26. Murray T, Hilditch TE, Bolster AA, Elliott AT. Perfusion lung scanning in pulmonary hypertension. Nucl Med Comm 1995; 16: 621–622

27. Mallol J, Diaz RV. Particle size and its mathematical distribution in six human albumin macroaggregate (MAA) kits. Nucl Med Comm 1997; 18: 87–88

28. Norenberg JP, Hladik WB III. Radiopharmaceuticals for pulmonary imaging. In: Henkin RE, Boles MA, Dillehay GL, Halama JR, Karesh SM, Wagner RH, Zimmer AM (eds). Nuclear Medicine. Mosby, St Louis, 1996: 1362–1381

29. Callahan RJ, Swanson DP, Petry NA, Beightol RW, Vaillancourt J, Dragotakes SC. A multi-institutional in vitro evaluation of commercial ^{99m}Tc macroaggregated albumin kits. J Nucl Med Technol 1986; 14: 206–209

30. Robinson MS, Colas-Linhart NC, Guiraud-Vitaux FM, Petiet AM, Bok BD. Heterogeneous distribution of technetium-99m-labeled microspheres in rat lungs: microautoradiographic evidence and dosimetric consequences. J Nucl Med 1997; 38: 650–654

31. Malone LA, Malone JF, Ennis JT. Kinetics of technetium 99m labelled macroaggregated albumin in humans. Br J Radiol 1983; 56: 109–112

32. Marcus CS, Mason GR, Kuperus JH. Pulmonary imaging in pregnancy: maternal risk and fetal dosimetry. Clin Nucl Med 1985; 10: 1–4

33. Berke RA, Hoops EC, Kereiakes JC, Saenger EL. Radiation dose to breast-feeding child after mother has ^{99m}Tc-MAA lung scan. J Nucl Med 1973; 14: 51–52

34. Ahlgren L, Ivarsson S, Johansson L, Mattsson S, Nosslin B. Excretion of radionuclides in human breast milk after the administration of radiopharmaceuticals. J Nucl Med 1985; 26: 1085–1090

35. Morrell NW, Nijran KS, Jones BE, Biggs T, Seed WA. The underestimation of segmental defect size in radionuclide lung scanning. J Nucl Med 1993; 34: 370–374

36. Palla A, Tumeh SS, Nagel JS, Meyerowitz MF, Goldhaber SZ, Holman BL. Detection of pulmonary perfusion defects by single photon emission computed tomography (SPECT). J Nucl Med Allied Sci 1988; 32: 27–32

37. Corbus HF, Seitz JP, Larson RK, Stobbe DE, Wooten W, Sayre JW, Chavez RD, Unguez CE. Diagnostic usefulness of lung SPET in pulmonary thromboembolism: an outcome study. Nucl Med Comm 1997; 18: 897–906

38. Vanninen E, Tenhunen-Eskelinen M, Mussalo H, Toyry J, Laitinen T, Ahonen E, Lansimies E. Are three-dimensional surface-shaded SPET images better than planar and coronal SPET images in the assessment of regional pulmonary perfusion. Nucl Med Comm 1997; 18: 423–430

39. Almquist HM, Palmer J, Jonson B, Wollmer P. Pulmonary perfusion and density gradients in healthy volunteers. J Nucl Med 1997; 38: 962–966

40. Coakley AJ. Timing of VQ ventilation perfusion scanning. Eur J Nucl Med 1995; 22: 1099–1100

41. Knipping HW, Bolt W, Ventrath H, et al. Eine Neue Methode zur Prüfung der Herz- und Lungenfunktion die regionale Funktionsanalyse in der Lungen und Herzklinik mit Hilfe des Radioaktiven Edelgases Xenon 133 (isotopen-thorakographie). Deutsch Med Wochenschr 1955; 80: 1146–1147

42. The PIOPED Investigators. Value of the ventilation/perfusion scan in acute pulmonary embolism. Results of the prospective investigation of pulmonary embolism diagnosis (PIOPED). JAMA. 1990; 263; 2753–2759

43. McNeil BJ, Holman BL, Adelstein J. The scintigraphic diagnosis of pulmonary embolism. JAMA 1974; 227: 753–756

44. Alderson PO, Biello DR, Khan AR, Barth KH, McKnight RC, Siegel BA. Comparison of 133Xe single-breath and washout imaging in the scintigraphic diagnosis of pulmonary embolism. Radiology 1980; 137: 481–486

45. Bunow B, Line BR, Horton ME, Weiss GH. Regional ventilatory clearance by xenon scintigraphy: a critical evaluation of two estimation procedures. J Nucl Med 1979; 20: 703–710

46. Secker-Walker RH. Pulmonary physiology, pathology, and ventilation-perfusion studies. J Nucl Med 1978; 19: 961–968

47. Alderson PO, Biello DR, Sachariah KG, Siegel BA. Scintigraphic detection of pulmonary embolism in patients with obstructive pulmonary disease. Radiology; 1981; 138: 661–666

48. Alderson PO, Lee H, Summer WR, Motazedi A, Wagner HN Jr. Comparison of Xe-133 washout and single-breath imaging for the detection of ventilation abnormalities. J Nucl Med 1979; 20: 917–922

49. Alderson PO, Secker-Walker RH, Forrest JV. Detection of obstructive pulmonary disease: relative sensitivity of ventilation-perfusion studies and chest radiography. Radiology 1974; 112: 643–648

50. Kipper MS, Alazraki N. The feasibility of performing 133Xe ventilation imaging following the perfusion study. Radiology 1982; 144: 581–586

51. Atkins HL, Robertson JS, Croft BY, Tsui B, Susskind H, Ellis KJ, Loken MK, Treves S. Estimates of radiation absorbed doses from radioxenons in lung imaging. J Nucl Med 1980; 21: 459–465

52. Prohovnik I, Metz CD, Atkins HL. Radiation exposure to human trachea from Xenon-133 procedures. J Nucl Med 1995; 36: 1458–1461

53. Goris ML, Daspit SG, Walter JP, McRae J, Lamb J. Applications of ventilation lung imaging with 81m Krypton. Radiology 1977; 122: 399–403

54. Atkins HL, Susskind H, Klopper JF, Ansari AN, Richards P, Fairchild RG. A clinical comparison of Xe-127 and Xe-133 for ventilation studies. J Nucl Med 1977; 18: 653–659

55. Hastings DL, Jeans SP, Wall WHJ, Hall BJ, Miller DE. The effect on diagnostic quality of using dual isotope imaging for 81mKr ventilation and 99mTc-MAA perfusion lung scanning. Nucl Med Comm 1995; 16: 281–289

56. Schor RA, Shames DM, Weber PM, Dos Remedios LV. Regional ventilation studies with 81mKr and Xe-133: a comparative analysis. J Nucl Med 1978; 19: 348–353

57. Newman SP. Therapeutic aerosols. In: Clarke SW, Pavia D (eds). Aerosols and the Lung: Clinical and Experimental Aspects. Butterworth, London 1984: 197–224

58. O'Callaghan C, Barry PW. The science of nebulised drug delivery. Thorax 1997; 52: S31–S44

59. Bennet WD, Smaldone GC. Human variation in the peripheral air-space deposition of inhaled particles. J Appl Physiol 1985; 59: 1603–1610

60. Smaldone GC, Messina MS. Flow limitation, cough, and patterns of aerosol deposition in humans. J Appl Physiol 1985; 59: 515–520

61. Taplin GV, Poe ND. A dual lung scanning technic for evaluation of pulmonary function. Radiology 1965; 85: 365–368

62. Pircher FJ, Temple JR, Kirsch WT. Distribution of pulmonary ventilation determined by radioisotope scanning. Am J Roentgenol 1965; 94: 807–814

63. Alderson PO, Biello DR, Gottschalk A, Hoffer PB, Kroop SA, Lee ME, Ramanna L, Siegel BA, Waxman AD. Tc-99m-DTPA aerosol and radioactive gases compared as adjuncts to perfusion scintigraphy in patients with suspected pulmonary embolism. Radiology 1984; 153: 515–521

64. White PG, Hayward MWJ, Cooper T. Ventilation agents – what agents are currently used? Nucl Med Comm 1991; 12: 349–352

65. Dolovich MB, Cockcroft DW, Coates G. Aerosols in diagnosis: ventilation, airway penetrance, epithelial permeability, mucociliary transport and airway responsiveness. In: Moren F, Dolovitch MB, Newhouse MT, Newman SP (eds). Aerosols in Medicine, Principles, Diagnosis and Therapy. Elsevier Science Publishers, 1993: 195–234

66. Mountford PJ, Hall FM, Wells CP, Coackley AJ. Breast-milk after a Tc-99m DTPA aerosol/Tc-99m MAA lung study. J Nucl Med 1984; 25: 1108–1110

67. Mackie A, Hart GC, Ibbett DA, Whitehead RJS. Airborne radioactive contamination following aerosol ventilation studies. Nucl Med Comm 1994; 15: 161–167

68. Belton IP, Burford D, Early MY. A risk assessment of multiple use of an aerosol system compared with single use for lung ventilation scans. Nucl Med Comm 1997; 18: 680–685

69. Burch WM, Sullivan PJ, McLaren CJ. Technegas – a new ventilation agent for lung scanning. Nucl Med Comm 1986; 7: 865–871

70. Mackey DWJ, Burch WM, Dance IG, Fisher KJ, Willett GD. The observation of fullerenes in a Technegas lung ventilation unit. Nucl Med Comm 1994; 15: 430–434

71. Strong JC, Agnew JE. The particle size distribution of technegas and its influence on regional lung deposition. Nucl Med Comm 1989; 10: 425–430

72. Lloyd JJ, James JM, Shields RA, Testa HJ. The influence of inhalation technique on Technegas particle deposition and image appearance in normal volunteers. Eur J Nucl Med 1994; 21: 394–398

73. James JM, Lloyd JJ, Leahy BC, Church S, Hardy CC, Shields RA, Prescott MC, Testa HJ. ^{99m}Tc-Technegas and krypton-81m ventilation scintigraphy: A comparison in known respiratory disease. Br J Radiol 1992; 65: 1075–1082

74. Sullivan PJ, Burke WM, Burch WM, Lomas FE. A clinical comparison of technegas and xenon-133 in 50 patients with suspected pulmonary embolism. Chest 1988; 94: 300–304

75. James JM, Herman KJ, Lloyd JJ, Shields RA, Testa HJ, Church S, Stretton TB. Evaluation of ^{99m}Tc technegas ventilation scintigraphy in the diagnosis of pulmonary embolism. Br J Radiol 1991; 64: 711–719

76. Cook G, Clarke SEM. An evaluation of Technegas as a ventilation agent compared with krypton-81m in the scintigraphic diagnosis of pulmonary embolism. Eur J Nucl Med 1992; 19: 770–774

77. James JM, Lloyd JJ, Leahy BC, Shields RA, Prescott MC, Testa HJ. The incidence and severity of hypoxia associated with ^{99m}Tc-Technegas ventilation scintigraphy and ^{99m}Tc-MAA perfusion scintigraphy. Br J Radiol 1992; 65: 403–408

78. Burch WM. Evidence for the long-term biological distribution of Technegas particles. Nucl Med Comm 1993; 14: 559–561

79. Lusted L.B. Introduction to Medical Decision Making. C.C. Thomas Publisher, Springfield, Illinois 1968

80. Schwartz WB. Decision analysis. A look at the chief complaints. N Engl J Med 1979; 300: 556–559

81. Hull RD, Raskob GE. Low Probability Lung Scan Findings: A Need for Change. Ann Intern Med 1991; 114: 142–143

82. Moser KM. Venous Thromboembolism. Am Rev Respir Dis. 1990; 141: 235–249

83. Bone RC. The Low Probability Lung Scan: Potentially Lethal Reading. Arch Int Med 1993; 153: 2621–2622

84. Gray HW, Bessent RG. Pulmonary embolism exclusion: A practical approach to low probability using the PIOPED data. Eur J Nucl Med 1998; 25: 271–276

85. Sox HC, Blatt MA, Higgins MC, Marton KI. Medical Decision Making. Butterworths, 1988

86. Tversky A, Kahneman D. Judgement under Uncertainty: Heuristics and Biases. Biases in judgements reveal some heuristics of thinking under uncertainty. Science 1974: 185: 1124–1131

87. Stein PD, Terrin ML, Hales CA, Palevsky HI, Saltzman HA, Taylor Thompson B, Weg JG. Clinical, Laboratory, Roentgenographic and Electrocardiographic Findings in Patients with Acute Pulmonary Embolism and no pre-existing Cardiac or Pulmonary Disease. Chest 1991; 100; 598–603

88. Freitas JE, Sarosi MG, Nagle CC, Yeomans ME, Freitas AE, Juni JE. Modified PIOPED Criteria Used in Clinical Practice. J Nucl Med 1995; 36; 1573–1578

89. Bryant GD, Norman GR. Expressions of probability: Words and Numbers. New Engl J Med 1980; 302: 411

90. Gray HW, McKillop JH, Bessent RG. Lung scan reports interpretation by clinicians. Nuc Med Commun 1993; 14: 989–994

91. Sostman HD, Coleman RE, DeLong DM, Newman GE, Paine S. Evaluation of revised Criteria for Ventilation Perfusion Scintigraphy in Patients with Suspected Pulmonary Embolism. Radiology 1994; 193; 103–107

92. Freeman LM. The Low Probability VQ Lung Scan: Can its Credibility Be Enhanced? J Nucl Med 1996; 37: 582–584

93. Lubsen J. Essentials of Bayesian Diagnostic Reasoning. Netherlands J Med 1995; 47: 252–259

94. Sox HC. Probability Theory in the Use of Diagnostic Tests. Ann Int Med 1986; 104; 60–66

95. Griner PF, Mayewski RJ, Mushlin AI, Greenland P. Selection and interpretation of Diagnostic Tests and Procedures. Ann Int Med 1981; 94, 4 (Part 2): 553–600

96. Urokinase Pulmonary Embolism Trial Study Group: Urokinase pulmonary embolism trial phase 1 results. A cooperative study. JAMA 1970; 214: 2163–2172

97. De Nardo GL, Goodwin DA, Ravasini R, et al. The Ventilatory Lung Scan in the Diagnosis of Pulmonary Embolism. N Engl J Med 1970; 282: 1334–1336

98. McNeil BJ. A Diagnostic Strategy Using Ventilation Perfusion Studies in Patients Suspect of Pulmonary Embolism. J Nucl Med 1976; 17: 613–616

99. McNeil BJ. Ventilation-Perfusion Studies and the Diagnosis of Pulmonary Embolism: Concise Communication. J Nucl Med 1980; 21: 319–323

100. Biello DR, Mattar AG, McNight RC, et al. Ventilation Perfusion Studies in Suspected Pulmonary Embolism. Am J Roentgenol 1979; 133: 1033–1037

101. Carter WD, Brady TM, Keyes JW, et al. Relative Accuracy of Two Diagnostic Schemes for Detection of Pulmonary Embolism by Ventilation Perfusion Scintigraphy. Radiology 1982; 145: 447–451

102. Cheely R, McCartney WH, Perry JR, et al. The Role of Non-invasive Tests Versus Pulmonary Angiography in the Diagnosis of Pulmonary Embolism. Am J Med 1981; 70: 17–22

103. Alderson PO, Biello DR, Sachariah KG, et al. Scintigraphic Detection of Pulmonary Embolism in Patients with Obstructive Pulmonary Disease. Radiology 1981; 138: 661–666

104. Spies WG, Burstein SP, Dillehay GL, et al. Ventilation Perfusion Scintigraphy in Suspected Pulmonary Embolism: Correlation with Pulmonary Angiography and Refinement of Criteria for Interpretation. Radiology 1986; 159: 383–390

105. Rosen JM, Biello DR, Siegal BA, et al. Kr-81m ventilation imaging: Clinical utility in suspected pulmonary embolism. Radiology 1985; 154: 787–790

106. Sullivan DC, Coleman RE, Mills SR. Lung Scan Interpretation: Effect of Different Observers and different Criteria. Radiology 1983; 149: 803–807

107. Biello DR, Mattar AG, Osei-Wusu A, et al. Interpretation of indeterminate lung scintigrams. Radiology 1979; 133: 189–194

108. Hull RD, Hirsh J, Carter CJ, et al. Pulmonary angiography, ventilation lung scanning and venography for clinically suspected pulmonary embolism with abnormal perfusion lung scan. Ann Int Med 1983; 98: 891–899

109. Hull RD, Hirsh J, Carter CJ, et al. Diagnostic value of ventilation perfusion lung scanning in patients with suspected pulmonary embolism. Chest 1985; 88: 819–828

110. Hull RD, Raskob GE. Low probability lung scan findings: a need for change. Ann Int Med 1991; 114: 142–143

111. Lowe VJ, Bullard G, Coleman RE. VQ lung scan probability category distribution in university and community hospitals. J Nucl Med 1993; 34: 17P

112. Neumann RD, Sostman HD, Gottschalk A. Current status of ventilation perfusion imaging. Semin Nucl Med 1980; 10: 198–217

113. Gottschalk A, Juni JE, Sostman HD, et al. Ventilation-perfusion scintigraphy in the PIOPED study. Part 2. Evaluation of the scintigraphic criteria and interpretations. J Nucl Med 1993; 34: 1119–1126

114. Stein PD, Terrin ML, Hales CA, et al. Clinical, laboratory, roentgenographic and electrocardiographic findings in patients with acute pulmonary embolism and no pre-existing cardiac or pulmonary disease. Chest 1991; 100: 598–603

115. Stein PD, Coleman RE, Gottschalk A, et al. Diagnostic utility of ventilation perfusion lung scans in acute pulmonary embolism is not diminished by pre-existing cardiac or pulmonary disease. Chest 1991; 100: 604–606

116. Sostman HD, Gottschalk A. Prospective validation of the stripe sign in ventilation perfusion scintigraphy. Radiology 1992; 184: 455–459

117. Quinn DA, Thompson BT, Terrin ML, et al. A prospective investigation of pulmonary embolism in women and men. JAMA 1992; 268: 1689–1696

118. Stein PD, Athanasoulis C, Alavi A, et al. Complications and validity of pulmonary angiography in acute pulmonary embolism. Circulation 1992; 85: 462–468

119. Stein PD, Terrin ML, Gottschalk A, et al. Value of ventilation/perfusion scans versus perfusion scans alone in acute pulmonary embolism. Am J Cardiol 1992; 69: 1239–1241

120. Lesser A, Leeper KV, Stein PD, et al. Diagnosis of acute pulmonary embolism in patients with chronic obstructive pulmonary disease. Chest 1992; 102: 17–22

121. Stein PD, Gottschalk A, Henry JW, et al. Stratification of patients according to prior cardiopulmonary disease and probability assessment based on the number of mismatched segmental equivalent perfusion defects. Chest 1993; 104: 1461–1467

122. Stein PD, Henry JW, Gottschalk A. The addition of clinical assessment to stratification according to prior cardiopulmonary disease further optimises the interpretation of ventilation perfusion lung scans in pulmonary embolism. Chest 1993; 104: 1472–1476

123. Worsley DF, Alavi A, Aronchic JM, et al. Chest radiographic findings in patients with acute pulmonary embolism. Observations from the PIOPED study. Radiology 1993; 189: 133–136

124. Worsley DF, Kim CK, Alavi A, et al. Detailed analysis of patients with matched ventilation perfusion defects and chest radiographic opacities. J Nucl Med 1993; 34: 1851–1853

125. Stein PD, Henry JW, Gottschalk A. Mismatched vascular defects. An easy alternative to mismatched segmental equivalent defects for the interpretation of ventilation perfusion lung scans in pulmonary embolism. Chest 1993; 104: 1468–1472

126. Patil S, Henry JW, Rubenfire M, et al. Neural network in the clinical diagnosis of acute pulmonary embolism. Chest 1993; 104: 1685–1689

127. Worsley DF, Alavi A, Palevsky HI. Role of radionuclide imaging in patients with suspected pulmonary embolism. Rad Clinics N Am 1993; 31: 849–858

128. Worsley DF, Palevsky HI, Alavi A. A detailed evaluation of patients with acute pulmonary embolism and low or very low probability lung sacn interpretations. Arch Int Med 1994; 154: 2737–2741

129. Worsley DF, Alavi A. Comprehensive analysis of the results of the PIOPED study. J Nucl Med 1995; 36: 2380–2387

130. Tourassi GD, Floyd CE, Sostman HD, et al. Artificial neural network for diagnosis of acute pulmonary embolism: Effect of case and observer selection. Radiology 1995; 194: 889–893

131. Stein PD, Henry JW, Relyea B. Untreated patients with pulmonary embolism. Outcome, clinical and laboratory assessment. Chest 1995; 107: 931–935

132. Stein PD, Henry JW, Gopalakrishman D, et al. Asymmetry of the calves in the assessment of patients with suspected acute pulmonary embolism. Chest 1995; 107: 936–939

133. Stein PD, Hull RD, Pineo G. Strategy that includes serial non-invasive leg tests for diagnosis of thromboembolic disease in patients with suspected acute pulmonary embolism based on data from PIOPED. Arch Int Med 1995; 155: 2101–2104

134. Henry JW, Relyea B, Stein PD. Continuing risk of thromboembolism among patients with normal pulmonary angiograms. Chest 1995; 107: 1375–1378

135. Henry JW, Stein PD, Gottschalk A. Pulmonary embolism among patients with a nearly normal ventilation/perfusion lung scan. Chest 1996; 110: 395–398

136. Stein PD, Relyea B, Gottschalk A. Evaluation of individual criteria for low probability interpretation of ventilation/perfusion lung scans. J Nucl Med 1996; 37: 577–581

137. Gottschalk A, Stein PD, Henry JW, et al. Can pulmonary angiography be limited to the most suspicious side if the contralateral side appears normal on the ventilation/perfusion lung scan. Chest 1996; 110: 392–394

138. Henry JW, Stein PD, Gottschalk A, et al. Scintigraphic lung scans and clinical assessment in critically ill patients with suspected acute pulmonary embolism. Chest 1996; 109: 462–466

139. Worsley DF, Alavi A, Palevsky HI, et al. Comparison of diagnostic performance with ventilation perfusion lung imaging in different patient populations. Radiology 1996; 199: 481–483

140. Stein PD, Goldhaber SZ, Henry JW, et al. Arterial blood gas analysis in the assessment in suspected acute pulmonary embolism. Chest 1996; 109: 78–81

141. Gottschalk A. Patient stratification by cardiopulmonary status in the diagnosis of pulmonary embolism. J Nucl Med 1996; 37: 570–572

142. Gottschalk A, Stein PD, Henry JW, et al. Matched ventilation perfusion and chest radiographic abnormalities in acute pulmonary embolism. J Nucl Med 1996; 37: 1636–1638

143. Stein PD, Henry JW, Gottschalk A. Small perfusion defects in suspected pulmonary embolism. J Nucl Med 1996; 37: 1313–1316

144. Stein PD, Relyea B, Gottschalk A. Evaluation of individual criteria for low probability interpretation of ventilation-perfusion lung scans. J Nucl Med 1996; 37: 577–581

145. Breslaw BH, Dorfman GS, Noto RB, et al. Ventilation/perfusion scanning for prediction of the location of pulmonary emboli: Correlation with pulmonary angiographic findings. Radiology 1992; 185(P): 180

146. Miniati M, Pistolesi M, Marini C, et al. Value of Perfusion Lung Scan in the Diagnosis of Pulmonary Embolism: Results of the Prospective Investigative Study of Acute Pulmonary Embolism Diagnosis (PISA-PED). Am J Respir Crit Care Med 1996; 154: 1387–1393

147. Alderson PO, Martin EC. Pulmonary Embolism: Diagnosis with Multiple Imaging Modalities. Radiology 1987; 164: 297–312

148. Wellman HN. Pulmonary Thromboembolism: Current Status Report on the Role of Nuclear Medicine. Semin Nucl Med 1986; 4: 236–274

149. Perrier A, Junod AF. Has the diagnosis of pulmonary embolism become easier to establish? Respiratory Medicine 1995; 89: 241–251

150. Stein PD, Willis PW, Dalen JE. Importance of Clinical Assessment in Selecting Patients for Pulmonary Angiography. Am J Cardiol 1979; 43: 669–671

151. Price L, Dunn M. Editorial: Are Modifications Necessary in the Performance of Pulmonary Angiography. Chest 1985; 88: 1–2

152. Kipper MS, Moser KM, Kartman KE, et al. Longterm follow up of patients with suspected pulmonary embolism and a normal lung scan. Chest 1982; 82: 411–415

153. Hull RD, Raskob GE, Coates G, et al. A new non-invasive management strategy for patients with suspected pulmonary embolism. Arch Int Med 1989; 149: 2549–2555

154. Hull RD, Raskob GE, Coates G, et al. Clinical validity of a normal perfusion lung scan in patients with suspected pulmonary embolism. Chest 1990; 97: 23–26

155. Sostman HD, Neuman RD, Gottschalk A. Evaluation of Patients with Suspected Venous Thromboembolism. In: Sandler MP, Patton JA, Coleman RE, Gottschalk A, Wackers FJTh, Hoffer HB (eds.). Diagnostic Nuclear Medicine. 3rd Edition. Williams and Williams, 1996: 585–612

156. McDougall IR, Goris ML, Kriss JP. Pulmonary Embolism (letter). Ann Int Med 1978; 88: 711

157. McNeill BJ, Bettman MA. The diagnosis of pulmonary embolism. In: Coleman RW, Hirsh J, Marder V, Salyman EW (eds). Haemostasis and Thrombosis. JB Lippincott, Philadelphia 1982: 857–871

158. Alderson PO, Rujanavech N, Secker-Walker RH, et al. The role of 133Xe ventilation studies in the scintigraphic detection of pulmonary embolism. Radiology 1976; 120: 633–640

159. Van Beek EJR, Tiel-van Buul MMC, Hoefnagel CA, et al. Reporting of perfusion/ventilation lung scintigraphy using an anatomical lung segment chart: a prospective study. Nucl Med Comm 1994; 15: 746–751

160. Neumann RD, Sostman HD, Gottschalk A. Current status of ventilation perfusion imaging. Semin Nucl Med 1980; 10: 198–217

161. Morrell NW, Nijran KS, Jones BE, et al. The underestimation of segmental defect size in radionuclide scanning. J Nucl Med 1993; 34: 370–374

162. Alderson PO, Doppman JL, Diamond SS, et al. Ventilation perfusion lung imaging and selective pulmonary angiography in dogs with experimental pulmonary embolism. J Nucl Med 1978; 19: 164–171

163. Alderson PO, Biello DR, Sachariah G, et al. Scintigraphic Detection of Pulmonary Embolism in Patients with Obstructive Pulmonary Disease. Radiology 1981; 138: 661–666

164. Kim CK, Worsely DF, Alavi A. "Ventilation (V)/Perfusion (Q)/chest X-ray" match is less likely to represent pulmonary embolism if Q is only "decreased" rather than "absent". J Nucl Med 1993; 34: 17P

165. Kotlyarov EV, Ruppel WF, Reba RC. Interpretation of perfusion lung scan based on presence and absence of "stripe sign". Invest Radiol 1983; 18: 515

166. Alderson PO, Dzebelo NN, Biello DR. Serial lung scintigraphy: utility in diagnosis of pulmonary embolism. Radiology 1983; 149: 797–802

167. Gottschalk A, Juni JE, Sostman HD, et al. Ventilation-perfusion scintigraphy in the PIOPED study. Part 2. Evaluation of the scintigraphic criteria and interpretations. J Nucl Med 1993; 34: 1119–1126

168. Isawa T, Taplin GV, Beazell J, et al. Experimental Unilateral Pulmonary Artery Occlusion. Acute and Chronic Effects on Relative Ventilation and Perfusion. Radiology 1972; 102: 101–109

169. De Berg JC, Pauwels EKJ. Lung scintigraphy: it could have been easier. Eur J Nucl Med 1993; 20: 93–95

170. Greenspan RH, Ravin CF, Polansky SM, McLoud TC. Accuracy of the chest radiograph in diagnosis of pulmonary embolism. Invest Radiol 1982; 17: 539–543

171. Rosenow EC III, Osmundson PJ, Brown ML. Pulmonary Embolism. Mayo Clin Proc 1981; 56: 161–178

172. Herlev Hospital Study Group. Diagnostic Decision Process in Suspected Pulmonary Embolism. Lancet 1979; 1: 1336–1338

173. ACCP Consensus Committee on Pulmonary Embolism. Opinions Regarding the Diagnosis and Management of Venous Thromboembolic Disease. Chest 1996; 109: 233–237

174. Li DK, Seltzer SE, McNeil BJ. VQ Mismatches Unassociated with Pulmonary Embolism: Case report and review of the Literature. J Nucl Med 1978; 19: 1331–1333

175. Van Beek EJR, Tiel-van-Buul MMC, Buller HR, et al. The Value of Lung Scintigraphy in the Diagnosis of Pulmonary Embolism. Eur J Nucl Med 1993; 20: 173–181

176. British Thoracic Society Standards of Care Committee, Suspected acute pulmonary embolism: a practical approach. Thorax. 1997; 52: S1–S24

177. Freeman LM. The Low Probability VQ Lung Scan: Can its Credibility Be Enhanced? J Nucl Med 1996; 37: 582–584

178. Hansell DM. Spiral Computed Tomography and Pulmonary Embolism: Current State. Clin Radiol 1997; 52: 575–581

179. Michel BC, Seerden RJ, Rutten FFH, et al. The Cost-Effectiveness of Diagnostic Strategies in Patients with Suspected Pulmonary Embolism. Health Economics 1996; 5: 307–318

180. Stein PD, Hull RD, Saltzman HA, et al. Strategy for Diagnosis of Patients with Suspected Pulmonary Embolism. Chest 1993; 103: 1553–1559

181. Gray HW, McKillop JH, Bessent RG. Lung scan reporting language: what does it mean? Nuc Med Com 1993; 14: 1084–1087

182. Wheeler HB, Andeson FA Jn, Cardullo PA, et al. Suspected deep vein thrombosis. Arch Surg 1982; 117: 1206–1209

183. Hull RD, Rascob G, Ginsberg J, et al. A non-invasive strategy for the treatment of patients with suspected pulmonary embolism. Arch Intern Med 1994; 154: 289–297

184. Huisman MV, Buller HR, Ten Cate JW, Vreeken J. Serial impedance plethysmography for suspected deep venous thrombosis in outpatients: The Amsterdam general practitioners study. N Engl J Med 1986; 314: 823–828

185. Smith LL, Iber C, Sirrs S. Pulmonary embolism: confirmation with venous duplex US as adjunct to lung scanning. Radiology 1994; 191: 143–147

186. Goodman LR, Lipchick RJ. Diagnosis of acute pulmonary embolism: time for a new approach. Radiology 1996; 199: 25–27

187. Bounameaux H, De Moerloose P, Perrier A, et al. D-dimer testing in suspected venous thromboembolism: an update. Q J Med 1997; 90: 437–442

188. Perrier A, Bounameaux H, Morabia A, et al. Contribution of D-dimer plasma measurement and lower-limb venous ultrasound to the diagnosis of pulmonary embolism: a decision analysis model. Am Heart J 1994; 127: 624–635

189. Goldhaber SZ, Simons GR, Elliot CG, et al. Quantitative plasma D-dimer levels among patients undergoing pulmonary angiography for suspected pulmonary embolism. JAMA 1993; 270: 2819–2822

190. Stein PV, Hull RD, Pineo G. Strategy That Includes Serial Non-invasive Leg Tests for Diagnosis of Thromboembolic Disease in Patients with Suspected Acute Pulmonary Embolism Based on Data From PIOPED. Arch Intern Med 1995; 155: 2101–2104

191. Oudkerk M, Van Beek EJR, Van Putten WLJ, et al. Cost-effectiveness analysis of various strategies in the diagnostic management of pulmonary embolism. Arch Intern Med 1993; 153: 947–954

IV.2 Echocardiography in pulmonary embolism – transthoracic, transoesophageal, and intravascular ultrasound

G. Görge, Ch. Bruch, R. Erbel

Introduction

Acute massive pulmonary embolism (PE) is an often missed but significant disease, with an estimated 2,000 cases diagnosed per 1,000,000 inhabitants in the western countries each year. The estimated prevalence of acute PE among 51,645 hospitalised patients was 1% and PE in hospitalised patients contributed to or caused death in 0.2% [1]. The incidence of clinically unrecognised PE has not diminished during three decades, despite advances in non-invasive diagnosis. Even fatal PE is not diagnosed in 51–70% of cases confirmed by the post mortem [2]. However, in most patients dying from PE in the hospital, co-morbid disease is present and many have a poor prognosis even before PE [3]. However, few other acute illnesses exist that take such a high death toll in patients already in the hospital.

It has been estimated that most deaths occur during the first two hours after the initial event. Therefore, rapid diagnosis and the prompt initiation of appropriate therapy are crucial for the prognosis of the patients. Unfortunately, the present diagnostic strategies are often time-consuming and also often require transportation of the patients to other wards or diagnostic facilities.

Clinical diagnosis

The clinical diagnosis of PE is often cumbersome (see Chapter II). The reason is that most clinical signs are variable and non-specific. The low oxygen content in acute massive PE, the low cardiac output, and bronchoconstriction explain most of the clinical symptoms [4, 5].

Physical examination

Tachycardia and shortness of breath are found most often. Intermitted tachyarrythmias may also be signs of recurrent embolic events. Pleuritic pain and hemoptoe are usually late signs and found most often in patients with impaired left ventricular function. The same is true for the occurrence of pulmonary infiltrates [6]. Although the source of embolism is most often the venous system of the legs and the groin, clinical signs of venous thrombosis are often absent in patients with PE. During the clinical examination, a gallop-rhythm over the right heart and a pronounced second heart sound with punctum maximum over the pulmonary valve may be found.

Electrocardiogram

The electrocardiogram is usually inconclusive, because tachycardia and non-specific ST-segment changes are found most frequently, while a shift towards the right axis or an incomplete or complete right bundle branch block is found in less than 1/3 of cases. The ECG, however, is important to exclude other diseases with a similar clinical presentation, especially acute myocardial infarction [6].

Blood gas analysis

Blood gas analysis under room air is usually not impaired in smaller PE. However, a pO_2 of > 65 mmHg under room air excludes a $> 50\%$ obstruction of the pulmonary circulation with a probability of 85% [7].

Chest X-rays

The chest X-ray is also non-specific for the diagnosis of PE. It is useful to enhance the specificity of the ventilation-perfusion scans of the lungs and to exclude a pneumothorax or other pulmonary diseases as causes of the symptoms [6].

Pulmonary angiography

Angiography is an invasive method that gives a rapid and complete image of the entire pulmonary circulation, yet it need not be performed in all patients with suspected PE to establish the definitive diagnosis (as described in Chapter IV.3).

While the value of angiography in the detection of a complete obstruction is uniformly accepted, the imaging of partially occluded vessel segments has been prone to misinterpretation [8, 9]. Flow in pulmonary arteries may be assessed using intravascular ultrasound probes [10]. As a contour method, angiography cannot be adequate in the visualisation of soft, wall-adherent thrombus formation. For this indication, angioscopy is the gold standard [11].

Computed tomography

A relatively new but very promising technique in the diagnosis of patients with PE is spiral CT [12–14] or contrast enhanced electron beam computed tomography (EBCT) [15, 16]. These techniques are discussed in Chapter IV.6 and IV.7.

D-dimer

The identification of D-dimer in a whole blood assay by bispecific antibodies with epiotopes for portions of the D-dimer and erythrocytes allows the identification of patients with venous thrombosis of any location [17–20]. Thus, although large prospective trials are not published as yet, the estimation of D-dimer allows for categorisation of patients with and without venous thrombus (see Chapter II).

Venous compression and Duplex sonography

Non-invasive leg tests for venous thrombosis have been discussed in Chapter III.1. It should be remembered that a negative non-invasive leg test does not exclude acute PE.

Scintigraphic assessment

As discussed in Chapter IV.1, lung scintigraphy is highly sensitive for PE and perfusion scans allow exclusion of the disease. However, the specificity of lung scintigraphy is rather low. These findings underline the need for a rapid bedside diagnostic test, that allows visualisation of pulmonary emboli and the assessment of the right ventricular afterload.

Echocardiography in pulmonary hypertension

Transthoracic echocardiography usually makes it possible to determine non-invasively the pulmonary artery pressure, the right ventricular volumes and function, and thus the hemodynamic consequences of a pulmonary embolus [21]. Transesophageal echocardiography has the additional advantage of directly identifying pulmonary artery embolism in a high percentage of patients [22, 23]. Thus, echocardiography, as a bedside technique, makes the diagnosis of a PE easier and faster [24, 25]. Patients identified as having hemodynamically relevant embolic events can be treated early by full-dose heparin and, if needed, by thrombolytic agents.

Intravascular ultrasound (IVUS) is a new invasive echo-based technique allowing imaging of the lumen and the vessel wall in patients with various forms of pulmonary hypertension [10, 26, 27].

Transthoracic echocardiography(TTE)

Transthoracic echocardiography is available around the clock in most hospitals [28]. Unlike other imaging devices in pulmonary hypertension, the echo console can be brought to the patient, not the patient to the machine. Transthoracic echocardiography can directly show thrombus forma-

G. Görge, Ch. Bruch, R. Erbel

tion within the right heart chambers or the pulmonary arteries or thrombus in transit. Acute and chronic pulmonary hypertension can be distinguished by the thickness of the right ventricular free wall (thinned in acute, hypertrophic in chronic pressure overload) and by estimation of the pulmonary artery systolic pressure (see below) [21, 24]. In acute PE without previous obstruction of the pulmonary circulation, maximum pressures almost never exceed 35–40 mmHg. The reason is that the relatively muscle-weak right ventricle cannot obtain higher pressures acutely.

TTE has the advantage of being-non invasive. The echo-transducer (usually 2.25–5 MHz) is placed in the 4th or the 5th left intercostal space, at the apex of the heart, and positioned in the jugular in some patients, for suprasternal images. The apical four chamber view is the most valuable, because it allows estimation of the size of the right and left heart chambers and estimation of the gradient over the tricuspid valve by continuous Doppler examination. Pulmonary emboli can be seen either directly or indirectly.

Direct echocardiographic signs of pulmonary hypertension are (Figs. 1a–c):

- Thrombus in the pulmonary artery or arteries
- Thrombus in the heart itself or thrombus "in transit"

Indirect echocardiographic signs of pulmonary hypertension are (Figs. 2a–c):

- Elevated pulmonary artery pressure in patients with tricuspid insufficiency
- Dilatation of the right atrium, with or without dilatation of the right ventricle
- Compression of the left ventricle
- Paradoxical motion of the septum
- Increased isovolumetric relaxation time of the right ventricle
- Shortening of the pulmonary artery acceleration time
- Hypertrophy of the right ventricle in primary pulmonary hypertension or in recurrent embolic events.

The estimation of the systolic pulmonary artery pressure is calculated as follows:

Systolic pulmonary artery pressure $= 4 \cdot V^2_{max} + 10$ mmHg

("Plus 10 mmHg" is the estimated right atrial pressure. In case of exact measurements of the right atrial pressure, e. g. in case of a central venous line, this value should be used.)

In case of poor signal quality, the addition of echo-contrast agents injected into a peripheral vein or a

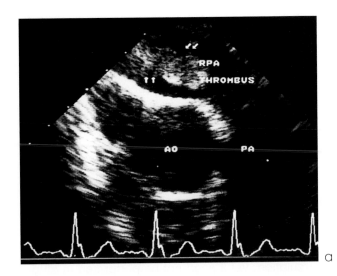

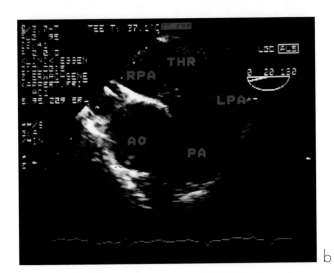

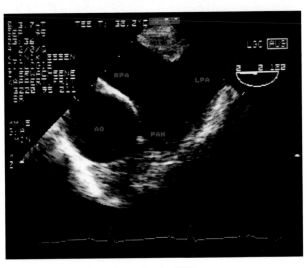

Fig. 1a–c. Transesophageal echo (TEE) images in a patient with PE, resuscitation and prolonged cardiogenic shock. Upper image: The pulmonary (PA) bifurcation and the aorta (AO) are shown. **(a)** In the right PA (RPA) a free-floating, highly mobile thrombus is indicated by the arrows. After thrombolytic therapy, the thrombus gets smaller **(b)** and is finally completely resolved **(c)**. (Modified with permission from [36]).

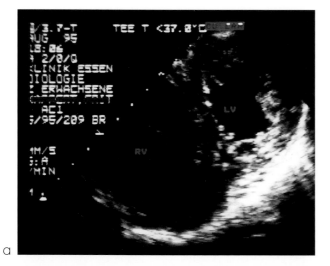

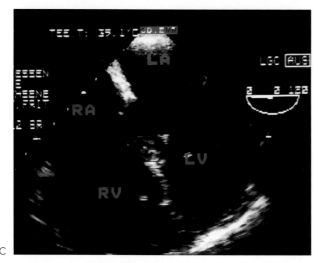

Fig. 2a–c. Effects of thrombolytic therapy on right and left ventricle dimensions assessed by TEE (Same patient as in Figure 1c). In the acute setting **(a)**, massive dilatation of the right ventricle (RV) and small, hypercontractile left ventricle (LV). Shortly after thrombolysis, the right ventricle becomes smaller, and the left ventricle shows improved filling **(b)**. **(c)** Same dimensions of the left and right ventricle (LV, RV) and the left and right atria (LA, RA) several days later. (Modified with permission from [46]).

central catheter will improve the Doppler signal quality in most patients.

Beside the estimation of systolic pulmonary artery pressure by tricuspid regurgitation, the diagnostic value of the "right ventricular isovolumetric relaxation time", and the "acceleration time" (AcT) have been estimated in patients with pulmonary artery embolism. Table 1 gives an overview of the results of various groups that compared echo parameters to invasive pressure measurements [24, 25].

Dilatation of the right ventricle can be found in 71–100% of patients with acute PE (Figs. 2a, b and c). Compression of the left ventricle is found in 38%, and paradoxical movement of the septum in 42% of patients with acute PE. Additionally, enlargement of the right pulmonary artery can be found in 72% of all patients with otherwise proven PE [29, 30]. The suprasternal approach allows the best visualisation of the pulmonary artery. In a comparative study of patients with proven PE, a tricuspid peak regurgitant velocity > 2.5 m/sec was found in 84% of cases, compared to 10% in the control group. An enlarged right ventricle (> 25 mm) was found in 67% of all patients with PE but only in 11% of all controls. The values for echocardiographic septum motion abnormalities were 42% versus 9%, respectively. A typical S1-Q3 ECG pattern was found in only 30% of all patients with PE [31].

No signs of elevated pulmonary artery pressure excludes any form of massive PE, but not minor ones. However, the latter patient group is characterised by a good short-term prognosis. In a recent survey in a total of 1,001 consecutive patients with suspected PE, the role of echocardiography for decision-making was compared to other techniques. Echocardiography was the most frequently performed diagnostic procedure (74%). Lung scan or pulmonary angiography were performed in 79% of clinically stable patients but much less frequently (32%) in those with circulatory collapse at presentation. Overall in-hospital mortality rate ranged from 8.1% in the group of stable patients to 25% in those presenting with cardiogenic shock and to 65% in patients necessitating cardiopulmonary resuscitation [32]. The finding or exclusion of right ventricular afterload stress by echocardiography has a high prognostic value. A total of 317 patients with clinically suspected PE were prospectively evaluated by echocardiography for the presence of right ventricular afterload stress and right heart or pulmonary artery thrombi by Kasper et al. Objective confirmation of PE by lung scan or pulmonary angiography was obtained in 164 patients (52%). The presence of deep venous thrombosis (DVT) was established in 90 of 158 pa-

Table 1. Comparison of Doppler echocardiographic pressure measurements versus invasive measurements in patients with pulmonary hypertension (SPAP = systolic pulmonary artery pressure, MPAP = mean pulmonary artery pressure). For details, see text.

Author	Patients (n =)	Technical success	Pressure estimated	r =	Standard error (mmHg)
Tricuspid regurgitation					
Yock [49]	62	87%	SPAP	0.93	8
Chan [50]	50	72%	SPAP	0.87	8
Hamer [51]	51	61%	SPAP	0.96	6.8
Gallet [52]	24	71%	SPAP	0.91	5.4
Torbicki [53]	72	24%	SPAP	0.92	7.7
Tramarin [54]	100	30%	SPAP	0.66	11.9
Isovolumetric relaxation time (RV)					
Hatle [55]	48	100%	SPAP	0.84	n. a.
Chan [50]	50	22%	SPAP	0.87	11
Torbicki [53]	70	84%	SPAP	0.70	8.8
Tramarin [54]	100	61%	SPAP	0.61	8.5
Acceleration time					
Kitabatake [56]	48	100%	MPAP	−0.88	n. a.
Matsuda [57]	67	100%	MPAP	−0.75	7.9
Von Bibra [58]	70	100%	MPAP	−0.77	17.4
Chan [50]	50	88%	MPAP	−0.85	10
Gallet [52]	24	71%	MPAP	−0.68	8.4
Torbicki [53]	72	97%	MPAP	−0.72	8.3
Morera [59]	68	97%	SPAP	−0.98	5.2
Migueres [60]	66	91%	MPAP	−0.73	n. a.
Tramarin [54]	100	97%	MPAP	−0.65	8
Sajkow [61]	81	84%	SPAP	−0.96	3.9

Modified from [24]

tients (57%) who underwent phlebographic or Doppler sonographic studies. Right ventricular afterload stress was diagnosed in 87 patients (27%). Objective confirmation of PE and diagnosis of DVT was more common in patients with right ventricular afterload stress than in those without (83% versus 40% and 46% versus 22%). This was also true for the detection of thrombi in the right heart and major pulmonary arteries (12 patients versus 1 patient; P < 0.001) as well as for the in-hospital mortality from venous thromboembolism (13% versus 0.9%; P < 0.001). One-year mortality from PE was 13% in patients with right ventricular afterload stress at presentation compared with only 1.3% in those without [33]. Therefore, transthoracic echocardiography allows for rapid decision-making and risk stratification in patients with suspected PE.

In summary, transthoracic echocardiography is a very reliable, safe, and easy-to-use method for both diagnosis and risk stratification in patients with PE.

Transoesophageal echocardiography (TEE)

The main advantages of transoesophageal echocardiography is the direct imaging of thrombi. Examples are shown in Figures 2a and b. The reason is the superior image quality due to imaging from the oesophagus [23, 25]. Therefore, TEE is most useful in patients with impaired transthoracic echo quality or inconclusive TTE results, ventilated patients, and patients under resuscitation. The disadvantage is the semi-invasive nature of TEE, requiring local anaesthesia and sometimes sedation of patients.

Thrombus can be found in the right atrium, the right ventricle, sometimes trapped in the Chiari-network, or at the tricuspid or pulmonary valve. Most often, however, thrombi are found at the bifurcation of the pulmonary artery or the right or left pulmonary artery. In a larger European co-operative study of 119 patients with right-sided thrombi the morphologic appearance was described as follows:

Type A = Long, thin, extremely mobile snakelike thrombi

Type B = Less mobile, non-specific clots

PE was found in 89% of patients with type A morphology. One third of patients died during the first 24 hours. Mortality was highest in type A lesions, with 27% in patients with acute surgery and 54% in patients with conservative treatment. However, the selection of patients for either surgery or medical treatment had been biased. In type B thrombi, 40% of patients had PE, but none had been fatal [34].

Value of contrast sonography

Echo contrast is sometimes useful to enhance the signal quality of the tricuspid regurgitation signal during transthoracic echocardiography, and to assess right to left shunting due to an open foramen ovale. Patients with an open foramen ovale have more lung perfusion deficits at a given pulmonary artery pressure [35]. Additionally, echo contrast is useful during TEE in suspected thrombus formation in the right pulmonary artery, giving a negative contrast in wall-adherent thrombus formation.

Use of echocardiography in decision-making, overall management of PE, and follow-up

A proposal for a decision flow chart with echocardiography as branch-point in patients with suspected PE is made in Diagram 1.

In all suspected cases, a bolus injection of 5,000–10,000 units of heparin to prevent further thrombus formation is indicated, if no contraindications for full-dose anticoagulation (see below) exist. The next steps are blood-gas analysis and ECG, usually readily available on every hospital ward. A normal blood gas analysis under room air excludes massive PE, but not PE resulting in less than 50% obstruction of the pulmonary arteries. The ECG is important to exclude other differential diagnosis, especially acute myocardial infarction. For diagnosis and management of patients with suspected PE, echocardiography allows for differentiation of patients with and without pulmonary hypertension. In patients without signs of pulmonary pressure elevation, PE is not excluded, but they represent a patient group with a very favourable short-term prognosis under full dose intravenous heparin. In this patient group, the further diagnostic work-up (ventilation-perfusion scans, venous Doppler, D-dimer, spiral CT/EBCT scans) can be done during the next hours. Transportation should be safe in this subgroup of patients. Patients with very high pulmonary artery pressures are unlikely to have an isolated acute episode of PE, rather than primary pulmonary hypertension or recurrent episodes of PE.

In a limited number of patients, thrombi in transit or intracardiac thrombi can be found by TTE and TEE. In these patients, the definitive diagnosis of PE is made and the necessary therapeutic steps can be taken. An angiogram is not necessary in all patients.

A Swan-Ganz catheter is usually not indicated as first-line diagnostic tool. The main impact of the Swan-Ganz catheter lies in monitoring of the effect of treatment. The invasive hemodynamical monitoring by a Swan-Ganz catheter allows for the calculation of cardiac output (best performed by the Fink principle but not by thermodilution in patients with tricuspid regurgitation) and monitoring of pulmonary artery pressures.

Treatment

In patients with cardiogenic shock, surgery with direct embolectomy might be the most beneficial approach, although no prospective and randomised studies exist as yet. In patients with impaired cardiac output without shock, thrombolysis is the best approach. Most centres recommend a total dose of 100mg rt-PA (tissue plasminogen activator), although positive studies exist also for streptokinase and urokinase, either as short or long-term infusion. Additionally, favourable results have been reported by use of mechanical fragmentation devices or the combination of both. Acute interventions like ultrasound thrombolysis or balloon angioplasty are highly experimental. The use of mechanical fragmentation devices depends on a catheterisation laboratory and a skilled invasive physician and will therefore be limited to a very small number of patients with acute PE.

Monitoring

The effects of treatment can be monitored clinically, by invasive monitoring or by repeated echocardiographic examinations. In selected cases, the resolution of the thrombus itself can be monitored by repeated TEE, as shown in Figures 1a, b and c

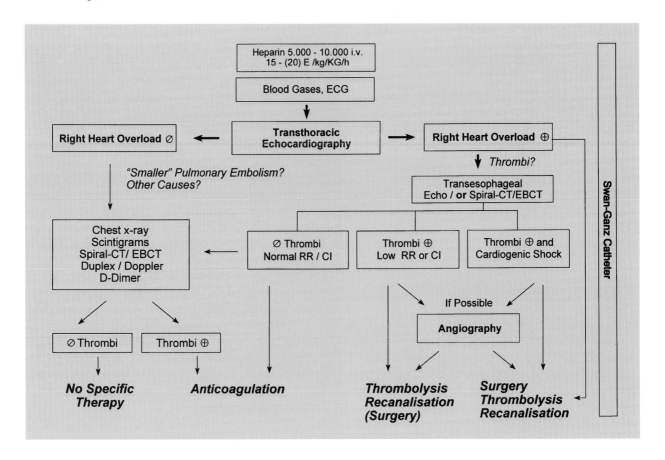

[36]. The estimations of the gradient over the tricuspid valve allows the assessment of pulmonary artery pressures, and the right ventricular morphology normalises in patients with successful treatment, as depicted in Figures 2a, b and c [36].

Intravascular ultrasonography (IVUS) in PE

While TTE and TEE have already found their place in the diagnosis of PE, IVUS in patients with PE is still experimental.

Intravascular ultrasound (IVUS) has evolved from a research tool into an intrinsic part of modern invasive cardiology. The development of intravascular or intracardiac echo systems dates back to the 1950s (for an in-depth review see [37, 38]). In the beginning, distance measurements in blood vessels or the heart were the main purpose of single or multi-element systems. In the late 1960s and early 1970s no one believed that transcutaneous echocardiography would ever be able to provide images of the human heart in enough detail for clinical decision-making purposes.

For use in blood vessels, catheters were miniaturised further. An echo device for use in blood vessels must combine high frequency to provide sufficient resolution with a penetration of 2–10 mm. The frequencies used at present are usually in the range of 10–40 MHz. Higher frequencies cause excessive reflection from erythrocytes.

At present, two different systems are in use. Mechanical systems consist of a drive shaft and a single, rotating imaging crystal within a catheter sheath or a fixed crystal with a rotating mirror at the end of the catheter. In contrast, electronic scanners use multi-element crystals mounted on the outside of a catheter without any moving parts. The advantage of the mechanical systems is the superior image quality in smaller vessels, because the zone of irregular echo propagation near the crystal lies within the catheter. The disadvantage is non-uniform rotational distortion ("NURD") which may occur due to bending-induced friction of the drive shaft, leading to image distortion. Electronic scanners offer a greater potential for electronic image optimisation or use of combination devices such as PTCA balloons on IVUS catheters [39].

Both catheter types are connected to various echo consoles for image generation and storage. Catheter diameters for use in coronary arteries are in the range of 2.9–3.5 French (1 French = 0.33 mm) and up to 10 French for peripheral vessels and intracardiac imaging with frequencies be-

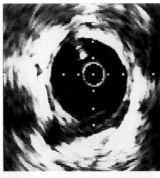
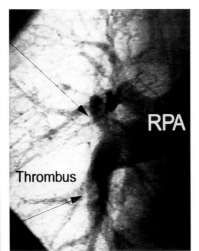
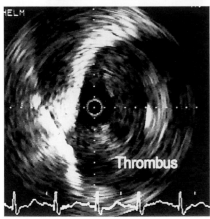

Fig. 3. Comparison of pulmonary arteries with acute thrombus and normal parts of the pulmonary circulation (RPA = right pulmonary artery) by intravascular ultrasound (IVUS) and angiography. IVUS provides cross-sectional images of the lumen (black area) and the vessel wall. The central structure with the "corona" represents the imaging catheter (3.5 French diameter, 30 MHz mechanical catheter). The distance between two dots equals 1 mm. The very bright spot in the upper IVUS image at 11 o'clock is the echo of the guide-wire. The angiogram shows a filling defect in the lower lobe and normal perfusion in the upper lobes. The arrows indicate the position of the IVUS catheter. The upper IVUS image shows a normal pulmonary artery, with a very thin wall surrounded by lung tissue. The lower IVUS image shows the small lumen around the catheter (black area) surrounded by normal vessel wall from 8 – 11 o'clock. The rest of the PA is filled by thrombus with echo-dense and echo-lucent areas. (Modified with permission from Görge G, Erbel R. Intravascular ultrasound in the pulmonary circulation. In: Erbel R, Roelandt JRTC, Ge J, Görge G (Eds.). Intravascular Ultrasound. Martin Dunitz, London, 1998 (1st ed.): pp 261 – 265).

tween 10 and 40 MHz. The IVUS catheters are guided into the pulmonary circulation over guide-wires or guiding catheters.

While the value of angiography in the detection of a complete obstruction is uniformly accepted, the imaging of partially occluded vessel segments has been prone to misinterpretation. As a contour method, angiography cannot be adequate in the visualisation of soft, wall-adherent thrombus formation; furthermore, cross-sectional imaging of the entire vessel wall is impossible. Intravascular ultrasound (IVUS) is, in contrast, a technique allowing imaging of the lumen and the vessel wall. A typical example is shown in Figure 3.

IVUS can help to identify the various causes of pulmonary hypertension. In patients with acute pulmonary hypertension, without failure of the left heart, the cause is often acute massive PE. The role of IVUS as a tomographic method in addition to angiography and other tomographic techniques is:

- Assessment of vessel wall motion
- Imaging of small pulmonary arteries (diameter 1.5 – 3 mm) to assess the vessel wall changes in patients with pulmonary hypertension without thromboembolic events
- Visualisation of thin, wall-adherent, or "soft" thrombus, not visible by angiography
- Imaging of venous vessels for occurrence of thrombi

Results of IVUS studies in pulmonary circulation

Pandian and Porter described the role of IVUS in patients with various pulmonary artery diseases and the response of the pulmonary circulation in patients with chronic heart failure [40, 41]. Kravitz examined a patient with pulmonary atherosclerosis, not visualised by angiography [42]. A detailed description of pulmonary anatomy by IVUS has been reported recently by Kawano et al. [43]. In patients with different degrees of pulmonary hypertension, he found a three-layered appearance of the pulmonary vessels in comparison to the monolayer appearance found normally. Additionally, he also had evidence of a plaque-like structure in one patient.

Our group reported first the IVUS findings in acute PE. It was possible to cross complete obstructions and to identify both wall-adherent and free-floating thrombi [26]. Tapson et al. reported their initial experience with IVUS in a canine model of PE, and found a higher sensitivity of IVUS for detection of residual thrombus in comparison to angiography [44, 45]. Scott et al. reported their initial experience with IVUS in three patients with acute massive PE [46]. Ricou et al. were the first to report on a larger series of IVUS in patients with recurrent thromboembolic disease. Again, IVUS was

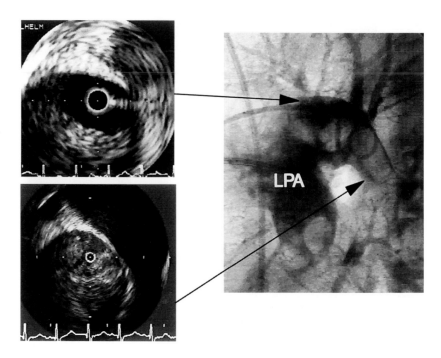

Fig. 4. Angiography and IVUS of the left pulmonary circulation (LPA = left pulmonary artery). Upper IVUS figure: bright guide-wire echo at 3 o'clock, normal lumen around the catheter, thrombus formation from 4 – 10 o'clock. The lower figure shows two types of thrombus: very mobile and "worm-like" around the IVUS catheter from 2 – 12 o'clock superimposed to more echo-dense" material from 3 – 8 o'clock. (Modified with permission from Görge G, Erbel R. Intravascular ultrasound in the pulmonary circulation. In: Erbel R, Roelandt JRTC, Ge J, Görge G (Eds.). Intravascular Ultrasound. Martin Dunitz, London, 1998 (1st ed.): pp 261-265).

superior to angiography in revealing wall-adherent thrombus formation [47]. We reported on a larger series of patients with IVUS after acute massive PE [10]. IVUS was superior to angiography for the identification of residual thrombus formation (Fig. 4). But beside these interesting findings, IVUS in the pulmonary circulation still has significant shortcomings:

- IVUS is an invasive method and the positioning of IVUS catheters in the pulmonary circulation is often cumbersome
- IVUS catheters with small crystals and high frequencies are not designed for use in the larger pulmonary arteries. Therefore, farfield is limited and assessment of the proximal circulation is difficult
- Present IVUS catheters are not steerable. Thus, their position cannot be controlled in the pulmonary circulation
- Because of the difficulties in steering the catheter, only a limited number of vessels in the pulmonary circulation can be examined

Despite these shortcomings, IVUS has already proved to be useful in the diagnosis of acute and chronic thromboembolic disease in animal models and patients. Sensitivity for the detection of thrombi seems to be superior to angiography.
The limitations in farfield penetration and steerability could be overcome by steerable IVUS catheters

and forward-viewing catheters that will allow orientation within the venous circulation with less fluoroscopy [48]. If indwelling IVUS catheters similar to the Swan-Ganz-catheters were available, IVUS-based examination of pulmonary circulation could be a potential bedside technique. Furthermore, the combination of pressure, Doppler, steerability, IVUS, and angioscopy should be the aim for the future, allowing for complete morphologic and functional assessment of the pulmonary circulation.

Conclusion

Echocardiography has become a very important non-invasive diagnostic tool in patients with suspected PE. Transthoracic echocardiography can distinguish patients with or without hemodynamically significant PE. Appropriate treatment or further diagnostic strategies can be based on the echo findings. In addition to transthoracic echocardiography, transoesophageal echo allows for superior image quality and often direct visualisation of the thrombus. In the future, invasive cross-sectional intravascular ultrasound will help in the differential diagnosis in patients with unclear causes of pulmonary hypertension.

References

1. Stein PD, Henry JW. Prevalence of acute PE in a general hospital. Chest 1995; 108: 978–981

2. Stein PD. Diagnosis and management of PE. Curr Opin Cardiol 1996; 11 (5): 543–549

3. Mandelli V, Schmid C, Zogno C, Morpurgo M. "False negatives" and "false positives" in acute PE: a clinical-postmortem comparison. Cardiologia 1997; 42 (2): 205–210

4. McIntyre KM, Sasahara AA. The hemodynamic response to PE in patients without prior cardiopulmonary disease. Am J Cardiol 1974; 28: 288–294

5. Elliot CG. Pulmonary physiology during PE. Chest 1992; 101, 4: 163S–171S

6. Stein PD, Terrin ML, Hales CA, Palevsky HI, Saltzman HA, et al. Clinical, laboratory, roentgenographic, and electrocardiographic findings in patients with acute PE and no pre-existing cardiac or pulmonary disease. Chest 1991; 100: 598–603

7. Stein PD, Coleman RE, Gottschalk A, Saltzman HA, Terrin ML, Weg JG. Diagnostic utility of ventilation/perfusion lung scans in acute PE is not diminished by pre-existing cardiac or pulmonary disease. Chest 1991; 100: 604–606

8. Benotti JR, Grossmann W. Pulmonary angiography. In: Grossman W (ed). Cardiac catheterization and angiography. Lea and Febiger, 3rd edition, Philadelphia 1985: 213–226

9. Marsh JD, Glynn M, Torman HA. Pulmonary angiography: application in a new spectrum of patients. Am J Med 1983; 75: 763–769

10. Görge G, Schuster S, Ge J, Meyer J, Erbel R. Intravascular ultrasound in patients with acute PE after treatment with intravenous urokinase and high-dose heparin. Heart 1997; 77 (1): 73–77

11. Uchida Y, Oshima T, Hirose J, Sasaki T, Morizuki S, Morita T. Angioscopic detection of residual pulmonary thrombi in the differential diagnosis of PE. Am Heart J 1995; 130 (4): 854–859

12. Van Rossum AB, Pattynama PM, Ton ER, et al. PE: validation of spiral CT angiography in 149 patients. Radiology 1996; 201 (2): 467–470

13. Van Erkel AR, Van Rossum AB, Bloem JL, Kievit J, Pattynama PM. Spiral CT angiography for suspected PE: a cost-effectiveness analysis. Radiology 1996; 201 (1): 29–36

14. Remy-Jardin M, Remy J, Deschildre F, et al. Diagnosis of PE with spiral CT: comparison with pulmonary angiography and scintigraphy. Radiology 1996; 200 (3): 699–706

15. Teigen CL, Maus TP, Sheedy PF II, et al. PE: diagnosis with contrast-enhanced electron-beam CT and comparison with pulmonary angiography. Radiology 1995; 194 (2): 313–319

16. Teigen CL, Maus TP, Sheedy PF II, Johnson CM, Stanson AW, Welch TJ. PE: diagnosis with electron-beam CT. Radiology 1993; 188 (3): 839–845

17. Perrier A. Noninvasive diagnosis of PE. Haematologica 1997; 82 (3): 328–331

18. Turkstra F, Van Beek EJ, Ten Cate JW, Büller HR. Reliable rapid blood test for the exclusion of venous thromboembolism in symptomatic outpatients. Thromb Haemost 1996; 76 (1): 9–11

19. Veitl M, Hamwi A, Kurtaran A, Virgolini I, Vukovich T. Comparison of four rapid D-Dimer tests for diagnosis of PE. Thromb Res 1996; 82 (5): 399–407

20. De Moerloose P, Desmarais S, Bounameaux H, et al. Contribution of a new, rapid, individual and quantitative automated D-dimer ELISA to exclude PE. Thromb Haemost 1996; 75 (1): 11–13

21. Kasper W, Meinertz T, Kersting F, Löllgen H, Limbourg P, Just H. Echocardiography in assessing acute pulmonary hypertension due to PE. Am J Cardiol 1980; 45: 567–572

22. Nixdorff U, Erbel R, Drexler M, Meyer J. Detection of thrombembolus of the right pulmonary artery by transesophageal two-dimensional echocardiography. Am J Cardiol 1988; 61: 448–449

23. Wittlich N, Erbel R, Eichler A, et al. Detection of central pulmonary artery thrombemboli by transesophageal echocardiography in patients with severe PE. J Am Soc Echocardiogr 1992; 5: 515–524

24. Erbel R, Drozdz J, Ge J, et al. Bildgebende Verfahren in der Kardiologie: Akute und chronische pulmonale Hypertonie. Internist 1994; 35 (11): 1039–1055

25. Erbel R, Wittlich N, Schuster S, Görge G, Ge J. Assessment of PE. Int J Card Imaging 1993; 9 (Suppl. 2): 39–49

26. Görge G, Erbel R, Schuster S, Ge J, Meyer J. Intravascular ultrasound in diagnosis of acute PE [letter]. Lancet 1991; 337 (8741): 623–624

27. Ricou F, Nicod PH, Moser KM, Peterson KL. Catheter-based intravascular ultrasound imaging of chronic thromboembolic pulmonary disease. Am J Cardiol 1991; 67 (8): 749–752

28. Schuster S. Transesophageal echocardiography in intensive care units. Herz 1993; 18 (6): 361–371

29. Bouvier JL, Bénichiou M, Antar M, et al. Echocardiographic detection of right sided intracavitary thrombi in acute PE. Arch Mal Coeur Vaiss 1987; 80: 10: 1441–1446

30. Kasper W, Geibel A, Tiede N, Hofmann T, Meinerzt T, Just H. Die Echokardiographie in der Diagnostik der Lungenembolie. Herz 1989; 14: 82–101

31. Nazeyrollas P, Metz D, Jolly D, et al. Use of transthoracic Doppler echocardiography combined with clinical and electrocardiographic data to predict acute PE. Eur Heart J 1996; 17 (5): 779–786

32. Kasper W, Konstantinides S, Geibel A, et al. Management strategies and determinants of outcome in acute major PE: results of a multicenter registry [see comments]. J Am Coll Cardiol 1997; 30 (5): 1165–1171

33. Kasper W, Konstantinides S, Geibel A, Tiede N, Krause T, Just H. Prognostic significance of right ventricular afterload stress detected by echocardiography in patients with clinically suspected PE. Heart 1997; 77 (4): 346–349

34. European Working Group on Echocardiography. The European Cooperative Study on the clinical significance of right heart thrombi. Eur Heart J 1989; 10 (12): 1046–1059

35. Miller RL, Das S, Anandarangam T, et al. Relation between patent foramen ovale and perfusion abnormalities in acute PE. Am J Cardiol 1997; 80 (3): 377–378

36. Bruch C, Othman T, Görge G, et al. Intensive medical monitoring with transesophageal echocardiography in fulminant PE. Deutsch Med Wochenschr 1996; 121 (25–26): 829–833

37. Bom N, Lancee CT, Van Egmond FC. An ultrasonic intracardiac scanner. Ultrasonics 1972; 10: 72–76

38. Bom N, Roelandt J (eds). Intravascular ultrasound. Kluwer Academic Publishers, Dordrecht, The Netherlands, 1989

39. Ten Hoff H. Scanning mechanisms for intravascular ultrasound imaging: a flexible approach [Thesis]. Erasmus University, Rotterdam, 1993: p 59

40. Porter TR, Taylor DO, Fields J, et al. Direct in vivo evaluation of pulmonary arterial pathology in chronic congestive heart failure with catheter-based intravascular ultrasound imaging. Am J Cardiol 1993; 71 (8): 754–757

41. Porter TR, Taylor DO, Cycan A, et al. Endothelium-dependent pulmonary artery responses in chronic heart failure: influence of pulmonary hypertension. J Am Coll Cardiol 1993; 22 (5): 1418–1424

42. Kravitz KD, Scharf GR, Chandrasekaran K. In vivo diagnosis of pulmonary atherosclerosis. Role of intravascular ultrasound. Chest 1994; 106 (2): 632–634

43. Kawano T. Wall morphology of the pulmonary artery: Intravascular ultrasound imaging and pathological evaluations. Kurume Med J 1994; 41 (4): 221–232

44. Tapson VF, Davidson CJ, Gurbel PA, Sheikh KH, Kisslo KB, Stack RS. Rapid and accurate diagnosis of pulmonary emboli in a canine model using intravascular ultrasound imaging. Chest 1991; 100 (5): 1410–1413

45. Tapson VF, Davidson CJ, Kisslo KB, Stack RS. Rapid visualization of massive pulmonary emboli utilizing intravascular ultrasound. Chest 1994; 105: 888–890

46. Scott PJ, Essop AR, al-Ashab W, Deaner A, Parsons J, Williams G. Imaging of pulmonary vascular disease by intravascular ultrasound. Int J Card Imaging 1993; 9 (3): 179–184

47. Ricou F, Ludomirsky A, Weintraub RG, Sahn DJ. Applications of intravascular scanning and transesophageal echocardiography in congenital heart disease: tradeoffs and the merging of technologies. Int J Card Imaging 1991; 6 (3–4): 221–230

48. Görge G, Ge J, Haude M, Baumgart D, Buck T, Erbel R. Initial experience with a steerable intravascular ultrasound catheter in the aorta and pulmonary artery. Am J Card Imaging 1995; 9 (3): 180–184

49. Yock PG, Popp RL. Noninvasive estimation of right ventricular systolic pressure by Doppler ultrasound in patients with tricuspid regurgitation. Circulation 1984; 70: 657–662

50. Chan KL, Currie PJ, Seward JB, et al. Comparison of three Doppler ultrasound methods in the prediction of pulmonary artery pressure. J Am Coll Cardiol 1987; 9, 3: 549–554

51. Hamer HPM, Takens BL, Posma JL, Lie KL. Noninvasive measurement of right ventricular systolic pressure by combined color-coded and continuous-wave Doppler ultrasound. Am J Cardiol 1988; 61, 8: 668–671

52. Gallet B, Saudemont JP, Bourdon D, et al. Evaluation of pulmonary arterial hypertension by Doppler echocardiography in chronic respiratory insufficiency. Arch Mal Coeur Vaiss 1989; 82 (9): 1575–1583

53. Torbicki A, Skwarski K, Hawrylkiewicz I, Pasierski T, Miskiewicz Z, Zielinski J. Attempts at measuring pulmonary arterial pressure by means of Doppler echocardiography in patients with chronic lung disease. Eur Respir J 1989; 2 (9): 856–860

54. Tramarin R, Torbicki A, Marchandise B, Laaban JP, Morpurgo M. Doppler echocardiographic evaluation of pulmonary artery pressure in chronic obstructive pulmonary disease. A European multicentre study. Working Group on Noninvasive Evaluation of Pulmonary Artery Pressure. European Office of the World Health Organization, Copenhagen. Eur Heart J 1991; 12 (2): 103–111

55. Hatle L, Angelsen BAJ, Tromsdal A. Non-invasive estimation of pulmonary artery systolic pressure with Doppler ultrasound. Br Heart J 1981; 45, 2: 157–165

56. Kitabatake A, Inoue M, Asao M, et al. Noninvasive evaluation of pulmonary hypertension by a pulsed Doppler technique. Circulation 1983; 68: 302–309

57. Matsuda M, Sekiguchi T, Sugishita Y, Kuwako K, Iida K, Ito I. Reliability of non-invasive estimates of pulmonary hypertension by pulsed Doppler echocardiography. Br Heart J 1986; 56, 2: 158–164

58. Von Bibra H, Ulm K, Klein G, Sebening H, Blömer H. Die Diagnose der Pulmonalen Hypertonie mittels gepulster Dopplerechokardiographie. Zeitschr Kardiol 1987; 76, 3: 149–158

59. Morera J, Hoadley SD, Roland JM, et al. Estimation of the ratio of pulmonary to systemic pressures by pulsed-wave Doppler echocardiography for assessment of pulmonary arterial pressures. Am J Cardiol 1989; 63 (12): 862–866

60. Migueres M, Escamilla R, Coca F, Didier A, Krempf M. Pulsed Doppler echocardiography in the diagnosis of pulmonary hypertension in COPD. Chest 1990; 98 (2): 280–285

61. Sajkov D, Cowie RJ, Bradley JA, Mahar L, McEvoy RD. Validation of new pulsed Doppler echocardiographic techniques for assessment of pulmonary hemodynamics. Chest 1993; 103 (5): 1348–1353

IV.3 Pulmonary angiography: technique, indications and interpretations

M. Oudkerk, E. J. R. van Beek, J. A. Reekers

Introduction

Pulmonary angiography has developed over a period of nearly 70 years, and has become a safe method for the assessment of patients with clinically suspected pulmonary embolism (PE). It has proven its superior diagnostic accuracy, and has gained widespread acceptance as the reference method. Nevertheless, its invasive nature has led to the investigation of many non-invasive techniques, as described in other chapters of this work. In this chapter, the main technique, interpretation and pit-falls will be described. It is our firm belief that, when the described precautions are taken, pulmonary angiography is safe and will remain an important final diagnostic test in the management of patients with suspected PE.

History of the technique

Forssmann is credited with the first successful introduction of a catheter into the right atrium when he performed an experiment on himself in 1929 [1]. Subsequently, he was able to visualise the right heart chambers and the pulmonary artery using a 20% sodium iodide solution in dogs [1]. It took nearly another 25 years before Bolt and co-workers were able to perform selective pulmonary angiography, i.e. with catheter positioned through the heart into the pulmonary artery [1].

Several advances were essential in the development of pulmonary angiography as it is being performed today, such as the development of safe catheter introduction by Seldinger, the development of rapid imaging equipment (film-changers) followed by progressive improvements in digital subtraction angiography and the ever safer contrast agents and catheter and guide-wire materials. These improvements have led to pulmonary angiography being a safe procedure. In fact, this increased safety is supported by data in the literature, when comparing studies which were published during the period of 1960–1980 [2–5] with those that were published during this decade [6–11] (Table 1). A more detailed description of safety and pitfalls may be read in the next chapter.

Indications/contraindications

Indications for performing pulmonary angiography differ with the availability of non-invasive diagnostic tests, the clinical status of the patient and the necessity of an absolute diagnosis. It is generally accepted that pulmonary angiography is the method of choice in the following patient categories:

1. Patients with suspected PE in whom non-invasive diagnostic tests fail to prove the presence or absence of PE (see the chapter of diagnostic strategies).
2. Patients with suspected PE in whom there is an increased risk of major or fatal bleeding complications, such as those who are recovering from recent neurosurgery. If the perfusion lung

Table 1. Complication rates of pulmonary angiography in patients with suspected PE in studies before and after 1990.

Study	Year	Patients	Deaths	Non-fatal complications
Before 1990				
Dalen et al. [1]	1967	367	1	4
Sasahara et al. [3]	1973	310	0	6
Bell and Simon [4]	1976	176	1	2
Mills et al. [5]	1980	1350	3	30
Total		2203	5 (0.2%)	42 (1.9%)
After 1990				
Stein et al. [6]	1992	1111	5*	9
Van Rooij et al. [7]	1995	211	0	0
Hudson et al. [8]	1996	1434	0	4
Van Beek et al. [9]	1996	150	0	3
Zuckerman et al. [10]	1996	547	0	5
Nilsson et al. [11]	1998	707	0	1
Total		4160	5* (0.12%)	22 (0.5%)

* = If severely ill patients with compromised circulation are deducted, only one patient died as a direct result of pulmonary angiography (0.02%).

scan is not normal, pulmonary angiography is the technique of choice to reach an absolute indication for anticoagulant therapy (or alternatively to introduce a vena cava filter).

3. Patients in whom the diagnosis of chronic pulmonary thromboembolism and pulmonary hypertension is made. As described in Chapter VI.3, pulmonary angiography is the method of choice, both for performing invasive pressure measurements and for ascertaining the extent of thrombi and the potential for thromboendarterectomy.

4. Patients in whom interventional therapy is contemplated, such as those who suffer from (sub) massive central pulmonary emboli (as described in Chapters VI.3 and VI.4).

5. Furthermore, nuclear medicine facilities are not available in some hospitals. This has led these hospitals to perform pulmonary angiography on all patients with suspected PE [7].

6. Finally, pulmonary angiography may be performed where there is a need (either as a matter of opinion or for medicolegal purposes) to obtain an absolute indication for the institution of anticoagulant therapy.

Contraindications for pulmonary angiography have declined over the years. No absolute contraindications currently exist, although several relative contraindications should be noted (Table 2).

Some extra measures may be required to reduce the risks in these patients.

1. Allergy to iodine containing contrast agents: with a previously documented allergic reaction to contrast agents, patients should have prophylactic steroid and antihistamines prior to the procedure.

2. Impaired renal function: the present contrast agents and the use of digital subtraction angiography have resulted in less nephrotoxicity and the ability to use less contrast agents. Hence, impaired renal function is no longer considered an absolute contraindication. Nevertheless, renal function should be monitored in these patients following angiography and dialysis equipment should be available if one is to perform angiography in these patients. In patients who suffer from severe renal insufficiency prior to angiography, dialysis should be scheduled following the procedure.

3. Left bundle branch block: this is not a contraindication, but extra care must be taken. During passage of the catheter through the right heart, a total ventricular block may develop. Hence, it is advised that a pacemaker be on stand-by during the procedure.

4. Severe congestive heart failure: this increases the risks of complications, largely as a result of volume overload during the injection of con-

trast agent. It is advised that patients should preferably be treated for their heart failure during 24 hours prior to angiography. If this is insufficient or not feasible, angiography should be undertaken using an amended contrast injection scheme consisting of a longer duration of linear rise, reduced amounts of contrast and more selective catheterisation.

5. Severe pulmonary hypertension (mean pulmonary artery pressure > 40 mm/Hg): this situation increases the risks of complications, but with the reduced amounts of contrast and longer duration of linear rise this is well within reasonable limits. Several studies have reported on the safety of pulmonary angiography in large patient groups with pre-existing pulmonary hypertension [8, 12, 13]. Furthermore, as described in Chapter VI.3, pulmonary angiography is an essential part of planning for thromboendarterectomy.

6. Right-sided endocarditis: this poses the risk of septicaemia and septic embolism during catheter manipulation. Pulmonary angiography should be carried out if other diagnostic techniques have failed to offer an adequate diagnosis and the bleeding risks are deemed too large.

7. Anticoagulated state or thrombocytopenia: these are mainly of concern for hematomas at the puncture site. In patients who are heparinised while awaiting angiography, the heparin pump should be stopped once the patient is prepared in the angiography suite. If pulmonary emboli are proven, the pump can be restarted and aPTT monitoring will be required to assess the need for additional heparin adminis-

Table 2. Relative contraindications for pulmonary angiography.

- Documented previous iodinated contrast allergy
- Renal failure
- Congestive heart failure
- Ventricular ectopy or left bundle branch block
- Severe pulmonary hypertension (mean PAP > 40 mmHg)
- Right-sided endocarditis
- Anticoagulated state or thrombocytopenia
- Pregnancy

tration. In patients with thrombocytopenia between 30 and 100 × 1012/l, no additional measures are required. For those with thrombocytopenia of less than 30 × 1012/l a dose of 6 to 12 units of thrombocytes may be required if bleeding at the puncture site cannot be controlled within 20 to 30 minutes.

8. Pregnancy is not an absolute contraindication (as discussed in Chapter VII.2). However, lead shielding of the abdomen, the preferential use of the brachial route and radiation hygiene are advised.

Albeit these contraindications are relative, they are usually part of the decision not to perform pulmonary angiography. However, the general condition of the patient is mostly the deciding factor, as demonstrated in two recent studies where pulmonary angiography could not be performed in 10%–20% of patients who were scheduled for the procedure [6, 9].

Patient monitoring during the procedure

Patients who are entering an angiography suite to undergo pulmonary angiography need to be monitored, while at the same time several items should be available at all times. First, it is imperative that oxygen can be obtained freely, since many patients have hypoxemia. An oxymeter may be useful, but is not essential since it has relatively little influence on patient management at the time of angiography. Second, an automated blood pressure and pulse measurement device is advised which can do rapid readings, i. e. one reading per minute, during the procedure.

The use of electrocardiography during the procedure is debated. Rhythm disorders do occur during passage of the catheter through the right heart chambers. This is further enhanced if one uses a guidewire. However, if electrocardiography prior to the procedure does not show a left bundle branch block or ventricular extrasystoles, one could decide to dispense with the electrocardiography monitoring and rely on blood pressure, pulse and oxymeter readings only. In virtually all patients some rhythm abnormalities occur, but these mainly consist of ventricular extrasystoles, which respond to short interruption of catheter manipulation. It is rather essential that radiologists who perform pulmonary angiography are capable of recognising the main electrocardiographic rhythm disorders and know how to treat them and to reassure the patient.

Common catheter-induced rhythm and conduction abnormalities during pulmonary angiography

A wide variety of rhythm and conduction abnormalities may be induced by catheter irritation and manipulation during passage of the catheter through the right atrium and ventricle into the pulmonary artery. The following most commonly occurring abnormalities are listed.

Sinus rhythm:
The normal situation. The atrial rate is by definition between 60 and 110 beats per minute and 'normal-appearing' P-waves should follow each discharge of the sino-atrial node. The P-wave is usually followed by a normal AV-conduction, QRS-complex and T-wave (Fig. 1).

a) Tachycardia
Sinus tachycardia: a sinus rate above 110 beats per minute with normal P-waves. This is innocent and is usually caused by anxiety (Fig. 2).
Atrial tachycardia: atrial rate is between 120–180 per minute, usually with a 1:1 atrioventricular response (Fig. 3).

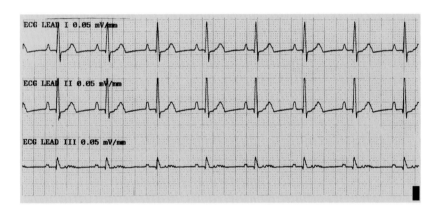

Fig. 1. Sinus rhythm chartspeed 25.0 mm/s.

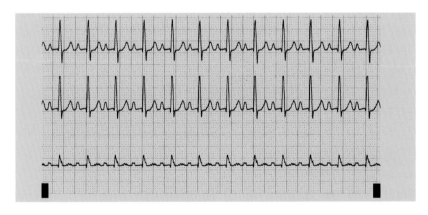

Fig. 2. Sinus tachycardia.

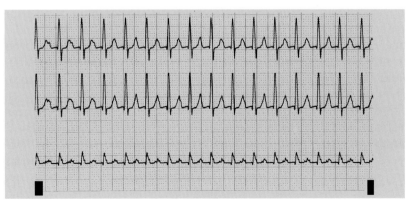

Fig. 3. Atrial tachycardia.

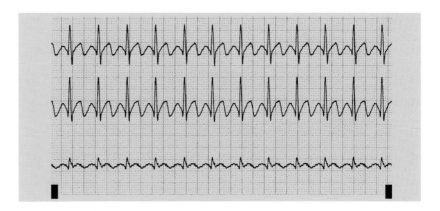

Fig. 4. Atrial flutter.

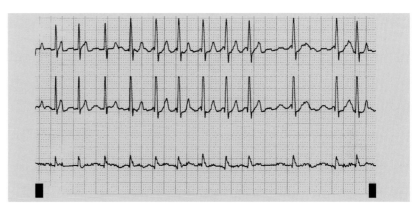

Fig. 5. Atrial fibrillation.

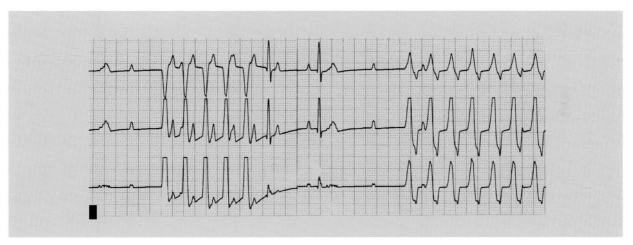

Fig. 6. Ventricular tachycardia.

Atrial flutter: regular rate between 260 and 350 per minute, usually with a 2:1 atrioventricular response (Fig. 4).

Atrial fibrillation: rapid irregular atrial rate approximately between 450 and 600 per minute with irregular often rapid ventricular response often between 130 and 160 per minute (Fig. 5).

Ventricular tachycardia: three or more ventricular extrasystoles in a row. It may be intermittent or sustained. The rate is rapid, essentially regular 150 to 200 per minute (Fig. 6).

b) Extrasystole

Atrial extrasystole: premature P-waves, with a configuration which is different from the normal P-wave and usually followed by a normal QRS-complex (Fig. 7).

Ventricular extrasystole: premature ventricular discharge with abnormal QRS and T-wave morphology. When they arise in the right ventricle, they have a left bundle branch block configuration (Fig. 8).

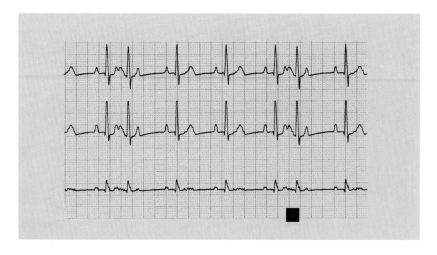

Fig. 7. Atrial extrasystole.

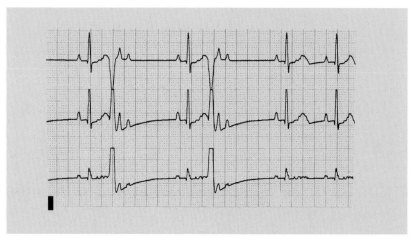

Fig. 8. Unifocal ventricular extrasystole.

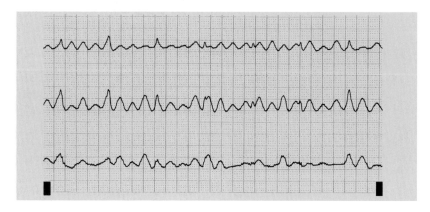

Fig. 9. Ventricular fibrillation.

c) Cardiac arrest:
Ventricular fibrillation: rapid (150–400/mmin) irregular, shapeless QRST modulations of variable amplitude associated with unrecognisable blood pressure and no cardiac output (Fig. 9).

d) Bradycardia
Second-degree AV-block: occasionally a P-wave is blocked. If the AV-block is advanced only a few P-waves are conducted to the ventricles (Fig. 10).

Complete atrioventricular block: complete electrical dissociation of the atria and ventricles. The ventricular rate is usually slower than the atrial rate, which often is normal (Fig. 11).

e) Bundle branch block
Right branch block: QRS complex exceeds 0.12 s with depressed ST-segment and asymmetrically inverted T-wave (Fig. 12).
During passage of the catheter through the right atrium to the tricuspid valve, mechanical stimula-

140

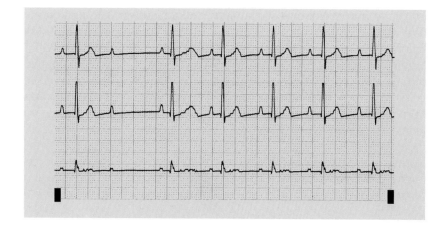

Fig. 10. Second degree atrio ventricular block.

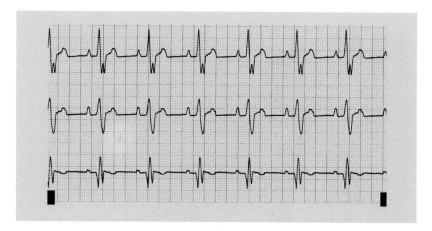

Fig. 11. Complete atrio ventricular block.

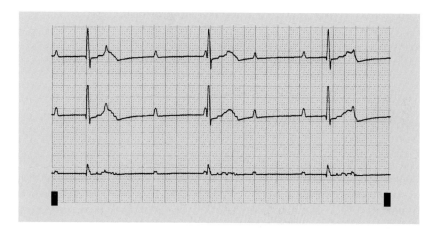

Fig. 12a. Right bundle branch block (RBBB).

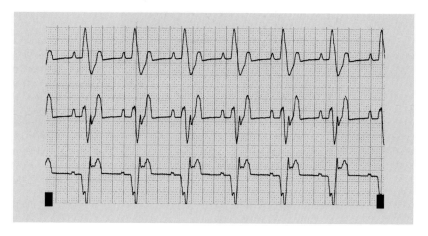

Fig. 12b. Left bundle branch block (LBBB).

tion may induce atrial extrasystoles, or tachycardia: atrial tachycardia, atrial flutter or atrial fibrillation. In the majority of cases this is transient, and terminates after stopping catheter manipulation. If atrial flutter or fibrillation persists the rapid ventricular rate may be slowed down by use of Beta-adrenergic blocking agents (isoptin IV – slowly injected 1 – 5 mg). Rarely electrical cardioversion is indicated.

During manipulation of the catheter in the area of the tricuspid valve irritation of the wall may cause bundle branch block, or bradycardia due to second-degree AV-block or complete AV-block. These conduction disturbances are usually temporary, but if sustained, atropine 0.5 – 1.0 mg i. v. may restore A-V node conduction. Occasionally temporary transvenous right ventricular pacing is indicated.

Manipulation of the catheter within the right ventricle may irritate the wall causing ventricular extrasystoles, which are innocent or short bursts of ventricular tachycardia which usually terminate after cessation of catheter manipulation.

Sustained ventricular tachycardia, which occurs very rarely, requires triggered electrical cardioversion. Ventricular fibrillation may occur, but is frequently self-terminating. However, if it persists this requires immediate electrical defibrillation (200 – 400 Joule).

Crossing the tricuspid valve with the catheter may occasionally induce right bundle branch block, which spontaneously reverts to normal conduction.

Materials

It is imperative that modern materials are used to decrease the chances of complications. A standard pigtail catheter, or a modification thereof, is generally used. The Grollman shaped or Church shaped catheters, when used complementarily, will allow central and selective catheterisation of both pulmonary arteries in all patients, also without guide-wire use (Fig. 13). The size of catheters may vary from 5F to 7F, depending on the manufacturer [14]. Size is relatively unimportant in the case of venous access. Therefore larger sizes can be used (7F) for increased torque control, higher flow rates and more stable catheter position. Balloon catheters have been described as helpful in guiding the catheter by flow, especially in patients with a large right atrium/ventricle. In our experience these catheters do not have a place in the majority of patients, since catheterisation is usually achieved without difficulty. Nevertheless, they may be beneficial in patients in whom amended contrast injections are required for fear of right ventricular overload. Balloon occlusion angiography may be able to reduce the total amount of contrast used in these patients [7].

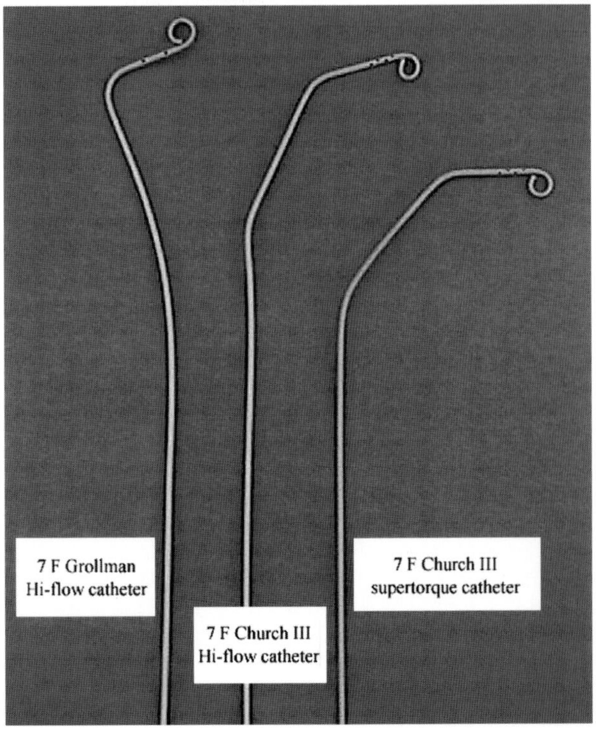

Introducer sheaths are quite comfortable for patient and examiner but not strictly required in the great majority of patients, since we are dealing with a vena puncture with a low-pressure system, which reduces the chance of pericatheter bleeding.

Guidewires may be used, but should be of atraumatic material. The Rotterdam group uses no guidewires at all, while the Amsterdam series have used 0.038 inch hydrophilic guidewires [9, 15]. When using guidewires, care must be taken not to perforate the heart (the atrial appendix is most at risk), while the pulmonary arterial tree is vulnerable for intima lesions. The latter may result in subintimal contrast injection, as shown in Figure 14.

7 F Grollman
Hi-flow catheter

7 F Church III
supertorque catheter

7 F Church III
Hi-flow catheter

Fig. 13a. Three 7F pulmonary artery catheters. The combined use of the Grollman and Church catheter shapes is always successful even without the use of guidewires.

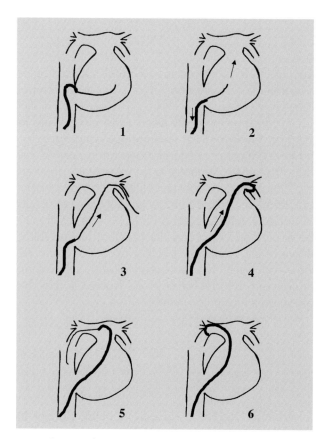

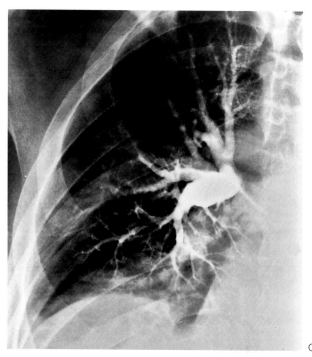

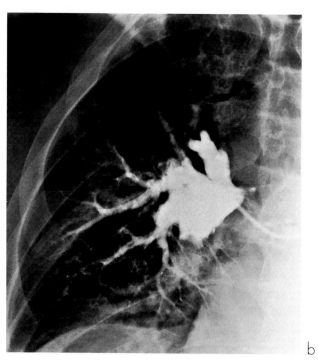

Fig. 13b. Guidewire steered catheter passage through right heart to pulmonary vessels. **1.** Pigtail catheter position in right atrium; guidewire through tricuspid valve. **2.** Stretching of the catheter by advancing guidewire. **3.** Guidewire passing pulmonary valve through conus pulmonaris deep into left pulmonary artery. **4.** Stretched catheter advanced over guidewire to left pulmonary artery; guidewire withdrawal, reshaping of catheter to pigtail configuration. Position for selective pulmonary angiography. **5.** Slight catheter withdrawal into conus pulmonaris and 180 degrees turning of pigtail position; stretching of catheter by guidewire, which is advanced deep into the right main pulmonary artery. **6.** Catheter advanced over guidewire. Guidewire withdrawal and reshaping of catheter to pigtail configuration; position for selective right pulmonary angiography.

Low-osmolar contrast agents should be used for pulmonary angiography. It has been shown that both ionic and non-ionic agents lead to a slight increase in pulmonary arterial pressure after injection, but the increase is slight and reversible [16–18]. Although the safety of all the available low-osmolar contrast agents has been shown, non-ionic agents are generally preferred due to better tolerance by the patient, reduced cough reflex and less nausea, which all contribute to better images on the basis of less patient movement [16–18]. A minimum of 300 mg Iodine/ml is required for optimal opacification of the pulmonary arterial tree.

Fig. 14a, b. Subintimal contrast injection into the right pulmonary artery **(a)**. Note that the proximal artery is abnormally distended, while the side-holes of the catheter give insufficient filling of peripheral branches. One second later **(b)**, there is contrast extravasation into the perivascular space of the interstitium. (Reprinted with permission: E. J. R. van Beek, P. M. M. Kuyer, J. A. Reekers. Dissection of pulmonary artery as a complication of pulmonary angiography. Röfo 1993;158:599-600).

X-ray equipment

Fast film exchange systems are increasingly being replaced by digital subtraction angiography units. The spatial resolution of conventional cut film remains superior to that of digital subtraction angiography. However, recent studies suggest that the added use of cinematic review and work station manipulation are beneficial for the interpretation of pulmonary angiography. These benefits are noticeable in terms of interobserver variation, adequacy of opacification of smaller branches and diagnostic performance [15, 19, 20]. Hence, it is warranted that digital subtraction angiography should replace cut film angiography as the method of choice for arteriography of the pulmonary arteries. It should be noted that 1024 × 1024 matrix imaging is preferred if digital subtraction is overtaking conventional film pulmonary embolism.

Cine arteriography has been used extensively in cardiac imaging. In pulmonary angiography, however, most procedures have been carried out by radiologists. Recently, a Swedish study showed that cine arteriography produced high diagnostic accuracy and a low number of inconclusive results in patients with suspected PE [21]. This result may be explained in part by the fact that filming takes place at 25 frames/s, which makes a dynamic review possible. In the latest digital subtraction equipment, images at 6 to 12 frames/s may be obtained with similar results.

Technique

It was previously suggested that intravenous digital subtraction angiography could adequately depict or exclude pulmonary emboli [22]. This would have the benefit of peripheral contrast medium injection (hence no transcardiac catheterisation). Initially, a sensitivity of 75 %–100 % and a specificity of 96 %–100 % were obtained, but these figures used lung scintigraphy as reference method [22]. Subsequently, it was shown that intravenous contrast is diluted to the extent that segmental and subsegmental branches are insufficiently opacified, and a sub-optimal sensitivity and specificity were obtained, which does not allow the diagnosis of pulmonary emboli to be made or refuted with certainty [23, 24]. Hence, it should be stressed that intra-arterial injection of contrast medium centrally and selectively into the pulmonary arteries is a prerequisite for adequate interpretation of pulmonary angiography.

Although a brachial, jugular and femoral venous approach may be applied, the latter is the entry site of choice. The right femoral vein has the additional benefit of nearly straight approach to the vena cava and right atrium, whereas a relatively sharp angle may be present where the left iliac vein enters the inferior vena cava. The femoral vein is generally located directly medial to the artery (sometimes the vein may actually be posterior to the artery). Following local anaesthesia using 1 % lidocaine-HCl, the femoral vein is punctured. This is best achieved by asking the patient to perform a Valsalva manoeuvre, which causes the vein to distend, and/or by positioning the patient in anti-Trendelenburg position. Subsequently, the Seldinger technique is employed and the pigtail catheter is advanced over the wire.

In case a non-guidewire passage of the heart is chosen, the Church catheter can directly pass the tricuspid valve by turning it clockwise at the level of the valve through the cusps; then, after a 2 cm advancement, a 180° anti-clockwise turn will bring it straight for the pulmonary valve, at which moment a 5 cm advancement will position the catheter central in the pulmonary artery confluens. If one decides to use a guidewire, the pigtail catheter is turned so that the end-hole faces anteromedially. The guidewire will easily pass through the tricuspid valve into the right ventricle. The next part of the manoeuvre consists of withdrawing catheter and wire to straighten the catheter. Once this is achieved, the catheter can be repositioned to let the end-hole face upward, and the guidewire may now be passed through the pulmonary valve into the pulmonary trunk. Once the catheter is moved forward over the guide-wire, a trial injection of contrast should be administered by hand to check for large central emboli. If central emboli are seen on fluoroscopy, it is advised that a full X-ray series be obtained with contrast injection in the right ventricle. However, if the trial injection does not reveal central emboli, the wire and catheter may be advanced into the right or left pulmonary artery. Care must be taken, because early branching of the left or right upper lobe artery

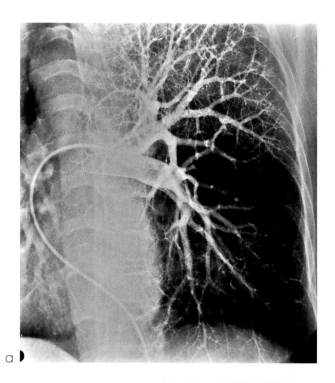

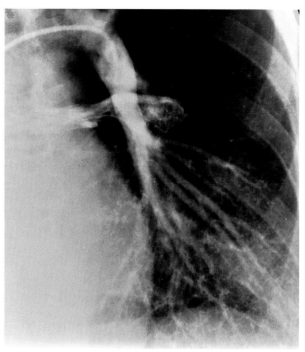

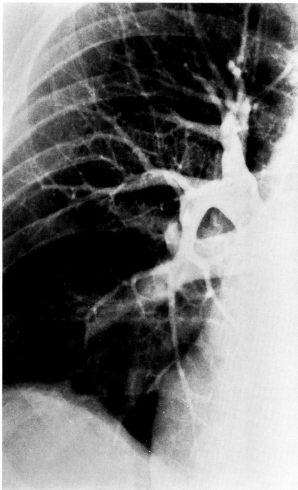

Fig. 16. Early capillary and venous filling as a result of wedging of tip of the catheter in a small side branch of the pulmonary artery. The resultant image may suggest arteriovenous malformation if not adequately recognised. (Reprinted with permission: E.J.R. van Beek, N.G.M. van 't Hullenaar, J.A. Reekers. Pseudo-arteriovenous malformation of the lung: a report of two cases. Eur Radiol 1993;3:264-265.)

may occur (Fig. 15), which could result in insufficient opacification of these lobes. Furthermore, a small bolus injection must be given prior to obtaining a full radiographic series to ascertain that the catheter tip is positioned adequately and is not wedged into a small side branch (Fig. 16) or in a subintimal position (Fig. 14).

Using an injection into the main pulmonary artery, adequate opacification of all segmental and subsegmental branches is usually obtained. However, in patients with atelectasis or with pain-related splinting of the diaphragm, inadequate visualisation of the lower lobe branches may occur, which may even suggest the presence of large emboli (Fig. 17a). In these patients, it is necessary to perform more selective catheterisation and injection of contrast to depict these branches (Fig. 17b). Also, an inadequate injection protocol can mimic a major pulmonary embolism (Fig. 17c).

Contrast injection should be performed using an automated injector system. A linear rise of 0.5 s is advised to reduce catheter recoil. Thereafter, 30–40 ml of contrast is given at a rate of 15–25 ml/s at a pressure of 600–1000 PSI (42–70 kg/cm^2). Timing depends on the circulatory dynamics and capillary resistance. In patients

Fig. 15a, b. Early branching of **(a)** left upper lobe artery and **(b)** right upper lobe artery.

145

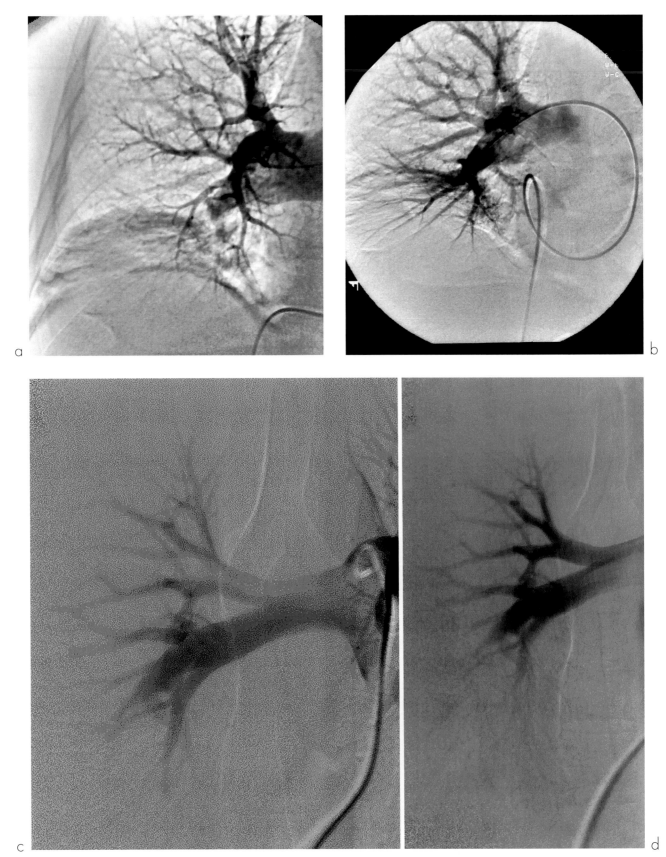

Fig. 17a–d. Patients with atelectasis of the right lower lobe with raised diaphragm. Injection into the right pulmonary artery shows cutoff of the right lower lobe artery **(a)**. Subsequent more selective injection into the right lower lobe artery shows normal vasculature without evidence of PE **(b)**. A contrast filling defect is seen in the right ascending upper lobe artery **(c)**. This was caused by an insufficient injection protocol of 15 ml/s x 2 s. Complete filling of the artery after optimal injection of 22 ml/s x 2 s **(d)**.

with pulmonary hypertension, lesser amounts are administered more selectively to prevent acute right ventricular overload (see below). Similarly, if contrast injections are performed in lobar or segmental arteries, the total amount of contrast is reduced to 10–15 ml/s for two seconds.

Besides the central AP view, a minimum of two radiographic series per lung is required. The standard projections used are anterior-posterior, and 20° to 50° left and right posterior oblique for the left and right lung, respectively [25]. Before each series these projection angles should be optimised in each patient during fluoroscopy, which visualises the contours of the vessels. However, in some patients additional series are required, especially if more selective angiography is needed in non-opacified segments.

Rotational angiography may open further diagnostic capabilities to pulmonary angiography. To present vessel overlap, two rotational views should be taken from the left and the right lung respectively by selective catheterisation. Optimal views can be taken from –40° (LAO) to +50° (RAO) projection for the right and +40° (RAO) to –50° (LAO) for the left lung. The best trade-off between number of projection views and rotation speed is a 10° per second rotation with a film-shot at every

10°. Masks should be taken from lateral to medial rotation. Contrast medium injection should start at medial position, digital subtraction should start from medial to lateral position. The total breath-holding will take 20 seconds i. c. 9 s masks, 2 seconds standstill and injection, 9 seconds digital subtraction. A volume of 75 ml contrast medium with a flow of 15 ml/s will provide a good vascular contrast filling. Timing of contrast medium injection and optimal breath-holding are crucial for successful, high quality images.

Only one mask per subtraction image is available for each projection angle, which makes the examination quite motion-sensitive. More consistent results are acquired without the use of subtraction. However, in this case higher contrast volumes are needed for satisfactory results. A further disadvantage of rotational angiography is the lack of a complete dynamic phase per projection angle and the different flow phases between the different projections. Therefore a good evaluation of lung perfusion is not possible with this technique. Although the different projection angles can be very helpful for subsegmental PE detection, in practice the best technical results are acquired in patients who can co-operate optimally.

Anatomy

The pulmonary trunk originates from the right ventricle at the level of the infundibulum. The trunk divides into a left and a right pulmonary artery. The left artery runs a more or less straight upwards and then anterior oblique course, whereas the right is in a more caudal position and traverses underneath the aortic arch in a more horizontal plane. Subsequently, the pulmonary arteries divide into three lobar arteries. The upper lobe arteries originate first, and may actually divide off within the mediastinum. The middle lobe and lingular lobe arteries stem from the descending part of the main right and left pulmonary arteries, respectively. The segmental distribution is analogous to the lung segment chart as shown in Chapter 4.1 (Fig. 18). Rotational views give good insight into the different projections of the pulmonary arteries depending on the beam angle (Fig. 19).

It is important to recognise anatomical variation, which is mainly related to left vena cava, atrial septum defects or patent foramen ovale. Some examples are demonstrated in Figure 5. Even rarer anomalies are an aberrant course of vessels as in

pulmonary sling, or aberrant vascular supply to lung segments as in pulmonary sequestration.

Hemodynamic measurements are an integral part of pulmonary angiography. Nevertheless, some people feel that they may be omitted, since echocardiography is presently able to adequately measure pressures non-invasively (see Chapter IV.2). If one decides to perform pressure measurements, it is valuable to determine right atrial, right ventricular and pulmonary artery pressure. The latter is most important, since it may signal pulmonary hypertension, which implies that one uses a linear rise of up to 1 s and injects less contrast agent (we prefer 30 ml at 15 ml/s). Alternatively, one could resort to super-selective catheterisation of lobar or segmental arteries, where an occlusion balloon may be used to further reduce the amount of contrast injected. These measures will reduce the risks of acute right ventricular overload in patients with pulmonary hypertension [12, 13].

The criteria for acute PE were defined over 30 years ago [2, 26]. Large studies have consistently used them, and demonstrated that these criteria

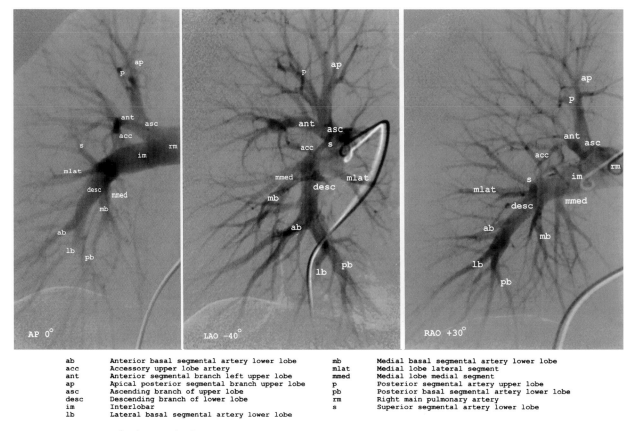

ab	Anterior basal segmental artery lower lobe	mb	Medial basal segmental artery lower lobe
acc	Accessory upper lobe artery	mlat	Medial lobe lateral segment
ant	Anterior segmental branch left upper lobe	mmed	Medial lobe medial segment
ap	Apical posterior segmental branch upper lobe	p	Posterior segmental artery upper lobe
asc	Ascending branch of upper lobe	pb	Posterior basal segmental artery lower lobe
desc	Descending branch of lower lobe	rm	Right main pulmonary artery
im	Interlobar	s	Superior segmental artery lower lobe
lb	Lateral basal segmental artery lower lobe		

Fig. 18a. Anatomy of right arterial pulmonary tree.

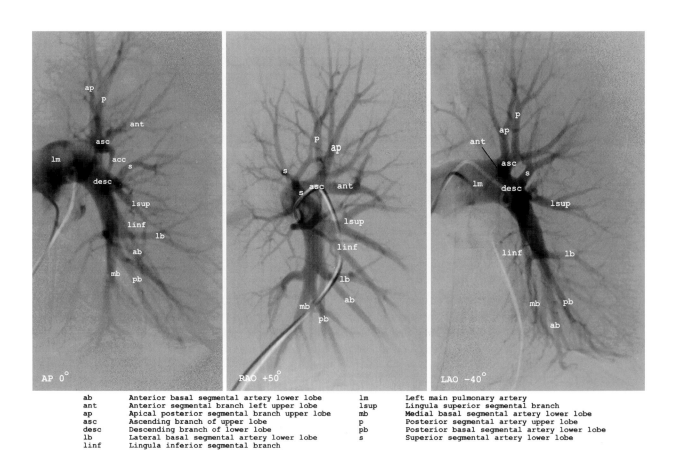

ab	Anterior basal segmental artery lower lobe	lm	Left main pulmonary artery
ant	Anterior segmental branch left upper lobe	lsup	Lingula superior segmental branch
ap	Apical posterior segmental branch upper lobe	mb	Medial basal segmental artery lower lobe
asc	Ascending branch of upper lobe	p	Posterior segmental artery upper lobe
desc	Descending branch of lower lobe	pb	Posterior basal segmental artery lower lobe
lb	Lateral basal segmental artery lower lobe	s	Superior segmental artery lower lobe
linf	Lingula inferior segmental branch		

Fig. 18b. Anatomy of left arterial pulmonary tree.

are valid. There are direct angiographic signs of PE, which are complete obstruction of a vessel (preferably with concave border of the contrast column) or a filling defect [2, 6, 27]. These criteria have been shown to be reliable in various studies which assessed intra- and interobserver variation [6, 15, 28]. More recently, it was demonstrated that the same criteria may be applied in digital subtraction angiography with equally good observer agreement [15, 19, 20]. However, one should be aware of the fact that the reliability of pulmonary angiography decreases with diminishing calibre of the vessels, i. e. the interpretation becomes much more difficult after the subsegmental level [28]. Another factor which influences diagnostic accuracy of pulmonary angiography is related to patient selection. In 140 patients who were referred for pulmonary angiography after a non-diagnostic lung scan had been obtained, the kappa values of cut-film angiography ranged between 0.28 and 0.59, while this increased to a range of 0.66–0.89 if digital subtraction angiography was used [15]. Nevertheless, these values were lower than those obtained in non-selected patient populations [6, 28], possibly because underlying pulmonary and cardiac diseases had a negative influence on the interpretation of images.

Indirect signs of PE may be slow flow of contrast media, regional hypoperfusion and delayed or diminished pulmonary venous flow. One should be aware that these signs could direct one's attention to a specific region, but they cannot be used for diagnostic purposes. None of these signs have been validated, and one should not diagnose PE in the absence of direct angiographic signs.

Chronic pulmonary thromboembolism may be diagnosed by pulmonary angiography, and is identifiable for several reasons [29]. Thrombi will be adherent to the vessel wall and will not move during the series of images. Secondly, signs of revascularisation are usually present, such as collateral vessels and stenotic lesions. In fact, it may be difficult to distinguish chronic pulmonary thromboembolism from inflammatory lesions like Takayasu's arteritis (see Chapter IV.4). Finally, the results of incomplete thrombus resolution may lead to complete obstruction, webs, bands and irregularity of the vessel wall [29]. It may be difficult to visualise emboli or adequate flow in partially occluded vessels [30]. Super-selective catheterisation will usually resolve this problem.

Pulmonary hypertension may develop as a result of (sub)massive PE. This phenomenon occurs if more than 50 % of the total peripheral pulmonary vascular bed is obstructed [31]. Prolonged pulmonary hypertension will show an increase in capillary flow resistance. This can be evaluated in pulmonary angiography by a prolonged capillary phase, and If this is noted during examination evaluation of pulmonary pressures delayed arterial washout is obligatory. Normal pressure values (systolic/diastolic) in mm Hg are: right circulation: right atrium 6–8 mm Hg, right ventricle 30/7 mm Hg, pulmonary artery 30/14 mm Hg; left circulation: left atrium 10–15 mm Hg and left ventricle 145/12 mm Hg.

PE scoring systems

Several attempts have been made to quantify the degree of pulmonary vascular obstruction. The main aim was to develop some form of objective scoring for the assessment of effectiveness of fibrinolytic therapy in large clinical trials, such as those described in Chapter VI.2.

The Miller index, which was developed in Europe, is based on the size and number of filling defects and contrast flow [32]. The presence of one or more filling defects is scored with one point, giving a maximum of 16 points (9 on the left and 7 on the right). The presence of a filling defect proximal to segmental branches is scored as equal to the segmental branches arising distally. A slightly impaired flow in 1/3 of each lung accounts for one point, delayed flow in 1/3 of each lung sores one point, and no contrast flow scores 3 points for each 1/3 of each lung. Due to the difficulty of measuring flow, most centres score only the filling defects [33].

The Walsh scoring system was developed in the urokinase-streptokinase PE trials [34]. This scoring system only takes central to segmental branches into consideration, but does not account for more peripheral perfusion defects. Neither the Miller index nor the Walsh system separated the elements of clot size and degree of occlusion.

The latest scoring system, which was developed by Simon et al., separated clot size and degree of occlusion and yielded a true quantitative score which was a measure for severity of occlusion of the pulmonary vascular tree [35].

None of the scoring systems mentioned have gained widespread acceptance. This is partly due to the relative subjectivity of scoring, its time-consuming nature, and finally its lack of clinical impact.

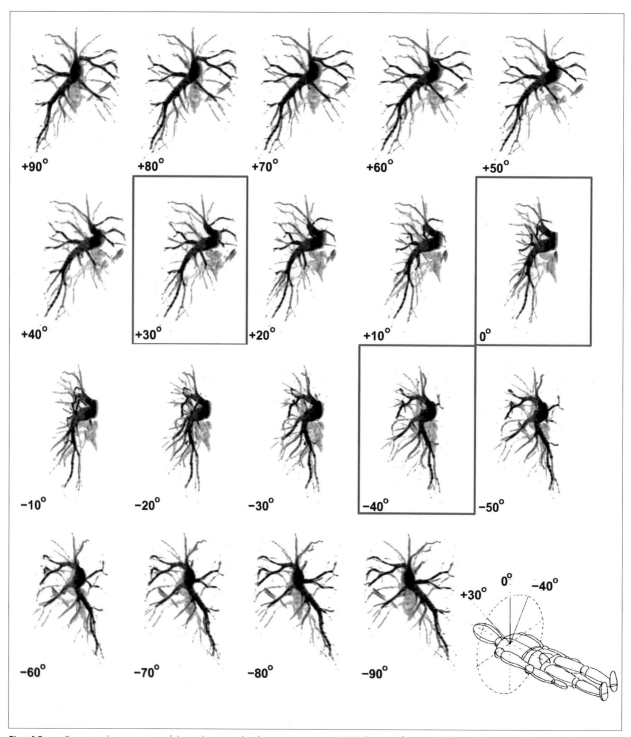

Fig. 19a. Rotational projections of the right arterial pulmonary tree over 180 degrees from +90 lateral view to −90 lateral view; the marked projections are the standard views used in arterial pulmonary angiography.

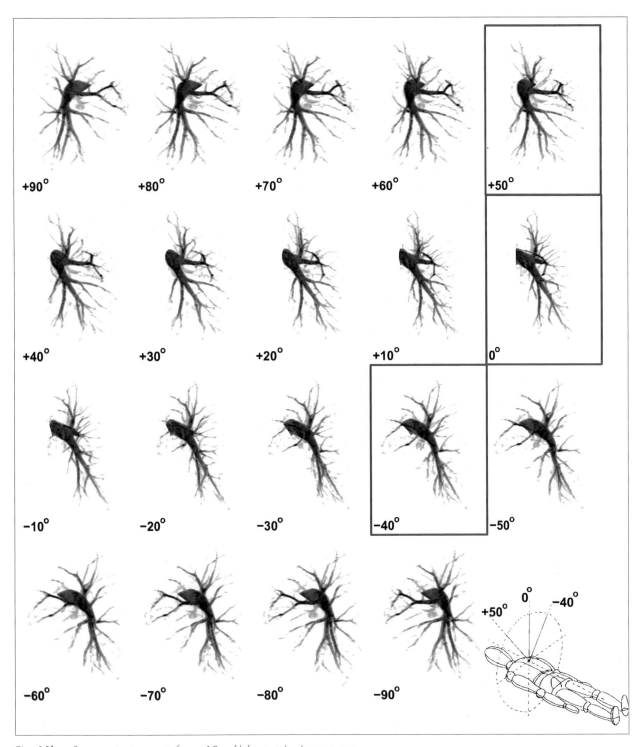

Fig. 19b. Same projections as in figure 19a of left arterial pulmonary tree.

Anatomic distribution of PE

Pulmonary emboli vary greatly in size, and distribution of emboli may be important for other, less-invasive modalities. An overview of pulmonary embolism at the different anatomic locations and levels in the pulmonary tree is given in figures 20 to 25. In one study in 76 patients with proven pulmonary emboli, emboli were located exclusively in subsegmental arterial branches in 23 (30%) patients [36]. In the PIOPED study, 6% of all patients who underwent pulmonary angiography had their emboli limited to subsegmental vessels [37]. Similarly, in a selected group of 140 patients who underwent angiography following a non-diagnostic lung scan, the largest emboli were in subsegmental vessels in 3 out of 20 patients (15%) in whom PE was proven [9].

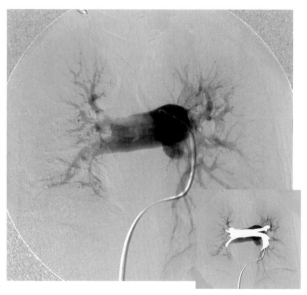
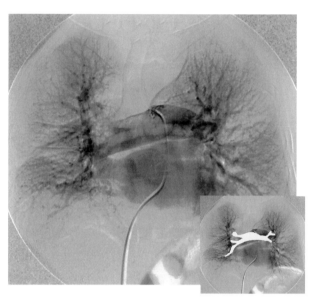

a   b

Fig. 20a, b. Central pulmonary emboli.
The large central emboli extend to both upper and lower lobe arteries **(a, b)**. Both patients were in deceptively good clinical condition, therefore this diagnostic outcome was totally unexpected. One patient showed almost no perfusion of the lower lobes **(b)** (see inserts for delineation of emboli extension (white pasting).

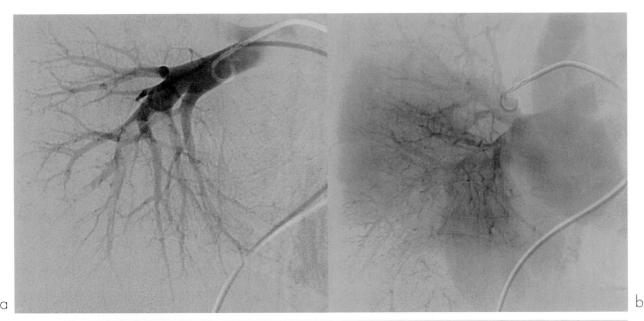

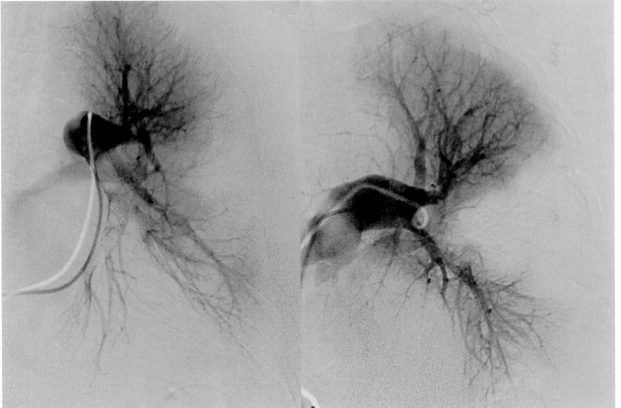

Fig. 21a–d. Occluding segmental pulmonary emboli.
Selective angiography of the right lower lobe artery (bypassing the ascending upper lobe artery) reveals a large embolus in RAO projection. Only partial occlusion is seen of the medial basal segmental artery **(a)**. The posterior and lateral basal segmental arteries show complete occlusion leading to a wedge-shaped perfusion defect in the corresponding segmental areas **(b)**. Selective angiography of the left main pulmonary artery shows a cut-off of the lower lobe and inferior longula arteries in RAO projection **(c)** a subtle outline of contrast medium along the embolus can be noticed. Two large wedge-shaped perfusion defects are seen corresponding with the lower lobe and inferior longula arteries except for the segment of the superior longula artery in AP projection **(d)**.

M. Oudkerk, E. J. R. van Beek, J. A. Reekers

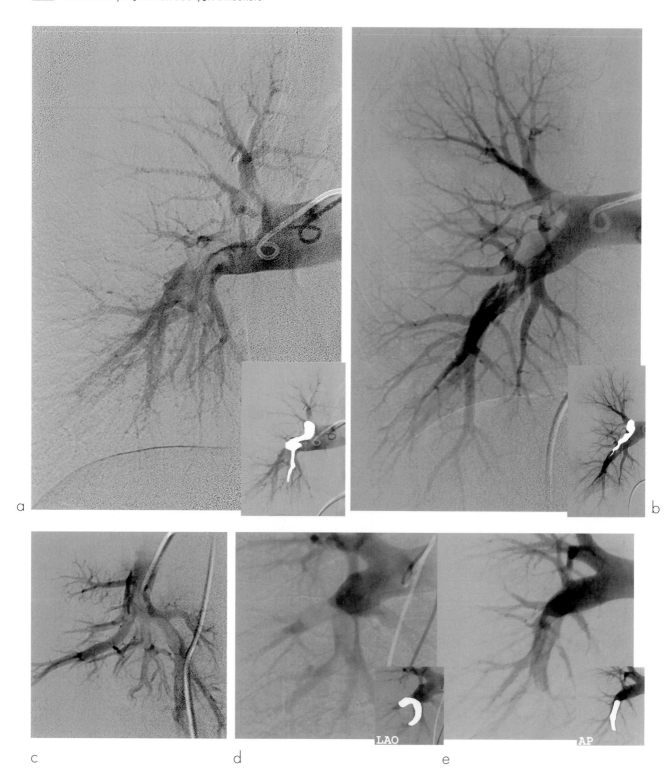

a

b

c　　　　　　　　　　d　　　　　　　　　　e

Fig. 22a–d. (Sub) segmental emboli of right lower and middle lobe arteries.

Selective angiography of the right main pulmonary artery shows a large embolus attached to the centre wall of interlobar pulmonary artery in RAO projection **(a)**. Although the thrombus extends along the ascending upper lobe artery and the superior segmental artery of the lower lobe, these vessels still show good filling. Only the lateral segment of the lower lobe shows complete cut-off and partial filling respectively (see insert).

Such large emboli in the same position, sliding over right upper, medial and lower lobe segmental arterial ostia often do not cause cut-off arteries and show normal enhancement of all segmental arteries **(b)**. The lateral branch of the medial lobe artery and the superior segment of the lower lobe artery seem to originate on the surface of the embolus.

Superselective angiography of the right lower lobe arterial segment reveals in LAO projection a casting of the emboli in all sub-segments except the anterior basal artery without any arterial cut-off **(c)**. The shape of the embolus can differ depending on the projection angle. A saddle embolus in the right medial and descending branch of the right lower lobe pulmonary artery in horseshoe LAO projection and linear AP projection configuration **(d)**, this causes the so called tramline configuration.

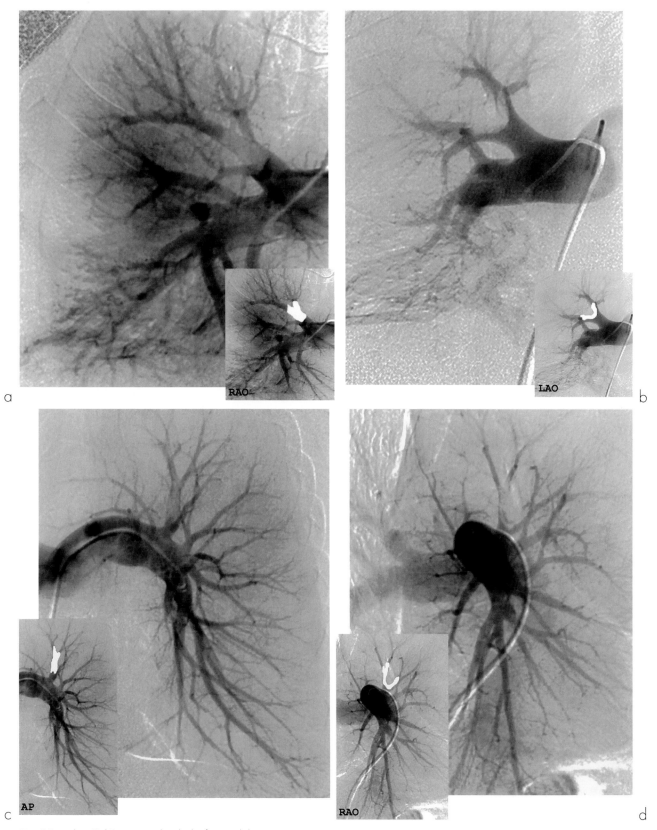

Fig. 23a–d. (Sub) segmental emboli of upper lobe arteries.
Selective angiography of right main pulmonary artery reveals extensive pulmonary emboli in upper and lower lobes. The anterior segmental upper lobe artery shows a separate branching directly from the interlobar artery. The apical and posterior segmental branches show a linear-shaped embolus in RAO projection (**a**) but a saddle embolus in LAO projection (**b**): Another example of separate branching of the left upper lobe segmental arterial branches. The anterior upper lobe branch originates directly from the descending left pulmonary artery. A linear filling defect is shown in the apical and posterior segmental upper lobe arteries in AP projection (**c**). In RAO projection a saddle embolus is seen over the crossing of these arteries (**d**).

155

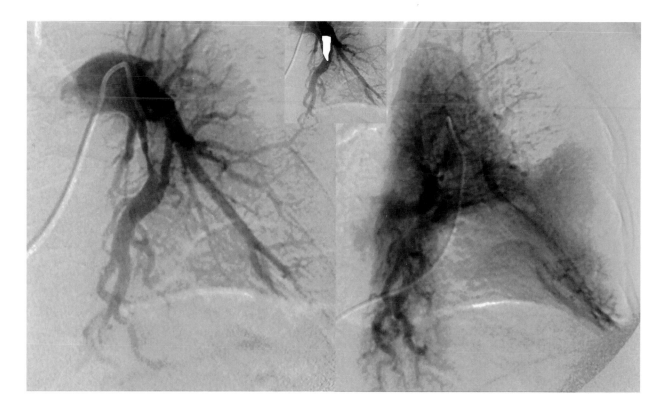

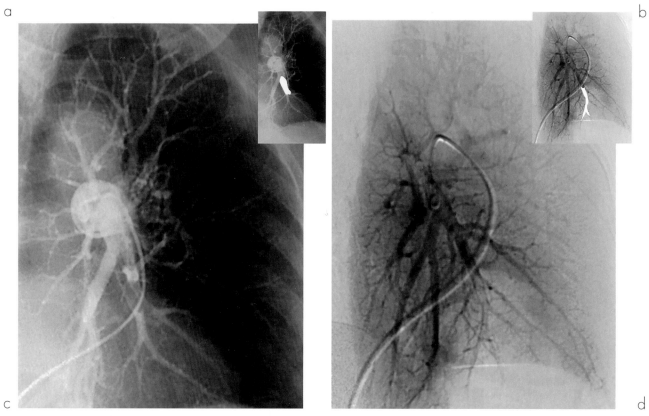

Fig. 24a–d. (Sub)segmental emboli of longula and left lower lobe arteries.
Selective angiography of the descending left pulmonary artery shows several vessel cut-offs in AP projection of the inferior longula, lateral, anterior and posterior basal arteries. Only the left medial basal segmental artery is still opacified **(a)**. Corresponding wedge-shaped perfusion defects are shown in the perfusion phase in RAO projection **(b)**. Selective angiography in RAO projection of the left lower lobe segmental arteries show a typical "tramline" of contrast medium attenuation along the posterior basal segmental artery **(c)**. An orthogonal branching half-way along this vessel causes a sharp white circular contrast enhancement with a central filling defect, nicely depicted in this non-subtracted image. Filling defects with "tramline" demarcation are seen in the anterior basal (sub)segmental artery of the left lower lobe at selective angiography in RAO projection **(d)**.

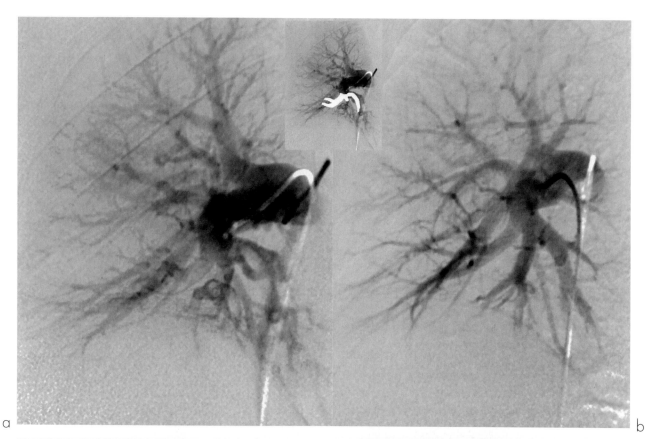

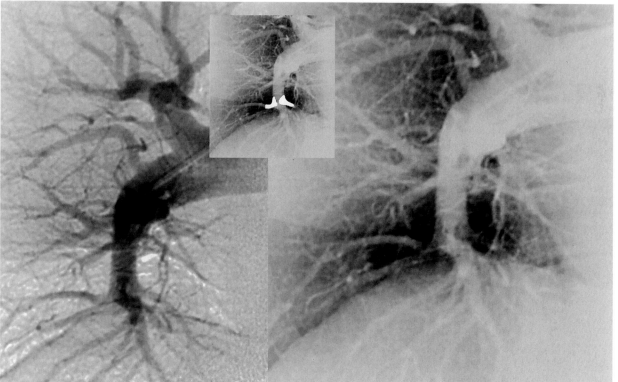

Fig. 25a–d. The selective angiography in LAO projection of the descending pulmonary artery shows a typical casting of emboli and/or thrombi in the lower lobe segmental arteries together with an elevated right diaphragm **(a)** (see insert). Repeat angiography one month later shows no filling defects after anticoagulant therapy **(b)**. Circumscribed filling defects, rounded, firmly attached to the descending right pulmonary artery wall are demonstrated at selective angiography in AP projection **(c)**. The lower lobe segmental arteries are curved by the elevated right diaphragm **(d)**, the anterior and medial basal segments show renewed opacification after 1 cm. The round shape protruding in the lumen and the fixation to the vessel wall and restoration of peripheral flow fit the diagnosis of chronic (sub)segmental emboli. Note that the cause of abnormal vessel orientation can be missed at subtractive images.

Reference method

Pulmonary angiography is generally regarded as the reference method for the diagnosis and (maybe more importantly) the exclusion of PE. Since angiography is the reference method, the sensitivity and specificity of this technique cannot be formally evaluated. This does not mean that pulmonary angiography is infallible.

The clinical validity of a normal pulmonary angiogram was assessed in five well-designed studies [6, 9, 37–39]. Anticoagulants were withheld in 840 patients with clinically suspected PE in whom a normal pulmonary angiogram was obtained. All patients were followed up for a minimum of 3 months. Recurrent thromboembolic events were demonstrated in 16 patients (1.9%; 95% CI: 1.4%–3.2%), and three of these were fatal events (0.3%; 95% CI: 0.09%–1.08%). Hence, it is regarded as safe clinical practice to withhold anticoagulants in patients with chest symptoms and a normal pulmonary arteriogram.

From these data, assuming PE was already macroscopically present at the initial examination, it may be concluded that the sensitivity of pulmonary angiography is in the region of 98%. Similarly, the specificity is thought to be between 95% and 98%. This figure is slightly lower than the sensitivity due to other illnesses which may mimic the criteria for pulmonary emboli, such as obstruction of a pulmonary artery by a mass (see Chapter IV.4).

References

1. Ludwig JW. Heart and coronaries – the pioneering age. In: Rosenbusch G, Oudkerk M, Amman E. Radiology in medical diagnostics – evolution of X-ray applications 1895–1995. Blackwell Science, Oxford, 1995: 213–224

2. Dalen JE, Brooks HL, Johnson LW, et al. Pulmonary angiography in acute PE: indications, techniques, and results in 367 patients. Am Heart J 1971; 81: 175–185

3. Sasahara AA, Hyers TM, Cole CM, et al. The urokinase PE trial. Circulation 1973; 47: 1–108

4. Bell WR, Simon TL. A comparative analysis of pulmonary perfusion scans with pulmonary angiograms. Am Heart J 1976; 92: 700–706

5. Mills SR, Jackson DC, Older RA, et al. The incidence, etiologies, and avoidance of complications of pulmonary angiography in a large series. Radiology 1980; 136: 295–299

6. Stein PD, Athanasoulis C, Alavi A, et al. Complications and validity of pulmonary angiography in acute PE. Circulation 1992; 85: 462–468

7. Van Rooy WJJ, den Heeten GJ, Sluzewski M. PE: diagnosis in 211 patients with use of selective pulmonary digital subtraction angiography with a flow-directed catheter. Radiology 1995; 195: 793–797

8. Hudson ER, Smith TP, McDermott VG, et al. Pulmonary angiography performed with iopamidol: complications in 1434 patients. Radiology 1996; 198: 61–65

9. Van Beek EJR, Reekers JA, Batchelor D, Brandjes DPM, Peeters FLM, Büller HR. Feasibility, safety and clinical utility of angiography in patients with suspected PE and non-diagnostic lung scan findings. Eur Radiol 1996; 6: 415–419

10. Zuckerman DA, Sterling KM, Oser RF. Safety of pulmonary angiography in the 1990s. J Vasc Intervent Radiology 1996; 7: 199–205

11. Nilsson T, Carlsson A, Mare K. Pulmonary angiography: a safe procedure with modern contrast media and technique. Eur Radiol 1998; 8: 86–89

12. Perlmutt LM, Braun SD, Newman GE, Oke EJ, Dunnick NR. Pulmonary arteriography in the high-risk patient. Radiology 1987; 162: 187–189

13. Nicod P, Peterson K, Levine M, et al. Pulmonary angiography in severe chronic pulmonary hypertension. Ann Intern Med 1987; 107: 565–568

14. Grollman JH, Gyepes MT, Helmer E. Transfemoral selective bilateral pulmonary arteriography with a pulmonary artery seeking catheter. Radiology 1970; 96: 102–104

15. Van Beek EJR, Bakker AJ, Reekers JA. Interobserver variability of pulmonary angiography in patients with non-diagnostic lung scan results: conventional versus digital subtraction arteriography. Radiology 1996; 198: 721–724.

16. Saeed M, Braun SD, Cohan RH, et al. Pulmonary angiography with iopamidol: patient comfort, image quality and hemodynamics. Radiology 1987; 165: 345–349

17. Tajima H, Kumazaki T, Tajima N, Ebata K. Effect of iohexol and diatrizoate on pulmonary arterial pressure following pulmonary angiography. Acta Radiol Scand 1988; suppl 29: 487–490

18. Smit EMT, van Beek EJR, Bakker AJ, Reekers JA. A blind, randomized trial evaluating the hemodynamic effects of contrast media during pulmonary angiography for suspected PE – ioxaglate vs iohexol. Acad Radiol 1995; 2: 609–613

19. Johnson MS, Stine SB, Shah H, Harris VJ, Ambrosius WT, Trerotola SO. Possible pulmonary embolus: evaluation with digital subtraction versus cut-film angiography -prospective study in 80 patients. Radiology 1998; 207: 131–138

20. Hagspiel KD, Polak JF, Grassi CJ, Faitelson BB, Kandarpa K, Meyerovitz MF. PE: comparison of cut-film and digital pulmonary angiography. Radiology 1998; 207: 139–145

21. Nilsson T, Carlsson A, Mare K, et al. Validity of pulmonary cine arteriography for the diagnosis of PE. Eur Radiol 1998 (in press)

22. Piers DB, Verzijlbergen F, Westermann CJJ, Ludwig JW. A comparative study of intravenous digital subtraction angiography and ventilation perfusion scans in suspected PE. Chest 1987; 91: 837–844

23. Musset D, Rosso J, Petiptretz P, et al. Acute PE: diagnostic value of digital subtraction angiography. Radiology 1986; 166: 455–459

24. Pond GD, Ovitt TW, Capp MP. Comparison of conventional pulmonary angiography with intravenous digital subtraction angiography for pulmonary embolic disease. Radiology 1983; 147: 345–350

25. Johnson BA, James AE. Oblique and selective pulmonary angiography in diagnosis of PE. AJR 1973; 118: 801–808

26. Bookstein JJ. Segmental arteriography in PE. Radiology 1969; 93: 1007–1012

27. Hull RD, Hirsh J, Carter CJ, et al. Pulmonary angiography, ventilation lung scanning, and venography for clinically suspected PE with abnormal perfusion lung scan. Ann Intern Med 1983; 98: 891–899

28. Quinn MF, Lundell CJ, Klotz TA, et al. Reliability of selective pulmonary arteriography in the diagnosis of PE. Am J Radiol 1987; 149: 469–471

29. Moser KM, Auger WR, Fedullo PF, Jamieson SW. Chronic thromboembolic pulmonary hypertension: clinical picture and surgical treatment. Eur Respir J 1992; 5: 334–342

30. Miller GAH, Sutton GC, Kerr IH, Gibson RV, Honey M. Comparison of streptokinase and heparin in treatment of isolated acute massive PE. Br Med J 1971; 2: 681–684

31. Görge G, Schuster S, Ge J, Meyer J, Erbel R. Intravascular ultrasound in patients with acute PE after treatment with intravenous urikinase and high-dose heparin. Heart 1997; 77: 73–77

32. Walsh PN, Greenspan RH, Simon M, et al. An angiographic severity index for PE. Circulation 1973; 47(suppl 2): 11–101

33. Simon M, Sharma GVRK, Sasahara AA. An angiographic method for quantitating the severity of PE. Internat Angiol 1984; 3: 389–392

34. Marsh JD, Glunn M, Torman HA. Pulmonary angiography: application in a new spectrum of patients. Am J Med 1983; 75: 763–769

35. Oser RF, Zuckerman DA, Gutierrez FR, Brink JA. Anatomic distribution of pulmonary emboli at pulmonary angiography: implications for crosssectional imaging. Radiology 1996; 199: 315

36. Value of the ventilation-perfusion scan in acute PE: results of the Prospective Investigation of PE Diagnosis (PIOPED). JAMA 1990; 263: 2753–2759

37. Cheely R, McCartney WH, Perry JR, et al. The role of noninvasive tests versus pulmonary angiography in the diagnosis of PE. Am J Med 1981; 70: 17–22

38. Novelline RA, Baltarowich OH, Athanasoulis CA, et al. The clinical course of patients with suspected PE and a negative pulmonary arteriogram. Radiology 1978; 126: 561–567

39. Henry JW, Relyea B, Stein PD. Continuing risk of thromboemboli among patients with normal pulmonary angiograms. Chest 1995; 107: 1375–1378

IV.4 Pulmonary angiography – safety and complications

T. P. Smith

Pulmonary angiography is an invasive procedure and therefore is not without complications. A number of reports, some from our own institution, have emphasised the potential complications [1, 2]. These potential complications have resulted in a reluctance to perform pulmonary angiography in many centres. This reluctance can be demonstrated in a study by Cooper et al who surveyed 126 hospitals in the United Kingdom and found that 47,000 V/Q scans were performed over a one year interval compared to only 490 pulmonary angiograms (1 %) despite the availability of angiography in most centres [3]. This compares to our own centre where the figures are much higher (13 %).

Based on our own experience and published data, complications of pulmonary angiography can be divided into 2 main categories relative to the performance of pulmonary angiography with a number of subcategories:

- Complications of catheter placement
  - puncture site difficulties
  - pulmonary embolism (PE) from pelvic/caval thrombus
  - vessel/cardiac injury or perforation
  - cardiac arrhythmias
- Complications of contrast injection
  - contrast related issues
  - cardiopulmonary alteration

Although this list is certainly not inclusive of every possible complication, it serves as a basis for discussion.

A complication is most often defined as that which alters the patient's expected course or requires any form of additional therapy. Complication rates for diagnostic pulmonary angiography are often listed as major and minor complications. The former are those requiring extensive therapy. The latter are less clearly defined and consist of those that require minimal therapy, often within the angiographic site even allowing the study to be completed.

Complications from the larger published series are summarised in Table 1. Many of the complications of pulmonary angiography presented here are based on publications in these series. As is often the case, it proved to be quite difficult to compile data from such varied sources. Reporting standards varied considerably. Many studies were retrospective and provided little or no follow up information. There were obvious differences in the technical aspects among studies and in patient populations. Finally, there have been technical advances over the years, which have altered virtually all radiographic diagnostic procedures, and pulmonary angiography is no exception. However, with these studies one can certainly note trends and grasp an overall picture of the complications of pulmonary angiography. Of the recent reports that gave both major and minor complications, the overall complication rate appears to be around 6 % [4, 5]. However, in both of these series, minor complications made up 5 % (Table 1).

Table 1. Review of pulmonary angiography complications in larger series.

Study	Number of angiograms	Cardiac perforation myo/ endocardial injury	Cardiac arrhythmia	Cardiac arrest	Contrast reaction	Chest pain	Respiratory arrest	Death
Dalen [30]	367	2	2	0	3	0	0	1
Stein [6]	122	1	5	0	1	1	1	0
Mills [1]	1,350	20	11	5	11	NA	NA	3
Cheely [31]	248	2	mentioned	1	0	0	0	0
Goodman [77]	350	0	1	1	unknown	0	0	0
Perlmutt [2]	1,432	NA	15	5	NA	5	5	2
Stein [4]	1,111	4	6	0	18	4	4	3
Van Beek [28]	150	1	unknown	0	0	0	0	0
Zuckerman [5]	547	0	2	0	22*	2	2	0
Hudson [10]	1,434	0	7	0	3	2	2	0

* = Includes nephrotoxicity and one case of respiratory bronchospasm from contrast.

NA = not available

Complications of catheter placement

Puncture site complications

Pulmonary angiography is most often performed from a femoral venous route. If this is precluded, access can also readily be achieved from the brachial or jugular venous routes. Puncture site complications include infection, hemorrhage, thrombosis and arteriovenous fistula formation.

Only one of the available series noted a wound infection at the venous entry site. Stein et al reported one minor wound infection in a total of 122 pulmonary angiograms (0.8 %) consisting of a mild purulent discharge 3 days following the procedure [6]. None of the other studies reported infections, however the follow-up in many of these studies is markedly limited. One could probably infer that the rate of access infection in follow up would be similar for the venous system when compared to the arterial system for diagnostic angiography. Published reports for arterial infections demonstrate extremely low rates. Messina et al reviewed vascular complications in patients undergoing interventional and diagnostic cardiac catheterisations [7]. Following a total of 6,912 procedures, 106 complications occurred in 101 patients, none of which were related to infection although the authors do suggest prophylactic antibiotics for indwelling sheaths or for patients experiencing tissue injury due to massive bleeding

into surrounding tissues. In a survey by Hessel et al, radiologists reported on complications of 118,591 examinations and infection was only noted for peripheral venography [8]. More recently, Fruhwirth et al found no deep wound infections following 11,833 diagnostic catheterisation procedures from the femoral artery, but 9 (0.3 %) following 3577 interventional procedures [9].

Patients who are undergoing pulmonary angiography are at risk for puncture site hemorrhage. In 1,111 patients from the Prospective Investigation of Pulmonary Embolism Diagnosis (PIOPED) study, Stein et al. reported eleven hematomas (1 %), 2 requiring transfusion [4]. There were no complications related to puncture site hemorrhage in the series of 1,434 patients reported from our centre by Hudson et al. [10]. These low numbers are not unexpected when one looks at the published arterial studies. In the survey by Hessel et al., hemorrhage following arterial puncture occurred in only 0.26 % of transfemoral and 0.68 % of transaxillary accesses [8].

One could postulate that bleeding would be a problem in selected patients requiring anticoagulation for suspected PE. This is of questionable significance as Wilson et al. found no relationship to coagulation parameters and hematoma formation in patients undergoing transfemoral arteriography [11]. However, Zuckerman et al. reported one patient (0.2 %) as becoming hypotensive and requiring transfusion after pulmonary angiography and this patient was receiving therapeutic levels of anticoagulants [5]. It has been shown that central access procedures can be performed in patients with disorders of hemostasis and those patients most likely to experience bleeding have severe thrombocytopenia (platelet count < 6,000/ml) [12].

Thrombosis of the access site has only been reported in one of the larger pulmonary angiography series. Stein et al. reported one symptomatic iliofemoral vein thrombosis in a total of 122 pulmonary angiograms (0.8 %) which was treated locally and with heparinisation without sequelae [6]. As with wound infections however, many studies do not have adequate follow up to allow reporting of later developing complications. In addition, earlier studies would have required either the development of symptoms or contrast venography for diagnosis compared to the non-invasive techniques available today. Most data concerning venous thrombosis are in patients with indwelling venous catheters, children with small vessels relative to catheter size, and in patients receiving inferior vena caval filters. Hammerer reviewed 700 heart catheterisations in children and infants and found occlusive thrombosis in 7 of 468 cases (0.7 %) [13]. Koksoy et al. correlated the risk factors in central venous catheter-related thrombosis [14]. One of the factors to reach statistical significance was the number of vein punctures, in that patients with two or more punctures were more likely to show thrombosis as compared to only one puncture. Whether the same technical considerations can be applied to short-term diagnostic venous catheterisation is unknown. Nolewajka et al. had 10 patients in their series with temporary transvenous cardiac pacers placed via a femoral route for 3 days or less [15]. Three (30 %) of these patients developed iliofemoral thrombosis. Kantor et al. found common femoral vein thrombosis in 7 of 17 patients (41 %) following placement of the Greenfield filter when using a 24 French introducer [16]. In a prospective evaluation, Mewissen et al. found thrombosis following insertion of the same filter to be somewhat less with 10 of 51 patients (20 %) having thrombus by sonography [17]. In addition, they found the rate of thrombosis to be greater with multiple dilations of the access site versus a single dilation with a balloon and the rate to be higher from the left common femoral vein than the right. In addition, thrombus was found in only 1 of 7 internal jugular veins (14 %).

Coupled with its low likelihood for symptoms following thrombosis, the internal jugular vein has been recommended by some as the primary site for filter placement. Whether this extrapolates to diagnostic pulmonary angiography is still unknown. Certainly the 24 F introducer is not equivalent to the 5 to 7 F catheters most often used for pulmonary angiography. However, McCowan et al. found 2 of 20 patients (10 %) to have deep venous thrombosis (DVT) following placement of the much smaller (9 F) Simon nitinol filter [18].

Arteriovenous fistulae (AVF) presumably occur when both the artery and vein are punctured and could theoretically occur when the vein is the target access just as with the artery although it has not been problematic in larger pulmonary angiography series. Messina et al. in their large series of patients undergoing interventional and diagnostic cardiac catheterisations found only 1 AVF in 106 complications [7]. In the survey by Hessel et al., AVF were noted in 0.01 % of transfemoral and 0.02 % of transaxillary accesses [8]. There was a single AVF (0.008 %) in the diagnostic arterial procedures reported by Fruhwirth et al. [9]. Finally, McCann et al. reviewed arteriovenous fistulas requiring surgical intervention from 16,350 cardiac catheterisations (0.0004 %) performed at our centre over a five year interval [19]. They concluded that most of these fistulas were small, hemodynamically insignificant and closed spontaneously without need for intervention.

In general, access site complications for pulmonary angiography are relatively rare and consist mostly of hematomas in the reported series. However, few series present the extensive long term follow up that would be necessary to record such complications as thrombosis, infection, or even AVF. Hematomas present as acute problems and would be more easily detected in the angiographic suite or by short term follow up.

PE from pelvic/caval thrombus

Although this has been questioned by recent publications, it is still widely believed that most pulmonary emboli originate in the venous system of the legs, pelvis, and inferior vena cava [20]. One of the most widely utilised studies for DVT is sonography, which has little utility in the pelvis and caval vein. Therefore one would expect to encounter thrombus within the pelvic venous system and inferior vena cava in a proportion of patients (Fig. 1) This has even caused some to avoid the femoral access [21]. If venography is not performed prior to catheter placement from the common femoral vein to the right atrium, thrombus could theoretically be dislodged by catheterisation causing PE. Ferris et al. found inferior vena caval

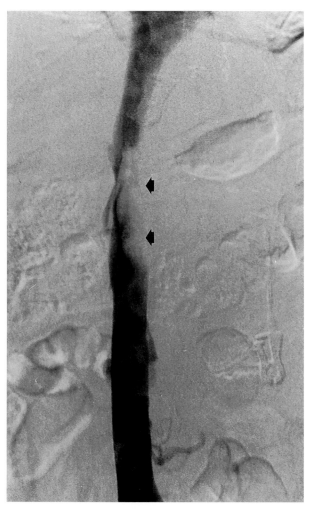

Fig. 1a. Inferior vena cavagram performed prior to pulmonary angiography demonstrates unexpected thrombus in the inferior vena cava (arrows).

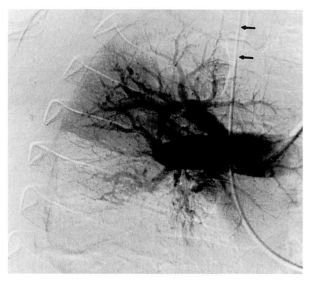

Fig. 1b. The right internal jugular vein was used as an alternative access (arrows). Angiography demonstrates findings consistent with chronic PE.

thrombus in 6 of 18 patients who had documented PE [22]. Others who performed cavography for inferior vena cava filter placement following pulmonary angiography positive for embolic disease, however have not substantiated these findings [23]. Therefore, although this complication is conceivable, it is much more theoretical than real. Stein et al. reported a single case of iatrogenic PE in 122 angiograms (0.8 %) and the source of the thrombus was presumed to be from the catheter [6]. Catheter thrombosis must be avoided in all situations but is particularly dangerous when angiography is performed for pulmonary arteriovenous malformations, in which there is in effect a left to right shunt.

Stein et al. found two clinically unsuspected iliac vein thromboses in 122 pulmonary angiograms preventing passage of the catheter (1.6 %) [6]. We did not encounter any problems stemming from caval thrombosis in our series of 1,434 pa-

tients [10]. Small amounts of contrast material were injected after femoral venous access in the initial patients in the PIOPED study [24, 25]. The pelvic system and inferior vena cava were visualised fluoroscopically to determine patency. However, due to difficulties with variability among techniques and investigators, this portion of the study was discontinued after the initial patients. Grollman states in his review article in 1992 that he has only rarely encountered unsuspected thrombus in the inferior vena cava during pulmonary angiography and he successfully and safely demonstrated such thrombus by angiography [26]. However, he does not routinely perform cavography prior to pulmonary angiography. We and most others agree with this approach [27]. In a patient with caval thrombosis, it is possible to catheterise safely around the thrombus. This may be clinically necessary in certain selected cases such as inferior vena cava filter placement, if thrombolysis is to be performed, if no other access is available, etc. However, for diagnostic pulmonary angiography in the presence of pelvic or caval thrombus, we use an alternative route such as the internal jugular vein if at all possible (Fig. 1).

Vessel and cardiac injury or perforation

Anytime catheterisation of a vessel occurs, one must be concerned with intimal injury or even perforation. Injury to the pelvic veins, inferior vena cava or pulmonary artery is theoretically possible. Subintimal contrast stain was reported in 4 of

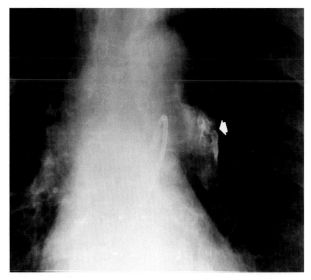

Fig. 2. Chest radiograph in a patient following pulmonary angiography. A pigtail catheter is still located in the left pulmonary artery. There is subintimal contrast in the left pulmonary artery representing a small stain (arrow). The angiogram was negative for PE and the patient had no untoward events related to the arterial injury.

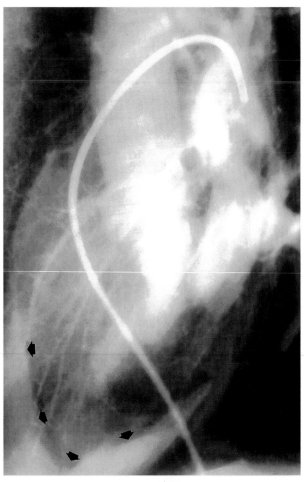

Fig. 3. Lateral view of the late phase of a pulmonary angiogram using an NIH-type catheter. During passage of the catheter through the heart there was myocardial perforation. There is a persistent contrast collection (arrows) surrounding the cardiac silhouette. Angiography was completed without difficulty and the patient remained asymptomatic.

1,111 cases (0.4%) by Stein et al. [4] (Fig. 2). One patient (0.7%) in the series by Van Beek had a pulmonary artery dissection and 2 patients had contrast extravasation [28]. However, none of these patients suffered any untoward events related to the arterial injury.

One of the historical worries with pulmonary angiography was for cardiac perforation (Fig. 3). In a review of 241 studies, Ranniger et al. found 2 cases of injection into the pericardium and 3 into the myocardium [29]. Dalen et al. had two cardiac perforations in their series of 367 patients [30]. Mills et al. reported cardiac perforation in 14 patients (1%) with endocardial or myocardial injury in an additional 4 [1]. Cheely et al. reported 1 right ventricular perforation (0.4%) which required surgical repair in 248 pulmonary angiograms [31]. Marsh et al. reported 1 patient in whom perforation of the right ventricle by the angiographic catheter resulted in cardiac tamponade which was initially managed by pericardiocentesis but subsequently required limited thoracotomy [32].

None of these perforations were fatal. However, Bell and Simon reported a single death from cardiac perforation during pulmonary angiography for the Urokinase Pulmonary Embolism Trial in a patient with known cardiomyopathy [34]. Death occurred 3 days after the procedure and was presumed to be due to cardiac perforation during pulmonary angiography on clinical grounds. All of these perforations (where the technical details were reported) occurred with catheters which were straight in configuration. Given these complications, a transfemoral pulmonary artery – seeking pigtail catheter was developed by Grollman in 1970 and various modifications in the design have been made since [33, 35]. Since the development of these catheters, the rate of cardiac perforation has significantly decreased. Hudson et al. noted none in their series of 1,434 pulmonary angiograms all performed with pigtail catheters [10]. Pigtail catheters are not without their own complications. The catheter can become entangled in the chordae tendineae of the tricuspid valve or even become knotted [36]. As recently as 1992, 3 cardiac perforations (2.6%) occurred in 114 pulmonary angiograms reported by Bernard et al. [37]. The authors elude to using pigtail catheters, but this was not definitely stated in the report. However, the perforations were not clinically apparent.

In summary, injury to pelvic veins, inferior vena cava, heart, or pulmonary arteries is quite rare with the techniques used today. When such injury does occur, it is most often of no clinical significance.

Cardiac dysrhythmias

Cardiac dysrhythmias occur during the performance of pulmonary angiography from either catheter manipulation or during contrast injection The latter very rarely occurs, it is short lived, and has neither been reported or been problematic in any of the larger available series. Cardiac dysrhythmias are quite common with passage of catheters through the right heart. Although pulmonary angiography has been performed for quite some time and these dysrhythmias are well known to interventionists, most information is derived from flow-directed balloon-tipped hemodynamic monitoring catheters, which are inserted at the bedside. These catheters were introduced in 1970, and due to the very large number inserted world-wide most data related to catheterisation of the pulmonary arteries through the right heart originate from these series. Recently, there has been some heated discussion as to whether pulmonary artery cathetherisation results in increased survival [38, 39]. Despite great debate over whether such catheters resulted in increased patient survival, complications of such catheterisation including significant cardiac dysrhythmias during insertion were not a major concern.

There are a number of studies available regarding rhythm disturbances during bedside pulmonary artery catheterisation. In 1983 Boyd et al. published a prospective study of complications of 500 consecutive patients receiving 528 catheters and found potentially life threatening arrhythmias (ventricular tachycardia) in 8 (1.5%); 6 responded to intravenous lidocaine while 2 required cardioversion [40].

Shah et al. prospectively studied 6,245 pulmonary artery catheterisations and dysrhythmias occurred in 72% of cases [41]. The vast majority however were transient premature ventricular (68%) or atrial (1%) depolarisations which responded to change in catheter position. Only 3% resulted in persistent premature ventricular contractions and all of these responded to intravenous lidocaine administration. Three patients developed right bundle branch block, none necessitating treatment. One patient out of 113 patients

with pre-existing left bundle branch block developed complete heart block necessitating a pacing catheter. Damen and Bolton reported on a prospective analysis of 1,400 pulmonary artery catheterisations and found much the same results, where dysrhythmias occurred in 67% overall, with supraventricular arrhythmias in 11 (0.8%), ventricular arrhythmias in 930 (66%), right bundle branch block in 2 (0.1%), and complete heart block in 1 (0.07%) [42]. Only 3 of the ventricular arrhythmias did not resolve spontaneously following catheter repositioning and these 3 responded to intravenous lidocaine.

The same dysrhythmias occur during the placement of angiographic catheters for pulmonary angiography and consist of supraventricular and ventricular arrhythmias with the possible induction of heart block. The major difference between bedside and angiographic catheters however consists of the construction of the catheter and its method of placement. Angiographic catheters are often larger and are usually made of stiffer material accounting for their radiopacity and torquability. Their method of placement also differs as they are usually placed over a guidewire or manoeuvred through the heart by torquing the catheter, both methods utilising fluoroscopy. The stiffer material and use of a guidewire should theoretically result in a greater number of dysrhythmias. However, as most such arrhythmias respond to catheter repositioning, usually advancement into the pulmonary artery or being pulled from the ventricle into the atrium or into the vena cava, fluoroscopy should theoretically aid such repositioning resulting in fewer serious dysrhythmias. Concerning catheter placement, Van Rooij et al. performed pulmonary angiography in 211 patients using a flow-directed balloon catheter in an effort to decrease problematic cardiac dysrhythmias and continuously monitored the ECG in 104 of these patients [43]. No patients required therapeutic intervention for dysrhythmia. Of the 104 patients with continuous monitoring, 22 (21%) had one to seven premature ventricular contractions without sustained tachycardia in any patient. To that end, balloon occlusion angiography of the pulmonary system has been shown to be quite valuable particularly as an adjunct to standard selective catheter techniques [44]. However, flow directed catheters have been shown to induce false aneurysms and rupture of the pulmonary artery during balloon occlusion angiography has been reported [45, 46].

In the larger series, Mills et al. reported the largest number of significant cardiac events from catheter manipulation [1]. A total of 16 events (1.2%) were reported including 11 arrhythmias (0.8%)

requiring treatment and 5 cardiac arrests (0.4%). The arrhythmias consisted of ventricular tachycardia, ventricular fibrillation, right bundle branch block, complete heart block, paroxysmal atrial tachycardia, and bradycardia although the numbers for each are not provided. The authors also state that cardiopulmonary arrest occurred in 5 patients as a result of catheter manipulation and all patients were resuscitated and pulmonary angiography subsequently completed although further details are not provided. Dalen et al. reported 2 cases of atrial fibrillation in 367 patients (0.5%) which were treated medically and returned to normal sinus rhythm within 24 hours [30]. The Urokinase Pulmonary Embolism Trial Investigators reported 5 arrhythmias in a total of 310 pulmonary angiograms (1.6%) [47] and Novelline et al. reported 4 in a total of 302 (1.3%) [48]. Stein et al. reported one of the largest rates that 4 patients experienced dysrhythmias during in a total of 122 angiograms (3%) [6]. In the PIOPED study, there were 9 cases of arrhythmia in 1,111 patients (0.8%), all converted spontaneously or promptly responded to medication [4]. However, two of the deaths in this series appear to be, at least in part, related to cardiac dysrhythmias encountered at pulmonary angiography. In one of these patients electromechanical dissociation occurred with the catheter in the right ventricle although no arrhythmia was noted and the mechanism of events were reported to be unclear. The second patient had a catheter in the right ventricle when ventricular tachycardia occurred which was reverted but respiratory arrest and hypotension occurred soon after and the patient died 24 hours after catheterisation. In the series of Hudson et al. consisting of 1,434 pulmonary angiograms, 8 patients (0.6%) had significant cardiac dysrhythmias

requiring treatment [10]. In 6 patients (0.4%) treatment with intravenous lidocaine was successful and pulmonary angiography was completed [10]. In 2 patients (0.1%) ventricular arrhythmia recurred during each catheter manipulation despite medical therapy and the procedure was selectively discontinued. All of these patients left the angiography suite in sinus rhythm and had no further cardiac rhythm disturbances during 48 hours of follow up.

Overall, although cardiac dysrhythmias appear to occur frequently during catheter manipulation for pulmonary angiography, they are for the most part self limited and respond well to catheter repositioning. Medical treatment appears to be necessary in only approximately 1% of patients or less and virtually all patients appear to respond well. Although quite rare, complete heart block has been produced in patients with a pre-existing left bundle branch block when a right block is induced by catheter manipulation. It is the practice of many to place either a temporary transvenous or external cardiac pacing device in all patients with pre-existing left bundle branch blocks or even those patients known to have pre-existing ventricular arrhythmias [27]. More recent literature does not altogether support the necessity of such a manoeuvre. In the series of Hudson et al. of over 1,400 patients, it was our practice to place an external device in all patients with left bundle branch block [10]. The device was not activated in any of these patients. However, the ease with which an external pacing device can be placed has tended to make its use in selected cases relatively routine, mostly for pre-existing right bundle branch block, particularly if the block has developed relatively recently.

Complications of contrast injection

Contrast related issues

Pulmonary angiography, as it has been in the past and is currently performed, requires the use of iodinated contrast material. These agents certainly are not without risk. Contrast, which is rapidly injected, as with pulmonary angiography, can cause intimal dissection depending on catheter position. In addition, contrast injection for pulmonary angiography has been associated with some benign dysrhythmias. These complications are discussed above. Additional complications asso-

ciated with contrast material injection can be further divided loosely into those associated with contrast injection anywhere in the vascular system and those associated more specifically with pulmonary angiography. The former consists mostly of contrast induced nephrotoxicity and allergic reactions. The latter consists mostly of hemodynamic alterations associated with contrast injection into the pulmonary vascular bed. There are in general two types of contrast agents: high osmolar ionic agents and low osmolar non-ionic agents and there are some variations between these two.

Early pulmonary angiography, like all angiography, was performed with high osmolar ionic contrast agents. More recently, it has become preferable to perform pulmonary angiography with the low osmolar agents. This has to do with several factors including less hemodynamic alterations with the non-ionic low osmolar agents (see following section), a decrease in contrast media associated nephrotoxicity and the potential for fewer severe contrast media reactions.

Contrast media associated nephrotoxicity is a common cause for hospital acquired acute renal failure. In general there is variability concerning contrast nephrotoxicity based on the criteria chosen to denote renal insufficiency and the nature of the study. Several risk factors are usually given for the development of contrast associated nephrotoxicity including pre-existing renal insufficiency and contrast volume. As pulmonary angiography can require relatively large contrast volumes and may be performed in very ill patients, the potential for contrast associated nephrotoxicity is certainly possible. The incidence of contrast associated nephrotoxicity in patients with pre-existing renal insufficiency varies widely but certainly occurs. In two studies involving 330 patients, the incidence of the development of significant nephrotoxicity, when the serum creatinine level exceeded 2.25–2.5 mg/dl, varied between 17% and 20% [49, 50]. It also appears as though there is a correlation between volume of contrast material and nephrotoxicity. Manske et al. evaluated 59 insulin dependent diabetics undergoing coronary angiography and found the incidence of nephrotoxicity to be 26% when less than 30 ml was giving compared to 79% when more than 30 ml was given [51]. Low osmolar non-ionic contrast material appears to be associated with less nephrotoxicity even in the azotemic patient. Rudnick et al. randomised 1,196 patients undergoing coronary angiography to receive high osmolar ionic agents or low osmolar non-ionic agents [52]. They found the risks of nephrotoxicity to be equal when there was no pre-existing renal insufficiency, but in the azotemic patient the risk was 7% in the high osmolar ionic group versus 4% in the low osmolar non-ionic group. These numbers rose to 12% and 27% respectively when the underlying insufficiency was coupled with diabetes mellitus. Although most cases of contrast media associated nephrotoxicity are largely reversible by medical therapy, acute renal failures are certainly not without associated morbidity and mortality [53].

Contrast associated nephrotoxicity does occur with pulmonary angiography. However, many of the studies did not produce adequate follow up either in length of time or laboratory analysis to determine the renal effects of contrast administration. Only two of the major studies consistently followed serum creatinine levels. Stein et al., reporting on patients in the PIOPED study, found 10 patients (0.9%) who developed increased serum creatinine levels which required treatment not including dialysis, and 3 patients (0.3%) who developed renal failure requiring dialysis [4]. In the former group, 5 patients had previously normal creatinine values, which increased to levels ranging from 2.1 to 5.9 mg/dl, and 5 patients with previously abnormal creatinine levels (1.5 to 2.7 mg/dl) developed a further increase. Two of the three patients requiring dialysis had baseline renal insufficiency with serum creatinine levels of 2.4 and 2.7 mg/dl. All patients in this series received high osmolar ionic contrast material. Zuckerman et al. in their series of 547 pulmonary angiograms using low osmolar non-ionic media had 11 patients (2.6%) with contrast media associated nephrotoxicity defined as an elevation in baseline serum creatinine of 50% or greater 2–3 days after the procedure [5]. Ten of the 11 patients had underlying renal insufficiency and all but one patient had a return of their creatinine level to baseline 2–3 weeks following the procedure. It is unclear whether any of these patients (including the final one who did not return to baseline) required dialysis.

Adverse reactions to the injection of contrast material are well know and can generally be classified as idiosyncratic or non-idiosyncratic. Idiosyncratic reactions are not dose dependent and are anaphylactoid in nature. Non-iodiosyncratic reactions are volume dependent and are the result of chemotoxic or hyperosmolar properties of the contrast. It is no longer disputed that both idiosyncratic and non-idiosyncratic reactions are occurring less often with low osmolar non-ionic agents. Palmer et al. in a series of 109,546 patients, Wolf et al. in a series of 600 patients, and Katayma et al. in a series of 337,647 patients, reported an overall incidence of all adverse reactions to high osmolar ionic contrast media of 3.8%, 4.17%, and 12.66%, respectively, compared to 1.2%, 0.69%, and 3.13%, respectively, for low osmolar non-ionic media [54–56]. Katayama et al. reported severe reactions and very severe reactions in 0.22% and 0.04% of patients with high osmolar ionic media compared to 0.04% and 0.004% with low osmolar non-ionic media, respectively [56]. In addition, the same study showed a significantly lower subsequent reaction rate to low osmolar non-ionic contrast media in patients who had had prior contrast reactions and those with a history of asthma or other allergies (besides contrast material) were less likely to have a severe adverse reaction to low osmolar non-ionic contrast material when compared to high osmolar ionic media [56].

Certainly, many of the above principles of contrast hold true for pulmonary angiography, but the exact comparison is difficult. Compared to patients undergoing excretory urography and CT (on which most of the contrast studies are based), the numbers of patients undergoing pulmonary angiography are relatively small and therefore the overall numbers of patients with contrast media associated nephrotoxicity and adverse reactions are small. In addition, many of these patients are already hospitalised and have received appropriate prophylactic measures for their underlying azotemia or known contrast media sensitivity. Pulmonary angiography also differs in that the contrast material is injected directly into the pulmonary arteries and at a very rapid rate. To that end, it has been anecdotally noted that severe idiosyncratic reactions to contrast material in the arterial system are quite rare, although deaths have been reported even with low osmolar non-ionic agents [57, 58]. Certainly the volume of contrast and its rate of injection for pulmonary angiography influences non-idiosyncratic reactions to contrast. To that end, where non-idiosyncratic reactions are concerned, probably the most striking advantage for the low osmolar non-ionic agents has been the lessening of contrast agent-induced coughing during pulmonary angiography [59, 60]. High osmolar ionic agents produce well known discomfort to the patient stimulating a marked coughing response. The discomfort is thought to be largely mediated by the hyperosmolarity and high viscosity of the ionic agents. Besides being uncomfortable for the patient, uncontrollable coughing can significantly degrade image quality. Smith et al. in a randomised study of 25 patients each receiving at least one injection with an ionic (diatrizoate sodium meglumine) and non-ionic (ioxaglate) agent showed a significant difference in the coughing response with the non-ionic agent [59]. In addition, they compared the quality of the images between the two agents and noted no differences between agents when coughing was excluded prompting the authors to recommend the use of non-ionic agents for pulmonary angiography. In addition to contrast-induced coughing, many of the cardiopulmonary alterations (see following section) may in fact be based on non-idiosyncratic adverse contrast reactions.

Idiosyncratic reactions to contrast are reported in most series of pulmonary angiography (Table 1).

Dalen et al. reported 3 cases of bronchospasm and 1 of anaphylaxis in 367 consecutive patients undergoing pulmonary angiography [30]. Mills et al. reported 11 minor contrast reactions in 1,350 patients (0.8%) but these were not defined further [1]. Stein et al. reported 16 patients (1.4%) with minor contrast reactions consisting of urticaria, itching, or periorbital oedema [4]. A single patient had bronchospasm most likely related to a severe contrast reaction requiring intubation. All of these series utilised high osmolar ionic contrast material. In the series by Hudson et al. of 1,434 patients who underwent pulmonary angiography with low osmolar non-ionic contrast material, minor contrast reactions consisting of urticaria occurred in only 2 patients (0.1%) and a single patient (0.1%) had a severe reaction requiring intubation [10]. Zuckerman et al. also using low osmolar non-ionic media reported one patient (0.2%) with bronchospasm following angiography which required intubation [5]. None of the reported deaths from pulmonary angiography can be specifically traced to an idiosyncratic reaction to contrast material. However, as discussed below, contrast definitely results in hemodynamic alterations and the mechanisms responsible for both idiosyncratic and non-idiosyncratic reactions are so unclear that it becomes difficult to separate the cause and effect relationships.

Based on limited data, contrast reactions with pulmonary angiography appear to be somewhat greater than the same reactions encountered with routine intravenous contrast administration. Reduction of these adverse reactions must involve careful patient assessment prior to the angiogram and appropriate prophylaxis when possible. This includes the routine use of low osmolar non-ionic agents. For pulmonary angiography, there are probably only two disadvantages for the non-ionic agents: their reported increased thrombogenicity and cost. Concerning the former, reports are available noting the increased incidence of thrombus formation during angiography when using low osmolar non-ionic agents. This has been particularly reported during cardiac catheterisation [61]. In addition, a recent study where patients were randomised to ionic and non-ionic agents for cerebral angiography found a significantly higher incidence of clot formation with low osmolar non-ionic media [62]. Although this has not been reported with pulmonary angiography, one must be cognisant of this problem when the low osmolar non-ionic agents are used. Cost is certainly a consideration in the overall picture of contrast usage. However, given the relatively small number of pulmonary angiograms related to other contrast procedures and the clear advantages gained by using the non-ionic low osmolar agents, their exclusive usage in pulmonary angiography is recommended and justified.

Hemodynamic and respiratory alterations

It is generally well known that the introduction of hyperosmolar contrast material into the pulmonary circulation results in a number of cardiovascular reflexes including systemic hypotension and a change in cardiac rate [63]. Hemodynamic alterations, including those which are life threatening, have been reported during and shortly following pulmonary angiography. It may however be difficult at times to separate whether this represents a severe adverse contrast reaction as described above or a different process altogether. However, due to their importance in the consideration of complications related to pulmonary angiography, they will be discussed here as a separate section. Patients undergoing pulmonary angiography have been reported to have a variety of hemodynamic alterations including systemic hypotension, increased pulmonary arterial pressures, and cardiopulmonary collapse. Systemic hypotension can be due to a number of causes including idiosyncratic adverse contrast reactions as reported above. Transient hypotension has been reported to occur with contrast injection due to peripheral vasodilation. It has been postulated that these systemic hypotensive reactions may be a reflection of reduced aortic pressure by the temporary decrease in pulmonary blood flow to the left heart. Many patients who are undergoing pulmonary angiography may be dehydrated resulting in a relative state of hypotension. Obviously this state needs correction if possible not only from a cardiovascular perspective, but also from one of contrast associated nephrotoxicity. Finally, physiologic reflex syncope (vasovagal) occurs during pulmonary angiography as with many other procedures. Such a reflex occurred in 2 patients (0.1%) in the series by Hudson et al. and were successfully treated with intravenous fluids in both with the addition of atropine sulfate in 1 [10]. Stein et al. reported 2 cases of physiologic reflex syncope in 122 consecutive pulmonary angiograms (1.6%) one requiring no treatment and the second treated medically [6].

Pulmonary artery pressures tend to increase after the injection of contrast material. The reasons for this increase in pressure remain unclear although a number of theories exist. Contrast material in the pulmonary vascular system causes arterial constriction, venous constriction, or both, resulting in increased arterial pressure [64, 65]. Hypertonic solutions tend to produce changes in red blood cells such as aggregation and crenation, which can result in capillary blockage and increased pulmonary pressures [66]. Data also supports that increased pressures may be related to contrast viscosity [67]. Finally, the volume of the injection alone may be responsible for increased pressures [68]. As would be expected with the above theories, the increase in pressures following the injection of high osmolar ionic contrast material tend to be greater than those with low osmolar non-ionic media [69, 70]. Smith et al. prospectively evaluated pulmonary artery pressures during pulmonary angiography performed with low osmolar non-ionic contrast media in 116 consecutive patients and found there was a small but statistically significant rise in pulmonary artery pressure after injection of low osmolar non-ionic contrast material [71]. The authors concluded that such a rise was unlikely to be of clinical significance. Pitton et al. confirmed the findings that bolus injection of non-ionic low osmolar contrast media caused no major hemodynamic effects even in patients with severe chronic thromboembolic pulmonary hypertension [72]. Since the hyperviscosity theories for elevated pulmonary artery pressures following pulmonary angiography would not apply as readily to low osmolar contrast media, it may be true that rapid increases in volume alone could be responsible for the rise in pulmonary pressures although this cannot be stated with certainty.

Increases in pulmonary artery pressure during angiography generated much interest in early reports. Death from pulmonary angiography was attributed to the sequelae of pulmonary hypertension [1, 30, 32]. Severe underlying pulmonary hypertension presumably places the right heart in an extremely compromised state such that any sudden increase in pulmonary pressure results in right heart decompensation and possibly death. Marsh et al. reported a single death in a series of 106 patients (1%) [32]. This patient had pulmonary artery systolic pressure of 70 mmHg. Moses et al. had a similar experience in their series of 298 pulmonary angiograms where 2 patients with severe obstruction of their pulmonary vasculature died shortly after injection although the authors did not necessarily attribute these deaths to the procedure itself [73]. Two deaths occurred in the series of Stein et al. of 122 consecutive pulmonary angiograms [6]. However, neither of the 2 deaths encountered was judged to be directly caused by pulmonary angiography. In more recent series, Stein et al. reported 5 deaths related to pulmonary angiography [4]. Three of those deaths variably

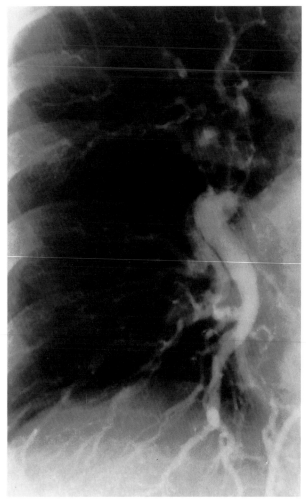

Fig. 4. View of right pulmonary artery approximately 20 seconds into pulmonary angiography. Contrast remains within the right pulmonary artery demonstrating very slow flow. The pulmonary artery and right ventricular end diastolic pressures were elevated. This patient suffered severe cardiopulmonary complications and died from pulmonary angiography.

followed the injection of high osmolar ionic contrast material. The other 2 deaths were probably related to consequences of catheter placement as noted in the section on dysrhythmias. The most quoted work on the subject of death from pulmonary angiography is that of Mills et al. [1]. In 1980, they reported on 3 deaths from pulmonary angiography, all in patients with pulmonary hypertension and right ventricular end diastolic pressures equal to or greater than 20 mmHg (Fig. 4). This prompted the authors to eventually recommend that pulmonary angiography should not be performed in such patients [74]. However, not all agreed that pulmonary artery hypertension posed a significant risk for pulmonary angiography. Nicod et al. performed pulmonary angiography in 67 consecutive patients with moderate to severe

primary pulmonary hypertension or hypertension secondary to chronic thromboembolic occlusion of the pulmonary artery where the average pulmonary artery systolic pressure was 74 mmHg and 14 patients had right ventricular end diastolic pressures of 20 mmHg or greater [21]. Despite marked elevation of right sided pressures, there were no deaths attributable to pulmonary angiography.

If the association of increased right heart pressures and cardiac failure were to hold true, the rate of mortality from pulmonary angiography should decrease with low osmolar non-ionic agent since they result in significantly less elevation in pulmonary pressure than high osmolar ionic agents as discussed above. Perlmutt et al. reported 1,434 patients who underwent pulmonary angiography, 388 (27%) of which had pulmonary arterial hypertension defined as greater than 40 mmHg. Two deaths occurred in this series, both in patients with severe pulmonary hypertension (greater than 70 mmHg) [2]. Hudson et al. compared an identical size population at the same institution using low osmolar non-ionic contrast material [10]. Pulmonary arterial hypertension defined as a systolic pressure greater than or equal to 40 mmHg was found in 402 patients (28%) and a systolic pulmonary artery pressure of 70 mmHg or greater was found in 99 patients (7%). Although these numbers exceeded that of Perlmutt et al., no deaths were attributable to pulmonary angiography prompting the authors to conclude that pulmonary angiography is safer with non-ionic, low osmolar contrast agents [2]. Combining the two recent series of Hudson et al. and Zuckerman et al., a total of 1,981 pulmonary angiograms were performed using low osmolar non-ionic contrast material without mortality [5, 10]. These findings lend credence to the idea that pulmonary angiography is safer with low osmolar non-ionic agents, although further investigation is still warranted.

A number of patients experience respiratory insufficiency and/or cardiac arrest following pulmonary angiography. Despite using low osmolar non-ionic contrast material, Zuckerman et al. had 2 patients (0.4%) develop respiratory distress during the procedure requiring intubation and 1 patient developed respiratory insufficiency 3 hours after pulmonary angiography [5]. Hudson et al. also had 2 patients (0.1%) who developed respiratory distress during angiography and required ventilatory support [10]. Certainly these could represent idiosyncratic adverse reactions to contrast material (see above) or the result of increased volume in already compromised patients, but the precise etiology cannot be determined.

Zuckerman et al. found a statistically significant relationship between the occurrence of minor complications and the presence of underlying pulmonary disease [5]. Moderate to severe pulmonary hypertension was correlated with major complications which occurred in 5 patients including groin hematoma, bronchospasm and respiratory insufficiency. As expected, there was a statistically significant association between complications and patients with a poor physical status as graded according to the American Society of Anesthesiology criteria. It is certainly conceivable that minor degrees of respiratory insufficiency developed in patients in other series, but due to the necessity of little or no therapy in the immediate angiography period, these may not have been reported.

Respiratory insufficiency and possibly some cardiac decompensation could certainly be based on the volume of fluids given to patients during angiography. Often a relatively large amount of fluid including contrast material, angiographic flush solutions and intravenous support fluids are necessary. As many of these patients are already severely compromised, additional intravascular volumes could be deleterious. Although this is certainly possible and probably does occur, it has not been reported as the etiology for acute respiratory insufficiency in any of the series reviewed here. Interestingly, Zuckerman et al. reviewed 547 consecutive patients who underwent pulmonary angiography and analysed their complications [5]. In their series, no statistically significant difference was noted for patient age or for volume of contrast material used. Finally, there are unusual situations where respiratory failure can be due to other causes, again often due to the difficulty with the clinical diagnosis of PE and the need to perform angiography in compromised patients. Acute respiratory failure has been reported in patients being treated with amiodarone for arrhythmias [75, 76]. Obviously, care should be taken prior to pulmonary angiography in all patients and their respiratory status must be fully evaluated prior to angiography.

Cardiac arrest has been reported with pulmonary angiography. The exact etiology is unclear. Ranniger et al. had 2 patients with cardiac arrest in their series of 241 patients [29]. A single patient suffered from cardiogenic shock in the series of Dalen et al. of 367 consecutive patients [30]. Five patients in the series by Mills et al. had cardiac arrest, which was thought to be related to catheter manipulation [1]. All 5 recovered and angiography was performed. It is interesting to note that in the series of Zuckerman et al. of 547 consecutive pulmonary angiograms and that of Hudson et al. of 1, 434 pulmonary angiograms, cardiac arrest was not given as a complication [5, 10]. As mentioned previously the cardiovascular effects of low osmolar non-ionic contrast material are less than those with the high osmolar ionic agents. Since these two studies used the former, it is interesting to speculate that the difference in contrast agents accounted for the lack of cardiac complications. However, this can only be inferred from the existing data.

Summary

Overall, pulmonary angiography is a very safe procedure. Even in light of the above review of major and minor complications, the most striking general feature is the safety with which pulmonary angiography can be performed. Technical refinements including the use of better imaging systems, pigtail catheters, and low osmolar non-ionic contrast media appear to enhance the safety of pulmonary angiography. Certainly the addition of better imaging equipment and patient monitoring adds to this safety although this is difficult to quantify. Much effort is currently underway to diagnose PE using less invasive techniques. Although the advancement of these techniques must be encouraged, reluctance to perform pulmonary angiography based on a perceived high complication rate is totally unfounded. When performed by experienced interventionists using modern equipment and techniques, pulmonary angiography should be viewed as a reasonable and safe diagnostic procedure, which greatly outweighs the potential complications of inadequate use of anticoagulant therapy.

References

1. Mills SR, Jackson DC, Older RA, et al. The incidence, etiologies, and avoidance of complications of pulmonary angiography in a large series. Radiology 1980; 136: 295–299

2. Perlmutt LM, Braun SD, Newman GE, et al. Pulmonary arteriography in the high-risk patient. Radiology 1987; 162: 187–189

3. Cooper TJ, Hayward MWJ, Hartog M. Survey on the use of pulmonary scintigraphy and angiography for suspected pulmonary thromboembolism in the UK. Clinical Radiology 1991; 43: 243–245

4. Stein PD, Athanasoulis C, Alavi A, et al. Complications and validity of pulmonary angiography in acute pulmonary embolism. Circulation 1992; 85: 462–468

5. Zuckerman DA, Sterling KM, Oser RF. Safety of pulmonary angiography in the 1990s. J Vasc Intervent Radiol 1996; 7: 199–205

6. Stein MA, Winter J, Grollman JH. The value of the pulmonary-artery-seeking catheter in percutaneous selective pulmonary angiography. Radiology 1975; 114: 299–304

7. Messina LM, Brothers TE, Wakefield TW, et al. Clinical characteristics and surgical management of vascular complications in patients undergoing cardiac catheteization: interventional versus diagnostic procedures. J Vasc Surg 1991; 13: 593–600

8. Hessel SJ, Adams DF, Abrams HL. Complications of angiography. Radiology 1981; 138: 273–281

9. Fruhwirth J, Pascher O, Hauser H, Amann W. Lokale gefasskomplikationen nach iatrogener femoralarterienpunktion. Wien Klin Wochenschr 1996; 108: 196–200

10. Hudson ER, Smith TP, McDermott VG, et al. Pulmonary angiography using low osmolar nonionic contrast material: complications in 1432 patients. Radiology 1996; 198: 61–65

11. Wilson NV, Corne JM, Given-Wilson RM. A critical appraisal of coagulation studies prior to transfemoral angiography. Br J Radiol 1990; 63: 147–148

12. Doerfler ME, Kaufman B, Goldenberg AS. Central venous catheter placement in patients with disorders of hemostasis. Chest 1996; 110: 185–188

13. Hammerer I. Das risiko der herzkatheter-untersuchung. Eine retrospektive auswertung der komplikationen nach 700 untersuchungen. IV. Gefasskomplikationen. Padiatr Padol 1979; 14: 405–414

14. Koksoy C, Kuzu A, Erden I, Akkaya A. The risk factors in central venous catheter-related thrombosis. Aust N Z J Surg 1995; 65: 796–798

15. Nolewajka AJ, Goddard MD, Brown TC. Temporary transvenous pacing and femoral vein thrombosis. Circulation 1980; 62: 646–650

16. Kantor A, Glanz S, Gordon DH, Sclafani SJA. Percutaneous insertion of the Kimray-Greenfield filter: incidence of femoral vein thrombosis. Am J Roentgenol 1987; 149: 1065–1066

17. Mewissen MW, Erickson SJ, Foley WD, et al. Thrombosis at venous insertion sites after inferior vena caval filter placement. Radiology 1989; 173: 155–157

18. McCowan TC, Ferris EJ, Carver DK, Molpus WM. Complications of the nitinol vena caval filter. J Vasc Intervent Radiol 1992; 3: 401–408

19. McCann RL, Schwartz LB, Pieper KS. Vascular complications of cardiac catheterization. J Vasc Surg 1991; 14: 375–381

20. Stein PD, Hull RD, Pineo .: Strategy that includes serial noninvasive leg tests for diagnosis of thromboembolic disease in patients with suspected acute pulmonary embolism based on data from PIOPED. Arch Intern Med 1995; 155: 2101–2104

21. Nicod P, Peterson K, Levine M, Dittrich H, Buchbinder M, Chappuis F, Moser K. Pulmonary angiography in severe chronic pulmonary hypertension. Ann Int Med 1987; 107: 565–568

22. Ferris EJ, Athanasoulis CA, Clapp PR. Inferior venacavography correlated with pulmonary angiography. Chest 1971; 59: 651–653

23. Gray RK, Buckberg GD, Grollman JH. The importance of inferior vena cavography in placement of the Mobin-Uddin vena caval filter. Radiology 1973; 106: 277–280

24. The PIOPED Investigators. Value of the ventilation/perfusion scan in acute pulmonary embolism. Results of the prospective investigation of pulmonary embolism diagnosis. JAMA 1990; 263: 2753–2759

25. Greenspan RH. Pulmonary angiography and the diagnosis of pulmonary embolism. Progress Cardiovasc Dis 1994; 37: 93–106

26. Grollman KJ. Pulmonary Angiography. Cardiovasc Intervent Radiol 1992; 15: 166–170

27. Newman GE. Pulmonary angiography in pulmonary embolic disease. J Thorac Imag 1989; 4: 28–39

28. Van Beek EJR, Reekers JA, Batchelor DA, et al. Feasibility, safety and clinical utility of angiography in patients with suspected pulmonary embolism. Eur Radiol 1996; 6: 415–419

29. Ranniger K. Pulmonary arteriography: a simple method for demonstration of clinically significant pulmonary emboli. Am J Roentgenol 1969; 106: 558–562

30. Dalen JE, Brooks HL, Johnson LW, Meister SG, Szucs MM, Dexter L. Pulmonary angiography in acute pulmonary embolism: indications, techniques, and results in 367 patients. Am Heart J 1971; 81: 175–185

31. Cheely R, McCartney WH, Perry JR, et al. The role of noninvasive tests versus pulmonary angiography in the diagnosis of pulmonary embolism. Am J Med 1981; 70: 17–22

32. Marsh JD, Glynn M, Torman HA. Pulmonary angiography: application in a new spectrum of patients. Am J Med 1983; 75: 763–770

33. Grollman JH, Gyepes MT, Helmer E. Transfemoral selective bilateral pulmonary arteriography with a pulmonary-artery-seeking catheter. Radiology 1970; 96: 202–204

34. Bell WR, Simon TL. A comparative analysis of pulmonary perfusion scans with pulmonary angiograms. Am Heart J 1976; 92: 700–706

35. Mills CS, Van Aman ME. Modified technique for percutaneous pulmonary angiography. Cardiovasc Intervent Radiol 1986; 9: 52–53

36. Winrow D, Beckmann CF, Lacomis JM, et al. Entanglement of a pigtail catheter by the chordae tendineae of the tricuspid valve during pulmonary angiography. Cardiovasc Intervent Radiol 1996; 19: 275–277

37. Bernard SA, Jones BM, Stuckey JC. Pulmonary angiography in a non-teaching hospital over a 12-year period. Med J Australia 1992; 157: 589–592

38. Pulmonary Artery Catheter Consensus Conference Participants: Pulmonary artery catheter consensus conference: consensus statement. Crit Care Med 1997; 25: 910–925

39. Connors, Jr., AF, Speroff T, Dawson NV, et al. The effectiveness of right heart catheterization in the initial care of critically ill patients. JAMA 1996; 276: 889–897

40. Boyd KD, Thomas SJ, Gold J, et al. A prospective study of complications of pulmonary artery catheterizations in 500 consecutive patients. Chest 1983; 84: 245–249

41. Shah KB, Rao TLK, Laughlin S, et al. A review of pulmonary artery catheterization in 6,245 patients. Anesthesiology 1984; 61: 271–275

42. Damen J, Bolton D. A prospective analysis of 1400 pulmonary artery catheterizations in patients undergoing cardiac surgery. Acta Anaesthesiol Scand 1986; 30: 386–392

43. Van Rooij WJJ, dee Heeten GJ, Sluzewski M. Pulmonary embolism: diagnosis in 211 patients with use of selective pulmonary digital subtraction angiography with a flow-directed catheter. Radiology 1995; 195: 793–797

44. Ferris EJ, Holder JC, Lim WN, et al. Angiography of pulmonary emboli: digital studies and balloon occlusion cineangiography. Am J Roentgenol 1984; 142: 369–373

45. Ferretti GR, Thony F, Link KM, et al. False aneurysm of the pulmonary artery induced by a swan-ganz catheter: clinical presentation and radiologic management. Am J Roentgenol 1996; 167: 941–945

46. Sumita S, Ujike Y, Namiki A, et al. Rupture of pulmonary artery induced by balloon occlusion pulmonary angiography. Intensive Care Med 1995; 21: 79–81

47. The Urokinase Pulmonary Embolism Trial: A National Cooperative Study. Circulation 1973; 47 (Suppl II): II–38–45

48. Novelline RA, Baltarowich OH, Athanasoulis CA, et al. The clinical course of patients with suspected pulmonary embolism and a negative pulmonary arteriogram. Radiology 1978; 126: 561–567

49. Moore RD, Steinberg EP, Powe NR, et al. Nephrotoxicity of high osmolality versus low osmolality contrast media: randomized clinical trial. Radiology 1992; 182: 649–655

50. Barrett BJ, Parfrey PS, Vavasour HM, et al. Contrast nephropathy in patients with impaired renal function: High versus low osmolar media. Kidney Int 1992; 41: 1274–1279

51. Manske CL, Sprafka JM, Strony JT, et al. Contrast nephropathy in azotemic diabetic patients undergoing coronary angiography. Am J Med 1990; 89: 615–620

52. Rudnick MR, Goldfarb S, Wexler L, et al. Nephrotoxicity of ionic and nonionic contrast media in 1196 patients: a randomized trial. Kidney Int 1995; 47: 254–261

53. Levy EM, Viscoli CM, Horwitz RI. The effect of acute renal failure in mortality. A cohort analysis. JAMA 1996; 275: 1488–1494

54. Palmer FG. The RACR survey of intravenous contrast media reactions. Final report. Australs Radiol 1988; 32: 426–428

55. Wolf GL, Arenson RL, Cross AP. A prospective trial of ionic vs nonionic contrast agents in routine clinical practice: comparison of adverse effects. Am J Roentgenol 1989; 152: 930–944

56. Katayama H, Yamaguchi K, Kozuka T et al. Adverse reaction to ionic and nonionic contrast media. Report from the Japanese Committee on the Safety of Contrast Media. Radiology 1990; 175: 621–628

57. Grollman JH. Complications of pulmonary arteriography. Sem Intervent Radiol 1994; 11: 113–120

58. Baltaoglu F, Balkanci F, Tirnaksiz B. Fatal reaction after intraarterial injection of nonionic contrast medium. Am J Roentgenol 1994; 162: 231

59. Smith DC, Lois JF, Gomes AS, et al.: Pulmonary arteriography: comparison of cough stimulation effects of diatrizoate and ioxaglate. Radiology 1987; 162: 617–618

60. Saeed M, Braun SD, Cohan RH, et al. Pulmonary angiography with iopamidol: Patient comfort, image quality and hemodynamics. Radiology 1987; 165: 345–349

61. Bashore M, Davidson CJ, Mark DB, et al. Iopamidol use in the cardiac catheterization laboratory: a retrospective analysis of 3,313 patients. Cardiology 1988; 5: 4–8

62. Sato E, Saito I, Tama Contrast Media Study Group. Risk of clot formation with ionic and nonionic contrast media in cerebral angiography. Acad Radiol 1996; 3: 925–928

63. Agarwal JB, Baile EM, Palmer WH, et al. Reflex systemic hypotension due to hypertonic solution in pulmonary circulation. J App Physiol 1969; 27: 251–255

64. Binet L, Burstein M. Sur les effets cardiovasculaires du serum salé hypertonique. C R Séances Soc Biol Fil 1953; 147: 1997–2000

65. Eliakim MD, Rosenberg SZ, Braun K. Effect of hypertonic saline on the pulmonary and systemic pressures. Circ Res 1958; 6: 357–362

66. Read R, Meyer M. The role of red cell agglutination in arteriographic complications. Surg Forum 1959; 10: 472–475

67. Tajima H, Kumazaki T, Ito K, Tajima N, Gemma K, Ebata K. Effect of an iso-osmolar contrast medium on pulmonary arterial pressure at pulmonary angiography. Acta Radiol 1991; 32: 134–136

68. Krovetz LJ, Benson RW, Neumaster T. Hemodynamic effects of isotonic 67 solutions rapidly injected into the heart and great vessels. Am Heart J 1967; 73: 525–533

69. Tajima H, Kumazaki T, Tajima N, Ebata K. Effect of iohexol and diatrizoate on pulmonary arterial pressure following pulmonary angiography. Acta Radiol 1988; 29: 487–490

70. Almen T, Aspelin P, Levin B. Effect of ionic and nonionic contrast medium on aortic and pulmonary arterial pressure. Invest Radiol 1990; 25: 519–443

71. Smith TP, Lee VS, Hudson ER, et al. Prospective evaluation of pulmonary artery pressures during pulmonary angiography performed with low osmolar nonionic contrast media. J Vasc Intervent Radiology 1996; 7: 207–212

72. Pitton MB, Düber C, Doz P, et al. Hemodynamic effects of nonionic contrast bolus injection and oxygen inhalation during pulmonary angiography in patients with chronic major-vessel thromboembolic pulmonary hypertension. Circulation 1996; 94: 2485–2491

73. Moses DC, Silver TM, Bookstein JJ. The complementary roles of chest radiography, lung scanning, and selective pulmonary angiography in the diagnosis of pulmonary embolism. Circulation 1974; 49: 179–188

74. Mills SR, Jackson DC, Sullivan DC, et al. Angiographic evaluation of chronic pulmonary embolism. Radiology 1980; 136: 301–308

75. Malden ES, Tartar VM, Gutierrez FR. Acute fatality following pulmonary angiography in a patient on an amiodarone regimen: a case report. Angiology 1993; 44: 152–155

76. Wood DL, Osborn MJ, Rooke J, et al. Amiodarone pulmonary toxicity: report of two cases associated with rapidly progressive distress syndrome after pulmonary angiography. Mayo Clinic Proc 1985; 60: 601–603

77. Goodman LR, Putman CE. Diagnostic imaging in acute cardiopulmonary disease. Clin Chest Med 1984; 5(2): 247–264

IV.5 The value of pulmonary angiography in the differential diagnosis of pulmonary embolism

E. J. R. van Beek, J. A. Reekers

Introduction

Pulmonary embolism (PE) is a frequently occurring diagnostic challenge. Generally, as discussed elsewhere in this book, the first diagnostic test will consist of perfusion-ventilation lung scintigraphy. A normal perfusion lung scan adequately excludes the presence of PE, and oral anticoagulants may be safely withheld [1–3]. The other end of the spectrum of lung scintigraphic findings consists of a high probability lung scan, i. e. one or more segmental or larger perfusion defects with locally normal ventilation, where it is acceptable to start treatment with anticoagulants [4–7].

However, in patients with a high probability lung scan finding, PE will be shown by pulmonary angiography in approximately 90%, hence, other diagnoses may be present and patients should undergo angiography when the diagnosis remains controversial given the patient's clinical signs and symptoms [6, 7]. Furthermore, when a patient has an increased bleeding risk and a more certain diagnosis is required, pulmonary angiography should still be carried out in spite of a high probability lung scan.

Pulmonary angiography should be performed according to the techniques described in Chapter IV.3 of this book. It is important to realise that selective catheterisation of lobar or even segmental branches may be required if pulmonary arteries do not show adequate opacification. Furthermore, digital subtraction angiography should preferably be used, since this may facilitate better interpretation and reduces the amount of intravenous contrast required [8, 9]. Several pitfalls in the catheterisation technique as well as in the interpretation of the images exist, and one has to be aware of potential complications (Fig. 1). The essential pitfalls and the safety aspects of the procedure are dealt with in Chapters IV.3 and IV.4.

The aim of this chapter is to show that, although pulmonary angiography is primarily used for the exclusion or demonstration of PE, other important

diagnoses may be encountered. We have attempted to categorise these various conditions and have included several examples of alternative findings, which are equally important for the management of these patients.

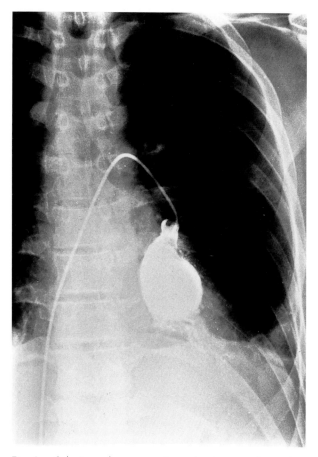

Fig. 1. Selective pulmonary angiography showing subintimal contrast injection and subsequent contrast extravasation. The patient recovered without long-term sequelae.

E. J. R. van Beek, J. A. Reekers

Pulmonary embolism

Acute pulmonary embolism

Patients with clinical signs suggestive of PE will have the diagnosis confirmed in approximately 30%–40% [10–14]. Pulmonary angiography remains the reference standard, although other non-invasive tests like lung scintigraphy, tests for deep leg vein thrombosis and blood tests may reduce the need for angiography considerably [5, 6, 15–17]. However, the fact that pulmonary angiography is now increasingly reserved for the more difficult patients may have implications for the findings on pulmonary angiography [8, 18]. Hence, it may be more difficult to identify the presence or absence of PE in patients with non-diagnostic lung scan results, especially if sub-segmental embolism has occurred or if coexisting lung disease renders the interpretation of the pulmonary arterial system more cumbersome [8, 18].

The findings of pulmonary angiography in patients with PE vary from sub-segmental filling defects or cut-off of vessels to large filling defects (Fig. 2) [10, 11, 14, 19]. In massive PE these filling defects are relatively easy to detect, or a tramline phenomenon may be visible (Fig. 3). However, small emboli require detailed radiographic series in multiple projections and segmental injections in order to become visible.

Chronic PE

Chronic pulmonary thromboembolism involving the major pulmonary arteries is recognised as a cause of pulmonary hypertension in increasing numbers of patients [20]. The recognition of this entity has become more important, since it has become clear that surgical therapy is feasible with good long-term results [21, 22].

In patients with suspected chronic pulmonary thromboembolism, lung scintigraphy tends to under-estimate the severity of central vessel obstruction and the degree of pulmonary hypertension [23]. Hence, pulmonary angiography is manda-

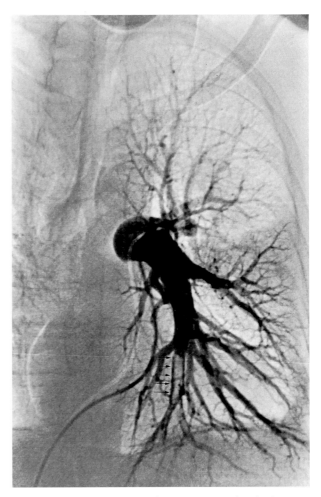

Fig. 2. Large filling defect (arrow) in right descending branch of pulmonary artery

Fig. 3. Selective angiogram showing segmental and subsegmental "tram-line" effect (arrows) as a result of non-occlusive emboli in postero- and mediobasal segments of the left lung.

176

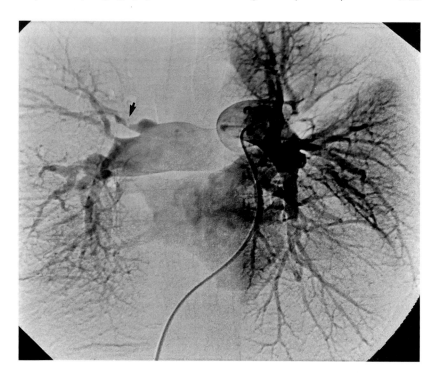

Fig. 4. Pulmonary angiogram of young woman with non-diagnosed post-partem pulmonary embolism. She developed pulmonary hypertension. Note revascularisation stenosis in right upper lobe (arrow), enlarged pulmonary artery and multiple cut-off and irregular vessels throughout. The image shows late arterial phase with early opacification of pulmonary veins and left atrium.

tory to properly assess chronic thromboembolism, both to visualise the arterial system and for performing pulmonary arterial pressure measurements. It should be noted that the main pulmonary arteries down to the segmental vessels need to be clearly visualised, since this eventually determines the potential for thrombus accessibility in patients where a surgical approach (i. e. endarterectomy) is sought. The subsegmental vessels are generally not amenable to surgical dissection, and are therefore not important in the work-up of these patients [24].

Patients may be referred for pulmonary angiography in the work-up of an acute episode suggesting PE. More frequently, they gradually develop dyspnea, which gradually progresses with increasing pulmonary arterial pressure and right ventricular dysfunction [24]. Lung scintigraphy usually reveals (persistent) segmental or larger perfusion defects, which are frequently bilateral [25].

The findings of pulmonary angiography include: webs, bands, pouches, vascular irregularities and cut-off or narrowed vessels (Fig. 4) [24].

Other types of embolism

The findings discussed above were related to venous thromboembolism. However, particles other than venous clots may embolise to the lungs. In particular, bone marrow following long bone fractures, tumour particles, drug crystals and fibres (i. e. in intravenous drug addicts), and air embolism (both iatrogenic, but also following road traffic accidents with open wounds and large vein lacerations) may be indistinguishable from thromboemboli [26–28]. The clinical setting will usually disclose the type of emboli one is dealing with.

An important diagnosis, which may be adequately visualised by echocardiography, is the intracardiac (usually right atrial) thrombus mass, which may in fact be "embolus in transit" [29]. This type of thrombus may arise following the introduction of long-term indwelling catheters or pacemaker wires, or it may arise due to inadequate contractibility of the atrium as in atrial fibrillation. The catheter may dislodge such clots, causing massive PE or obstruction of the right ventricular outflow tract [30]. Hence, if one cannot advance the catheter past the right atrium, injection of contrast medium may be required to demonstrate the obstruction. Obviously, in the presence of a right atrial thrombus the procedure should be abandoned.

Infectious diseases

Any infection will lead to an inflammatory response, consisting of a local increase of blood flow and also an increase of permeability of the venous capillaries and venules. The effects of an inflammatory response may be visible during angiography. Several clinical entities may resemble PE, and many of these are infectious by nature.

Pneumonia

There are three major subtypes of pneumonia, which are described in detail in the standard textbook [28]: lobar pneumonia (initial airspace disease), bronchopneumonia (peribronchial spread) and interstitial pneumonia (within interstitium). The most important factor of any pneumonia is the resultant hyperemia. Furthermore, with airspace disease and atelectasis the alveolar oxygen pressure will decrease and the autoregulation mechanism of the lung will divert blood flow to other, well ventilated lung regions. This will often lead to lung scintigraphic abnormalities, usually of a non-diagnostic category. Finally, a lobar pneumonia may be visible as a consolidation on the chest radiograph, which may in turn resemble a pulmonary infarction [31, 32].

Pulmonary angiography may reveal the hyperemia of the lung segment without evidence of actual occlusion of pulmonary artery branches (Fig. 5). This is in contrast with a pulmonary infarction, where the typical findings of PE will be seen.

Pleuritis

Similar to pneumonia, pleuritis will result in hyperemia of the pleura cavity, and usually gives rise to pleural effusion due to the capillary leak that occurs [28]. The symptoms of pleuritis may very closely resemble PE: pain related to breathing with a (sub)acute onset and a pleural rub on physical examination. Chest radiography will usually show a pleural effusion, which may be small in the early stages. Lung scintigraphy is often non-diagnostic, due to the effusion and reduced blood flow to the lower lobes as a result of splinting as a reaction to pain.

Pulmonary angiography is usually normal, but occasionally the pleuritic hyperemia may be evident (Fig. 6). This is the result of anastomoses between the pulmonary and bronchial arterial circulation, which become more prominent due to increased demand of the hyperemic pleura.

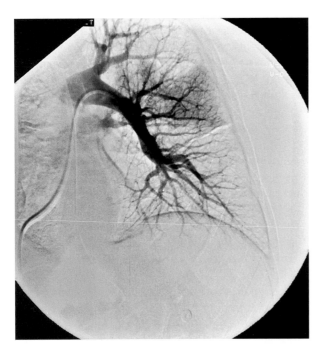

Fig. 5. Selective angiogram showing hyperemia of basal segment left upper lobe and volume loss lower lobe. The chest X-ray showed infiltrative changes 3 days after the angiogram.

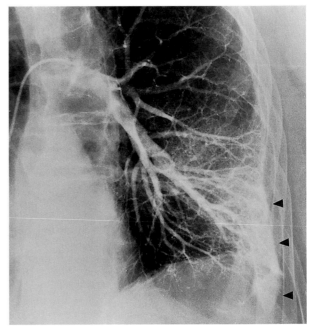

Fig. 6. Patient with systemic lupus erythematosus who developed pleuritic chest pain. The chest X-ray revealed small pleural effusion. Pulmonary angiography shows extensive hyperemia of visceral and parietal pleura (arrow heads) without evidence of pulmonary embolism.

Fibrosing mediastinitis

Fibrosing mediastinitis is a rare disorder, which may result from chronic infection by such organisms as histoplasmosis and tuberculosis, while most often no etiologic substrate is demonstrated (idiopathic fibrosing mediastinitis) [28, 33]. The complications of fibrosing mediastinitis affect the oesophagus and pericardium in particular, and patients may present with hematemesis [34]. Less frequently, the fibrosis causes superior vena cava obstruction or obstruction of the pulmonary arteries and veins when signs and symptoms of PE may predominate [28, 33].

Airways diseases

Atelectasis

Atelectasis is the result of bronchial obstruction by any cause. The effect is obstruction of air flow, and the trapped air is slowly absorbed leading to the collapse of the alveolar walls. Eventually, the overall volume of the affected lung segment is severely diminished with total collapse of lung parenchyma.

Atelectasis is commonly seen in patients who are considered at risk for PE, i. e. following surgery, and in those where the diagnosis of thromboembolism is more difficult, i. e. patients with chronic obstructive pulmonary disease [28]. Finally, atelectasis may be seen in the course of PE, usually as plate atelectasis, or may be rather indistinguishable from pulmonary infarction [28, 31, 32]. Since both perfusion and ventilation are affected in these areas, patients will often be referred for pulmonary angiography if the symptoms suggest a diagnosis of PE.

Angiography will reveal the diagnosis as a result of volume loss. The arteries are more tortuous than normal and are relatively close together ("bunched"), as shown in Figure 7. Furthermore, compensatory hyperinflation of the normal lung segments will result in an abnormally widespread configuration of arterial branches (Fig. 7). One has to take care that selective and even superselective angiography is performed to rule out small, subsegmental emboli in these patients.

Emphysema

Emphysema is a disease that affects the septa and alveolar walls. As a result of progressive destruction, the airspace becomes increased while the effective membrane for gas exchange becomes diminished [28]. In the work-up of PE, emphysema shows a relatively common pattern: lung scintigraphy shows combined ventilation and perfusion ab-

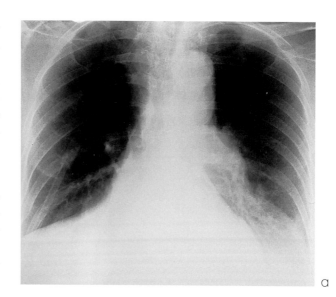

a

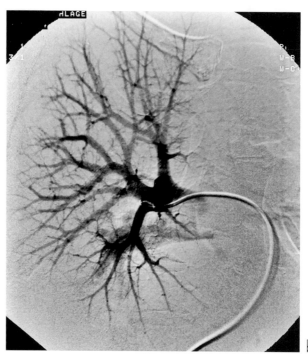

b

Fig. 7a, b. Patient with right lower lobe atelectasis (a). The corresponding angiogram depicts wide spread arteries of upper and middle lobe due to hyperinflation with diminished opacification of the lower lobe (b).

179

normalities, and patients will often be referred for angiography.

Angiography may reveal several signs, which are dependent on the extent of emphysema. In bullous emphysema (Fig. 8), an area of persistent oligemia with pulmonary arterial branches stretched around the bulla may be seen. Smaller areas with oligemia and early tapering of distal arterial branches may be detected in emphysematous lung areas without bullae.

Pulmonary fibrosis

A great number of disorders may cause fibrotic changes of the lungs, such as: (chronic) inflammatory reactions (i. e. sarcoidosis, pneumocystis carinii pneumonia), (chronic) exposure to small particles (i. e. pneumoconiosis), collagen vascular diseases (i. e. systemic sclerosis, SLE, rheumatoid arthritis), and neoplasms [28].

Patients with lung fibrosis generally exhibit a progressive diminution of lung function with increasing dyspnea. However, regularly, patients may ex-

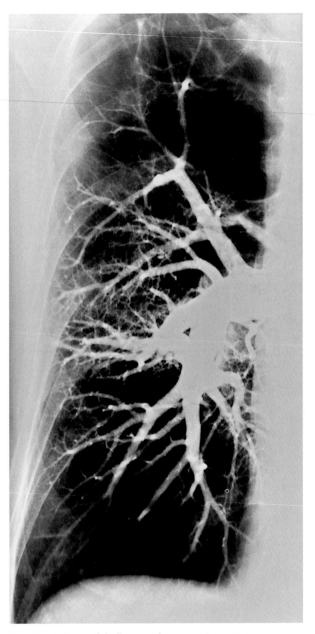

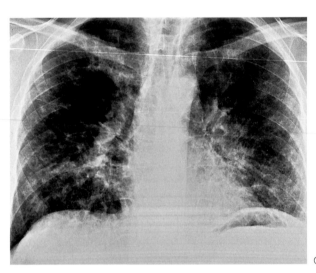

a

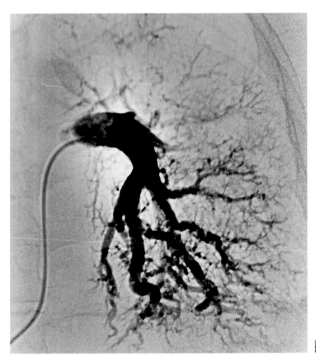

b

Fig. 8. Patient with bullous emphysema. Note arteries running around bullae. This patient had concomitant infiltrate, which may be recognised due to focal hyperemia.

Fig. 9a, b. Patient with end-stage sarcoidosis (a). Corresponding angiogram reveals extensive vascular changes, notably increased tortuosity, irregularity, pruning, and signs of volume loss in lower lobe (b).

perience more acute episodes of chest symptoms, which results in work-up for suspected PE. In these patients, a lung scan is nearly always abnormal without clear high probability findings. Hence, angiography is frequently performed in these patients.

Several findings may be evident: tortuous arteries with irregular vessel wall may be striking, as shown in a patient with sarcoidosis (Fig. 9), pruning of arterial branches, and sometimes hyperemia where the inflammatory component is still active (Fig. 10).

Miscellaneous disorders

Pulmonary hypoplasia and the acquired hypoplastic lung of the Swyer-James (or Macleod's) syndrome are both rare conditions, which may present at pulmonary angiography [28, 35 – 37]. Pulmonary arterial hypoplasia usually becomes clinically apparent during childhood, and several types have been documented which usually lead to early progressive dyspnea and death. Type III survives to adulthood and may present with hemoptysis [28]. There is normal ventilation with absence of a pulmonary artery or pulmonary arterial branch [28 – 35]. In Swyer-James' syndrome there is a hyperlucent lung on plain chest radiography. Pulmonary angiography reveals that, in contrast with congenital pulmonary hypoplasia, the pulmonary arterial system is present, albeit diminutive [28, 36, 37].

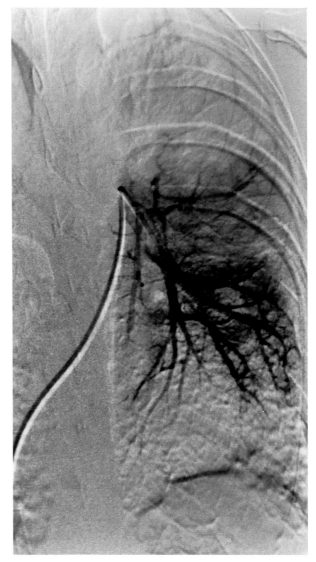

Fig. 10.   Patient with fibrosing alveolitis and acute increase in dyspnea. There is extensive hyperemia, especially in the lingular lobe, which proved active alveolitis.

Pleural disease

Pneumothorax

A pneumothorax, especially of a spontaneous nature, is one of the main differential diagnoses for patients with suspected PE. Pneumothoraces may develop spontaneously, but may also be related to pre-existent pulmonary diseases, such as bullous emphysema, carcinoma or infections. In general, chest radiography will be able to detect pneumothorax, however, small or anterior pneumothoraces may be difficult to detect.

In these instances, a patient may inadvertently be referred for lung scintigraphy, which will demonstrate a combined perfusion-ventilation defect. Angiography will show that there is an increased distance of the pulmonary arterial tree from the chest wall, and furthermore, will enhance the actual edge of lung parenchyma in relation to the chest wall.

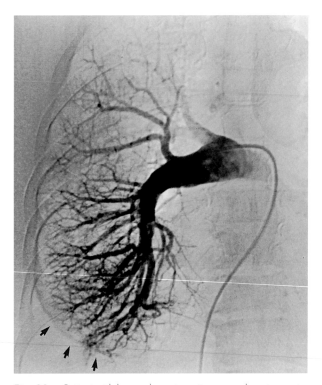

Fig. 11. Patient with known breast carcinoma and acute onset dyspnea. The angiogram shows pleural effusion (arrows) and compression atelectasis of right lower lobe.

Pleural effusion

Pleural effusions are frequently seen in pleuritis, pleuropneumonia, heart failure, disseminated malignant disease, infectious diseases just below the diaphragm and in patients with PE. In the work-up of patients with non-diagnostic lung scan findings, pleural effusions often show their nature by the laterally ascending fluid level, which will usually be accompanied by a compression atelectasis (Fig. 11).

Vascular disorders

Anatomical variants

A variety of anatomical variants exist, which may be discovered as part of the work-up of a patient with clinically suspected PE. Most of these variants will have little or no clinical impact on the management of these patients. More severe anatomical abnormalities, like left pulmonary artery sling, are usually detected at an early age due to tracheal compression with wheezing, stridor and/or recurrent pulmonary infections [38]. It should be noted that the pulmonary artery may have an earlier branching than normal, resulting in lobar arteries arising in the mediastinum. This variety is of importance, since Swan-Ganz catheters may inadvertently be malpositioned in these patients.

Finally, with sequestration, the pulmonary arterial supply to a lung may be derived entirely or in part from the systemic circulation [39–42]. Often an abnormal vascular structure will be recognised on initial chest radiography, however, this may be difficult to detect in some cases. In these patients, pulmonary angiography will reveal absence of the left or right pulmonary artery or its branches. It is important to note that no true cut-off arterial branches will be seen, and that a late film may demonstrate filling of the lung or lung segment, indicating a systemic vascular supply. An aortogram will reveal the true extent, although occasionally the pulmonary arterial supply may be derived from the coronary arteries [39]. Patients with one of these anomalies may require surgery or endovascular treatment, especially if severe hemoptysis is their main presenting symptom.

Congenital heart disease

The main congenital heart anomalies that are of interest in this context are the septal defects of the atrium (ASD) and ventricular septum (VSD).

An ASD of substantial size is usually detected at an early age due to shunting, and Eisenmenger's reaction may occur. These patients virtually never present themselves with suspected PE, and the diagnosis of ASD is generally made without pulmonary angiography. However, a small ASD may remain clinically silent. In these patients, the catheter

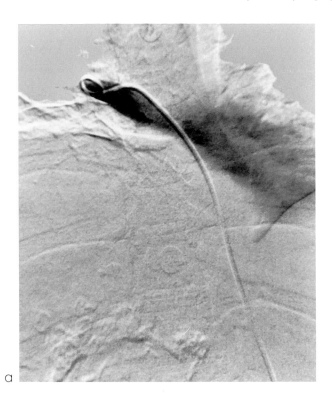

a

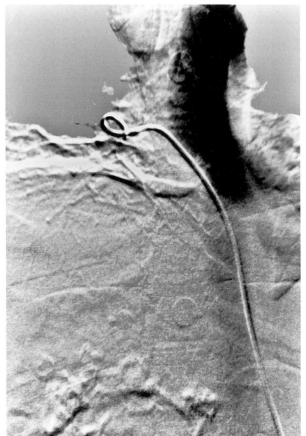

b

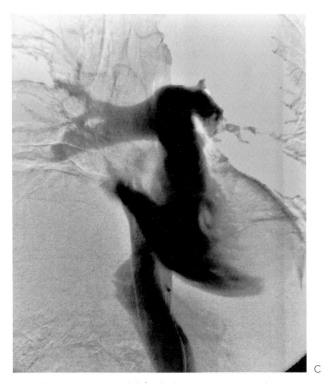

c

may inadvertently pass through the atrial septum to the left atrium. Contrast injection will then reveal rapid filling of the atrium and left ventricle, and subsequently the aorta will opacify. Sometimes, an ASD may be part of more extensive vascular anomalies, such as a left sided vena cava inferior (Fig. 12).

A patent foramen ovale (PFO) is another cause of inadvertent passage of the catheter to the left heart chambers. The prevalence of PFO in the normal population is estimated to be 27%–35% [43]. Patients with PFO who develop deep vein thrombosis (DVT) may present either with PE or with systemic embolism (i.e. stroke) or both [44]. In fact, PE may result in a rapid rise of right ventricular and right atrial pressure, which in turn may lead to paradoxical embolism [45, 46]. Hence, due to its potential catastrophic sequelae, it is important to recognise a PFO. In patients who have proven PE and PFO, it may be necessary to use additional means of prevention, such as inferior vena cava filters, especially if pulmonary hypertension exists and a right to left shunt is demonstrated [43, 45].

A VSD rarely remains asymptomatic for a prolonged period of time. Nevertheless, in a young patient with chest symptoms one may encounter a small VSD. In these rare cases, pressure monitoring may reveal elevated pulmonary arterial and right ventricular pressure, and the catheter may enter the VSD during its passage of the right ventricle.

Fig. 12a – c. Patient with left-sided vena cava (note catheter to left of spine) and ASD in whom first contrast injection fills left atrium (a) and aorta (b). Repositioning of the catheter shows concomitant filling of pulmonary artery, left atrium and aorta (c).

Pulmonary vasculitis

Pulmonary vascular inflammation occurs in a wide variety of systemic collagen vascular diseases, such as Wegener's granulomatosis, systemic lupus erythematosus, Goodpasture's syndrome and microscopic polyarteritis [47, 48]. In most cases, the capillaritis leads to alveolar hemorrhage with resultant dyspnea and hemoptysis. The chest radiography will usually show diffuse, bilateral, alveolar infiltrates. Although these symptoms arise subacutely in most patients, more acute onset may be encountered. Hence, its clinical picture may resemble that of PE. Furthermore, lung scintigraphy often yields non-diagnostic findings as a result of both vascular and airspace disorders which accompany these diseases.

Some forms of pulmonary vasculitis are important in the setting of pulmonary angiography findings. These will be described in more detail. Most of the illnesses, however, will not lead to angiographic work-up, because other tests (i.e. fibreoptic bronchoscopy with broncho-alveolar lavage, carbon monoxide diffusion testing) and serum investigations will reveal the different etiology [47].

Systemic lupus erythematosus (SLE)

Systemic lupus erythematosus is an auto-immune rheumatic disease, commonly affecting young women, with a broad spectrum and complex immunopathology. Small arteries and capillaries are involved in approximately 30% of the patients [49]. In patients with SLE, a variety of pulmonary manifestations may occur, including acute alveolitis, interstitial pneumonitis, pulmonary hypertension (sometimes due to chronic venous thromboembolic disease), necrotising vasculitis, and pleural effusions [47, 50].

Often SLE will present with new, diffuse infiltrates and concomitant symptoms of (sub)acute onset, like dyspnea and hemoptysis [47, 51]. It may be difficult to distinguish these symptoms from true PE. Furthermore, patients with SLE are at increased risk of developing venous thromboembolic complications [52], in particular in those patients with a circulating lupus anticoagulant, or anticardiolipin antibodies. Hence, both signs of vasculitis and true pulmonary emboli may be encountered during pulmonary angiography.

Takayasu's arteritis

Takayasu's arteritis is a primary arteritis of unknown origin, which primarily affects the thoracic and abdominal aorta and its major branches. In approximately 50% of cases the pulmonary arteries are also affected [53–57]. Although the disease predominates in the Orient, it does have a world-wide distribution affecting mainly young women [57]. The disease pattern may be classified radiologically in four types, as proposed by Lupi [53]. Type IV is reserved for those patients that have involvement of the pulmonary arterial system. Although most patients will have both aortic and pulmonary involvement, some patients present exclusively with pulmonary arterial Takayasu arteritis [58, 59].

In patients with concomitant aortic and pulmonary arterial arteritis, the symptoms of the systemic circulatory insufficiency usually predominate. However, some patients will present with symptoms suggestive of PE [58, 60, 61].

The chest radiograph may be normal or may show a variety of signs, such as slightly prominent or narrowed pulmonary arteries, ill-defined infiltrates, cardiomegaly, pulmonary oligemia, rib notching or aortic abnormalities [54, 62]. The lung scan will show perfusion and ventilation defects due to infarction, secondary infections, and pulmonary hypertension. These defects may indicate both in high probability and non-diagnostic lung scan findings [63, 64].

The angiographic findings are mainly stenoses and occlusions, with occasional dilatation of the pulmonary trunk in those patients where pulmonary hypertension dominates (Fig. 13) [54, 55]. Furthermore, aneurysmal dilatation of the pulmonary artery may occur even in the absence of pulmonary hypertension [60]. The upper lobes are more commonly involved than the other lung zones, and the pulmonary trunk and lobar arteries are usually macroscopically normal [54, 55]. Communications between bronchial and pulmonary arteries and between coronary and bronchial arteries may occur as complications of the arteritis [58].

Behçet's disease

Behçet's disease is a systemic disorder, which is based on a vasculitis of unknown etiology [65, 66]. It primarily affects young adults between 20 and 40 years of age, with men twice as often involved, and is more common in people from Mediterranean, Middle Eastern and Japanese origin, although it has a world-wide distribution [67]. The patients may present with a wide range of ailments, but the major criteria are urogenital ulceration, erythema nodosum, thrombophlebitis, and ocular disease [66]. Less commonly there is involvement of the joints, gastrointestinal tract and central nervous system. Intrathoracic manifestations of Behçet's disease consist mainly of thromboembolism of the superior vena cava and other medias-

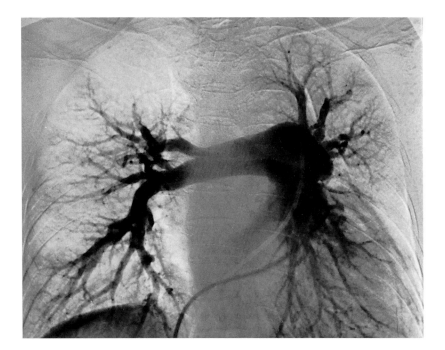

Fig. 13. 46-year-old female with 10 year history of shortness of breath and dizziness. Physical examination revealed different systolic blood pressures on left and right arms and multiple vascular bruits. She was diagnosed with Takayasu arteritis. The pulmonary angiogram shows multiple occlusions of pulmonary artery branch vessels in the upper lobe of right lung and in lingula segment of left lung (Courtesy of Dr. Ichiro Yamada, Department of Radiology, Tokyo Medical and Dental University, Japan).

tinal veins, aneurysms of the aorta and pulmonary arteries, pulmonary infarction and hemorrhage, and rarely myocardial or pericardial disease, cor pulmonale, and mediastinal and hilar lymphadenopathy [68]. In fact, Behçet's disease is the most frequent cause of pulmonary arterial aneurysms [69], which may lead to massive hemoptysis and ultimately death [70].

The diagnosis is usually made on clinical history, examination and serological and skin tests [71]. Chest radiography may reveal focal or diffuse opacities with variable clinical course, consolidation, pleural effusion, or sometimes lymphadenopathy [68]. Sudden hilar enlargement or the appearance of a parenchymal rounded opacity may be a sign of pulmonary arterial aneurysm development [68, 70].

Angiography is generally avoided in patients with Behçet's disease, because they are at increased risk of developing local and systemic complications, such as aneurysms or thromboembolism [66, 72, 73]. Lung scintigraphy is the test of choice, but will often merely indicate non-diagnostic findings, especially in pulmonary infarction and in patients with massive hemoptysis. However, since PE and infarction are frequent occurrences, pulmonary angiography may be performed either early in the disease with a presentation of PE or in cases where pulmonary hypertension or aneurysms have already occurred. Angiography may reveal pulmonary artery dilatation, aneurysms, and thromboembolism (both acute and chronic). Aneurysms may be missed al-

together due to complete thromboembolic occlusion or thrombosis.

The differential diagnosis is mainly that of Takayasu's arteritis, although the fact that mucocutaneous involvement is usually present in Behçet's disease makes distinction generally possible.

Pulmonary artery aneurysms

There are various types of pulmonary artery aneurysms. The congenital variants are exceedingly rare, and are often accompanied by other pulmonary abnormalities or congenital heart disorders [28]. Much more frequently, pulmonary artery aneurysms are acquired, such as in cases of pulmonary hypertension. Even then, the diagnosis is usually made by chest radiography and computed tomography, while pulmonary angiography is reserved for definitive pre-operative assessment.

Pseudo-aneurysms, which are the result of an intimal tear, may present with signs and symptoms suggestive of PE [74, 75]. The etiology of pseudoaneurysms may be infection [74], chest trauma [75, 76], or even following the introduction of Swan-Ganz catheters [77]. The importance of adequate diagnosis is related to the risk of further enlargement and fatal hemorrhage, and prompt surgical or preferably endovascular treatment is required [74].

185

Pulmonary arteriovenous malformations and fistulae

Direct connections between the arterial and venous vascular beds result in increased local flow and reduce the capability of the lungs to filter small particles from the blood stream. The connections may be large, i. e. artery to vein [78], or more at a capillary bed level [79]. Peripheral embolism may be the primary symptom [79]. These connections may be congenital in origin, and in these cases up to one third of patients will have multiple lesions [28]. In patients with hereditary hemorrhagic telangiectasia (Rendu-Osler-Weber disease), a dominant non-sex-linked hereditary disorder, multiple arteriovenous malformations may be observed in the lungs, but in more than half of the patients also in other organs, such as liver, kidneys, gastrointestinal tract and skin [28, 80, 81]. In acquired arteriovenous malformations, these may be traumatic in origin or the result of (chronic) inflammatory processes, such as pneumoconiosis. In general, the diagnosis is made on the clinical spectrum, where hemoptysis is a frequent symptom. The chest radiograph will often reveal a round or oval homogenous mass, which is sharply defined. The feeding artery and/or draining vein may be discernible. In some patients, symptoms of PE may be the presenting signs, and pulmonary angiography will reveal the true nature of these symptoms. However, some cases have been described where spontaneous embolisation of arteriovenous malformations have taken place [82], as shown in a patient with pneumoconiosis related arteriovenous malformation in Figure 14.

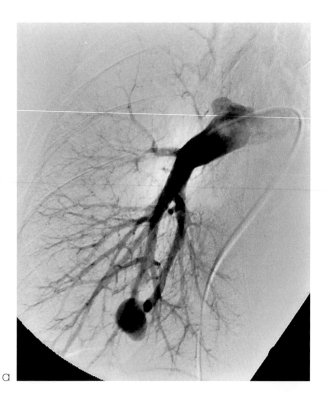

a

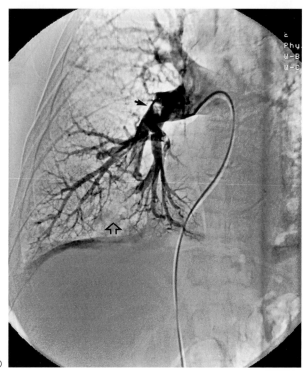

b

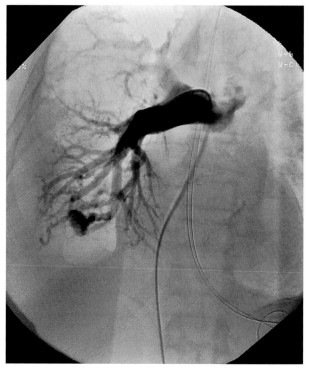

c

Fig. 14a–c. Patient with pneumoconiosis and known AVM **(a)**, who suffered acute chest pain. Pulmonary angiography showed major pulmonary embolism (arrow) and embolisation of the AVM **(b)**. Three weeks after heparin and oral anticoagulants the emboli have resolved, but the AVM is only revascularised incompletely **(c)**.

Neoplasms

Lung parenchymal malignancies

Both primary and secondary malignancies of the lungs may cause obstruction of blood flow to lung segments [28]. Furthermore, with (sub)acute obstruction of pulmonary arterial branches or bronchi, symptoms may simulate PE. Lung scintigraphy will often reveal perfusion and/or ventilation defects. As a result of local compression, focal thrombosis may occur, which is indistinguishable from thromboembolism. This is especially true of lymphomas and lymph node metastases, which tend to obstruct the large pulmonary artery branches in the mediastinum or at hilar level [83]. Although the diagnosis is made by other modalities, pulmonary angiography may be required for the exclusion of thromboembolism, especially since patients with malignant diseases are at increased risk of thrombotic disorders. Findings compatible with neoplasms may include: displacement of arterial branches (Fig. 15), cut-off of large branches (Fig. 16) or encasement of arteries (Fig. 17). Finally, pleuritis carcinomatosa will result in large amounts of pleural effusion (see above).

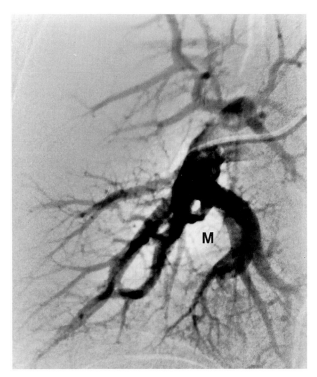

Fig. 15. Displaced lower lobe pulmonary artery in patient with metastatic oesophagus carcinoma (M).

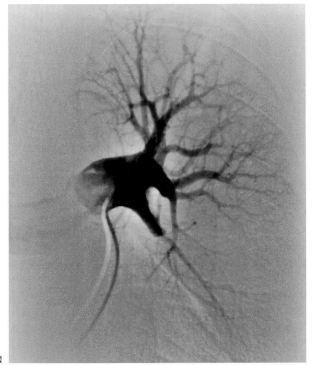

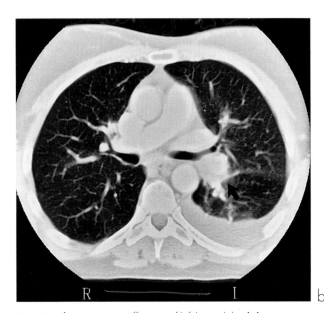

Fig. 16a, b. Large cut-off artery of left lower lobe (a) in patient with subsequently proven bronchus carcinoma (arrow) and corresponding CT scan (b).

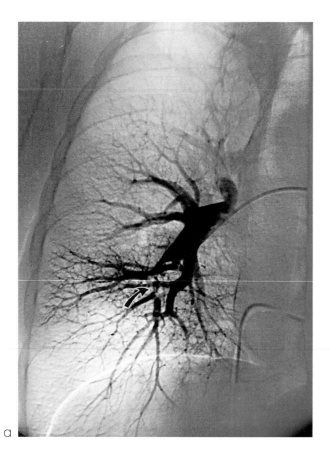

a

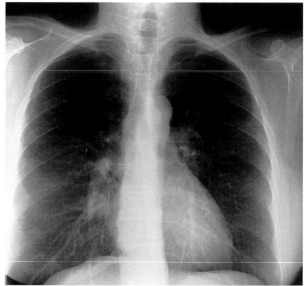

b

Fig. 17a, b. Encasement of right lower lobe arteries (arrow) **(a)** in patient with multiple lung metastases in left hilar and right perihilar region **(b)**.

Pulmonary artery sarcoma

These are rare tumours, which may arise from the intimal or muscular layers of the vessel wall. They are often located in the main pulmonary artery, and may present with signs and symptoms of PE [84–87]. At chest radiography a prominence of the hilum may be noted.

Pulmonary angiography will reveal a prominent filling defect with normal filling of the more distal branches [84–87]. Although this is a non-specific finding compared to PE, it is noteworthy that this filling defect does not respond to anticoagulant therapy, and no DVT will be present. Usually, it is a chance finding at surgery for intended thromboembolectomy or endarterectomy [85, 86, 88].

Myxoma

A right atrial myxoma may present with right ventricular obstruction or recurrent PE [89, 90]. Lung scintigraphy will often disclose one or more perfusion defects, however, the cardiac status of the patient will generally not improve with anticoagulant therapy. Cardiac ultrasonography is usually the first means of detecting an intra-atrial mass, which may in fact be indistinguishable from a thrombus mass [91].

In the event of pulmonary angiography in patients with myxoma, the first signs will be resistance to enter the right atrium or right ventricle. If this occurs, a trial injection of contrast will reveal an intraluminal filling defect within the heart chambers [92]. It is imperative that the procedure is discontinued at once, and (echo)cardiology work-up should be commenced. Alternatively, thrombolytic therapy may be given in the first instance, to try to dissolve any large thrombus mass that may be present.

Conclusions

Pulmonary angiography is still considered the reference standard for the diagnosis of PE. This chapter discussed some of the more common disorders, which may be discernible at angiography. Many of these findings are "by accident", but they should not be missed, since clinical management of patients may be severely affected by them. Hence, any radiologist who performs pulmonary angiography should be aware of them, and also of the implications during the procedure. Certainly, the literature has severely underemphasised this additional value of pulmonary angiography in this patient category.

References

1. Kipper MS, Moser KM, Kortman KE, Ashburn WL. Longterm follow-up of patients with suspected PE and a normal lung scan. Chest 1982; 82: 411–415

2. Hull RD, Raskob GE, Coates G, Panju AA. Clinical validity of a normal perfusion lung scan in patients with suspected PE. Chest 1990; 97: 23–2

3. Van Beek EJR, Kuyer PMM, Schenk BE, Brandjes DPM, Ten Cate JW, Büller HR. A normal perfusion lung scan in patients with clinically suspected PE: frequency and clinical validity. Chest 1995; 108: 170–173

4. Hull RD, Raskob GE, Coates G, Panju AA, Gill GJ. A new noninvasive management strategy for patients with suspected PE. Arch Intern Med 1989; 149: 2549–2555

5. Hull RD, Raskob GE, Ginsberg JS, et al. A noninvasive strategy for the treatment of patients with suspected PE. Arch Intern Med 1994; 154: 289–297

6. Stein PD, Hull RD, Saltman HA, Pineo G. Strategy for diagnosis of patients with suspected acute PE. Chest 1993;103:1553–1559

7. Van Beek EJR, Tiel-van Buul MMC, Büller HR, Van Royen EA, Ten Cate JW. The value of lung scintigraphy in the diagnosis of PE. Eur J Nucl Med 1993; 20: 173–181

8. Van Beek EJR, Bakker AJ, Reekers JA. Interobserver variability of pulmonary angiography in patients with non-diagnostic lung scan results: conventional versus digital subtraction arteriography. Radiology 1996; 198: 721–724

9. Hudson ER, Smith TP, McDermott VG, et al. Pulmonary angiography performed with iopamidol: complications in 1434 patients. Radiology 1996; 198: 61–65

10. Hull RD, Hirsh J, Carter CJ, et al. Pulmonary angiography, ventilation lung scanning, and venography for clinically suspected PE with abnormal perfusion lung scan. Ann Intern Med 1983; 98: 891–899

11. The PIOPED investigators. Value of the ventilation-perfusion scan in acute PE: results of the Prospective Investigation of PE Diagnosis (PIOPED). JAMA 1990; 263: 2753–2759

12. Hull RD, Raskob GE, Pineo GF, Brant RF. Low-probability lung scan: a need for change in nomenclature. Arch Intern Med 1995; 155: 1845–1851

13. Stein PD, Athanasoulis C, Alavi A, et al. Complications and validity of pulmonary angiography in acute PE. Circulation 1992; 85: 462–468

14. Van Beek EJR, Reekers JA, Batchelor D, Brandjes DPM, Peeters FLM, Büller HR. Feasibility, safety and clinical utility of angiography in patients with suspected PE and non-diagnostic lung scan findings. Eur Radiol 1996; 6: 415–419

15. Oudkerk M, Van Beek EJR, Van Putten WLJ, Büller HR. Cost-effectiveness analysis of various strategies in the diagnostic management of PE. Arch Intern Med 1993; 153: 947–954

16. Ginsberg JS. Management of venous thromboembolism. N Engl J Med 1996; 335: 1816–1828

17. Perrier A, Bounameaux H, Morabia A, et al. Diagnosis of PE by a decision analysis-based strategy including clinical probability, D-dimer levels and ultrasonography: a management study. Arch Intern Med 1996; 156: 531–536

18. Quinn MF, Lundell CJ, Klotz TA, et al. Reliability of selective pulmonary arteriography in the diagnosis of pulmonary embolism. Am J Roentgenol 1987; 149: 469–471

19. Bookstein JJ. Segmental arteriography in PE. Radiology 1969; 93: 1007–1012

20. Moser KM, Auger WR, Fedullo PF. Chronic major vessel thrombembolic pulmonary hypertension. Circulation 1990; 81: 1735–1743

21. Moser KM, Daily PO, Peterson KL, et al. Thromboendarterectomy for chronic, major-vessel thrombembolic pulmonary hypertension: immediate and long-term results in 42 patients. Ann Intern Med 1987; 107: 560–565

22. Jamieson SW, Auger WR, Fedullo PF, et al. Experience and results with 150 pulmonary thromboendarterectomy operations over a 29-month period. J Throac Cardiovasc Surg 1993; 106: 116–127

23. Ryan KL, Fedullo PF, David GB, Vasquez TE, Moser KM. Perfusion scans underestimate the severity of angiographic and hemodynamic compromise in chronic thromboembolic pulmonary hypertension. Chest 1988; 93: 1180–1185

24. Moser KM, Auger WR, Fedullo PF, Jamieson SW. Chronic thromboembolic pulmonary hypertension: clinical picture and surgical treatment. Eur Respir J 1992; 5: 334–342

25. D'Alonzo GE, Bower JS, Dantzker DR. Differentiation of patients with primary and thromboembolic pulmonary hypertension. Chest 1984; 85: 457–461

26. Chakeres DW, Spiegel PK. Fatal pulmonary hypertension secondary to intravascular metastatic tumor emboli. Am J Roentgenol 1982; 139: 997–1000

27. Ten Duis HJ. The fat embolism syndrome. Injury 1997; 28: 77–85

28. Fraser RG, Paré JAP, Paré PD, Fraser RS, Genereux GP (eds). Diagnosis of diseases of the chest. WB Saunders Co, Philadelphia, 1989

29. Farfel Z, Shechter M, Vered Z, Rath S, Goor D, Gafni J. Review of echocardiographically diagnosed right heart entrapment of pulmonary emboli in transit with emphasis on management. Am Heart J 1987; 113: 171–178

30. Waller BF, Dean PJ, Mann O, Rosen JH, Roberts WC. Right ventricular outflow obstruction from thrombus with small peripheral pulmonary emboli. Chest 1981; 79: 224–225

31. Moser KM. Venous thromboembolism. Am Rev Respir Dis 1990; 141: 235–239

32. Stein PD, Terrin ML, Hales CA, et al. Clinical, laboratory, roentgenographic and electrocardiographic findings in patients with acute PE and non preexisting cardiac or pulmonary disease. Chest 1991; 100: 598–603

33. Berry DF, Buccigrossi D, Peabody J, et al. Pulmonary vascular occlusion and fibrosing mediastinitis. Chest 1986; 89: 296–301

34. Camacho MT, Edelman M, Rozenblit A, McKitrick JC, Pinsker K, Fell SC. Mediastinal histoplasmosis causing massive hematemesis. J Thorac Cardiovasc Surg 1996; 111: 1283–1286

35. Kuo PH, Wu WD, Lee LN. A patient with haemoptysis and a smaller right lung. European Respiratory Journal 1996; 9: 847–849

36. Salmanzadeh A, Pomeranz SJ, Ramsingh PS. Ventilation-perfusion scintigraphic correlation with multimodality imaging in a proven case of Swyer-James (Macleod's) syndrome. Clin Nucl Med 1997; 22: 115–118

37. Mayeux I, Aubry P, Jounieaux V. Syndrome de Swyer-James ou Macleod ou poumon clair unilateral. Presse Medicale 1996; 25: 929–932

38. Vogl TJ, Diebold T, Bergman C, Dohlemann C, Mantel K, Felix R, Lissner J. MRI in pre- and postoperative assessment of tracheal stenosis due to pulmonary artery sling. J Comp Assist Tomogr 1993; 17: 878–886

39. Mehnert F, Lenz M, Fischer J. Fehlen der rechten Pulmonalarterie mit Kollateralversorgung der Lunge aus allen 3 Koronargefäßen. Röntgenpraxis 1996; 49: 4–7

40. Tagliente MR, Troise D, Milella L, Vairo U. Isolated anomalous origin of left pulmonary artery from the ascending aorta. Am Heart J 1996; 132: 1289–1292

41. Flisak ME, Chandrasekar AJ, Marsan RE, Ali MM. Systematic arterialization of lung without sequestration. Am J Roentgenol 1982; 138: 751–753

42. Hirai T, Ohtake Y, Mutoh S, Noguchi M, Yamanaka A. Anomalous systemic arterial supply to normal basal segments of the left lower lobe. A report of two cases. Chest 1996; 109: 286–289

43. Ward R, Jones D, Haponik EF. Paradoxical embolism. An underrecognized problem. Chest 1995; 108: 549–558

44. Stollenberger C, Slany J, Schuster I, et al. The prevalence of deep venous thrombosis in patients with suspected paradoxical embolism. Ann Intern Med 1993; 119: 461–465

45. Loscalzo J. Paradoxical embolism: clinical presentation, diagnostic strategies, and therapeutic consequences. Am Heart J 1986; 116: 879–885

46. Pell ACH, Hughes D, Keating J, Christie J, Susutth A, Sutherland GR. Brief report: fulminating fat embolism syndrome caused by paradoxical embolism through patent foramen ovale. N Engl J Med 1993; 329: 926–929

47. Green RJ, Ruoss SJ, Kraft SA, Berry GJ, Raffin TA. Pulmonary capillaritis and alveolar hemorrhage. Update on diagnosis and management. Chest 1996; 110: 1305–1316

48. Menon S, Isenberg DA. Small vessel vasculitides. In: Tooke JE, Lowe GD. A textbook of vascular medicine. London; Arnold, 1996: 295–313

49. Ansari A, Carson PH, Bates HD. Vascular manifestations of systemic lupus erythematosus. J Vas Dis 1986; 37: 423–432

50. Haupt HM, Moore GW, Hutchins GM. The lung in systemic lupus erythematosus. Am J Med 1981; 71: 791–798

51. Myers JL, Katzenstein AA. Microangiitis in lupus-induced pulmonary hemorrhage. Am J Clin Pathol 1986; 85: 552–556

52. Love PE, Santoro SA. Antiphospholipid antibodies: anticardiolipin and the lupus anticoagulant in systemic lupus erythematosus (SLE) and in non-SLE disorders. Ann Intern Med 1990; 112: 682–698

53. Lupi E, Sanchez G, Horwitz S, Gutierrez E. Pulmonary artery involvement in Takayasu's arteritis. Chest 1975; 67: 69–74

54. Yamato M, Lecky JW, Hiramatsu K, Kohda E. Takayasu's arteritis: radiographic and angiographic findings in 59 patients. Radiology 1986; 161: 329–334

55. Yamada I, Shibuya H, Matsubara O, et al. Pulmonary artery disease in Takayasu's arteritis: angiographic findings. Am J Roentgenol 1992; 159: 263–269

56. Park JH, Han MC, Kim SH, Oh BH, Park YB, Seo JD. Takayasu arteritis: angiographic findings and results of angioplasty. Am J Roentgenol 1989; 153: 1069–1074

57. Lupi-Herrera E, Sanchez-Torres G, Marcushamer J, Mispireta J, Horwitz S, Espino J. Takayasu's arteritis: clinical studies in 107 cases. Am Heart J 1977; 93: 94–103

58. Hayashi K, Nagasaki M, Matsunaga N, Hombo Z, Imamura T. Initial pulmonary involvement in Takayasu's arteritis. Radiology 1986; 159: 401–403

59. Nakabayashi K, Kurata N, Nangi N, Miyake H, Nagasawa T. Pulmonary artery involvement as first manifestation in three cases of Takayasu arteritis. Int J Cardiol 1997; 54 (suppl): S177–183

60. Kerr KM, Auger WR, Fedullo PF, Channick RH, Yi ES, Moser KM. Large vessel pulmonary arteritis mimicking chronic thromboembolic disease. American J Respiratory and Critical Care Medicine 1995; 152: 367–373

61. Ferretti G, Defaye P, Thony F, Ranchoup Y, Coulomb M. Initial isolated Takayasu's arteritis of the right pulmonary artery: MR appearance. Eur Radiol 1996; 6: 429–432

62. Berkmen YM, Lande A. Chest roentgenography as a window to the diagnosis of Takayasu's arteritis. Am J Roentgenol 1975; 125: 842–846

63. Cassling RJ, Lois JF, Gomes AS. Unusual pulmonary angiographic findings in suspected PE. Am J Roentgenol 1985; 145: 995–999

64. Suzuki Y, Konishi K, Hisada K. Radioisotope lung scanning in Takayasu's arteritis. Radiology 1973; 109: 133–136

65. Behçet H. Ueber rezidivierende, aphthoes, durch ein virus verursachte Geschwuere am Mund, am Auge und an den Genitalien. Dermatol Monatsschr 1937; 105: 1152–1157

66. Chajek T, Fainaru M. Behçet's disease. Report of 41 cases and a review of the literature. Medicine 1975; 54: 179–196

67. James DG. Behçet's syndrome. N Engl J Med 1979; 301: 431–432

68. Tunaci A, Berkmen YM, Gokmen E. Thoracic involvement in Behçet's disease: pathologic, clinical and imaging features. Am J Roentgenol 1995; 164: 51–56

69. Grenier P, Bletry O, Cornud F. Godeau P, Nahum H. Pulmonary involvement in Behçet's disease. Am J Roentgenol 1981; 137: 565–569

70. Gibson RA, Morgan H, Krausz T, Hughes GRV. Pulmonary artery aneurysms in Behçet's disease. Br J Radiol 1985; 58: 79–82

71. Park JH, Han MC, Bettmann MA. Arterial manifestations of Behçet's disease. Am J Roentgenol 1984; 143: 821–825

72. Koc Y, Güllü, Akpek G, et al. Vascular involvement in Behçet's disease. J Rheumatol 1992; 19: 402–410

73. Efthimiou J, Johnston C, Spiro SG, Turner-Warwick M. Pulmonary disease in Behçet's syndrome. Q J Med 1986; 58: 259–280

74. Ghaye B, Trotteur G, Dondelinger RF. Multiple pulmonary artery pseudoaneurysms: intrasaccular embolization. Eur Radiol 1997; 7: 176–179

75. Dillon WP, Taylor AT, Mineau DE, Datz FL. Traumatic pulmonary artery pseudoaneurysm simulating PE. Am J Roentgenol 1982; 139: 818–819

76. Kasai T, Kobayashi K. Bilateral pseudo-aneurysms of the pulmonary arteries by blunt chest injury. Intensive Care Medicine 1992; 18: 51–52

77. Labrunie E, Levy C, Paugam C, Augereau B, Tubiana JM. Pseudoaneurisme arteriel pulmonaire post-cathe-ter de Swan-Ganz traité par embolisation. Annales de Radiologie 1993; 36: 310–314

78. Aydogdu S, Ozdemir M, Diker E, Korkmaz S, Kutuk E, Goksel S. Fistulous connection between the left pulmonary artery and the innominate vein. Cath Cardiovasc Diagnosis 1996; 39: 80–81

79. Altstaedt HO, Thermann M, Raute-Kreinsen U. Angiomatous pulmonary arteriovenous fistula as a cause of recurrent peripheral arterial embolisms. Chirurg 1993; 64: 422–423

80. White RI Jr. Pulmonary arteriovenous malformations: how do we diagnose them and why is it important to do so? (editorial). Radiology 1992; 182: 633–635

81. Hagspiel KD, Christ ER, Schopke W. Hereditary hemorrhagic telangiectasis (Osler-Rendu-Weber disease) with pulmonary, hepatic and renal disease pattern. Fortschr Röntgenstr 1995; 163: 190–192

82. Clouston JE, Pais SO, White CS, Dempsey JE, Templeton PA. Pulmonary arteriovenous malformation: diagnosis and treatment of spontaneous thrombosis and recanalization. J Vasc Interv Radiol 1995; 143–145

83. Achong DM. Ventilation-perfusion mismatch caused by extrinsic compression of the pulmonary artery. Correlative imaging. Clin Nucl Med 1994; 19: 61–63

84. Cook DJ, Tanser PH, Dobranowski J, Tuttle RJ. Primary pulmonary artery sarcoma mimicking pulmonary thromboembolism. Can J Cardiol 1988; 4: 393–396

85. Madu EC, Taylor DC, Durzinsky DS, Fraker TD Jr. Primary intimal sarcoma of the pulmonary trunk simulating PE. Am Heart J 1993; 125: 1790–1792

86. Disler L, Manga P. Primary leiomyosarcoma of the pulmonary trunk. Int J Cardiol 1992; 35: 412–414

87. Casullo J, Lisbona A, Palayew MJ. General case of the day. Primary sarcoma of the pulmonary artery (chondrosarcoma). Radiographics 1992; 12: 401–404

88. Akomea-Agyin C, Dussek JE, Anderson DR, Hartley RB. Pulmonary artery sarcoma mimicking PE: successful surgical intervention. Ann Thorac Surg 1996; 61: 1536–1538

89. Zuber M, Evequoz D, Stulz P, Erne P. Right ventricular myxoma mimicking recurrent PE after primary ligament reconstruction. Vasa 1997; 26: 49–51

90. Anonymous. Case records of the Massachusetts General Hospital. Weekly clinicopathological exercises. Case 16–1194. A 57-year-old woman with a mass in the right atrium. N Engl J Med 1994; 330: 1143–1149

91. Waller BF, Dean PH, Mann O, Rosen JH, Roberts WC. Right ventricular outflow obstruction from thrombus with small peripheral pulmonary emboli. Chest 1981; 79: 224–225

92. Detrano R, Salcedo EE, Simpfendorfer C, Hodgman J. Digital subtraction angiography in the evaluation of right heart tumours. Am Heart J 1985; 109: 366–368

Acknowledgement: The cooperation of Springer Verlag GmbH & Co KG for allowing the use of figures 4, 5, 6, 8, 9, 11 and 17, which will appear in European Radiology, is gratefully acknowledged.

IV.6 Helical computed tomography and pulmonary thromboembolism

A. B. van Rossum, A. H. H. Bongaerts, P. K. Woodard

Introduction

This chapter will first discuss the historical background of the development of helical computed tomography (hCT) and review published studies relating to the CT evaluation of patients suspected of having pulmonary embolus (PE).

Next, the general design and function of the hCT scanner will be reviewed, followed by a description of scanning protocols designed for the detection of PE, including evaluation of secondary signs. The essence of the hCT method is direct visualisation of an embolus by identifying an intraluminal filling defect after the pulmonary arteries have been enhanced with iodinated contrast material. Secondary signs include the identification of the pulmonary parenchymal effects of emboli, such as pleural based areas of infarction, pleural effusions, and areas of differential perfusion.

A review of experimental (animal) studies and a description of diagnostic findings in human patients will be followed by a review of the data concerning the technical and diagnostic accuracy of hCT in the diagnosis of pulmonary emboli. Also discussed in this section will be the difficulties and pitfalls causing inaccurate, indeterminate, false positive and false negative examinations. Helical CT then will be compared with results of electron beam tomography and magnetic resonance imaging (MR) of PE.

Historical background

Development of the helical computed tomograph

Computed tomography (CT) was introduced into diagnostic radiology in 1973 by EMI Ltd [1]. In 1979 Godfrey Hounsfield and Allen Cormack were awarded the Nobel Prize in Physiology in Medicine for their contribution in the development of CT [2, 3]. Early CT scanners initially were used almost exclusively for imaging the head, because, according to Gould, the head was the only body part that could be held still throughout the very long scan time. Once the scan time (for one slice) was reduced below 5 seconds, extension to other parts of the body could be considered.

In the first generation scanner a rigid gantry maintained the relative position of the x-ray tube and detector, ensuring proper alignment. This 'gantry' moved in two directions [4]. First, a linear motion made 160 exposures per each motion. Next, one rotatory motion was made between each linear motion with the axis of rotation passing through the centre of the object. This resulted in a total of 28,800 measurements and a total scan time of nearly 5 minutes for one tomographic slice. The total examination time approached 40 to 50 minutes.

For the next generation, the pencil beam of the original EMI scanner was abandoned and a fan-shaped beam with multiple detectors was installed with as many as 30 detectors collecting the information from the fanned beam [4]. Although the movement of the x-ray tube together with the detector array remained both linear and rotatory, larger rotatory steps (up to 30°) were obtained, with the rotation equal to the x-ray fan angle. These motions were repeated until the full data set was acquired. This resulted in a further reduction of scan time for one tomographic slice, with each image acquired in 10–90 seconds.

The third generation used a much wider fan beam and many more detectors (up to 300) with the fan beam wide enough to encompass the entire width of the patient [4]. Thus, no linear movement was required. Only a continuous rotatory movement remained, reducing the scan time to 2 to 10 seconds. Still, the entire x-ray tube remained within the gantry while the detectors moved, fixed to the x-ray tube.

Fourth generation CT scanners were built in the late 1970's. A fixed ring of detectors completely surrounded the object with only the x-ray tube moving, rotating through an arc of 360°. Initially, this resulted in only a technical improvement, since it now became easier to calibrate the detectors [4, 5]. Yet, for each slice, the scanner had to be restarted, and the table moved. This incremental technique resulted in a scan time of approximately 2 seconds for each slice acquisition.

In 1988, the first continuously rotating scanner was installed in the Dr. Daniel den Hoed Clinic, Rotterdam, the Netherlands. However, the table could not yet move through the gantry during image acquisition. Shortly thereafter, table movement was made possible. Using a 12-second continuous scan, 10 images could be reconstructed by a 360° reconstruction algorithm. Because of the limited total scan time the total z-axis distance which could be covered was limited to 12 times the collimation width. For example, in order to cover the liver, a collimation of 10mm was used.

In 1989 the Somatom Plus scanner was introduced [6 – 11]. Employing slip ring techniques it now became possible to quickly and continuously move the x-ray tube through the gantry, while the detectors remained stationary. Advanced computer technology simultaneously allowed for continuous motion of the patient-table, thus transporting the body through the continuously radiating scanner, acquiring a data set representing the entire scanned volume. Further development of software packages allowed reconstructions of nearly any desired scan thickness and slice distances including overlapping slices. Scan time now was reduced to 1-second images. Using partial-view images together with interpolation techniques, scan time can even be reduced to sub-second levels [12, 13].

Thus, scanning time decreased from nearly 5 minutes to subsecond levels permitting the fast scanning and interpolation necessary for PE detection by hCT.

Some discussion remains with respect to the name of this up-to-date scanning technique [14]; originally called 'spiral' CT. However, 'helical' CT appears to be a preferable term, as 'spiral' implies a change in diameter in each turn [15]. More generically, the term 'continuous volume CT' has been proposed, but we propose to refrain from this generic term, since another up-to-date scanning technique (electron beam tomography) is also capable of generating a continuous volume data set. Therefore, in this chapter we will use the term 'helical computed tomography' (abbreviated 'hCT') in contrast to the more conventional (incremental) computed tomographic technique (cCT) and distinct from electron beam tomography (EBT), which will be discussed in Chapter IV.7.

History of (h)CT and pulmonary embolism

Sinner et al., in 1978, were the first to report on CT findings of pulmonary infarction, focusing on the parenchymal sequelae of pulmonary embolism (PE) [16]. In the early days of body CT, accidental discoveries of filling defects in pulmonary arteries were reported with anecdotal documentation of PE detection in patients being scanned for other indications. More recently, Verschakelen [17] and Winston [18] elaborated on this theme, discussing findings made with conventional and helical computed tomography respectively.

In addition, several authors have presented experimental data using mainly dogs [19 – 21]. It is not clear, however, who was the first to focus CT studies on direct visualisation of the emboli in the pulmonary arteries in the living human being.

The first report on direct visualisation of pulmonary artery filling defects was published in 1980 by Godwin [22]. The report describes three patients, in whom conventional CT was a logical and practical alternative to arteriography for different reasons in the diagnostic work-up. For one case, a then conventional General Electric 8000 scanner was used with a scan time of 4.8 sec. For the two other cases a 'special' General Electric CT scanner was used (not further specified in the article) which could perform a 'rapid sequence of up to twelve 2.4 second scans' which was called 'dynamic scanning.'

The first case concerned a 16-year-old girl with lupus erythematosus and exogenous Cushing syndrome admitted with onset of severe dyspnea. Pulmonary arteriography was believed to be very risky in this patient because of her obesity, hypoxemia, and probable pulmonary vasculitis. The second patient was a 48-year-old woman who fell and injured her right calf 4 weeks before admission for pleuritic chest pain and progressive dyspnea. PE was confirmed by pulmonary angiography and she underwent CT 15 days later to determine if it could show the central thrombi and provide a non-invasive method for following the resolution of central pulmonary emboli. The last case was a 64-year-old man with previous pulmonary thromboembolism. Despite long-term anticoagulation, his dyspnea had worsened. Because of his pulmonary hypertension, only selective pulmonary angiography was performed; evaluation of the central pulmonary arteries was attempted by CT.

In 1982, Sinner [23] published his material, consisting of 21 patients with a clinical suspicion of PE. Of these 21 patients, 17 were presumed to have PE based on clear-cut symptoms along with results of plain chest x-rays, isotope perfusion lung scans and CT scans, or evidence of a peripheral source as assessed by venography. In 2 cases, selective pulmonary angiography was performed verifying the presence of PE. Early generation scanners were used with scan times of 2.5 min, but 7 cases were scanned on a newer machine (General Electric T7800) with 4.8 second scanning time.

In this article [23] Sinner claimed that 'to [his] best knowledge' the cases represented the first imaging of pulmonary thromboembolism by CT. According to Sinner, during the Nordic Congress of Radiology this was a matter of extensive discussion. Sinner suggested that a series of examinations should be made by an independent institution in order to confirm his original findings. Still, according to Sinner, 'as a result of this stimulation, Godwin, Webb, Gamsu and Overfors, using a more refined scanner, confirmed (Sinner's) findings completely.'

A most important step forward was made in 1984, when Breatnach et al. published a case report demonstrating segmental PE [24]. However, up to 1988, sentiments remained doubtful about the potential assets of CT in the diagnosis of PE, and Chintapalli et al. concluded that 'although one would not choose CT as a primary modality for evaluating PE, an understanding of the CT appearance may lead to the diagnosis of thromboembolism when a different disease was suspected clinically' [25]. They based their conclusions on a study of 18 patients studied over a 5-year period. Most of the patients were evaluated for abnormal chest radiographic findings including hilar and pulmonary masses. The diagnosis of PE was established in 14 cases by angiography, biopsy, or surgery.

However, improvements in scanning techniques, as described before, provided for a more sophisticated experience and in 1992, Remy-Jardin et al. published their first prospective study comparing pulmonary angiographic findings with helical computed tomography tailored to visualise the pulmonary vessels [26]. This was described by Rubin et al. as 'the exciting discovery that hCT might provide an alternative means for diagnosing acute pulmonary embolism' [27]. This enthusiasm was reinforced by the publication by Teigen one year earlier, reporting on experience of EBT and PE [28] and was further reinforced by studies by Van Rossum et al. [29] and the work of Goodman et al. [30].

Gradually, patients were referred more often for rapid assessment of the pulmonary arterial tree if helical CT scanners were available and if the clinical condition of the patient did not allow for more 'extensive' diagnostic approaches. These initial directed examinations produced dramatic pictures of large thrombi within the pulmonary arteries, leading in turn to increased interest and additional referrals [31]. In addition, Tardivon et al. brought attention to the vascular and parenchymal alterations induced by chronic pulmonary disease [32].

Later, Sheedy et al. reported on the difficulty in recruiting patients for prospective studies containing a number of subjects large enough to achieve results of statistical significance [31]. Up to 1995, the precise place of hCT (and MRI) within the diagnostic work-up of patients suspected of acute PE was not well defined [33]. Sheedy et al. considered their recruitment problems 'to reflect the clinician's growing confidence in the CT method and a reluctance to subject their patients to multiple additional studies'. Furthermore, they reported that fast CT methods have been incorporated into the daily practice of the Mayo Clinics.

These developments led Goodman et al. to propose a new algorithm in which fast CT is used as the first diagnostic modality in patients suspected of acute PE after assessment of the presence or absence of deep venous thrombosis (DVT) by ultrasonography [34, 35]. This algorithm was discussed extensively in the Journal of Thoracic Imaging by Rubin [27] and Stein [36]. Stein, who has extensively studied the role of scintigraphy in the diagnosis of PE is reluctant to drop ventilation/perfusion scintigraphy in favour of fast CT scanning. Alternatively Sostman, working in the field of MRI and PE, has hypothesised that 'the most likely candidate for a single procedure for the detection of thromboembolic disease is MRI' [37].

In the same discussion, Remy-Jardin et al. expect CT to simplify the diagnostic guidelines in PE, but also emphasise that larger databases are required to provide more information on the accuracy of each imaging modality before making new recommendations [38]. Mayo believes that the new algorithm proposed by Goodman et al. will prove to be correct, but he also states that further technical developments are required before this approach is ready for general implementation [39]. Finally, Gefter and Palevsky conclude with the hope 'that we will not have to wait too long before identifying the optimal diagnostic approach to patients with suspected acute PE. Before accepting the proposed algorithm by Goodman et al., they ask for cost-effectiveness studies to be tested empirically [40].

Very recently two more comparative studies were published, again adding substantial information to this still expanding database in favour of fast computed tomography in the diagnosis of PE [41, 42].

So, although there is good evidence that helical CT can play a role in a diagnostic algorithm of PE, there remains some reluctance to give it a central role. There is a sentiment that available studies are not rigorous enough to base final decisions on. This is principally because of the concern that subsegmental pulmonary emboli may not be detected by hCT. To date, no clinical outcomes or cost-effectiveness studies have been performed using CT based algorithms. Also, little attention has been given to the application of hCT in the severity assessment of PE, although recently a first study on this subject was published [43].

Presently, while the exact position of fast CT imaging in the diagnostic algorithm for PE remains an issue of debate, in some centres, like the Mayo Clinic and in Montpellier, France [44], spiral CT has attained routine use.

Helical computed tomography protocol and the diagnosis of pulmonary embolus [45]

Direct visualisation of the embolus

Principles
As already described, scanning techniques have undergone a tremendous change over the past 20 years. Hardly any study is comparable with other studies with respect to image acquisition protocols. However, all studies had the same goals: optimal spatial resolution and contrast resolution. The final imaging parameters are determined by these concepts. The next discussion will illustrate how, in principle, for each patient, a tailored image acquisition protocol can be derived.

Protocol
First, a limited pre-contrast scan is obtained in order to demonstrate the location of the pulmonary artery trunk and the aortic root. Next, in order to estimate the required time delay between initiation of injection of contrast material and initiation of image acquisition, a time-density curve can be obtained, using contrast material parameters tailored to the specific patient. Finally, a dedicated contrast enhanced scanning protocol is used in order to visualise the pulmonary arterial tree. If desired, the study can be completed by a 'standard' CT of the chest in order to visualise the whole thorax, and to determine coincidental or alternative disease processes, which can explain the patient's complaints.

Spatial resolution
In order to acquire optimal resolution and to minimise partial volume effects, a small volume element (voxel) should be imaged while it is not moving.

Voxel size is determined by the chosen field of view in relation to matrix size, determining the in-plane resolution, and, independently, by the voxel depth, determined by the collimation width. Field of view and collimation should be as small as possible. In hCT, the relation between collimation width and table translation is expressed in pitch; a pitch of 1 means that the collimation width (for example 3mm) equals the table translation per gantry revolution (for example 3mm/revolution), pitch equalling table translation per gantry revolution divided by collimation.

Scan time can be expressed as a function of the distance to be covered (i.e. z-axis length) and the table speed; for example, if 15 cm are to be covered with a table speed of 5mm/sec, scan time will be 30 seconds.

Motion of the pulmonary arteries is primarily determined by respiration; so the ability of the patient to hold his or her breath will determine the length of time available for image acquisition. Ideally, respiration should be postponed, which can be done voluntarily, by asking a co-operative patient to hold his/her breath, or by interrupting respiration at a prefixed percentage of tidal volume. In patients on artificial ventilation the respirator can be stopped for a short while. If these options are not available, an effort to obtain images can be made by asking the patient to breathe very slowly and superficially.

Thus, the first step is to estimate the breathhold capacity of the patient, which indicates the time window for image acquisition. The second step is to decide the distance along the z-axis to be covered. In principle the level from just above the aortic arch down the tip of the diaphragms should be covered, but, ideally, as much of the lungs as possible should be included. Dividing the distance to be covered by the time window length results in the required table translation per second (revolution – supposing 1 revolution per second).

In view of the maximally allowed table speed, and in view of the disadvantages of a larger pitch, the collimation width can be chosen. The pitch should not exceed 2 in order to avoid reconstruction artifacts.

Some advocate a pitch of 1 (with 5 mm collimation) provided 3 mm incremental reconstructions are performed [46]. However, a dedicated study suggested that collimation down to 2 mm with a pitch of 2 [47] (i.e. 4 mm/revolution table speed) can improve visualisation of peripheral pulmonary arteries. The loss in table speed (from 5 to 4 mm per revolution) was compensated by subsecond (0.75 sec) revolution time. The mean number of *segmental* pulmonary arteries coded as 'analysable' per patient, in the first group (2 mm collimation, pitch 2), i.e. 18.6/20 or 93%, was significantly higher than that observed in the other group (3 mm collimation, pitch 1.7), i.e. 17/20 or 85%. The mean number of *subsegmental* branches analysable per patient was statistically higher using a scan protocol with 2 mm collimation and a pitch of 2 than using a protocol with 3 mm and a pitch 1.7 (5 mm/revolution table speed). Forty subsegmental pulmonary arteries were defined to be analysed; in the first group, 61% (24.6 of 40) of the subsegmental arterial bed was 'adequately' depicted; whereas in the other group this was only 37% (14.8 of 40).

Narrower collimation without sub-second scanning techniques may not permit adequate z-axis coverage in a single breathhold. However, if faster scanning methods are available, the substantial increase in visibility of segmental and subsegmental pulmonary arteries could provide improved detection of pulmonary emboli in these more distal order vessels.

Contrast resolution

The aim of contrast material administration is to use, over time, an optimal amount of contrast material to enhance the pulmonary arterial tree. Image acquisition time should coincide with the time during which the contrast enhancement is at its peak level; however, this peak level should not cause streak artifacts [48].

The time at which contrast reaches its peak level can be estimated by simply supposing a mean time required for all human beings for contrast material to reach the pulmonary artery trunk after start of injection into a peripheral vein. This will usually be an antebrachial vein. One can then shorten or lengthen this mean time depending upon the clinical condition of the patient. The delay can be estimated more precisely by injection (for example) of a 10 ml bolus of 0.5% magnesium sulfate (with 9 ml of normal saline) at the planned venous injection site, and the time measured until the patient reports a warm salty taste in his or her mouth. A variant of this method which does not require patient co-operation is the injection of a dye, for example 0.2 mg indocyanine dye, with time measured until the presence of the dye is detected by an ear oximeter.

More sophisticated is the method in which a small amount of iodinated contrast medium is injected (i.e. 15 to 20 ml) while the pulmonary arterial trunk and aortic root are scanned, acquiring multiple images at the same level over time (i.e. one image every 2 seconds for 20 to 30 seconds). This allows for a construction of the time-density curve (using available software), in which the increase in Hounsfield units, caused by the arrival of the iodinated contrast medium, is recorded as a function of time. The time delay between start of injection of contrast material and start of image acquisition is calculated as the time after start of contrast medium injection until time of peak enhancement in the pulmonary artery trunk plus the time of peak enhancement in the aortic root divided by two. By using this approach (and not the time to peak enhancement in the pulmonary artery trunk alone), one can be sure that at initiation of image acquisition there is peak enhancement throughout the pulmonary arterial tree, including the peripheral zones (which will be scanned first at initiation of image acquisition). This allows for a nearly exact determination of the delay required between start of injection and start of peak enhancement.

Newer software allows this process to be executed automatically with the scanner itself discovering the time of peak enhancement (i.e. the time at which nearly no increase in density is recorded) and starting scanning automatically.

The duration of the plateau of peak enhancement is determined by the time during which injection will be maintained. The peak level will be determined partially by the iodine concentration of the contrast material used, and the injection velocity. The injection velocity, if considered as a function of the required image acquisition time, is limited by the amount of contrast material which one is willing to administer. In the reported literature, injection velocities range from 2 ml/sec [49] up to 7 ml/sec [26, 50]. If one supposes a scan delay of 18 seconds, and a required acquisition time of 24 seconds, then, with an injection rate of 2 ml/sec, a total amount of 84 ml contrast material is required. If one does not want to apply more than 150 ml, using the same assumptions on scan delay and acquisition time, the maximum injection velocity allowed in this case is 3.5 ml/sec. In order to obtain such a fine-tuned contrast material administration, an automated power injector is an absolute requirement.

Some centres advocate having the arm of the patient, used for intravenous access, remain alongside the patient. This would prevent stagnation of venous flow at the brachio-thoracic junction and would permit supervision of the injection site, at least during the first few seconds. To our knowledge, there are no systematic studies concerning the effect of arm position on contrast material arrival in the thorax. Furthermore, if a time-density curve has been obtained with the arm in the same position as planned during the contrast-enhanced scan, any delay has been accounted for. In addition, having the arms of the patients outside the scanning field will improve image quality. Inspection of the injection site will also be possible with the arms above the head of the patient.

mA and kV

Our strategy is to use the smallest possible collimation combined with a relatively high pitch in order to cover as large a z-axis as possible with respect to the patient's breathholding capabilities. To do this a high mA is required to achieve a high image to noise ratio. Small collimation will increase image noise, and a high pitch will cause 'helical' artifacts (i.e. fine lines and a degraded slice profile, which can add to the intrinsic quantum noise) [39]. Thus, it is recommended to use the highest attainable mA settings [39]. The kilovoltage will be fixed by this parameter and the requirements of the tube, and may be 120 kV to 140 kV. Thus, in principle, for each patient, depending on his/her clinical condition, a scanning protocol can be tailored to optimise image quality (see Table 1).

Streak and motion artifacts

In imaging for pulmonary emboli streak artifacts caused by dense objects within the scanned plane are most destructive at the level of the superior vena cava. This is especially true at the level of the right pulmonary hilus, where streak artifacts can disrupt the opacification of smaller vessels. High densities of contrast in the superior vena cava may be avoided by using a relatively low concentration of contrast material. This, however, may decrease small vessel enhancement. Preferably, the artifact caused by dense contrast within the superior vena cava can be corrected by scanning in a caudo-cranial direction, giving time for the contrast material in the superior vena cava to dissipate. Also, it has been proposed that a saline push be used in order to clear the vena cava superior at the moment the scanner arrives at these levels [51].

Some centres use less concentrated contrast material, i.e. 24% or 30% iodinated contrast media, with the added advantage of preventing the overshadowing of small clots, but lower concentrations may require a higher injection rate. The lowest concentration reported for the evaluation of pulmonary arteries was 120 mg/l injected at a rate of 7 ml/sec [26, 38].

Scanning in the caudo-cranial direction also has the advantage that, if the patient cannot hold his/her breath, and is allowed to start quiet respiration, the areas which will start moving most, i.e. the lower lung zones, have already been scanned.

These factors are fixed, and we propose to use a 'full strength' (non-ionic) iodinated contrast material, with up to 60% iodine concentrations (with an injection velocity around 3ml/sec tailored to the patient's condition) [33, 52] while scanning in a caudo-cranial direction.

Image reconstruction and viewing

CT interpretation is best performed at a console, using cine-viewing to follow each vessel on consecutive images. Thus, filming all images does not appear to be useful or cost-effective.

It has been recommended to reconstruct the data volume in axial planes using a 180° linear interpolation algorithm [45, 53]. Reconstruction of overlapping sections is also recommended to improve longitudinal resolution and diminish partial volume effects [45, 54]. However, as Remy-Jardin remarked, based on her extensive experience [45], overlapping reconstructions may be less important for detecting (central) pulmonary emboli when scanning patients with 2mm collimation, although it may be worthwhile to use overlapping reconstructions when scanning with 5mm collimation. If

Table 1.   Review of parameters.

Time window	20 – 30 seconds*
Scan direction	caudo-cranial
Field margins	tip of lowermost diaphragm up to upper roof of aortic arch larger if condition of patients allows
Z-axis distance	12 – 16 cm*
Table speed	5 mm/sec (/revolution)*,**
Collimation	2 – 6 mm*,**
(pitch = table speed/collimation)	
Contrast material	
– concentration	30 – 60%
– non-ionic	
– scan delay	15 – 25 seconds*
– amount	80 – 150 ml*,**
– velocity	2 – 4 ml/sec*,**

mA: as high as possible up to 300 mA

kV: 120, 140 kV

*   = determined by patient's condition/constitution

** = determined by time window

These considerations have led to the following 'standard' protocols as proposed by Remy-Jardin:

	Eupneic patients		Dyspneic patients	
revolution/sec	1/1	0.75/1	1/1	0.75/1
collimation	3 mm	2 mm	5 mm	3 mm
table feed	5	4 mm/revolution	10	6 mm/revolution
pitch	1.7	2.0	2	2
z-axis coverage	10 cm	10 cm	10 cm	10 cm
breathhold duration	0 sec	20 sec	10 sec	12 sec

not routinely performed, overlapping reconstructions may be useful at the level of equivocal findings.

The window level and width may be adapted to the specific site under consideration, as has been studied by Brink [55]. Brink suggested a window setting equal to the measured mean density plus two standard deviations of the opacified mean pulmonary artery and a level equal to one half of this window [52]. However, Kuzo appears somewhat doubtful about alternating window level and width, since narrower windows can increase the conspicuity of artifacts caused by image noise, beam hardening, and motion [52].

In our experience, cine-viewing of the reconstructed axial images from a work station allows sufficient information; however, in a further study,

Remy-Jardin studied the usefulness of multiplanar reformations [56]. Thirty-nine consecutive patients were prospectively evaluated with hCT with respect to pulmonary embolic disease using ventilation perfusion scintigraphy, hCT and conventional (invasive) pulmonary angiography. Mutiplanar 2D reformations were systematically obtained along the main axis of 10 obliquely oriented pulmonary arteries known as potential sources of interpretative difficulties on axial images. The proper plane of reformation was selected (interactively) by a localising cursor positioned over the lateral view of a three-dimensional display obtained with a threshold view of – 300 Hu. Curved or tortuous vessels were analysed by 2 or 3 successive reformations for each segment of the arterial curvature. Obtaining all required views took approximately

30 minutes for each study. Reference was hCT itself, if there was clear evidence of (central) PE. If no emboli were found on hCT or if the result was indeterminate, patients underwent ventilation/perfusion scan (n = 9), or pulmonary angiography (n = 6).

Four patients were excluded (3 due to poor quality caused by motion, 1 with extensive coal worker's pneumoconiosis and hilar lymphadenopathy). Based on the axial hCT images, the population was divided into three groups; group 1 (n = 20) with hCT demonstrated presence of PE; group 2 (n = 6) without signs of PE on axial hCT images; and group 3 (n = 9) with uncertain interpretation.

The main role of MPR in group 1 (with clear signs of PE on axial hCT images) was to more precisely analyse the extent of thromboembolic disease. In group 2 ('clear' absence of embolic signs of axial hCT image) no additional information was provided by MPR. When the interpretation of the axial hCT images was doubtful, all questionable abnormalities were resolved by MPR excluding intraluminal filling defects. Although not further specified, the authors stated that no false-negative CT findings were observed.

Multiplanar reformation is a laborious exercise, but will become more feasible with improved work stations and software. As yet, the contribution could prove not be 'cost-effective'.

Interpretation
General rules
It is recommended to interpret hCT scans with precise knowledge of the conditions under which the examination has been obtained [45]. An effort should be made to identify all of the (sub)segmental levels during each examination [52]. In order to differentiate between arteries and veins, it may be helpful to display lungsettings and mediastinal window settings simultaneously on the work station at the same axial level. The segmental pulmonary arteries are always seen near the accompanying branches of the bronchial tree and are situated medial to the bronchi in the upper lobes, and lateral to the bronchi in the middle lobe, lingula, and lower lobes. The exceptions to this are the artery to the posterior subsegment of the left upper lobe, and the lingular arteries that can run independently for a short distance before joining with their bronchi [26, 52]. With these exceptions, the vessels that are not accompanied by bronchi are likely veins; furthermore, pulmonary veins have a more horizontal course and lead to the left atrium.

Image quality
First of all, image quality should be assessed before image interpretation. In the literature, however, no clear criteria concerning imaging quality can be found, although some studies assessed scored image quality. For example, Remy-Jardin et al. graded vascular opacification as poor (grade 1) when insufficient for the detection of filling defects, good (grade 2) when sufficient for the analysis of pulmonary arteries without a high degree of contrast enhancement, and excellent (grade 3) when demonstrating a high degree of vascular opacification [26, 57], However, no further specification of these qualifications was given, and, probably, they are very difficult to define.

In another study, Remy-Jardin et al. proposed that the (sub)segmental arteries be considered analysable when the vessel of interest was depicted without partial volume effects from the proximal to the distal portions on single or successive CT scans. The arteries were considered non-analysable when the vessel of interest was not confidently depicted on axial CT scans, owing either to the small size of the vessel and the subsequent presence of partial volume effects, or to anatomic variants [47].

Pulmonary embolism: yes or no
Negative cases should show good opacification of all pulmonary arteries to the subsegmental levels without any of the findings indicative of PE.

Clear demonstration of even one embolus is enough to make a definitive diagnosis of PE. Arteries are considered thromboembolic if they show signs of a modified Sinner's description [16], including 1) a complete filling defect or cutoff ('amputation sign') (Fig. 1; 2) or a partial filling defect (Fig. 2). Partial filling defects may be either central or marginal. Findings may consist of intraluminal areas of low attenuation surrounded by variable amounts of contrast medium ('railway track sign') (Fig. 3) and may have regular or irregular borders. These findings are caused by thromboembolic masses floating freely in the lumen. Alternatively one may see mural defects or peripheral areas of low attenuation (Fig. 4). Small (sub)segmental filling defects are called 'positives' only when a definite filling defect is seen on more than one axial image in which artifactual causes have not been excluded [52].

On reformatted images the most distinctive CT features for a perivascular abnormality are the absence of endoluminal irregularity and no abrupt narrowing of the arterial lumen at the level of these marginal areas of hypoattenuation [56].

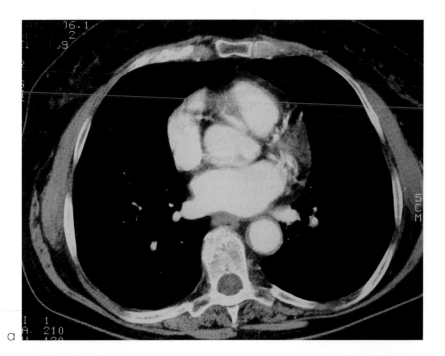

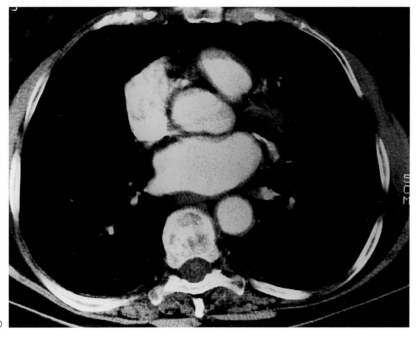

Fig. 1a–c. Three slices in one patient cranial to caudal.
(a) Normal enhancement of segmental arteries.
(b) and **(c)** Small emboli in left posterobasal branch at subsegmental level in lower slices.

Localisation
Several anatomic divisions of the arterial pulmonary tree have been proposed reflecting the variable (sub)segmental anatomy. Quite extensive descriptions of the pulmonary arterial tree can be found in dedicated studies of Jackson and Huber [58] and of Boyden [59]. Teigen et al. proposed a simplified nomenclature to be used for fast CT image analysis for PE (Table 2) [60].
The scheme was modified by Remy-Jardin for her first studies on helical CT and PE (Table 3) [26, 61].

A more refined description, adapted for (axial) fast CT images has recently been proposed by Remy-Jardin, modifying the Jackson-Huber and Boyden classification system (Table 4) [47]. Slight modifications to the naming of a few subsegmental arteries are proposed in the right and left upper lobes on the basis of the respective orientations of the vessels.
According to Remy-Jardin, rA1, in the right upper lobe, usually divides into two branches, an apical ramus rA1a and an anterior ramus rA1b; however, on axial images rA1a is located posteriorly

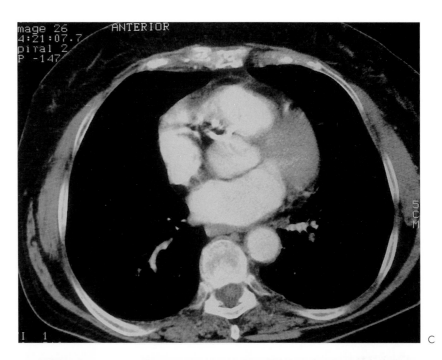

Fig. 1 c.

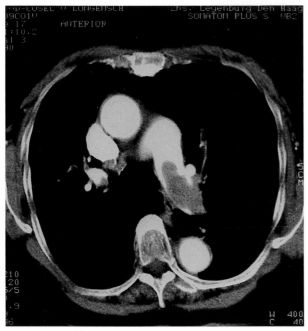

Fig. 2. Large thrombus left pulmonary artery.

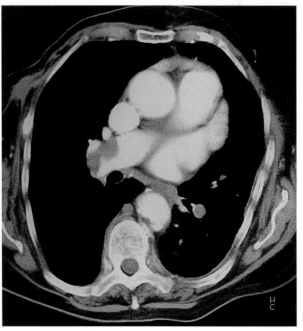

Fig. 3. Filling defect in right pulmonary artery extending into interlobar artery. Furthermore, embolus in left lower lobe artery.

relative to rA1b and therefore she proposes calling rA1a a posterior ramus, while rA1b retains its 'anterior' designation. Owing to the lateral location of rA2a relative to rA2b, rA2a is in fact called in this adapted scheme 'lateral', whereas rA2b remained recorded as the anterior ramus. Similarly, rA3a takes the name of 'lateral' ramus.

She also introduced a slightly modified nomenclature for the anterior segment of the left upper lobe coding 1A2a as 'lateral' and 1A2b as anterior

subsegmental arteries. Furthermore, due to the (usually) separate origin of the apical (1A1) and posterior (1A3) arteries (in contrast to the common origin of the bronchial trunk for the apical and posterior segments of the right upper lobe), separate numbers are attributed to these arteries, coding the subsegmental arteries in a similar manner as those of the right upper lobe.

We reviewed the current classification systems according to location of any possible pulmonary em-

201

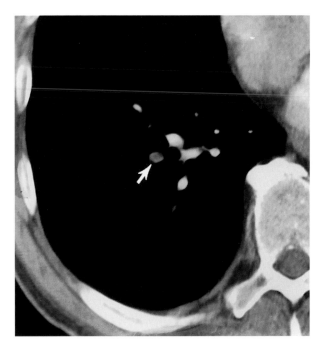

Fig. 4. Embolus in lateral basal segment branch artery of the right lower lobe (arrow). Note the lower attenuation of this vessel in comparison to the other basal segmental arteries.

Table 2. 12 zones [60].

c = central	
p = peripheral	
c = main pulmonary artery	

right lung

c	right pulmonary artery
c	anterior trunk
p	segmental vessels of right upper lobe
c	right interlobar artery
p	segmental vessels of the right middle lobe
p	segmental vessels of the right lower lobe

left lung

c	left pulmonary artery
c	left upper lobe trunk
c	segmental vessels of the left upper lobe
c	left descending trunk (interlobar artery)
p	segmental vessels of the left lower lobe

bolus; it will be clear that only great experience in viewing and interpreting the axial image, combined with great patience, will allow use of a detailed anatomic scheme. Quite possibly, the 15-zone scheme will prove to be the most suited for practical use.

Age of the embolus

Clinically, It will be important to differentiate between 'fresh' emboli ('acute') and 'older' ('chronic') emboli.

Emboli are considered acute if they completely or partially occlude the arterial lumen; i. e. centrally in the vascular lumen outlined by contrast material. However, they are more probably 'chronic' if the embolus is eccentric and contiguous with the vessel wall. Other characteristics of chronic emboli include evidence of recanalisation within an area of arterial hypo-attenuation, stenosis or webs of the involved pulmonary artery, or a reduction of more than 50% of the overall diameter [31, 60–62]. With smaller, peripheral emboli, however, it will be impossible to make this distinction.

Table 3. 15 zones [26, 61].

9 central vascular zones	6 peripheral vascular zones
pulmonary trunk	i. e. the segmental arteries of:
right main pulmonary artery	
left main pulmonary artery	
truncus anterior	
right interlobar artery	right upper segmentals
	right middle segmentals
left interlobar artery	culmen
	lingula
left upper lobe trunk	
right lower lobe artery	right lower segmentals
left lower lobe arteries	lower segmentals

Table 4. Nomenclature of bronchopulmonary anatomy [58, 59, 47].

	s	segmental artery	subsegmental artery	
Right upper lobe				
apical	S1	rA1	rA1a	apical
			rA1b	anterior
anterior	S2	rA2	rA2a	posterior
			rA2b	anterior
posterior	S3	rA3	rA3a	apical
			rA3b	posterior
Right middle lobe				
lateral	S4	rA4	rA4a	posterior
			rA4b	anterior
medial	S5	rA5	rA5a	superior
			rA5b	inferior
Right lower lobe				
apical	S6	rA6	rA6a+b	superomedial
			rA6c	lateral
medial	S7	rA7	rA7a	anterolateral
(paracardiac)			rA7b	anteromedial
anterior basal	S8	rA8	rA8a	lateral
			rA8b	basal
lateral basal	S9	rA9	rA9a	lateral
			rA9b	basal
posterior basal	S10	rA10	rA10a	laterobasal
			rA10b	mediobasal
Left upper lobe				
Upper division				
apicoposterior	S1+3	lA1	lA1a	posterior
= culmen			lA1b	anterior
		lA3	lA3a	lateral
			lAb3	posterior
anterior	S2	lA2	lA2a	lateral
			lA2b	anterior
(Slightly modified for CT)				
(See hereafter – left lung)				
Lower division				
(lingula)				
superior	S4	lA4	lA4a	posterior
			lA4b	anterior
inferior	S5	lA5	lA5a	superior
			lA5b	inferior
Left lower lobe				
apical	S6	lA6	lA6a+b	superomedial
			lA6c	lateral
anteriomedial	S7+8	lA7+8	lA7a	anterior
basal			lA7b	medial
			lA8a	lateral
			lA8b	basal
lateral basal	S9	lA9	lA9a	lateral
			lA9b	basal
posterior basal	S10	lA10	lA10a	laterobasal
			lA10b	mediobasal

Extent of the disease

Bankier recently studied two (modified) scoring systems for the staging of PE based on fast computed tomography findings [63]. These scoring systems were developed in the early 1970's by Walsh [64] and by Miller [65] and these scoring systems were more recently validated in several studies (Tables 5 and 6) [66–68]. The scoring systems are based on the number of vessels supposed to be underperfused because of obstruction or filling defects. As Bankier described, the Walsh score differentiates between complete obstruction and partial filling defects whereas the Miller system attributes the same value to both filling defects and obstructions. Furthermore, both systems were designed to evaluate pulmonary arteries up to the segmental level.

Miller originally suggested assessing the angiographic velocity of perfusion on the basis of a subjective evaluation. However, because velocity of perfusion cannot be assessed on hCT, Bankier omitted this factor from the scoring system.

In the Miller scoring system the scores range from a minimum of 0 to a maximum of 16. In Miller's scoring system the right pulmonary artery has 9 major segmental branches: 3 to the upper lobe, 2 to the middle lobe, 4 to the lower lobe. The left pulmonary artery has 7 major segmental branches: 2 to the upper lobe, 2 to the middle lobe and 3 to the lower lobe. The presence of obstruction or filling defects in any of these branches scores 1 point. Thus, the involvement of emboli of all the branches of the right pulmonary artery scores a maximum of 9 points and the left pulmonary artery a maximum of 7 points. The presence of an abnormality proximal to segmental branches scores a value equal to the number of segmental branches arising distally [63].

Bankier proposed the following modification of this system, using the 15 anatomic zones as defined before, for embolus localisation with fast CT: every positive peripheral zone will have a score equal to the number of segmental branches in a given lobe. The presence of a filling defect at the level of a proximal artery results in a score equal to the number of branches that arise distally. When a proximal artery is involved more peripheral emboli are not scored.

Bankier also used a modified Walsh score ranging from 0 to a maximum of 18, which, however, resulted in a very complex system of rules:

- the scores for abnormalities in both lungs are added to result in a maximum score of 18;
- abnormalities in a single segmental vessel may receive a total score not to exceed a value of 1, regardless of the type or number of abnormalities;
- abnormalities in a single lobar region may receive a total score not to exceed a value of 3 for the upper lobe, of 2 for the middle lobe or lingula, and of 4 for the lower lobe;
- obstructions in central anatomic regions receive scores according to the vessel involved;
- if the total score for the lung in question is greater than 4 without considering filling defects in the central region the central filling defects are ignored;
- all filling defects in a single central region, whether single or multiple, receive a score 3 if they are considered;
- if a single vessel contains both a filling defect and a obstruction only the obstruction is scored;
- the sum total of scores for all abnormalities in one lung must not exceed a value of 9.

Table 5. CT-modified Miller scoring system.

Embolus in	right	left
upper lobe artery	3	3
middle lobe artery	2	2 (lingula)
lower lobe artery	5	5
interlobar artery	7	7
truncus anterior		3 (to left upper lobe)
main pulmonary	10	10
truncus a. pulm.		20

Maximum possible score for involvement = 20

Table 6. CT modified Walsh scoring system.

Score	Obstruction
9	Main pulmonary artery
6	Intermediate artery
3	Lobar artery
2	Upper
4	Middle (or lingular)
1	Segmental
	Filling defect
3	Central region
2	Lobar/or lingular
1	Segmental

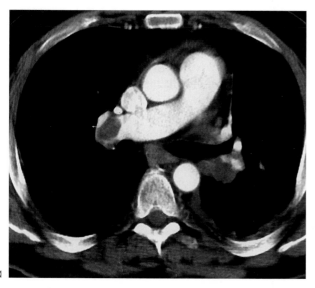
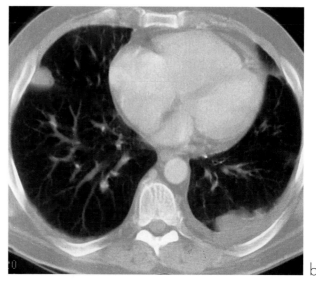

a   b

Fig. 5a, b. **(a)** Large emboli in right pulmonary artery and left lower lobe pulmonary artery. A small pleural effusion is present on the left. **(b)** The lung windows demonstrate several wedge-shaped peripheral infarcts, one in the right middle lobe and one in the left lower

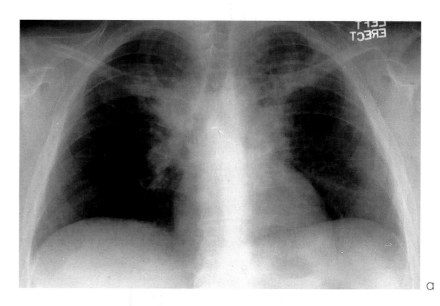

a

Fig. 6a, b. **(a)** Posterior-anterior chest radiograph demonstrating ground glass upper lobe opacities and enlarged hila in a patient with chronic pulmonary emboli and antiphospholipid antibody syndrome. **(b)** Lung windows on CT show the mosaic pattern caused by areas of differential perfusion. Areas of increased attenuation are regions of hyperperfusion and low-attenuation areas are regions of hyperperfusion. Note also that the vessels in the areas of hyperperfusion (arrows) are engorged and have a larger diameter than those in the hypoperfused regions. Some adenopathy of unknown etiology, possibly granulomatous disease, is also present and may contribute to the enlarged hila on the chest radiograph. (credit to P.K. Woodard, Mallinckrodt Institute of Radiology, Washington University Medical Center, and H.P. McAdams, Duke University Medical Center, Durham, USA).

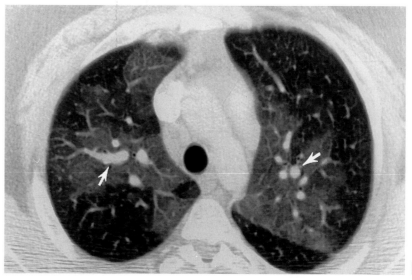

b

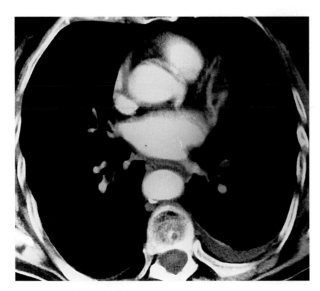

Fig. 7. Embolus in left lower lobe artery, extending into segmental artery with concomitant pleural effusion.

Remy-Jardin et al. also used the modified Miller scoring system in the follow-up of acute thromboembolic disease with spiral CT [61]. They proposed reducing the Miller score to the following degrees in the extent of pulmonary embolic disease: minor disease if the actual score was less than 25 % of the total possible score, moderate disease if the actual score was between 25 % and 50 % of the maximum possible score, and severe disease if the estimate score was larger than 50 % of the maximum possible score.

Bankier compared both scoring systems. The clinical condition of 31 patients with acute pulmonary disease was established, and patients underwent hCT, from which the extent of pulmonary embolic disease was estimated using the modified Miller and the modified Walsh scores [63]. Interobserver agreement was good for both scoring systems with values obtained by analysis of variance for repeated measurements for the Miller score of $r = 0.96$ and a slightly lower correlation coefficient (as could be expected in view of its complexity) for the Walsh score ($r = 0.85$). Correlations were studied between the two scores and arterial oxygen pressure, heart rate, and

right ventricular strain as assessed by echocardiography resulting in a quite complex analysis. This suggested that the modified scores can be used to distinguish mild from severe pulmonary embolic disease, but that the distinction between mild and moderate and between moderate and severe disease may be less confident. Miller scores of more than 10 and Walsh scores of more than 11 were indicative for marked clinical abnormalities.

A more widespread use of such staging systems may make investigational studies more comparable with respect to spectrum of disease of the patients. It can also help the physician in clinical practice to refine decision making. Maybe the modified Miller system is more practical than the more complex modified Walsh system.

Visualisation of secondary signs of pulmonary embolism

Visual inspection of parenchymal abnormalities
Viewing the images in the lungsetting (window level – 500 Hu, width 1,500 Hu) allows assessment of the lung-parenchymal sequelae, which might be associated with pulmonary emboli. This includes identification of a mosaic pattern caused by differential perfusion and infiltrates caused by either hemorrhage or infarction (Figs. 5 and 6).

Furthermore, secondary cardiac changes may be visible. Acute pulmonary emboli may cause dilatation of the right ventricle and right atrium, which may occur rapidly with the occurrence of large pulmonary emboli. In addition, in the case of chronic pulmonary emboli in which the pulmonary out-flow is obstructed over a period of time, right ventricular myocardial hypertrophy may occur.

Pleural effusion often accompanies acute pulmonary embolus but is a non-specific sign as it can occur in a number of clinical situations (Fig. 7).

Ventilation-perfusion protocol
No studies have been addressed to perfusion/ventilation characteristics using helical computed tomography (as has been done with Electron Beam Tomography (see Chapter IV.7).

Clinical experience

During the past 5 years, the fast CT features of pulmonary emboli have been described and comprehensive summaries have been published by Sheedy et al. [31] and Greaves [69]. Since hCT and EBT both produce comparable images with respect to direct visualisation of the embolus and its parenchymal sequelae some overlap in description with findings from hCT is inevitable. What follows are descriptions of the findings expected with acute and chronic pulmonary emboli.

Pulmonary artery findings

In the absence of pulmonary embolus on a good quality examination, homogeneous opacification of the pulmonary arteries is expected after administration of intravenous contrast material. This opacification is expected up to and beyond the subsegmental pulmonary artery branches. Emboli are considered to be acute if they are located centrally or eccentrically within the pulmonary artery lumen, outlined by contrast material, or if they completely occlude a vessel, presenting an abrupt interruption of the high density contrast column. Emboli are considered to be more chronic in nature if they are visible as eccentrically located filling defects contiguous with the wall of the vessel. These chronic pulmonary emboli often assume a crescent configuration, conforming to the curvature of the vessel. In addition, contrast channels within the embolus may indicate recanalisation.

Acute emboli appear in the larger, more central pulmonary arteries (main pulmonary artery, right and left main pulmonary arteries, and the upper lobe, lower lobe, middle lobe, and lingular arteries) as filling defects within the lumen surrounded or partially surrounded by the iodinated contrast material (Fig. 8). Larger clots in the main pulmonary artery or in the right or left pulmonary artery are often elongated tubular or serpiginous structures that appear similar to the intraluminal cast of the vein from which they originated, usually from the lower extremity (Fig. 2). These elongated clots can appear as so-called 'saddle emboli', with the thrombus lying across a vascular bifurcation with one end in each of two branches. These saddle emboli can be seen at the bifurcation of the main pulmonary artery or at the bifurcation of the lobar or even segmental branches.

If a vessel contains an embolus and it is completely obstructed, it may enlarge. The obstruction is only obvious because of the abrupt change of density

in an adjacent scan level, a lower level in the case of upper lobe emboli, and the upper level in the case of lower lobe emboli in vertically oriented branches (Figs. 1 and 4). Often it is possible to see opacification distal to a high grade obstruction indicating that blood (and contrast material) is flowing into the vessel beyond an obstruction, even with a high-grade obstruction. This so-called 'flow-by phenomenon' sometimes is more obvious when viewing horizontally oriented vessels on transaxial scans or vertically oriented vessels on sagittal and coronal reconstruction of the transaxial images.

If the embolus is located more peripherally in small subsegmentals or even branches of the subsegmental arteries, occluded vessels may be seen as dark dots adjacent to opacified vessels of similar size that do not contain clot (Fig. 4). As the branching vessels become smaller, it can be difficult to be confident that the vessel does or does not contain contrast material or alternately does or does not contain an occlusive filling defect. This would occur when the branches become 1–2 mm in diameter.

It is essential to differentiate between the appearance of acute and chronic pulmonary emboli. It is possible to do so in the larger, more central vessels out to the segmental branch levels. Beyond this, in the absence of more central characteristic appearing filling defects, an occlusion could be due to either an acute or a chronic process.

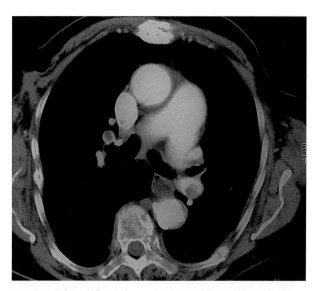

Fig. 8. Filling defect right upper segmental apical branch with filling defect in anterior branch and third filling defect in left interlobar artery.

A. B. van Rossum, A. H. H. Bongaerts, P. K. Woodard

Parenchymal abnormalities

On CT scans, the lung parenchyma supplied by an embolus may become oligemic with decreased flow. However, there is usually not a decrease in the number or calibre of vessels but a decrease in the density of the vessels with an associated decreased or inhomogeneous attenuation of the lung described as 'mosaic oligemia' (Fig. 6).

Bergin [70] et al. reported a disparity in vessel size, with vessels that are not perfused being collapsed and smaller with respect to neighbouring vessels in the same anatomic area which are perfused or when compared to the contralateral side at the same level. This report showed a significantly larger ratio of vessel size (right to left) in patients with chronic embolic disease (n = 17) (average 2.21 + 0.98 mm) than in patients with other diseases (n = 51) (average size 1.1 + 0.47 mm).

Remy-Jardin described the *mosaic pattern* as areas of ground-glass attenuation in patients with chronic pulmonary embolic disease, characterised by a 'sharp demarcation with lobular borders' [71]. This pattern is ascribed to differential perfusion: areas of hyperperfusion and oligemia. In the experience of Sheedy et al. this mosaic pattern does not seem to be as prevalent as observed by others [31] but it is definitely more common to find this pattern in chronic pulmonary embolus. This may be explained by observations made by Im [72] who, in an experimental study on pigs, found that the mosaic pattern was not associated with pulmonary artery obstruction (in 4 pigs) but with bronchial airway obstruction (in 4 other pigs).

Seemingly, coexistent small airway disease is required to cause this parenchymal pattern. Acute vascular occlusion results in reduced arterial carbon dioxide concentration in the affected lung, which has been associated with bronchoconstriction of small airways [73]. Airway trapping may then be expected in the affected areas of the lung due to this bronchoconstriction [74]. However, airway trapping as an isolated finding appeared not to be helpful in the distinction of airway disease from other causes of mosaic attenuation [74]. However, in patients with chronic thromboembolism, Remy-Jardin described bronchial dilatation in 64 % of areas where the pulmonary arteries had been occluded completely by an embolus [75].

Another parenchymal finding is haemorrhage, which may occur with or without infarction and appears as an area of ground-glass opacification or air space consolidation.

Peripheral densities that result from infarcts can vary in appearance [16]. The appearance most suggestive of an infarct is a wedge-shaped, or even rounded pleura-based density with their apexes directed toward the hilum (Figs. 5 and 9). The configuration may be irregular or polyhedral depending on the number and location of the involved vessels and supplied pulmonary lobules. The apex of the infarcted zone may be truncated if the lobules, immediately subtended by the embolus, are still perfused adequately by bronchial collaterals. The presence of a *vascular sign*, i. e. a thickened vessel leading to the apex of the opacity, increases the likelihood that the lesion represents an infarct [69].

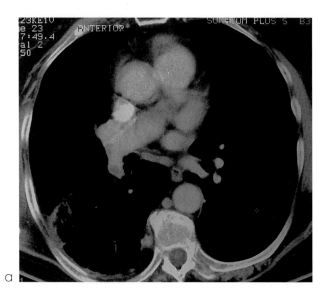
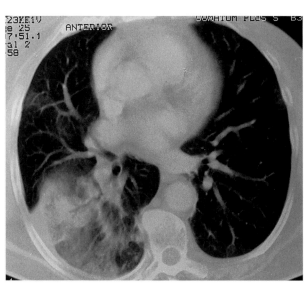

Fig. 9a, b. CT with suboptimal contrast enhancement. A pulmonary embolus is visible in the right lower lobe with wedge-shaped pleural-based area of consolidation, which was interpreted as a pulmonary infarct.

Pulmonary infarcts may contain central regions of low attenuation, which has been associated with preserved, uninfarcted secondary pulmonary lobules [76]. It is hypothesised that at the time of the embolic shower these unaffected lobules may not have been perfused; alternatively, the unaffected lobules may be supplied by retrograde flow from pulmonary veins or bronchial collaterals [69].

True cavitation is considered unusual and usually implies secondary infection or septic emboli [25, 69]. However, the observational basis for this last association is limited. McGoldrick did not find a case of cavitation in 58 angiographically proven (thus selected) pulmonary infarcts followed for 3 months or longer by serial chest radiography [77]. However, Gumes reported radiographic findings in 4 patients with septic embolic disease; all 4 patients had fever, positive blood culture, peripheral abscesses or endocarditis [25].

Infarcts may constrict and become atelectatic or parenchymal bands [77], but normally, healing of pulmonary infarcts occurs in 3 to 5 weeks [69], decreasing from the periphery while maintaining its original shape. This phenomenon is called the 'melting sign' [69]. The infarct eventually may resolve totally or leave a fibrotic scar with some associated thickening of adjacent pleura.

Cardiac changes

Changes in the heart, especially enlargement of the right ventricle and the right atrium and dilatation of the coronary sinus and dilatation of the inferior vena cava, may be seen especially with large acute pulmonary emboli or more commonly with long-standing pulmonary hypertension due to chronic pulmonary embolic disease.

Difficulties

Current clinical practice has revealed several difficulties and pitfalls [31, 45]. Difficulties may arise because of technical failure and factors associated with the condition of the patient, and may be caused by intrinsic anatomical and pathological properties.

Technical causes

Image quality strongly depends on contrast enhancement of the pulmonary arterial tree as described before. Any mistake in choosing the appropriate technical parameters may cause image acquisition without optimal contrast enhancement. The peripheral pulmonary zones are particularly vulnerable in this respect. If image acquisition is started too early the first slices will be acquired without optimal contrast enhancement. If image acquisition is started too late, the last images show suboptimal opacification of the peripheral pulmonary arterial tree. Thus, Teigen et al. reported 3 of 60 patients for whom the technical quality of the EBT images was considered less than optimal because of suboptimal enhancement of the upper lobe vessels secondary to the initiation of the scanning without adequate delay after injection of contrast material [49].

The effects of an improper timing of image acquisition with respect to contrast medium administration may be recognised when considering the overall opacification of the first slice with the level of enhancement of the last slices; with optimal timing, there should be no differences in 'brightness'. If the vessels in the first slices are brighter (or darker) than those in the last slices, something may have gone wrong [78]. In order to avoid misreadings due to pseudofilling defects, Remy-Jardin advises acquiring an additional data set over the involved area after proper modification of the start delay. Although this may appear 'overdone', it could help avoid additional diagnostic procedures.

As previously indicated, streak artifacts are to be avoided and several propositions have been made in this respect. These streak artifacts are most cumbersome at the level of the subclavian and brachiocephalic veins as well in the course of the superior vena cava.

Scanning at an increased pitch may cause an increase in helical artifacts, described as 'fine lines' and a degraded slice profile. This can add to intrinsic quantum noise. This is most problematic in large patients, or in those with large amounts of pleural effusions. To cope with this problem, implementation of a high milli-amperage is advised [39].

With small collimation, it usually is not possible to cover the lungs completely from apex to the lowermost basal portions due to the breathhold capacity of the patient (even with an increased pitch up to 2). Hence, the lung apices are not included in the data set with the theoretical possibility of not detecting emboli in this region.

It has been remarked that a high spatial frequency reconstruction algorithm may result in an artifactual high attention rim around vertically oriented arteries, which can mimic a central filling defect in vessels not optimally filled with contrast material [85, 79].

Patient-related factors

Motion artifacts can be caused by non-sustained apnea, shallow breathing or dyspneic breathing (gasping). In addition, variations in pulmonary blood flow between inspiration and expiration may cause heterogeneous pulmonary artery opacfication [45]. Furthermore, there may be changes in diameter and orientation of the pulmonary vasculature.

For vessels oriented along the z-axis, a change in orientation will have little consequence, since the vessel will remain orthogonal to the scan plane. However, vessels oriented more obliquely or even in-plane with respect to the axial images may change considerably in orientation, being displayed two or more times on consecutive slices. Because of obliquity some vessels may display an increased partial volume artifact. For this reason, during image interpretation, it is important to know if the breathhold was optimal, and, if not, whether the patient was breathing superficially or gasped during image acquisition. Without this information, artifacts secondary to displacement of vessels could go unnoted. Examining the same image at lungsettings can make motion artifacts more obvious, giving a further argument for simultaneous display of both lungsettings and mediastinal settings of the same image during cine-viewing.

Focal motion artifacts may be caused by the beating heart, which interferes with accurate depiction of paracardiac (lingular and middle lobe) segmental and subsegmental vessels running near the larger hilar pulmonary arteries.

Intrinsic causes

Intrinsic properties of the pulmonary arterial tree will inevitably cause difficulties in interpreting the images, despite optimal contrast enhancement and the absence of any motion artifact.

Altered blood flow

Abnormal venous inflow because of acute or chronic obstruction of systemic veins may cause delay and consequent suboptimal opacification of the pulmonary arteries. This is especially true if the scan delay between start of contrast administration and image acquisition has not been individualised for that particular patient. Poor opacification may also be caused by poor cardiac function. Shunting may also cause poor opacification of the pulmonary vasculature [45]. For example, Remy-Jardin described a 25-year-old man with a patent foramen ovale in whom suboptimal enhancement of the pulmonary vasculature was observed in two successive hCT studies [57]. Similarly, adaptations of the contrast medium application are required in patients with surgical anastomoses (Blalock, Waterston, Potts and Glenn).

Any cause of unilateral increased vascular resistance may lead to asymmetric pulmonary arterial opacification [45, 80]. Arterial resistance may be increased because of local diseases involving the pulmonary arteries, such as atelectasis or consolidation, or by mural diseases, such as vasculitis. In addition, increased arterial resistance has also been associated with larger amounts of pleural effusion. For instance, Remy-Jardin described a 21-year-old woman presenting with left sided chest trauma and suspected right-sided PE on hCT [26]. The asymmetry in arterial perfusion was explained by slow flow though the left basilar arteries because of the ipsilateral pleural effusion and posterior lung consolidation whereas the normally circulating right pulmonary arteries appeared 'abnormally' hypo-attenuated. Along these lines, Goodman explained two false-positive diagnoses of PE in patients with atelectasis, consolidation, and pleural effusion, observing spurious filling defects caused by slow flow, ipsilateral to the pleuroparenchymal changes [30]. In both cases, angiographic studies showed slow but unobstructed flow through the involved vessels.

In more advanced pulmonary parenchymal disease, systemic-pulmonary shunting may occur. This is particularly true in patients with extensive bronchiectasis in whom prominent bronchopulmonary and collateral circulation can develop. This collateral circulation has been reported to produce retrograde segmental flow from the systemic bronchial arteries into the pulmonary arteries [45]. Thus, in these patients, dilution of contrast medium may occur resulting in pseudo-filling defects, which may simulate emboli. This phenomenon has been previously reported on conventional pulmonary angiograms [45, 81]. One example of this, described by Remy-Jardin et al., is a 37-year-old woman with severe lung sarcoidosis. Findings included extensive fibrosis of both upper lungs, and a right upper lobe aspergilloma. There were hypoattenuated vascular sections in the right upper lobe in contrast to a high degree of vascular enhancement in the left upper lobe [45]. On conventional pulmonary angiography there was faint opacification of the right upper lobe pulmonary artery ascribed to systemic-to-pulmonary artery shunting.

Arterial resistance may also be increased in response to altered ventilation. Examples include bronchial disease, any cause of bronchiolitis, or disease at the alveolar level. In these cases, differential circulation and blood vessel opacification may arise if the disease does not uniformly affect both lungs, but is restricted to focal areas. This asymmetry can cause pseudo-filling defects, which can be falsely interpreted as PE. This misinterpretation may be avoided by simultaneously assessing the lungsettings of the axial image under consideration.

Also, with asymmetrical increased resistance in the pulmonary venous circulation, differential pulmonary arterial opacification may be observed [45]. Remy-Jardin presented a 63-year-old patient with tumour invasion of the left upper and lower pulmonary veins resulting in heterogeneous enhancement of the left interlobar pulmonary artery compared with optimal enhancement of the right interlobar pulmonary artery. At the level of the left lower lobe segmental arteries filling defects were ascribed to the impediment in pulmonary venous circulation rather than to pulmonary artery emboli.

Altered interfaces

Normally, there is excellent intrinsic contrast between the opacified pulmonary vessels and the surrounding air-filled lung parenchyma. However, with adjacent atelectasis or fluid-filled lungs, this contrast may be lost, causing loss of distinction of vessel contrast with respect to the surrounding tissue. In a less advanced state, partial volume averaging may occur between densities of the opacified vessels and the surrounding solidified tissues, causing apparent less dense vessel contrast which can result in false-positive interpretations.

Anatomical consideration

The anatomical nomenclature, as discussed above, supposes a more or less rigid anatomy, but numerous anatomic variants are supposed to be present in the origin and the calibre of these (sub)segmental vessels. Furthermore, the posterior segmental artery of the right upper lobe (rA3) is reported to be short, as can be seen in the apico-posterior segmental artery to the left upper lobe (lA1). Also, the anteromedial segmental arteries to the left lower lobe may be relatively small, thus causing difficulties in discerning any filling defect. Finally, vascular distortions and altered anatomy may result from (local) pathologic processes, more systematically, as in pulmonary fibrosis, or temporarily as with atelectasis or consolidation. Another approach is to repeat the examination, but now with a longer scan delay [45].

One of the most important and unavoidable difficulties is caused by partial volume averaging due to the fixed axial plane in which the images are to be acquired in relation to vessels not running in plane or orthogonal to the scan plane. The more they are in between these two ideal positions and the smaller the vessels, the more partial volume averaging will occur. This nearly always occurs in the anterior (sub)segmental vessels of both upper lobes, the (sub)segmental vessels of the lingula and of the medial and lateral middle lobe and the (sub)segmental vessels of the superior segment of the lower lobes. Image reformations are helpful but only for larger (segmental) vessels. Smaller (subsegmental) vessels will remain inadequately depicted, since the effect of the volume averaging will not be improved by reconstruction from an insufficient data set.

Remy-Jardin et al. estimate that between 4% and 7% of the pulmonary arterial branches, predominantly in the right middle lobe and lingula, are inadequately visualised with fast CT. The only remedy to this problem seems to be reduction in collimation [35].

Comparing 3 mm with 2 mm collimation (with a pitch of 1.7 and 2, respectively), Remy-Jardin observed in 40 patients (20 patients in each group), that for 40 subsegmental pulmonary arteries in the 2 mm group, 61% (24.6 of 40) of the subsegmental arterial bed was 'adequately' depicted; whereas in the 3 mm group this was only 37% (14.8 of 40) [47]. Thus, even with a reduced collimation, about 40% of the subsegmental arteries remained inadequately visualised (Table 7).

In the 2 mm collimation group the following subsegmental vessels remained very difficult to analyse. This was especially true in the upper lobes, anterior and posterior subsegmental arteries (rA2a+b, rA3a+b). The authors think this reflects the numerous anatomic variants in the origin and calibre of these vessels. All subsegmental vessels of the right middle lobe and lingula remained poorly visible, despite improved image acquisition: on average, these vessels were judged to be analysable in less than 50%. In the lower lobe the

Table 7. Subsegmental arteries [47].

Group A: 3 mm collimation   Group B: 2 mm collimation

Right upper lobe

Group	rA1a	rA1b	rA2a	rA2b	rA3a	rA3b
A	11 (50)	11 (55)	3 (15)	6 (30)	3 (15)	3 (15)
B	16 (80)	16 (80)	5 (25)	13 (65)	8 (40)	12 (60)

Upper division left upper lobe

Group	lA1a	lA1b	lA2a	lA2b	A3a	lA3b
A	10 (50)	6 (30)	5 (25)	9 (45)	7 (35)	17 (85)
B	10 (50)	15 (75)	9 (45)	12 (60)	7 (35)	14 (70)

Right middle lobe

Group	rA4a	rA4b	rA5a	rA5b
A	2 (10)	3 (15)	4 (20)	3 (15)
B	4 (20)	6 (30)	8 (40)	10 (50)

Lingula

Group	lA4a	lA4b	lA5a	lA5b
A	4 (20)	7 (35)	7 (35)	5 (25)
B	9 (45)	9 (45)	11 (55)	7 (35)

Right lower lobe

Group	rA6a+b	rA6c	rA7a	rA7b	rA8a	rA8b	rA9a	rA9b
A	9 (45)	4 (20)	9 (45)	12 (60)	8 (40)	11 (55)	3 (15)	7 (35)
B	019 (95)	15 (75)	13 (65)	14 (70)	11 (55)	16 (80)	10 (50)	13 (65)

Left lower lobe

Group	lA6a+b	lA6c	lA7a	lA7b	lA8a	lA8b	lA9a	lA9b
A	9 (45)	4 (20)	1 (5)	2 (10)	5 (25)	13 (65)	7 (35)	8 (40)
B	18 (90)	18 (90)	5 (30)	7 (35)	12 (60)	18 (90)	12 (60)	17 (85)

Group	lA10a	lA10b
A	14 (70)	17 (80)
B	17 (85)	19 (95)

paracardial subsegmental vessels, i.e. medial (right lower lobe) and anteromedial subsegmental arteries (left lower lobe) were judged analysable in about 50% of the cases. This may be caused by too many motion artifacts due to the beating heart. Also, difficulties appeared in evaluating the laterobasal subsegmental arteries. The other subsegmental vessels were found with a frequency of 70% or more with vertically oriented vessels being among the most accurately depicted arterial branches, as could be expected from our previous considerations. Borderline cases included the posterior ramus of the left upper lobe (70%) [47].

In this study segmental arteries were also studied systematically. Difficulties were reported in adequate depiction especially of the posterior segmental artery of the right upper lobe, the apicoposterior segmental artery of the left upper lobe, and the (antero)medial segmental arteries of the lower lobes. The mean number of segmental pulmonary arteries coded as not analysable per patient in the 3mm collimation group was 3/20 (15%) and was significantly less (i.e. 1.4/20, or 7%) in the 2 mm collimation group.

Ferretti also reported on image quality limited to the segmental level in 164 patients [42]. They also used the Boyden anatomical classification of the segmental arteries. Again, the segmental arteries of the middle lobe (104 of 164, or 63%) and lingula (84 of 164, or 51%) appeared to be nonanalysable in many cases. Also the segmental artery to the apex of the left upper lobe was reported non-analysable in 73 (45%) of cases. Considerable difficulties were reported in analysing the posterior segmental artery of the right upper lobe (30% non-analysable). All other segmental arteries were analysable in over 90% of the cases. Overall, 23 % of the segmental arteries were reported as non-analysable. The segmental arteries which could not be analysed most often had an oblique course with respect to the axial scan plane.

The same experience was reported by Goodman et al. [30], with segmental arteries in middle lobe and lingula being the most difficult to evaluate. They report that early in the course of the study (using 5 mm collimation and pitch 1) it became clear that subsegmental vessels could not be reliably identified on CT scans, and attempts to grade these vessels on CT scans were abandoned [30]. This may have led several other researchers not to include systematic analysis of subsegmental vessels.

In conclusion, only one study implemented a 2 mm collimation in image acquisition of the pulmonary arterial tree, resulting in some improvement in the consistency of visualising adequately the subsegmental vessels, but considerable difficulties were still encountered. Most other studies, using wider collimation, reported, more subjectively, the same difficulties and some authors even were discouraged from taking these vessels into consideration. The importance of this problem will be discussed when considering the clinical value of fast CT imaging in the diagnostic algorithm of PE.

Value of hCT

Technical accuracy

Indeterminate studies

Because of the just described difficulties, a considerable number of studies are reported to be indeterminate, not allowing firm conclusions on the presence or absence of pulmonary emboli. Remy-Jardin estimates that up to 10 % – 26 % of studies remain inconclusive [47]. Kuzo appears somewhat more optimistic, estimating these percentages to be 5 – 10 % [52].

However, detailed considerations of reported series appear to indicate a lower occurrence of indeterminate studies. Mayo, using 3 mm collimation and a pitch of 1.8 to 2.0, observed only 4 indeterminate studies in a series of 139 cases (3 %) [41], reported to be due to poor enhancement, poor signal-to-noise ratio or excessive patient motion. Remy-Jardin in the study on 39 patients to study the role of MPR in improving overall analysis, found poor images in 3 (8 %) of 39 studies, and these cases were excluded from further consideration. Finally, in a recent study Van Rossum found 10 of 123 cases to be inconclusive (8 %) [82].

In a more detailed study, Ferretti reported no overall technical failure [42]. However, only 2558 (78 %) of the 3280 (i. e. 164 cases, 20 segmental arteries per case) expected segmental arteries were adequately visualised.

Observer variability for assessment of the presence/absence of pulmonary emboli

Only few studies have explicitly addressed the issue of interpretation variability of helical CT studies for PE.

Goodman [30], in a study population of 20 subjects deduced from 37 eligible patients, found a 'modest' agreement between the two CT reviewers for the presence or absence of thrombi for each specific site (main – lobar – segmental vessels). The reviewers were in accordance in 14 of 20 right-sided and 16 of 20 left-sided lung vessels, giving, according to Goodman, a 75 % overall accordance.

Chartrand addressed this issue in a recent presentation, in a retrospective analysis of 60 patients with hCT for PE; each study was analysed by three independent radiologists with assessment of the presence or absence of central (main, lobar, and segmental) PE on axial images [83]. Interobserver variation was assessed on a per-patient, lobar and segmental basis. The 3 observers considered the CT scans positive for PE in 26, 22 and 21 patients and ambiguous in 2, 1 and 4 patients. Among 360 lobar and 1140 segments analysed, 93 and 183 respectively were considered positive by at least one observer. Agreement between 3 observers was good (kappa 0.64) for the detection of PE on a per-patient basis and good (k = 0.64) for the presence of PE at the lobar level. When individual segments were analysed, agreement was fair (k = 0.37) for the detection of PE.

In a more recent study of 139 subjects, Mayo found a concordant positive reading for PE in 42 cases, and a concordant indeterminate reading in 2 cases [41]. In 85 cases, both readers interpreted the hCT studies as negative for PE, thus obtaining 129 concordant readings. In one case, one reader scored the scan as positive, whereas the other reader concluded there was no indication for pulmonary emboli. In 5 cases one reader scored the studies as indeterminate, whereas the other reader again opted for the absence of pulmonary emboli. Finally, 4 cases were scored as negative by one reader, whereas the other reader scored one of these cases as positive and 3 cases as indeterminate. Recalculating these data resulted in a kappa of 0.85. The authors did not elaborate on the cause of these differences.

Van Rossum et al. determined the interobserver variability for three different observers with different experience in assessing hCT images for the presence or absence of PE, using the gamma statistics. The most experienced observer attained a kappa of 0.90 when compared with a less experienced observer, with a kappa of 0.82 compared to the least experienced observed [84].

Observer variability for extent of pulmonary embolic disease

In their extensive study of the modified Miller and Walsh scores, Bankier et al. addressed the interobserver variability of these scoring systems [63]. The results have been discussed here before. The Walsh score appeared to show more inter-observer variability than the Miller score, which has been ascribed to the more complex structure of the Walsh score.

Discussion

Only very few studies explicitly addressed the issue of interpretation variability and we even have to conclude that there is not enough scientific information to draw firm conclusions. The impression exists that 'since a positive diagnosis relies simply on identification of an intravascular filling defect, inter-observer variation will be likely to be similar to conventional pulmonary angiography' [15]. However, as discussed before, the occurrence of indeterminate studies increases with more peripheral location of pulmonary emboli and it is to be expected, as with conventional pulmonary angiography, that the observer variability will increase with more peripheral location of the emboli.

Further studies using 2 mm collimation and optimal scanning techniques are required to assess the extent of this problem.

Diagnostic accuracy

Several studies have been performed assessing the diagnostic accuracy of helical computed tomography. They all have more or less the same study design. Patients suspected of having PE are selected, most often after having had a ventilation/perfusion scintigraphy. This is followed by an hCT. In order to obtain a two-by-two table from which

the classical test parameters (sensitivity and specificity) are to be derived, a reference test is introduced, most often invasive pulmonary arteriography, but some also use a diagnostic ventilation perfusion scan as reference test (considering a negative ventilation/perfusion scan as indicative of the absence of PE, and a high probability ventilation/perfusion scan results as sufficient evidence to classify the patient as indeed having PE.

The first diagnostic accuracy study was published by Remy-Jardin et al. in 1992 [26]. Forty-two patients were included in this study; 32 were referred with a suspicion of PE, while 10 patients had unexplained pleuroparenchymal changes on chest radiographs. Apparently, all these patients were hospitalised; for example 19 had chronic lung disease, 3 cardiac disease, 4 patients had malignant disease, 7 had right ventricular failure, but no clear statement is made about in/out patient condition at inclusion. Scanning was performed with 5mm collimation and a pitch of 1. Invasive pulmonary arteriography was used as reference test (selective right and left pulmonary angiograms). The prevalence of PE in this population was 42% (18/42). There was only 1 false positive hCT and no false negative scan results were found, resulting in a sensitivity of 100% and a specificity of 96%. No mention is made of exclusion criteria, although inability to breathhold did not appear to be a reason for exclusion. No inconclusive scan results were found. Apparently, as Hansell recently remarked, ascribing later less favourable results to the 'exclusion of technically unsatisfactory hCTs in [this] initial study' [85].

Thus, a next study published in 1996 by the same group [57] reported on extended experience. A total of 75 patients were referred for invasive pulmonary angiography to assess the presence or absence of PE. All 75 patients underwent CT. Initially a collimation of 5mm and a pitch of 1 were used, but during the study, the protocol was adapted to 3 mm collimation with a pitch of 1.7. The available invasive pulmonary arteriography was used as reference test. The prevalence of PE was high, i. e. 57% (43/75) (as could be expected in view of the method by which these patients were selected, apparently having such a high 'pre-test' probability that an invasive diagnostic test seemed warranted). This time, some inconclusive scan results were reported: 3 studies were suboptimal and 7 studies were reported to be 'inconclusive' (although 'optimal'?). Nevertheless, all patients were used in a two by two table to calculate sensitivity as 91% (39/43) and specificity as 78% (25/32); there was only 1 false negative scan result (and 3 inconclusive scans of patients having

PE) but there were no false positive scan results (but 4 inconclusive scan results and 3 suboptimal scans in patients having no PE at pulmonary angiography).

Meanwhile, Goodman published his study in 1995 on (only) 20 patients [30]. The study started with 37 patients with unresolved ventilation/perfusion scans. 17 patients were excluded; 3 patients refused co-operation, but in 10 cases, hCT related reasons for exclusion were reported (7 had medical conditions that precluded performing the additional CT scan, 3 had catheter or equipment problems before CT study was completed; and, strangely, 3 were not identified (after inclusion?) as potential candidates; another patient was excluded from further consideration because CT scan revealed a large central tumour. HCT was performed with 5mm collimation and a pitch of 1. Selective invasive pulmonary arteriography was used as reference test (13 bilateral, 7 unilateral). A high prevalence (55% i.e. 11/20) was found. Due to the study design no inconclusive study results were reported (they apparently were excluded). Only 1 false positive case was found, resulting in a specificity of 89%; and 4 false negative cases (of whom 3 had isolated subsegmental PE), resulting in a sensitivity of 63%.

Van Rossum et al. published three studies with a comparable design, but a more 'liberal' use of reference test was chosen; this group differs from the others in that it accepts a normal ventilation/perfusion scan as conclusive evidence of the absence of PE, and a high-probability ventilation/perfusion scan as enough evidence to classify patients as having PE; only in inconclusive cases (low- and intermediate probability results) an invasive pulmonary arteriography is applied for outcome final classification.

Thus, in a first study [86] between November 1992 and October 1995, 195 patients were observed who underwent both ventilation/perfusion scintigraphy and hCT because of clinically suspected acute PE. Whenever available (in 56 cases), results of pulmonary angiography served as reference test, otherwise conclusive ventilation/perfusion scan results were used to classify patients according to their 'real' condition. 36 patients were excluded from further analysis because no such definite reference data became available. The hCT scan was performed with 5 mm collimation and pitch 1. Again, a high prevalence of PE was found, 68 patients being classified as having the disease (prevalence 68/149 = 45%). Of these (only) 15 were proven with invasive pulmonary angiography. In this study, no inconclusive hCT results were found (or reported). There were 4 false negative cases (Fig. 10) resulting in a sensi-

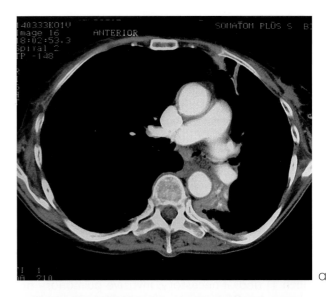

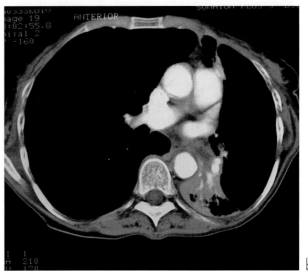

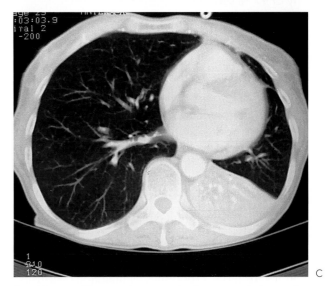

Fig. 10a–c. Patient with suspected pulmonary embolism and non-diagnostic lung scan. Normal enhancement of the pulmonary arteries, but atelectasis of the left lower lobe, which could explain the patient's complaints.

215

tivity of 94% (95% confidence interval 90.2–98%); and there were 3 false positive cases for a specificity of 96% (95% confidence interval 93–99.5%).

In the same year, the same group reported a larger study in 348 patients [87]. This study apparently was executed parallel with the previous study, since the observation period ran from August 1993 to January 1995. Patients were eligible if a clinician felt it necessary to refer a patient suspected of PE to undergo a ventilation perfusion scan. If the ventilation/perfusion scan was normal (in 172 cases) the patient was classified as having no pulmonary emboli and no further studies were performed. With all other results, patients were invited to undergo additional hCT (5 mm collimation, pitch 1) and, if necessary, invasive pulmonary angiography. 25 patients refused, 52 patients were excluded because they appeared to be anticoagulated for more than 48 hours, 20 because they had cardiac dysfunction, and 2 because of other reasons. Thus, the final (selected) study group consisted of 77 patients. If these patients had a high probability ventilation/perfusion scan and also a positive hCT scan, they were classified as having the disease and no further reference testing was felt necessary (35 cases); the remaining 42 cases underwent additional invasive pulmonary angiography. The prevalence of PE in the final study group was 52% (49/77). Finally, 1 of these 77 cases was excluded because the hCT scan was inconclusive. This complex study design resulted in 2 false negative cases and a sensitivity of 95% (37/39) and 1 false positive case with a specificity of 97% (36/37).

In a last study, the same group more systematically compared the diagnostic accuracy of a strategy which used all clinical (pre-test) information, including the chest radiography, combined with (only) ventilation perfusion scintigraphy, with a strategy which used the same pre-test information, but now combined with hCT findings (but without ventilation/perfusion findings) [82]; in 123 patients a prevalence of 43%, a sensitivity for the hCT strategy of 75% and a specificity of the same strategy of 90% was reported.

More recently, Mayo published a series of 139 patients with suspected PE who were referred to the imaging department [41]. HCT was used with 3mm collimation and a pitch of 1.8 or 2.0. Like the previous studies of Van Rossum the combination of a high probability ventilation/perfusion scan and hCT findings of PE was considered diagnostic of PE and no further imaging was performed (thus introducing the diagnostic test under investigation into the reference test). Again, the

combination of a very low probability or normal ventilation/perfusion scan and a hCT without findings of PE with a low clinical suspicion with concordant follow-up was considered sufficient to exclude PE. The decision to perform invasive pulmonary angiography was based upon the above considerations; all patients not having those combined hCT/ventilation/perfusion results were candidates for this more invasive investigation (thus introducing risk verification bias). Three patients were lost to follow-up. The prevalence of PE in this study group was 33% (46/139). Four hCT results were considered indeterminate but were included in the two by two table (1 as false negative, 3 as false positive). Thus, 6 cases were considered false negative with a sensitivity of 87% (40/46) and 5 cases were considered false positive with a specificity of 95% (88/93).

Finally, Ferretti studied a group of 502 eligible patients [42]. All these patients had clinical evidence of acute PE, and showed indeterminate ventilation/perfusion scintigraphy results and negative findings at ultrasonography for DVT. However 338 patients were not elected: 32 of these 338 patients had severe PE; the interval between clinical suspicion and hCT was considered too long (more than 72 hours) in 31 patients, 35 patients had contraindications for contrast medium, images obtained at ventilation/perfusion scintigraphy were considered insufficient in 19 patients, and for 10 patients no follow-up was possible. The remaining 164 patients thus both had (intermediate) ventilation/perfusion scintigraphy and hCT (5 mm collimation, pitch 1). Again, the hCT scan was included in the reference test, since 'invasive pulmonary angiography was indicated for patients whose clinicians did not consider the normal results of hCT to be accurate and therefore refused to withdraw anticoagulants'. Thus, invasive pulmonary angiography was performed in 15 of 123 patients with high clinical suspicion but normal hCT results. If hCT was positive, anticoagulant therapy was started (or continued) without further diagnostic testing. All patients who were considered as not having PE remained untreated and were followed for 3 months. One patient was lost to follow-up, 98 patients were re-examined by the investigators and 65 patients were assessed by a telephone call after 3 months. The prevalence of PE was 25% (40/164). The authors reported no indeterminate hCT results. Six studies were considered false negative, with a sensitivity of 85%; and 5 cases were considered false positive with a specificity of 96% (5/124).

During follow-up 6 thromboembolic events occurred (5.4%; 95% confidence interval: 1.9–

11%) and one of these was fatal (0.9%; 95% confidence interval: 0.02–5%).

It is clear from this description that it is hardly possible to compare, or even to pool, these studies in order to get an overall measure for the traditional test parameters. Patient selection varies between the studies, resulting in a wide range of prevalences, varying from 25% up to 57%. As has been discussed, collimation may have an important impact on the accuracy of hCT in the detection of PE; some studies used 5 mm collimation, others 3 mm, and one of these studies changed during the acquisition from 5 to 3 mm collimation. Finally, the reference test differs in a fundamental way between the studies; some studies use only invasive pulmonary angiography (with a resulting impact on patient selection); others combine ventilation/perfusion scintigraphy with pulmonary angiography and follow-up introducing the risk of verification bias. Finally, some studies have incorporated the test under investigation (i.e. hCT) into the reference test.

Due to these considerations we will not attempt to propose an overall estimate of sensitivity and specificity for hCT and we even conclude that this is not as yet possible. We even doubt that this will ever be possible, due to the inherent instability of these traditional parameters, since they are dependent on disease spectrum, and, by this mechanism, on prevalence (although this phenomenon is incidentally mentioned in textbooks on diagnostic epidemiology, these parameters remain widely accepted as the sole important test descriptors). This phenomenon may – partially – explain the differences in sensitivity and specificity between the available studies on the diagnostic accuracy of hCT in the diagnosis of PE.

	n	Prevalence	sensitivity	specificity
1/Ferretti	164	25%	85%	96%
2/Mayo	130	33%	87%	95%
3/Remy-Jardin 1992	42	42%	100%	96%
4/Van Rossum 1997	149	45%	94%	96%
5/Van Rossum 1998	123	45%	75%	90%
6/Van Rossum 1997	77	52%	95%	97%
7/Goodman	20	55%	63%	89%
8/Remy-Jardin 1996	75	57%	91%	78%

Thus, there is a tendency of the sensitivity and specificity to decrease with increasing prevalence. This may be due to the study design or to an inherent dependency of these classical parameters to depend (despite the common opinion of the contrary) on prevalence (since an increase in prevalence will – in most cases – be accompanied with a more 'full blown' disease spectrum).

Again, such a comparison should be considered as highly preliminary; no firm overall conclusions can be drawn from the available literature up to this date.

Alternative diagnoses

As will be apparent from the above presented data, the prevalence of PE in patients with discomfort suggesting this disease varies between 25 and 57% in the hCT/PE studies. In general, it is estimated that in clinical practice PE will be considered as an explanation in only one third of similar patients [89]. Thus it is very important to have a diagnostic modality which not only detects the presence of pulmonary emboli, but – in the absence of PE – will provide clues to other diseases which may cause the same clinical presentation. CT may provide alternative diagnoses in patients who do not prove to have PE, since it allows one – without additional data acquisition – to study the hilar and mediastinal structures and also, by simply changing window width and level settings, to visualise the pulmonary parenchyma.

Thus, in the study population of Ferretti [42] 124 suspected patients proved not to have PE. They reported an alternative diagnosis that could explain the clinical presentation in 18 of these 124 patients (14%); 10 patients were diagnosed as having infectious pneumonia; in 2 patients the complaints were ascribed to 'bronchial dilatation'; in 2 patients lung carcinoma was found; 2 patients had a pneumothorax and another 2 patients showed atelectasis, which was considered to be sufficient explanation for the complaints (Fig. 10). Of these 18 patients none had PE at 3-month follow-up.

In one of the studies reported by van Rossum [82] PE was considered not to be the cause of the signs and symptoms in 70 of 123 suspected patients. Alternative diagnoses were made in 41 of these 70 patients by other means than hCT. The largest group (17 cases) was considered to have pneumonia (Fig. 11) and in 13 cases the complaints were ascribed to an exacerbation of chronic obstructive lung disease; in 4 patients a malignancy was discovered and in another 4 patients ischemic heart disease was considered to cause the patient's discomfort; in 1 patient an aortic dissection was discovered (Fig. 12), and one patient had a rupture of the oesophagus; finally, in 1 patient, vertebral collapse was considered to explain the clinical picture. HCT detected 38 of these 41 alternative diagnoses, i.e. in 38 of 70 (54%) of 'unexplained' cases.

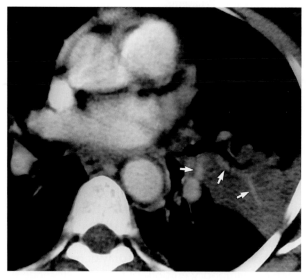

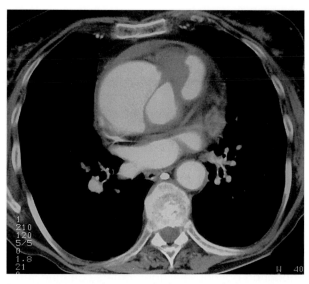

Fig. 11. Patient with suspected pulmonary embolism and non-diagnostic lung scan. Normal enhancement of the vessels. An alternative diagnosis of the left infiltrate with normal enhancing pulmonary artery along the bronchus (arrows).

Fig. 12. Patient with suspected pulmonary embolism and normal enhancing pulmonary arteries. A coincidental finding of aortic dissection in the aorta descendens was discovered. Patient was acutely operated but died shortly afterwards.

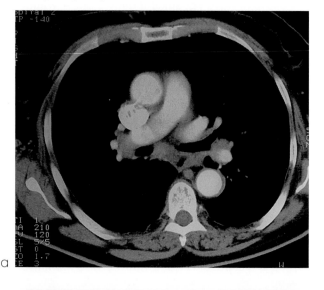

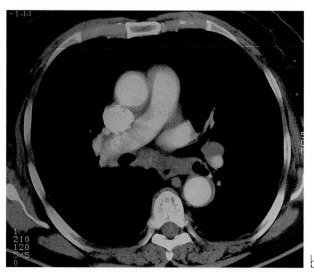

a

b

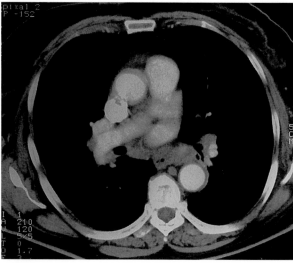

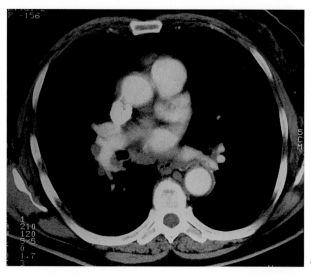

c

d

Fig. 13a-d. Four slices from cranial to caudal showing normal enhancement of the vessels with several hilar lymph nodes, which should not be confused with pulmonary embolism.

In another study by the same group, the (final) study group consisted of 77 cases, of whom 35 had a high probability scan and were considered to have PE [87]. hCT detected an alternative diagnosis in 24 of the 42 (57%) patients with a non-diagnostic ventilation/perfusion scintigram, which could explain the ventilation/perfusion scan defects. Again, the largest group was considered to have pneumonia (9 cases), while emphysema and pleural effusion were detected in 6 and 5 patients respectively. Other findings included empyema (1 case), lung fibrosis (1 case), lymphadenopathy (1 case, Fig. 13a–d) and diaphragmatic hernia (1 case).

Senac reported 10 alternative diagnoses in a group of 34 patients suspected of PE: pulmonary edema (3) causing their complaints, 4 lymphangitic carcinoma, and 3 pleural effusions; absence of PE was proven in these cases by pulmonary angiography [88].

Thus, in large studies, hCT seems to be able to offer an alternative diagnosis in up to 50% of patients with suspected PE, in whom this disease is subsequently excluded. Furthermore, contra-indications for treatment of PE may be detected, such as pathologic conditions with a high risk of hemorrhage or such as certain malignancies or vascular disorders.

Comparative value

cCT vs ventilation/perfusion scan

In 1998, van Rossum et al. published a retrospective study in order to compare the usefulness of ventilation perfusion scintigraphy with helical computed tomography [82]. From a database used in their first study [87] 123 cases were selected. All patients had undergone ventilation/perfusion scanning and hCT (5 mm collimation and pitch 1) but it is not made clear in their article what other selection criteria were used to choose these cases from the apparently larger study base. The final diagnosis in each patient was made by using the opinion of multiple expert readers; pulmonary angiography was the definite gold standard in 49 patients. In the remaining cases the ventilation perfusion scan was used as reference test; they hoped to avoid verification bias by having the ventilation/perfusion scan interpreted independently by different observers as challenged test and as reference test. In patients thus considered not to have PE, clinical follow-up was applied for final diagnosis. The prevalence of PE in this study was 43% (53/123).

The cases were presented to the observers twice; each time all clinical (pre-test) data were made available; but, randomly, each case was presented with the ventilation/perfusion images (but not with the hCT images), and, at an other time, with the hCT images (but not with the ventilation/perfusion images). With the hCT strategy, there were 10 inconclusive cases; sensitivity of the strategy, now including all pre-test diagnostic information, was 75% and specificity was reported as 90%. With the ventilation/perfusion strategy, there were 35 inconclusive cases; sensitivity of the strategy was 49% and specificity was reported as 75%. This difference was statistically significant (p value reported 0.007). The ventilation/perfusion strategy detected 21 of 41 (51%) alternative diagnoses, whereas the hCT strategy detected 38 of 41 (93%) alternative diagnoses, and this difference also was statistically significant (p < 0.001). Theoretically, ventilation/perfusion scintigraphy and hCT should be able to function equally well; although they are based on different manifestations of PE, with ventilation/perfusion scanning aimed at detecting perfusion defects (not matched by ventilation defects), while hCT primarily evaluates vascular filling defects, they – theoretically – appear to be sensitive to the same level of location of the emboli, i.e. at the lobar and segmental levels; since subsegmental perfusion defects are detectable with ventilation/perfusion scanning, it may even be expected that this test should be more accurate than hCT.

However, the main problem with ventilation/perfusion scanning is the large proportion of indeterminate test results. In the PIOPED study, 676 of 931 patients had intermediate (39%) or low probability (34%) ventilation/perfusion scan readings and only 41% with PE had a high probability scan result [89]. Although it is possible that the low incidence of inconclusive hCT scan results in the reported studies (see paragraph on technical accuracy of hCT) could be caused by a priori exclusion of these cases from reporting, it seems that the proportion of inconclusive results is substantially less, as suggested by the more elaborate comparison of hCT and ventilation/perfusion scintigraphy.

Interobserver agreement seems to be better with hCT than with ventilation/perfusion scintigraphy. Thus, Mayo reported a significantly higher agreement among CT readers compared to ventilation/perfusion scan readers (k statistic 0.85 vs 0.61) [41]. No other studies are available making this direct comparison.

Finally, there is a tendency in the literature showing that hCT will show an alternative diagnosis to explain the patient's discomfort more often than ventilation/perfusion scintigraphy. This is based on theoretical grounds and on the direct comparison by Van Rossum et al., who found that the ventilation/perfusion strategy detected 21 of 41 (51%) alternative diagnoses, whereas the hCT strategy detected 38 of 41 (93%) alternative diagnoses [82].

hCT vs EBT

No studies are available comparing hCT and EBT; considerations on this topic will be given in Chapter IV.7.

hCT vs MRI

Woodard et al. compared the accuracy of hCT and MRI for detecting PE in a canine model [90]. With knowledge of the pathologic findings an unblinded observer was able to identify 90% of the emboli imaged with CT and 68% to 91% of the emboli imaged by various MR techniques [91].

In 1996, Sostman et al. published the first article in which hCT and MRI were compared in the detection of PE in 53 patients [91]. They intended to perform a randomised study in which patients who were suspected clinically to have acute PE were eligible for enrolment into the study; unstable patients were excluded as were patients with contraindications for both MRI and hCT and if a confident diagnosis could not be established. It was defined that if pulmonary angiography was performed (available in 21 patients), its results would have priority over the ventilation/perfusion scan; but if only the ventilation/perfusion scan was available high probability and normal scan results were considered as conclusive for the presence or absence of PE respectively. HCT was performed with 5mm collimation, pitch 1; MRI was performed using a GRASS pulse sequence in a 1.5T MRI scanner.

A total of 310 patients were eligible during the study period of whom 257 were not included, most of them (116) due to the inability to schedule both examinations within the required period. Another large group of patients (64) were considered unstable, and in 54 other patients, no informed consent could be obtained. Thus, in the end, only 53 patients were included. No comparison was made between the eligible patients and the study group, so it is not clear if the finally selected group is representative for the total group of patients, but this seems very unlikely.

By study design, it was accepted that if a patient was not considered suited for one modality, he or she was selected for the other modality. Initial allocation showed that 31 patients were randomised to CT, and 22 to MRI. Because of contraindications, 9 were crossed over from CT to MRI, and 6 from MRI to CT. Twelve of these 53 patients were

recruited, but did not complete the study or 'for other reasons deemed ineligible'. Seven of these patients were randomised for MRI, 5 for CT. So in the end, apparently, the study base consisted of 41 subjects, of whom 23 had CT and 18 had MRI. Due to these complex events, the randomisation did not succeed. The authors report an overall prevalence of PE in the 53 subjects of 38% (20/53). From their report, it can be reconstructed (they do not mention this by themselves), that the prevalences in the subgroups were quite different. They reported that 'a total of 13 CT patients and 7 MRI patients had PE, whereas 15 CT patients and 18 MRI patients did not have pulmonary embolism'. Thus, the prevalence in the CT group was 13/28 or 46%, nearly twice as much as in the MRI group, in which the prevalence can be calculated as 7/25 or 28%. Thus, the groups are not comparable.

They used more or less experienced readers for both studies; they calculated sensitivity and specificity for each reader, and then calculated the average for these parameters. For example, the sensitivity for CT for the 5 readers varied from 62 to 92% with an average of 75%; a much larger range was observed for the sensitivity of MRI, from 14% to 86% with an average of 46%. Despite this large interobserver variability they propose an average sensitivity and specificity for hCT of 75% and 89% and for MRI of 46% and 90%, respectively.

Well-designed studies are needed before any conclusion is possible. Comparative studies should focus on the proportion of indeterminate studies with both techniques, the accuracy, and the proportion of alternative diagnoses made with hCT and MRI in order to assess their comparative value and their value in respect to ventilation/perfusion scintigraphy.

Theoretically, MRI may perform better, since, with the use of venous saturation, (reconstructed) MR images will more easily differentiate arteries from veins than CT. Furthermore, MRI will allow assessment of DVT in the lower extremities [92, 93], although some studies have been directed in the application of hCT in the diagnostic work-up of DVT [94, 95]. No comparative studies are available to assess directly which technique will be most valuable in this respect.

hCT vs Pulmonary Angiography

Axial tomographic imaging has an advantage over angiography. It may explain pulmonary arterial occlusion by extrinsic causes, as well as intravascular thrombus. Such a differentiation has been reported in the EBT PE literature, as will be dis-

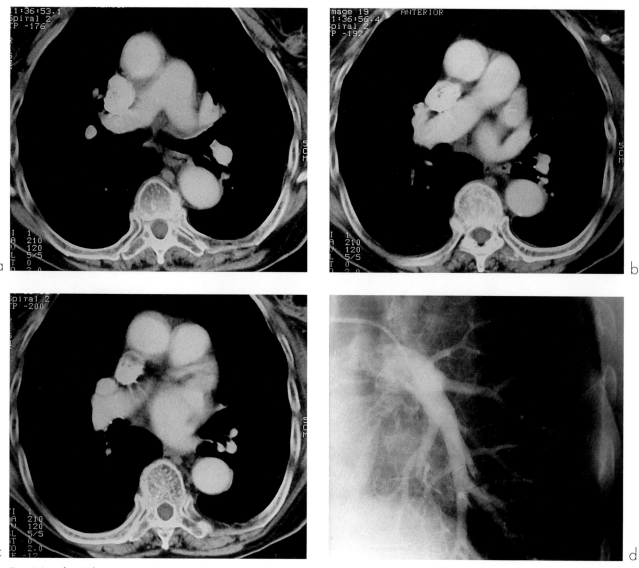

Fig. 14a–d. False negative CT scan at three levels without evidence of pulmonary embolism. The angiogram reveals filling defect in the lingular branch and left lower lobe.

cussed in the chapter on Electron Beam Tomography and Pulmonary Embolism. Other than this data, no observations have been found in the literature on helical CT and PE. However, hCT will perform in the same way as EBT in this respect. Thus, fast computed tomography may demonstrate false positive pulmonary angiography findings. However, as long as pulmonary angiography is considered the standard of reference, fast CT will never perform better.

The main issue in this respect is the accuracy of pulmonary angiography to detect subsegmental PE (see Chapter IV.3 and Fig. 14a–d). It is doubtful if even pulmonary angiography can be used as a 'gold' standard at this level, since the interobserver variability for subsegmental pulmonary emboli on pulmonary angiograms is reported to be considerable. In the PIOPED study the interreader agreement for subsegmental PE was reported to be only 66 % [96]. Quinn reported that 3 angiographers agreed on all main, lobar and segmental pulmonary emboli, but only on 13 % of subsegmental pulmonary emboli (2 of 15) [97]. More up-to-date hardware and software may improve visualisation of subsegmental PE by pulmonary angiography. Whether or not this technique is the most suitable reference test remains a subject of discussion. To date, however, no other reference test is available.

HCT may offer the chance to non-invasive follow-up in the assessment of thrombus resolution (Fig. 15). This could reduce the number of patients

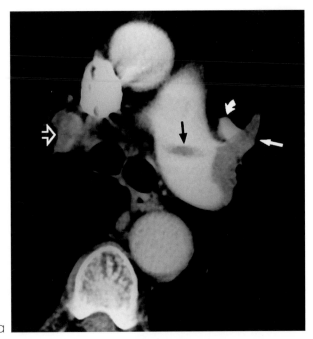
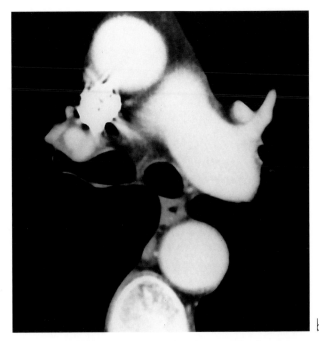

a   b

Fig. 15a, b. Use of CT in follow-up. **(a)** Multiple central filling defects, suggesting pulmonary embolism. **(b)** After 6 weeks of anticoagulation the thrombi have resolved.

who develop pulmonary hypertension or show these at risk at an earlier stage (see Chapter VI.3). Cost-effectiveness studies will be presented and considerations will be presented concerning the possible position of hCT in the diagnostic algorithm of patients suspected of PE (see Chapter VII.1).

References

1. Gould RG. Principles of Electron Beam Tomography. In: Stanford W, Rumberger J (eds). Ultrafast Computed Tomography in cardiac imaging: principles and practice. Futura Publishing 1992

2. Cormack AM. Respresentation of a function by its line integrals, with some radiological applications. J Appl Phys 1963; 34: 2722

3. Hounsfield GN. Computerized transverse axial scanning. Br J Radiol 1973; 46 (552); 1016–1022

4. Curry TS, Dowdey JE, Murry RC Jr (eds). Christensen's introduction to the physics of diagnostic radiology. Lea & Febiger, Philadelphia, 1984

5. Husband JES. Whole body computed tomography: general principles. In: Grainger RG, Allison DJ (eds). Diagnostic Radiology. Churchill Livingstone, London, 1992: 23–42

6. Crawford CR, King KF. Computed tomography with simultaneous patient translation. Med Phys 1990; 17: 967–982

7. Rigauts H, Marchal G, Baert AL, Hupke R. Initial experience with volume CT scanning. J Comp Assist Tomogr 1990; 14: 675–682

8. Herts BR, Einstein DM, Paushter DM. Spiral CT of the abdomen: artifacts and potential pitfalls. Am J Roentgenol 1993; 161: 1185–1190

9. Kalender WA, Seissler W, Klotz E, Vock P. Single breathhold spiral volumetric CT by continuous patient translation and scanner rotation. Radiology 1989; 137 (P): 414

10. Kalender WA, Seissler W, Klotz E, Vock P. Spiral volumetric CT with single breathhold technique, continuous transport, and continuous scanning rotation. Radiology 1990; 176: 181–183

11. Oudkerk M. CT of hilar adenopathy with 1 second and subsecond scan time. Radiology 1989; 173 (P): 452

12. Brink JA. Technical aspects of helical spiral CT. Radiol Clin N Am 1995; 33: 825–841

13. McCollough CH, Morin RL. The technical design and performation of ultrafast computed tomography. Radiol Clin N Am 1994; 32: 521–536

14. Kalender WA. Spiral or helical CT: right or wrong. Radiology 1994; 193: 583

15. Hansell DM, Padley SP. Continuous volume CT in pulmonary embolism; the answer or just another test. Thorax 1996; 51: 1–12

16. Sinner WN. Computed tomography patterns of pulmonary thromboembolism and infarction. J Comp Assist Tomogr 1978; 2: 395–399

17. Verschakelen JA, Vanwijck E, Bogaert J, Baert AL. Detection of unsuspected central pulmonary embolism with conventional contrast enhanced CT. Radiology 1993; 188: 847–850

18. Winston CB, Wechsler RJ, Salazar AM, Kurtz AB, Spirn PW. Incidental pulmonary emboli detected at helical CT: effect on patient care. Radiology 1996; 201: 23–27

19. Ovenfors CO. Diagnosis of peripheral pulmonary emboli by computed tomography in the living dog. Radiology 1981; 141: 519–523

20. Lourie GL. Experimental pulmonary infarction in dogs: a comparison of chest radiography and computed tomography. Invest Radiol 1982; 17: 224–232

21. Grossman ZD. Successful identification of oligaemic lung by transmission CT after experimentally produced acute pulmonary occlusion in the dog. Invest Radiol 1981; 16: 275–280

22. Godwin JD, Webb WR, Gamsu G. CT of pulmonary embolism. Am J Roentgenol 1980; 135: 691–695

23. Sinner WN. Computed tomography of pulmonary thromboembolism. Eur J Radiol 1982; 2: 8–13

24. Breatnach E, Stanley RJ. CT diagnosis of segmental artery pulmonary embolism; a case report. J Comp Assist Tomogr 1984; 8: 762–764

25. Chintapalli K, Thorsen MK, Olson DL, Goodman LR, Gurney J. CT of pulmonary thromboembolism and infarction. J Comp Assist Tomogr 1988; 12: 533–539

26. Remy-Jardin M, Remy J, Wattine L, Giraud F. Central pulmonary thromboembolism: diagnosis with spiral volumetric CT with single breathhold technique – comparison with pulmonary angiography. Radiology 1992; 185: 381–387

27. Rubin GD. Helical CT for the detection of acute pulmonary embolism: experts debate. J Thorac Imaging 1997; 12: 81–82

28. Teigen CL, Maus TP, Sheedy PF II, Johnson CM, Stanson AW. Pulmonary embolism: diagnosis with electron beam tomography. Radiology 1991; 181 (P): 338

29. Rossum AB van. Spiral volumetric CT in patients with clinical suspicion of pulmonary embolism. Radiology 1994; 193 (P): 262

30. Goodman LR, Curtin JL, Mewissen MW, et al. Detection of pulmonary embolism in patients with unresolved clinical and scintigraphic diagnosis: helical CT vs angiography. Am J Roentgenol 1995; 164: 1369–1384

31. Sheedy PF, Johnson CM, Welch TJ, Stanson AW, Breen JF, Mays TP. Fast CT of pulmonary embolism. Semin Radiol 1996; 17: 324–338

32. Tardivon AA, Musset D, Maitre S, et al. Role of CT in chronic pulmonary embolism; comparison with pulmonary angiography. J Comp Assist Tomogr 1993; 17: 345–351

33. Gefter WB, Hatabu H, Hollland GA, Gupta KB, Henschke CI, Palevsky HI. Pulmonary thromboembolism: recent developments in diagnosis with CT and MRI. Radiology 1995; 197: 561–574

34. Goodman LR, Lipchik RJ. Diagnosis of acute pulmonary embolism; time for a new approach. Radiology 1996; 199: 25–27

35. Goodman LR, RJ Lipchik, Kuzo RS. Acute pulmonary embolism: the role of CT imaging. J Thorac Imag 1997; 12: 83–86

36. Stein PD. Opinion response to acute pulmonary embolism, the role of CT. J Thorac Imag 1997; 12: 86–89

37. Sostman HD. Opinion response to acute pulmonary embolism, the role of CT. J Thorac Imag 1997; 12: 89–92

38. Remy-Jardin M, Artaud D, Deschildre F, Beregei JB. Opinion response to acute pulmonary embolism, the role of CT. J Thorac Imag 1997; 12: 92–95

39. Mayo JR. Opinion response to acute pulmonary embolism, the role of CT. J Thorac Imag 1997; 12: 95–97

40. Gefter WB, Palevsky HI. Opinion response to acute pulmonary embolism, the role of CT. J Thorac Imag 1997; 12: 100–102

41. Mayo JR, Remy-Jardin M, Muller NL, et al. Pulmonary embolism: prospective comparison of spiral CT with ventilation-perfusion scintigraphy. Radiology 1997; 205: 447–452

42. Ferretti, GR, Bosson JL, Buffaz PD, et al. Acute pulmonary embolism: role of helical CT in 164 patients with intermediate probability at ventilation-perfusion scintigraphy and normal results at Duplex US of the legs. Radiology 1997; 205: 453–458

43. Bankier AA, Janata K, Fleischmann D, et al. Severity assessment of acute pulmonary embolism with spiral CT: evaluation of two modified angiographic scores and comparison with clinical data. J Thorac Imag 1997; 12: 150–158

44. Lesnik A, Vernhet H, Bousquet C, Giron HM, Godard P, Senac J. The clinical suspicion of pulmonary embolism: a one year experience with spiral CT. Radiology 1997; 205 (P): 412

45. Remy-Jardin M, Remy J, Artaud D, Deschildre F, Fribourg M, Beregi M. Spiral CT of pulmonary embolism: technical considerations and pitfalls. J Thorac Imag 1997; 12: 103–117

46. Costello Ph. Optimal hCT pitch in detecting pulmonary embolism. Questions and Answers. Am J Roentgenol 1995; 165: 732–733

47. Remy-Jardin M, Remy J, Artaud D, Deschildre F, Duhamel A. Peripheral pulmonary arteries: optimization of the spiral CT acquisition protocol. Radiology 1996; 207: 157–163

48. Napel SA. Principles and techniques of three dimensional computed tomography angiography. In: Fishman EK. (ed). CT: principles, techniques and clinical applications. Raven Press 1995; 167–182

49. Teigen CI, Maus TP, Sheedy PF, et al. Pulmonary embolism; diagnosis with Electron Beam CT and comparison with pulmonary angiography. Radiology 1995; 194: 313–319

50. Rubin GD. Optimization of thoracic spiral CT: effects of iodinated contrast medium concentrations. Radiology 1996; 201: 785–791

51. Vogel N, Kauczor HU, Ries BG, Heussel C, Thelen M. Optimizing bolus enhanced spiral CT of the pulmonary arteries using a saline push. Radiology 1997; 205 (P): 412

52. Kuzo RS, Goodman LR. CT evaluation of pulmonary embolism: technique and interpretation. Am J Roentgenol 1997; 169: 959–965

53. Polacin A, Kalender WA, Marchal G. Evaluation of section sensitivity profiles and image noise in spiral CT. Radiology 1992; 185: 29–35

54. Kalender WA, Polacin A, Suss C. A comparison of conventional and spiral CT: an experimental study on the detection of spherical lesions. J Comp Assist Tomogr 1994; 18: 167–176

55. Brink JA, Horesh L, Heiken JP, Glazer HS, Wang G. Depiction of pulmonary emboli with hCT: optimatization of window width and level in a porcine model. Radiology 1995; 197 (P): 304

56. Remy-Jardin M, Remy J, Cauain O, Petyt L, Wannebroucq J, Beregi JP. Diagnosis of central pulmonary embolism with helical CT: role of 2D multiplanar reformation. Am J Roentgenol 1995; 165: 1131–1138

57. Remy-Jardin M, Remy J, Deschildre F, et al. Diagnosis of pulmonary embolism with spiral CT: comparison with pulmonary angiography and scintigraphy. Radiology 1996; 200: 699–706

58. Jackson CL ea. Correlated applied anatomy of the bronchial tree and lungs with a system of nomenclature. Dis Chest 1943; 9: 319–326

59. Boyden EA. Segmental anatomy of the lungs. McGraw-Hill 1955

60. Teigen CL, Maus Tp, Sheedy PF, Johnson CM, Stanson AW, Welch TJ. Pulmonary embolism diagnosis with Eletron Beam Computed Tomography. Radiology 1993; 188: 839–845

61. Remy-Jardin M, Louvegny S, Remy J, et al. Acute central thromboembolic disease; posttherapeutic follow-up with spiral CT. Radiology 1997; 203: 173–180

62. Auger WR, Fedullo PF, Moser KM, Buchbinder M, Peterson KL. Chronic major-vessel thromboembolic pulmonary artery obstruction: appearance at angiography. Radiology 1992; 182: 393–398

63. Bankier AA, Janata K, Fleischman D, et al. Severity assessment of acute pulmonary embolism with spiral CTt: evaluation of two modified angiographic scores and comparison with clinical data. J Thorac Imag 1997; 12: 150–158

64. Walsh PN. An angiographic severity index for pulmonary embolism. Circulation 1973; 47/48S: 101–107

65. Miller GA, Sutton GC, Kerr IH, Gibson RV, Honey M. Comparison of streptokinase and heparin in the treatment of isolated acute massive pulmonary embolism. Br Med J 1971; 2: 681–684

66. Schwarz F. Sustained improvement of pulmonary hemodynamics in patients at rest and during exercise after thrombolytic treatment of massive pulmonary embolism. Circulation 1985; 71: 117–123

67. Diehl, Meyer G, Igual J, et al. Effectiveness and safety of bolus administration of Alteplase in massive pulmonary embolism. Am J Cardiol 1992; 70: 1477–1480

68. Meneveau N, Bassand JP, Schiele F, et al. Safety of thrombolytic therapy in elderly patients with massive pulmonary embolism; a comparison with nonelderly patients. J Am Coll Cardiol 1993; 22: 1075–1079

69. Greaves SM. Pictorial essay: pulmonary thromboembolism: spectrum of findings in CT. Am J Roentgenol 1995; 165: 1359–1363

70. Bergin C, Rios C, King MA, Belezzuoli E, Luna J, Auger WG. Accuracy of high-resolution CT in identifying chronic pulmonary thromboembolic disease. Am J Roentgenol 1996; 166: 1371–1377

71. Remy-Jardin M, Remy J, Giraud F, Wattinne L, Gosselin B. CT assessment of ground glass opacity; semiology and significance. J Thorac Imag 1993; 8: 249–264

72. Im JG, Choi YW, Kim HD, Jeong YK, Han MC. Thin-section CT findings of the lungs: experimentally induced bronchial and pulmonary artery obstructions in pigs. Am J Roentgenol 1996; 167: 631–635

73. Austin J, Sagel SS. Alterations of airway caliber after pulmonary embolization in the dog. Invest Radiol 1972; 3: 135–139

74. Worthy SA, Muller NL, Hartman ThE, Swensen SJ, Padley SPG, Hansell DM. Mosaic attenuation pattern on thin section CT scans of the lung: differentiation among infiltrative lung, airway, and vascular disease as a cause. Radiology 1997; 205: 465–470

75. Remy-Jardin M, Remy J, Louveguy S, Artaud D, Deschildre F, Duhamel A. Airway changes in chronic pulmonary embolism: CT findings in 33 patients. Radiology 1997; 203: 355–360

76. Balakrishnan J, Meziane MA, Siegelman SS, Fishman EK. Pulmonary infarction: CT appearance with pathologic correlation. J Comp Assist Tomogr 1989; 13: 941–945

77. McGoldrick PJ, Rudd TG, Figley MM, Wilhelm JP. 'What becomes of pulmonary infarcts? Am J Roentgenol 1979; 133: 1039–1045

78. Remy-Jardin M. Spiral CT of pulmonary embolism. In: Remy-Jardin M et al. Spiral CT of the chest. Springer Verlag, Berlin, 1996: 202–230

79. Swensen SJ, Morin RL, Aughenbaugh GL, Leimer DW. CT reconstruction algorithm selection in the evaluation of solitary pulmonary nodules. J Comp Assist Tomogr 1995; 19: 932–935

80. Sagel SS, Greenspan RH. Nonuniform pulmonary arterial perfusion: pulmonary embolism? Radiology 1971; 111: 541–548

81. Bookstein JJ, Silver TM. The angiographic differential diagnosis of acute pulmonary embolism. Radiology 1974; 110: 25–33

82. Rossum AB van, Pattynama PMT, Mallens WMC, Hermans J, Heyerman H. Can helical CT replace scintigraphy in the diagnostic process in suspected pulmonary embolism: a retrospective-prolective cohort study, focussing on total diagnostic yield. Eur Radiol 1998; 8: 90–96

83. Chartrand-Lefebvre C, Howarth NR, Lucidarme O, Beigelman GI, Cluzel P, Grenier PA. Interobserver variation in the diagnosis of pulmonary embolism on spiral CT. Radiology 1997; 205 (P): 411

84. Rossum AB van, Erkele AR van, Persijn A van, et al. Accuracy of helical CT for acute pulmonary embolism: ROC analysis of observer performance related to clinical experience. Eur Radiol 1998; 8: 1160–1164

85. Hanssel DM. Review: helical CT and pulmonary embolism: current state. Clin Radiol 1997; 52: 575–581

86. Rossum AB van, Pattynama PMT, Tjin a Ton ER, et al. Pulmonary embolism: validation of spiral CT angiography in 149 patients. Radiology 1996; 201: 467–470

87. Rossum AB van, Treurniet FEE, Kieft GJ, Smith SJ, Schepers R. Role of hCT scanning in the assessment of patients with clinical suspicion of pulmonary embolism and an abnormal vp lung scan. Thorax 1996; 51: 23–28

88. Senac JP, Vernhet H, Bousquet C, et al. Pulmonary embolism: contribution of spiral x-ray computed tomography. J Radiol 1995; 76: 339–345

89. PIOPED investigators. Value of ventilation perfusion scan in acute pulmonary embolism. JAMA 1990; 263: 2753–2759

90. Woodard PK, Sostman HD, MacFall JR, et al. Detection of pulmonary embolism: comparison of contrast enhanced spiral CT and time of flight MR techniques. J Thorac Imag 1995; 10: 59–72

91. Sostman HD, Layish DT, Tapson VF, et al. Prospective comparison of hCT and MRI in clinically suspected acute pulmonary embolism. J Magn Reson Imag 1996; 6: 275–281

92. Bluemke DA, Wolf RL, Tani I, Tachiki S, McVeigh ER, Zerhouni EAI. Extremity veins: evaluation with fast spin-echo MR venography. Radiology 1997; 204: 562–565

93. Laissy JP, Cinqualbre A, Loshkajian A, et al. Assessment of deep venous thrombosis in the lower limbs and pelvis: MR venography vs duplex Doppler sonography. Am J Roentgenol 1996; 167: 971–975

94. Stehling MK, Rosen MP, Weintraub J, Kim D, Raptopoulos V. Technical note: spiral CT and venography of the lower extremity. Am J Roentgenol 1994; 163: 451–453

95. Baldt MM, Zontsich T, Stumpflen A, et al. Deep venous thrombosis of the lower extremity: efficacy of spiral CT venography compared with conventional venography in diagnosis. Radiology 1996; 200: 423–428

96. Stein PD, Athanasoulis C, Alavi A, et al. Complications and validity of pulmonary angiography in acute pulmonary embolism. Circulation 1992; 85; 462–468

97. Quinn MF, Lundell CJ, Klotz TA, et al. Reliability of selective pulmonary arteriography in the diagnosis of pulmonary embolism. Am J Roentgenol 1987; 149: 469–471

IV.7 Electron beam tomography and pulmonary thromboembolism

A. H. H. Bongaerts, P. F. Sheedy II

Introduction

Electron beam tomography (EBT) is a relatively new method of cross-sectional imaging which has recently been investigated for potential use in pulmonary embolism (PE). This chapter will give a historical account, detail scanning protocols and discuss diagnostic accuracy and pitfalls.

The chapter will conclude with a discussion of the relevant observations and some suggestions for future investigations.

Historical background

Development of the electron beam tomography scanner

EBT was developed in the early 1980s in an effort to produce a device capable of imaging moving cardiac structures [1] with the same spatial resolution as Computed Tomography (CT). In fact, EBT originally was termed CVCT for cardiovascular CT [2]. In 1984 an Imatron C-100 was installed at the University of Iowa to be used primarily for cardiovascular research purposes [3]. By 1993 22 of these scanners were operational in the United States of America, and there were approximately 45 scanners world-wide. In 1994, a partnership between the manufacturer of EBT technology (Imatron Inc., San Francisco) with Siemens International (Erlangen, Germany) resulted in the development and release of an upgraded EBT scanner, the C-150. Gradually, EBT began to be known as ultrafast computed tomography (UFCT). Later, with the development of the slip ring technique, image acquisition time of conventional computed tomography was reduced significantly also allowing for improved speed of scanning. Currently, a designation of 'fast CT' may refer to both ultrafast CT technology and spiral (helical) scanning.

X-rays are generated using a high voltage between a cathode and anode (tungsten); high-energy electrons collide against tungsten and due to interactions with the electrons of the tungsten atoms, X-rays emerge from the anode. In conventional computed tomography (CT), including rapid helical (spiral) CT, an X-ray tube revolves within a scanning gantry around the recumbent patient and is capable of acquiring images with scanning times of 1–2 sec or even 750 msec. It is probable that this need for motion of the X-ray tube will remain as a limiting factor in the ability to further reduce scan time.

In EBT, the electron beam generator is placed outside the CT scanning gantry; the electron beam is directed toward either one or four stationary tungsten target rings located to the side of and below the patient and it is directed radially along the target ring followed by generation of X-rays which are detected by a stationary detector ring located above the patient (Fig. 1). Therefore, there is no mechanical limitation to the scan speed and this combination of target and detector rings allows for highly efficient scanning which results in a minimal scan time of 100 msec for a single slice high resolution scan or a 50 msec multislice scan. The distinguishing feature of this design is the electron beam, which is located outside the scanning gantry itself. For this reason, the designation 'electron beam tomography' is more descriptive of this mode of computed tomography.

Until recently, the electron beam methodology allowed acquisition of a maximum of 40 scans (each of 100 msec) in one image acquisition scan

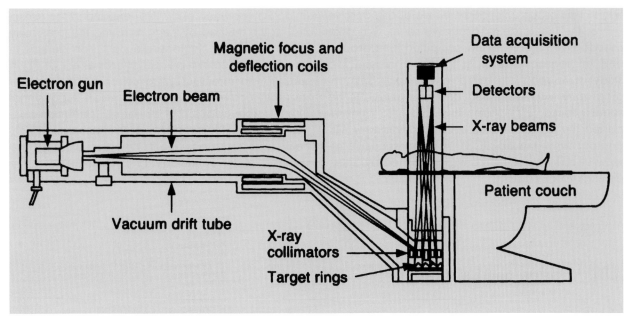

Fig. 1. Schematic representation of the electron beam tomograph.

protocol. A more recent upgrade extends the capacity to 120 consecutive contiguous scans allowing 1 scan run to cover both chest and abdomen with 6 mm thick slices or the chest alone or the abdomen alone with thinner contiguous slices (such as with PE studies often carried out with 40 to 80 contiguous 3 mm thick slices).

Electron beam technology now has been established in many clinical practices and much experience has accumulated in regard to various clinical applications. A review of the literature on EBT indicates that it can be used not only for cardiac imaging but for any application suitable for conventional computed tomography and especially for additional applications which take advantage of the uniqueness of the very short scan duration. EBT has been applied to study the airways, which can be done in a dynamic fashion [4], even in children [5, 6]. Other investigators have exploited the rapid imaging capability for study of movement in the extremities [7], enlarging the spectrum of EBT applications further. In 1989, a first publication regarding abdominal applications of EBT appeared [8] and a description of non-cardiac applications in the thorax was published.

Periodically, additional studies are conducted and described to call attention to the unique applications of EBT that might not be possible with conventional helical (spiral) CT. Among these studies are those focused on quantification of calcification in the coronary arteries [9], detection of PE [10], and dynamic airway studies [11]; also reports on oncologic applications [12], including metastatic

disease to the heart [13], and studies characterising liver lesions by their perfusion characteristics [14]. Finally, some experimental work has been done to study renal perfusion.

History of EBT and pulmonary embolism

In 1992 Geraghty et al. [15] reported on their experience with 7 mongrel dogs in which gelfoam pulmonary emboli were introduced and the pulmonary arteries subsequently studied with EBT to investigate the visibility of these emboli in the third and fourth (segmental) order pulmonary arteries. Stanford et al. [16] used artificial autologous (blood) clots to introduce PE into segmental vessels in an effort to confirm the results of Geraghty. Both studies confirmed the capability of the electron beam scanner to reveal PE down to the 3rd and 4th (segmental) pulmonary arteries.

A first study reporting a specific pathologic condition in a patient was published in 1991 by Minor et al., demonstrating biventricular thrombi and PE complicating idiopathic dilated cardiomyopathy [17]. In 1992, Rooholamin demonstrated intracardiac and proximal pulmonary artery thromboembolism in patients with cardiac tumours, using EBT [18]. Another dedicated study was published in 1995 by Jamali, using EBT in the management of pulmonary embolectomy [19].

In 1991, Teigen et al. [20] first reported results using EBT in the diagnosis of PE in clinical patients. This group extended their database and, in 1993, the first large retrospective series was published in 1993 comparing computed tomography and angiography [21]. In 1995, a prospective study comparing computed tomography and angiography was presented and published by the same groups [22]. Also, in 1993, Holland reported the first studies comparing pulmonary MR angiography and EBT [23]. A comprehensive review of EBT findings in PE was published by Sheedy et al. in 1996 [24].

In 1995, Hoffman et al. [25] expanded the potential of the method by demonstrating the possibility of using EBT to demonstrate perfusion defects in the lung indicating the peripheral effect of PE in addition to direct visualisation of an occluded or partially occluded vessel. Their results suggest that the possible addition of EBT-based perfusion studies enhances the sensitivity of this technique in detection of occlusions due to PE which were not detected directly by identifying a filling defect in the pulmonary artery.

EBT – Design and function

Design

In the electron beam scanner, as indicated in the previous section, the electron beam used to generate X-rays is located outside the gantry and external to the patient couch (Fig. 1). Instead of a movable X-ray source (rotating X-ray tube) as in conventional computed tomography, stationary tungsten target rings are located in the lower half of the gantry. Using magnetic fields, the electron beam is deflected rapidly along the tungsten target rings at 100 msec or 50 msec intervals. Between each sweep, an interscan delay of 8 msec occurs. In addition to these fixed exposure times, there is a fixed current in the electrode of 600 – 650 mAs with a fixed potential between the electron source and the tungsten target rings of 130 kVp. The distance between the electron source and the tungsten rings is approximately 7 feet. The trajectory of the electron beam is completely encased in a vacuum that must be maintained.

There are four tungsten target rings covering 210° of the gantry curvature beneath the patient. The target ring is quite a bit wider than with convention computed tomography with a target radius of 90 centimetres. Usually, (for PE studies), only one target ring is used during an imaging episode (the multislice capacity is used only for dynamic scanning such as with cardiac function, myocardial perfusion, or airway scanning). A collimator covers the target rings allowing for variable slice thicknesses of 1.5, 3.0, or 6.0 mm. In the upper half of the gantry two detector rings are located. In single slice mode the high resolution detector is used, containing 864 detector elements. For multislice mode two detector rings are available that can be configured to have the same amount of 432 detector elements each.

The rapid scan speed and short scan time requires a very fast data acquisition system. Scan data is temporarily stored before reconstruction commences. Initially the first C-100 release was only able to scan 20 levels during one acquisition. This was gradually increased to 40 scans and now it is possible to obtain 120 scans during one acquisition. Specific consoles and software allow first inspection of the images, and certain forms of data analysis, especially construction of time-density curves. The image data then can be exported to other workstations for further elaboration.

Function

EBT scanners offer several scanning modes. In single slice mode, only one target ring is activated and the high resolution detector ring is used to acquire scan data. Although each sweep for each level is performed at a 100 msec exposure, the actual exposure time can be prolonged by multiple scans of 100 msec at the same level, which results in an increase of signal to noise and a relative reduction of noise (or so-called graininess) on scan images. Scanning can also be carried out with continuous table motion allowing for continuous volume scanning (CVS mode, which is comparable to the conventional computed tomography helical or spiral scan technology).

In the multislice mode, 2, 3, or 4 target rings are activated and both detector rings are used. The signal of two adjacent elements in the high resolution detector ring are combined effectively to obtain the same number of detector rings (432) as in the adjacent ring. Thus, by using all four target rings and both detector rings, 8 scans can be obtained in 224 (50 msec + 8 msec + 50 msec +

8 msec + 50 msec + 8 msec + 50 msec) msec, as 2 slices are obtained for each target ring.

Subsequently, in multislice mode, depending on the sequence in which the target rings are activated, two submodes are available. In "movie mode", to follow the motion of a rapidly moving organ the same target ring is activated at the highest scan rate available, thus obtaining an image of the same level at the rate of 1 scan each 58 msec. Up to 15 scans can be obtained within one second at the same two levels which allows the construction of a "cine-movie" of the beating heart.

In the "flow mode", the target ring is activated but now a reasonable time level is introduced between each activation in order, for example, to follow the arrival, passage, and dilution of a contrast material bolus. In the intervening time another target ring can be imaging an adjacent level. For example, in the first second several target ring activations may be used in order to study the arterial time density curve, followed (if required) by an activation only after each second, in order to follow re-circulation and washout.

The single slice, high resolution, continuous volume mode is the optimum for evaluation of the anatomy of the pulmonary arteries.

EBT protocol and the diagnosis of pulmonary embolism

Direct visualisation of the embolus

Detection of PE depends on visualisation of the actual clot within a vessel. It is therefore necessary to opacify the flowing blood in the pulmonary arterial tree in order to see the clot as a filling defect in the vessel. The best chance to see such a clot is when the blood is densely opacified. Such opacification is achieved after determination of the circulation time from arm to the pulmonary arteries and scanning at that time.

When using the original C-100 EBT scanning software Teigen [21–23] first determined a circulation time with the use of magnesium sulfate to acquire the arm to tongue circulation time. Then, to opacify the pulmonary arteries, 80–100 ml of contrast material was used, injected at a rate of 2 ml/sec. Patients were usually asked to hold their breath as long as possible and then if necessary to slowly exhale toward the end of the 20 scan acquisition. Scanning was begun one circulation time plus 4–6 sec after the beginning of intravenous contrast material administration. Twenty contiguous 6 mm thick slices were obtained that began at the middle of the arch of the aorta. The to-

tal scanning time was 28 sec and the entire examination (including patient handling time) took 10–15 min. It should be noted that only the central 12 cm of the thorax were evaluated with this method and the lung apices and bases were excluded from the examination.

When the updated C-150 Evolution scanner became available, it was possible to obtain 40 contiguous scan levels in high resolution mode during a single acquisition with continuous table motion. A recent software upgrade of the C-150 Evolution scanner allowed for acquisition of more than 40 scan levels with continuous table motion so that most of the thorax could be included in a single examination. Alternately, it was possible to reduce the slice thickness from 6 mm to 3 mm and scan the same 12 cm volume of thorax but with better z-axis resolution. Next it was possible to obtain more than 40 levels so that a 3 mm slice thickness could be used to obtain contiguous scans over the thorax from the apices to the bases.

In this review we propose a protocol designed for the updated C-150 Evolution scanner. The aim of this protocol is to optimise data acquisition by a protocol tending to isotropic voxels [26, 27], in order to obtain 3D images comparable to MRI, since non-isotropy will provoke reconstruction artefacts.

Since the quality of the examination is largely determined by the density of the contrast material in the pulmonary arterial circulation, it is necessary to determine an accurate circulation time. The ability to do this was improved by utilising a small test dose of contrast material (15 ml) and a preview scan technique at the level of the right pulmonary artery. By this method it is possible to obtain a precise circulation time for the pulmonary artery and the aorta and to select the optimum time in which the pulmonary arteries and pulmonary veins will be maximally opacified.

At the level of the pulmonary trunk the systemic venous circulation time (SVCT) is determined in high-resolution mode (to avoid time loss due to switching between scan modes) using the single slice mode with slice thickness of 3 mm. The patient is asked to hyperventilate, and 10 sec after initiation of iv-contrast medium administration, image acquisition will be started and 20 100 ms scans will be obtained (at the same scan position) during 40 sec, at each alternate second. Twenty ml Omnipaque will be administered followed by 40 ml NaCl with a flow rate of 4 ml/sec. The circulation time is calculated by the Imatron software packet, obtaining time – density curves from the pulmonary artery and aorta. Usually, a circulation time between the pulmonary artery peak and the aorta peak is selected for commencement of scanning.

In this way, both the pulmonary arteries and pulmonary veins may be expected to be opacified for the duration of the examination.

Contrast material is injected at a rate of between 2–4 ml/sec. If 150 ml of contrast material is injected with an injection rate of, for example, 4 ml/sec a plateau phase is obtained of approximately 35 sec. Exposure time for each level is either 100 msec (one scan sweep) or 200 msec (two beam sweeps). In the continuous volume scan mode, an exposure time of 200 msec is used at a slice thickness of 3 mm and a table translation velocity of 13 mm/sec. A total scan time of 17 sec can cover a volume of almost 23 cm. If a shorter volume is scanned, a shorter scan time can be used. If patients are not able to hold their breath they are allowed to breathe quietly during image acquisition, though breath-holding is preferred.

A field of view of 300 mm is used, with a collimation of 3 mm and an effective slice thickness of 3 mm. Image reconstruction from the continuous volume set is at 3 mm increment, which results in 86 images (covering 26 cm). Using the same data, a second image set of 85 (86 − 1) images can be reconstructed now at the intervening positions, again at 3 mm increment. Both sets together (171 images) correspond to an image set of 1.5 mm incrementation which will enhance axial dynamic viewing due to very smooth transitions between the images. This will enable the inspection of the vessels between the images.

Visualisation of secondary signs of pulmonary embolism

Inspection of parenchymal abnormalities

Viewing the images as obtained by the above 'direct' imaging protocol, in lungsetting (window level −500 Hu, width 1,500 Hu) allows assessment of the lung-parenchymal sequelae, which may be associated with PE. These include identification of so-called mosaic alogemia and infiltrates that may be due to infarction. Furthermore, secondary changes may be visible in the heart, where dilatation of the right ventricle and right atrium occurs rapidly with the occurrence of large acute PE. In addition, in the case of chronic PE in which pulmonary outflow is obstructed over a period of time, right ventricular myocardial hypertrophy occurs.

Pleural effusion often accompanies acute PE but is a non-specific sign and can occur with many other clinical situations.

In addition, the scanning capabilities of EBT may also allow more dynamic studies of ventilation and perfusion of the lung parenchyma, using the multi-slice modes.

Ventilation protocol

Galvin [28] described a method to dynamically image the structures of the lung using EBT based on changes in parenchymal attenuation of X-ray during the respiratory cycle. For example, a series of 10 individual 100 msec scans may be obtained at 500 msec intervals acquired over 5 sec, as the patient forcibly inhales and exhales, with 3 mm slice thicknesses and a high-resolution reconstruction algorithm. No intravenous contrast medium is used. This 10-scan dynamic series is obtained at only 3 levels (near the aortic arch, through the carina, and at the lung bases). The mean attenuation for a specific region of interest is measured as a function of time, which is related to respiration, producing a curve showing the change in lung attenuation during the respiratory manoeuvre [29]. Each tissue compartment has its specific attenuation features (range of Hounsfield Units) and thus for each parenchymal compartment (interstitium, air-containing compartment) its function over time can be assessed (Fig. 2) [30, 31]. Theoretically, areas with underventilation – i. e. relatively less or no change in attenuation as a function of time/respiration – may be identified. Some experimental data is available, using this specific property of fast CT scanning to assess lung function [32]. However, no data on this subject is yet available in clinical cases of PE.

Perfusion protocol

Using intravenously administered contrast medium Hoffman et al. [26, 33] developed a method to use the rapid imaging properties of EBT to assess perfusion of lung parenchyma in an animal model. They proposed to acquire high temporal resolution images by sequentially activating each of the four target rings at selected points in time gated to the subject's ECG curve in order to obtain a parenchymal 'time-density' curve, which is now largely determined by the arrival and wash-out of the intravenously administered contrast medium. Scanning may be performed first at every heartbeat for 6 heartbeats, to assure acquisition of the peak of the contrast curve, and then at alternate heartbeats for the next 4 heartbeats to maximise the amount of the tail of the curve to be sampled. Using all 4 targets and the 2 detector rings with a slice thickness (maximum) of 8 mm and accounting for the 4 mm inter-target gap, an area of 76 mm can be covered during each image acquisition period (8*8 mm + 3*4 mm). Contrast medium was injected at a rate of 10 ml/sec over 2 sec. After display of the time-density curve, the image with peak enhancement was selected and subtracted

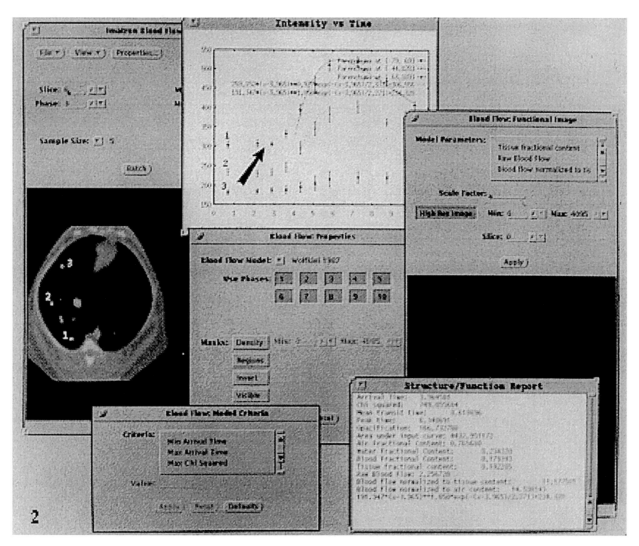

Fig. 2. A screen captured from the VIDA program for image analysis demonstrates the amount of information available from high-speed CT scanning in conjunction with a bolus intravenous injection of contrast medium. With EBT scanning, it is possible to follow a bolus of contrast material as it passes through the lung parenchyma and to use the intensity-time information from the main pulmonary artery and the parenchymal to evaluate regional air, blood, and tissue (parenchyma plus extravascular water) content as well as blood flow and transit time. (Arrow points to baseline of region number 1). Regional air content is calculated using the baseline information from the curve. The blood and tissue content of the non-air component is then calculated by a comparison of the area under the arterial curve and the area under the parenchymal curve. All parameters thus calculated can be colour coded and displayed as an overlay on the anatomic data. If both an HRCT and a high temporal resolution scan are acquired without intervening motion of the patient, and if lung volume is the same for the two scans, high resolution anatomy can be mapped together. Such data in combination with gas (xenon) washout curves open the door to a complete evaluation of structure-function correlates throughout the lung [30].

from the first image (acquired at first heartbeat, without any contrast enhancement). This allows for visual inspection of homogeneity of parenchymal enhancement due to arrival of contrast medium. Perfusion defects will reveal themselves by lack of enhancement in comparison to well-perfused areas.

Thus it seems possible to visualise both the actual PE and the sequelae, i. e. perfusion defects, which – theoretically – could be matched by ventilation characteristics of the same area. So far only animal models have been studied and this ventilation perfusion protocol has not been implemented in clinical practice.

Experimental data on EBT and pulmonary embolism

Both Geraghty et al. [15] and Stanford et al. [16] were concerned with whether EBT was able to depict PE in segmental pulmonary arteries. This is an important question, since, as will be discussed elsewhere in this book, fast conventional computed tomography appears to be able to depict PE in the first and second order pulmonary arteries with ease. In the absence of central PE the issue is raised if the presence of subsegmental emboli is clinically relevant. These questions still remain to be answered and in the meantime it appears important to determine the sensitivity of this new technique for the non-invasive detection of emboli in third and fourth order branches.

Geraghty studied 7 mongrel dogs in which PE was simulated by injecting gelfoam emboli, adapted in size to pass through the central pulmonary arterial vasculature and to lodge in the segmental arteries. Stanford used the same approach but now in 8 pigs using autologous blood clots. In both studies, the clot was marked by a silk suture, and after a direct EBT imaging protocol the animals were sacrificed and the thorax dissected so as to be compared with the electron beam images. In both studies, contrast medium was introduced by a central venous catheter lodging in the vena cava.

In the study of Geraghty 19 of 21 emboli had lodged in the 2nd to 4th generation pulmonary arteries and all of these emboli were identified unequivocally on the EBT images. Stanford studied the animals before and after injection of the autologous blood clot; these observers did not know if a scan was obtained before or after provocation of PE. In the 8 pre-embolic studies, no emboli were identified. In 7 of the 8 post-embolic images, emboli were correctly identified in the 3rd to 4th division pulmonary arteries. In the 8th study, no embolus was found on EBT. It was postulated that the autologous clot had fragmented prior to the scan. Both authors conclude that it appears possible to diagnose segmental PE by EBT.

Hoffman et al. [25] – as already indicated – focused on the hemodynamic consequences of PE, using the specific properties of the EBT to assess perfusion properties of the pulmonary parenchyma. Similarly to Stanford et al., they studied 14 pigs in which autologous blood clots were injected, designed to lodge in the segmental pulmonary arteries. Again, the clots were marked with a silk suture, and after the image acquisition, the animals were sacrificed and sectioned according to the EBT images. The perfusion protocol – already described in a previous section of this chapter – was used. The animals were scanned before and after installation of PE.

The authors reported an example of a sharply demarcated perfusion defect in the lower lobe of the left lung, corresponding to an embolus in the parent artery as demonstrated at autopsy study (Fig. 3) [34]. In the same animal, a sharply demonstrated perfusion defect in the right lower lobe was found, after embolism injection. However, the embolus could not be demonstrated at autopsy. Thus, in addition to locating the position of the 14 primary clots by EBT (which were confirmed at autopsy), functional (perfusion) imaging defined an additional 8 regions which presumably represented areas of decreased perfusion caused by clot fragmentation. Only 5 of the 22 clots identified by functional (perfusion) imaging were identified using a direct visualisation protocol. This study suggests that perfusion studies by EBT may considerably enhance the sensitivity of this diagnostic tool particularly in situations in which the clots fragment and move into the distalmost pulmonary arteries where they may not be visible as filling detects in the arteries.

It should be pointed out that these perfusion studies have not yet been added to clinical practice protocols.

Goldin et al. [35] studied the accuracy of EBT pulmonary angiography in the detection of pulmonary artery embolism in a porcine model. In 5 animals, under general anaesthesia, (sub)segmental pulmonary arteries were selectively catheterised and embolised with gelfoam pledgets. Conventional pulmonary angiography confirmed 21 emboli (upper lobe 3, right lower lobe 7, left lower lobe 11). Immediately after angiography 3 mm contrast enhanced EBT images were obtained, acquiring 40 cardiac-gated scans without breathholding. These were interpreted without knowledge of the results of pulmonary angiography. Eighteen (out of 21) emboli were identified with a reported sensitivity and specificity of 85% and 100%, respectively. According to the investigators, breathholding appeared unnecessary for detection of PE. They concluded that EBT pulmonary angiography is a highly sensitive method for the detection of up to segmental pulmonary artery embolism.

In conclusion, animal studies suggest that EBT is a sensitive tool in defining segmental PE; it may not be necessary to combine the standard imaging protocol with perfusion studies for detection of emboli up to segmental (fourth order) pulmonary ar-

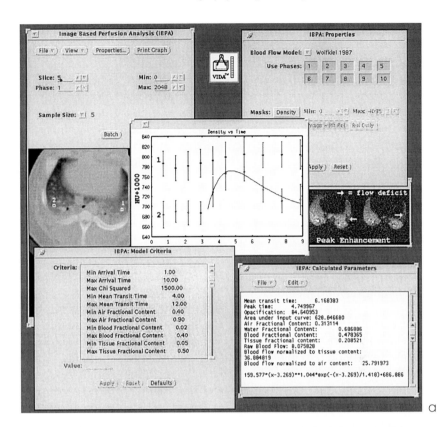

Fig. 3a. The above images are a montage taken from the computer screen depicting an image based perfusion analysis module of VIDA in which time intensity curves are used to evaluate tissue perfusion. In the case shown above, the peak of the parenchymal curve is compared with the area under the pulmonary arterial curve to evaluate a number of physiologic parameters including regional air content, tissue content, blood content, blood flow normalised to tissue content (ml/g parenchyma/min) or blood flow normalised to air content, mean transit time, arrival time, etc. Criteria can be set (lower left panel) such that only the image data is accepted from pixels representing lung parenchyma by throwing out pixels in which contrast arrives early (representing an artery) or late (representing a vein), etc. In this particular data set, flow in region 2 represented normal parenchymal perfusion, and flow in region 1 was found to represent an unperfused region [25].

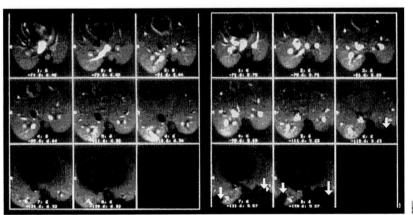

Fig. 3b. Shown left is a photographic image of the frozen section in which a clot was found and verified based upon the presence of the suture material which was passed through the clot at the time of injection [25]. On the right a sequence of images represents the eight sections scanned under protocol 3 for the same pig depicted in Figure 3a. Sectioning is from mid-chest to lung base going from top left to bottom right. Images are derived from the digital subtraction of the first time point from the time point where maximal parenchymal enhancement was found. These images represent parenchymal flow distribution prior to clot injection [25].

teries. Perfusion studies may improve diagnostic results in regard to the more peripheral (fifth order or greater) emboli in which small vessel occlusions may be present but difficult to detect because of the very small size of the involved vessels and the difficulty associated with determining whether or not they are actually opacified with contrast material as opposed to being occluded.

Clinical experience

During the past 5 years, the fast CT features of PE have been described and a comprehensive summary has been published by Sheedy et al. [24] and Greaves [36]. Since conventional CT (helical or spiral CT) and EBT both produce comparable images with respect to direct visualisation of the embolus and its parenchymal sequelae the reader is referred to the chapter on helical CT and PE for a detailed description of the vascular and parenchymal CT findings of (acute) PE.

Ventilation-perfusion characteristics

Although it is theoretically possible to study ventilation characteristics of areas supplied by arteries that contain PE using EBT, to our knowledge no such clinical studies are available. Only one animal study is available describing perfusion characteristics associated with embolic disease using EBT [25]. The technique and an example of the findings (Fig. 3) have been described in a previous section. They observe flow voids with a sharp edge in all 18 provoked pulmonary emboli. Whenever there was a flow void present which had poorly defined edges, the parenchymal abnormalities were found both before and after injection of the PE and were associated with regions of pulmonary edema. With pulmonary edema it is well documented that vessels are constricted locally so as to shunt blood to regions receiving better oxygenation [37].

Pictorial intermezzo

Optimum viewing methods

EBT examinations for possible PE are now usually comprised of 60–80 3 mm thick contiguous sections. Reviewing and interpretation of these images in the standard film format is cumbersome, laborious, and requires considerable expertise. Alternatively, rapid viewing of contiguous transaxial images on a standard workstation is an attractive, timesaving and arguably a more accurate method to evaluate such examinations. In this way, all images can be reviewed rapidly and repetitively from top to bottom and back again. In doing so, all vessels and its branches can be traced from origin

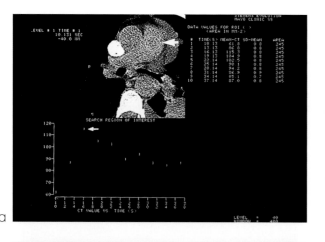
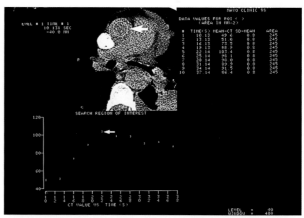
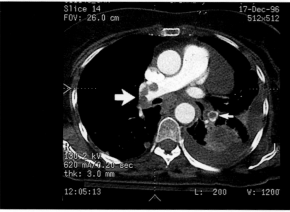
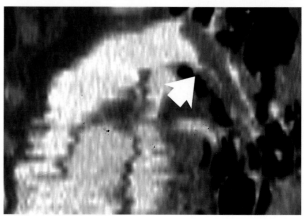

a b c d

Fig. 4a–d. Circulation time and PE. **(a)** Circulation time in the main pulmonary artery (large arrow) was 16 sec on the time density curve (small arrow). **(b)** Circulation time in ascending aorta (large arrow) was 22 sec on the time density curve (small arrow). **(c)** PE present in the artery to the left lower lobe (small arrow) and in the distal right main pulmonary artery extending into the right lower lobe artery (large arrow). **(d)** Curved sagittal reconstruction of the right pulmonary artery demonstrating elongated thrombus in the distal main pulmonary

to termination. Such viewing makes it easier to detect abrupt changes in density due to occlusion, easier to detect small filling defects, and certainly easier to accurately differentiate arteries from veins, which can be quite time-consuming if done from a film format. Simply, arteries come from the pulmonary artery at the hilum and veins enter into the left atrium. Also, rapid multilevel viewing on a workstation allows inspection of the images at a variety of window level and window width settings without the need to select one or more optimum settings for inspection in the film format.

Rapid multilevel viewing has become the viewing method of choice for most radiologists involved in interpretation of EBT examinations for possible PE. It should thus be noted that in a chapter or a written publication such as this one, viewing of photographs of selected images offers only a glimpse of a portion of the total examination. Reconstructions of transaxial images in the sagittal or coronal or in curve planar depictions does help but cannot substitute for the rapid multilevel real time viewing of all images at a variety of window and level settings. However, use of curved multiplanar reconstructions can assist in evaluating questionable density differences and in following vertically oriented vessels from origin to termination [38].

As indicated before, the EBT findings in PE may be categorised according to direct visualisation of PE, pulmonary parenchymal findings, and indirect signs (pleural, cardiac). The main features will be demonstrated in this section (Figs. 4–19).

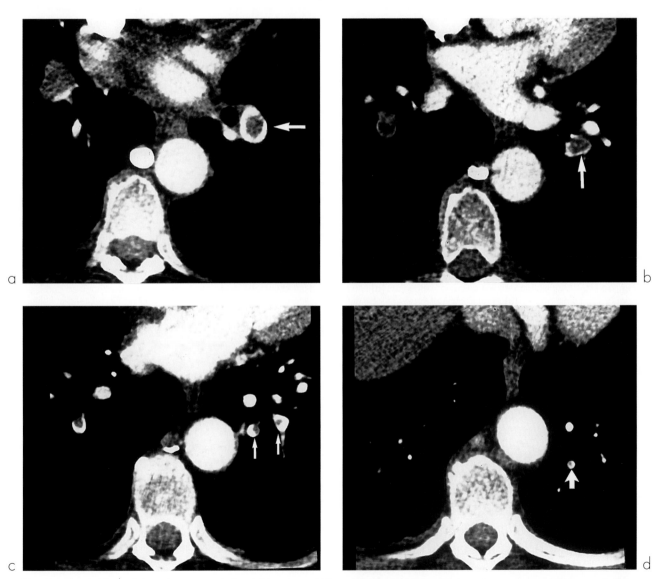

Fig. 5a–d.   Left lower lobe pulmonary embolus. **(a)** Intraluminal filling defect in the left lower lobe pulmonary artery (white arrow). **(b)** Embolus extends into segmental branch (large arrow). **(c)** Subsegmental branches (two white arrows) also contained emboli. **(d)** Small peripheral vessel beyond the subsegmental level (sub-subsegmental) contains embolus 1.5 mm in diameter (white arrow). Also noted, on the right side, is embolus in the right lower lobe pulmonary artery and segmental branches posteriorly **(a, b, c)**.

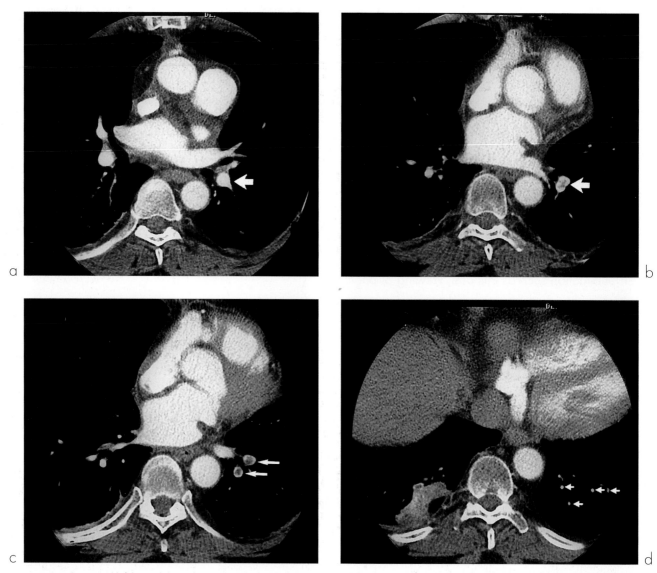

Fig. 6a–d. Distal left lower lobe pulmonary embolus. **(a)** Main trunk of left lower lobe pulmonary artery is normally opacified and is of normal size (white arrow). **(b)** At bifurcation of the lower lobe pulmonary artery, a filling defect is present straddling this bifurcation (white arrow). **(c)** This distal saddle embolus extends into two subsegmental branches (two white arrows). **(d)** More distal, in the periphery small vessels (sub-subsegmental) are opacified indicating incomplete obstruction (small white arrows). It is possible that other vessels in the area are not opacified because of occlusion.

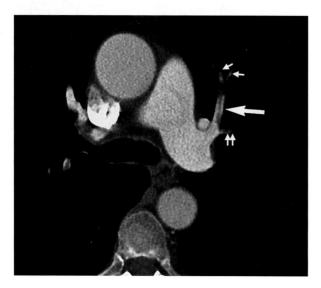

Fig. 7. Acute pulmonary embolus. Acute embolus located in the anterior segment of the left upper lobe pulmonary artery (large white arrow). Technically this larger branch is a subsegmental branch as the main trunk of the anterior segment artery is quite short and gives rise to a laterally extending, smaller subsegmental branch (two small arrows) which also contains embolus. More anteriorly, two sub-subsegmental branches are visible (small white arrows).

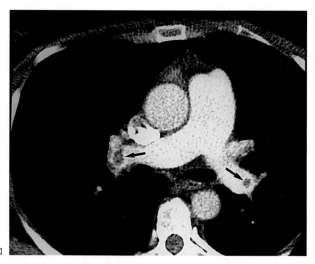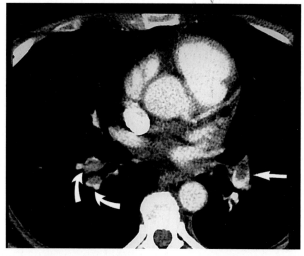

Fig. 8a, b. Acute pulmonary embolus. **(a)** Small filling defects are present in the distal portion of both the right main and left main pulmonary arteries (black arrows). **(b)** Larger component of the embolus on the left extends into the lobar branch (large white arrow) and on the right into two segmental branches (curved white arrows).

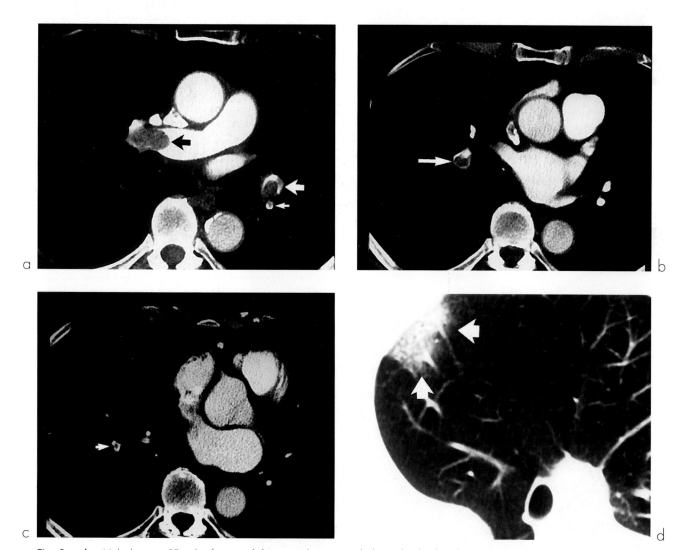

Fig. 9a–d. Multiple acute PE with infarction. **(a)** Large pulmonary embolus in distal right pulmonary artery (black arrow) and, partially occluding embolus in the left lower lobe artery (large white arrow) and in smaller superior segmental artery (small white arrow). **(b)** Main right pulmonary artery embolus extends into artery of the right lower lobe (white arrow). **(c)** Embolus extends into subsegmental branch of the right lower lobe (small white arrow). **(d)** On lung settings a pleural based density in the periphery suggests infarction, seen at lung settings (two white arrows).

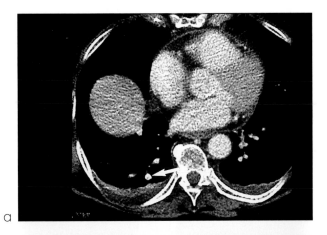

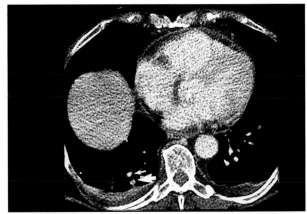

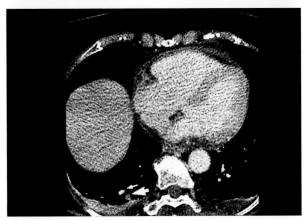

Fig. 10a–c. Small solitary peripheral pulmonary embolus.
(a) A subsegmental branch of the posterior basal segment in the right lower lobe is opacified with contrast material (white arrow).
(b) Two scan levels below **(a)**, a branch of the subsegmental branch harbours a filling defect (white arrow); immediately above is a normally opacified branch (small white arrow).
(c) Two scan levels below b) the posterior branch remains unopacified and occluded (white arrow) and the branch above those smaller is clearly opacified and therefore patent (small white arrow). This isolated peripheral pulmonary embolus is in at least one sub-subsegmental branch. Note additionally small bilateral pleural effusions.

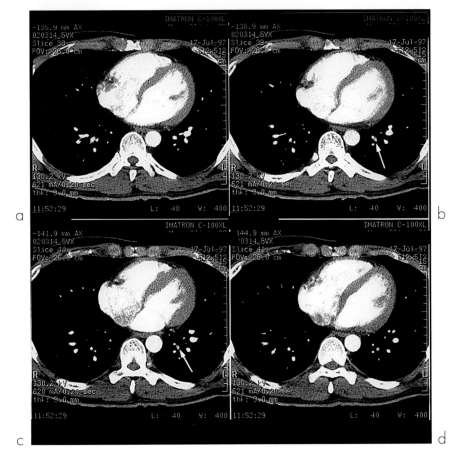

Fig. 11a–d. Tiny peripheral pulmonary embolus. Four contiguous 3 mm thick scan levels show opacification of all arteries and veins at these four levels except for a tiny embolus occupying a subsegmental branch on two consecutive levels (small white arrows on **(b)** and **(c)**. The finding is subtle but definite.

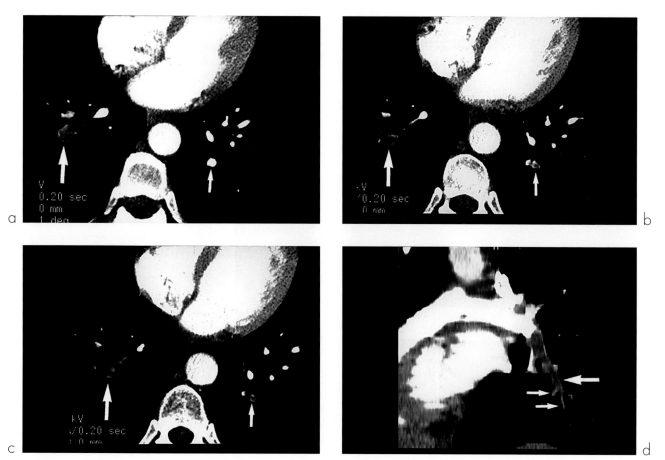

Fig 12a–d.   Acute embolus. **(a)** Scan through the lower lobes shows occlusion of the artery to the right lower lobe (large white arrow) and patent segmental artery in the left lower lobe (small white arrow). **(b)** Occlusion of segmental branch of the right lower lobe (large white arrow) and embolus at the bifurcation of a segmental branch in the left lower lobe (small white arrow). **(c)** Continuing occlusion of segmental branch in the right lower lobe (large white arrow) and embolus almost filling one of the subsegmental branches in the posterior left lower lobe with an adjacent smaller subsegmental branch being opacified and patent. **(d)** Curved planar semi-sagittal reconstruction of the right pulmonary artery and the right lower lobe pulmonary artery and the posterior basal segmental artery and two subsegmental branches showing embolus filling the left lower lobar (large white arrow) and segmental branch and extending into the subsegmental branches (two small arrows).

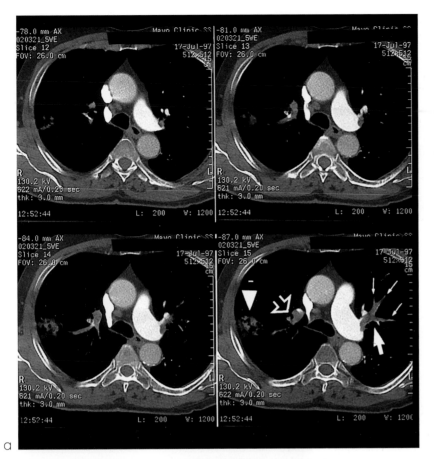

a

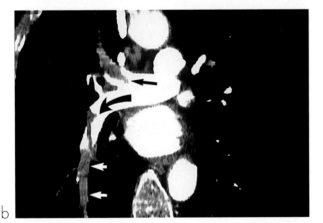

b

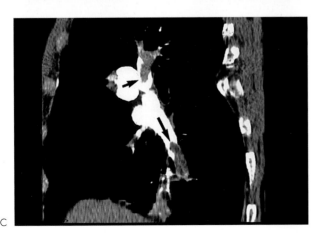

c

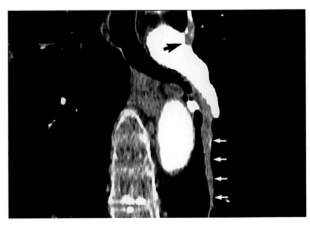

d

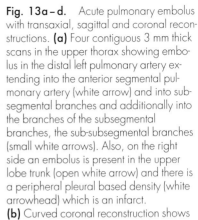

Fig. 13a–d. Acute pulmonary embolus with transaxial, sagittal and coronal reconstructions. **(a)** Four contiguous 3 mm thick scans in the upper thorax showing embolus in the distal left pulmonary artery extending into the anterior segmental pulmonary artery (white arrow) and into subsegmental branches and additionally into the branches of the subsegmental branches, the sub-subsegmental branches (small white arrows). Also, on the right side an embolus is present in the upper lobe trunk (open white arrow) and there is a peripheral pleural based density (white arrowhead) which is an infarct. **(b)** Curved coronal reconstruction shows embolus filling the right upper lobe artery (small black arrow) and an elongated thrombus extending into the lower lobar artery (curved black arrow) and eventually almost occluding the posterior basal segmental artery (two white arrows) and one of its subsegmental branches. **(c)** Curved sagittal reconstruction, also on the right side, shows embolus in the right upper lobe artery (small black arrow) extending into the segmental branches of that vessel, and good opacification of the lower lobar artery down to an occluding embolus in the posterior basal segmental branch on the right side with an associated peripheral infarct against the diaphragm. **(d)** A curved coronal reconstruction of the left side reveals embolus extending into the anterior segmental branch of the left upper lobe as seen in **(a)** and also an occlusive embolus in the posterior basal segmental artery extending into the subsegmental and probably to the sub-subsegmental level as well (small white arrows).

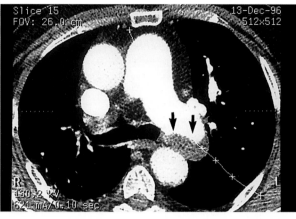
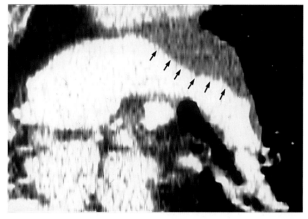

Fig. 14a, b. Chronic pulmonary embolus. Vertical reconstructions help differentiate acute from chronic PE findings. **(a)** A filling defect is present in the distal portion of the dilated left main pulmonary artery (two black arrows). **(b)** A curved coronal reconstruction reveals the filling defect to be eccentrically located and a mural thickening in the upper curve of the left pulmonary artery (small black arrows). This eccentric filling defect is due to chronic embolus, not acute embolus, which would appear as an intraluminal filling defect.

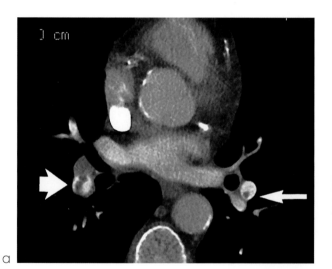
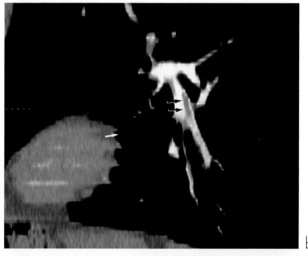
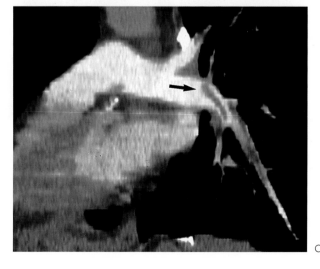

Fig. 15a–c. Acute pulmonary embolus (small and bilateral).
(a) Scan through the proximal lower lobe artery showing a moderate sized embolus in the artery to the right lower lobe (fat arrow) and a thin embolus in the proximal portion of the artery to the left lower lobe (white arrow). **(b)** A straight sagittal reconstruction reveals the thin embolus in the proximal lower lobe artery (tiny black arrows). **(c)** A curved sagittal reconstruction shows the left lower lobe embolus (black arrow) that was seen in **(a)** and **(b)** but to better advantage as occupying the left lower lobe artery and extending into the segmental and subsegmental branches.

241

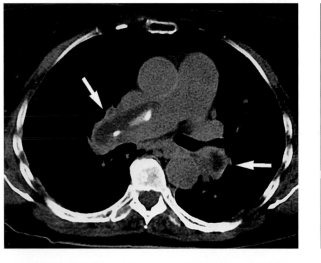
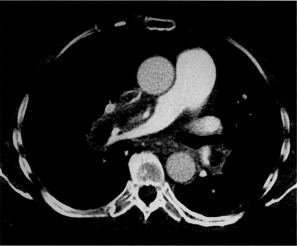

a   b

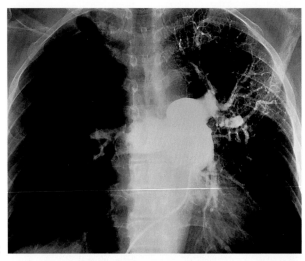

c

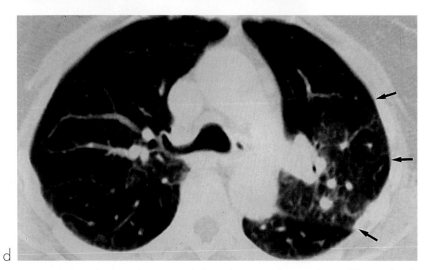

d

Fig. 16a–d. Chronic pulmonary embolus with mosaic oligemia due to differential perfusion. **(a)** Non-contrast scan at the level of the right pulmonary artery reveals partially calcified filling defect in the distal right pulmonary artery (white arrow) and filling defect, even on a non-contrast scan, in the proximal left lower lobe artery, which is dilated (white arrow). **(b)** Same scan level, with intravenous contrast material showing the filling defects seen in a) now outlined by iodinated contrast material. **(c)** Scan through the upper lobes at lung window settings showing differential density in the pulmonary parenchyma of the left upper lobe with increased density in the posterior division of the left lower lobe (black arrows) compared to the lower density of the pulmonary parenchyma in the anterior division of the left upper lobe. **(d)** Selective left pulmonary angiogram showing differential perfusion of the left upper lobe corresponding to the mosaic appearance seen in **(c)**.

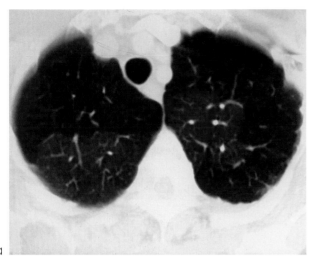
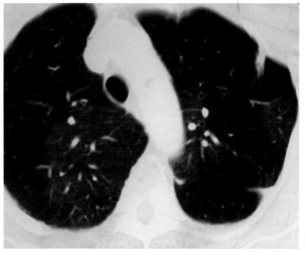

Fig. 17a, b. A more subtle appearance of the mosaic oligemia pattern. **(a)** In the posterior portion of the right upper lobe and in the apical portion of the left upper lobe is seen increased density compared to the adjacent lung. Also, the vascular structures within those areas of increased density seem to be slightly larger than those in the adjacent lung parenchyma. **(b)** Scan at a slightly lower level than **(a)** showing the differential density and the slightly increased size of the vascular structures compared to the adjacent parenchyma.

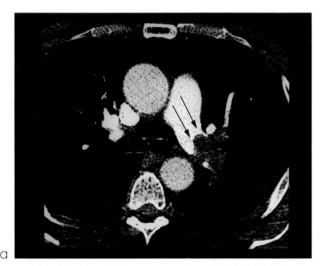
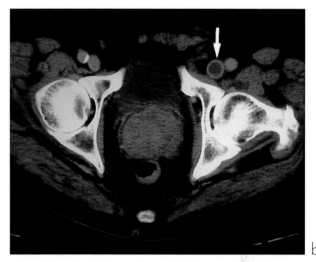

Fig. 18a, b. Acute pulmonary embolus and left femoral thrombosis. **(a)** Large occlusive filling defect present in the left pulmonary artery (black arrows) with almost total occlusion of the distal left pulmonary artery. **(b)** In the same patient a scan of the pelvis made immediately after the pulmonary scan reveals thrombus in the left femoral vein (white arrow) medial to the femoral artery. It is possible to compare the thrombus on the left side with a normal-appearing femoral vein on the right side.

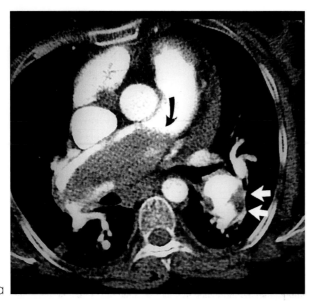 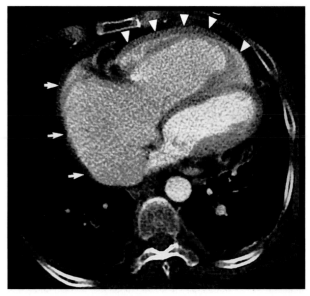

a
b

Fig. 19a, b. Chronic pulmonary embolus with cardiac enlargement. **(a)** Enlarged right pulmonary artery containing an eccentric filling defect within the lumen posteriorly (curved black arrow). Also noted is massive dilatation of the left lower lobe pulmonary artery with filling defect and evidence of recanalisation (two white arrows). **(b)** Massive cardiac enlargement with dilatation of right atrium (small white arrows) and moderate hypertrophy of the right ventricular myocardium (white arrowheads) and dilatation of the right ventricular chamber.

Value of EBT

Technical accuracy

No studies have been reported regarding inter- and intraobserver variability or reproducibility of EBT in the diagnosis of PE. Also, interstudy reproducibility has not been evaluated.

Diagnostic accuracy

Although sensitivity and specificity appear to be of limited value as indicators of the value of a diagnostic test [39], they are still widely used with respect to EBT for diagnosis of PE. The only two studies now available reporting the accuracy of EBT in the diagnosis of PE used only these classical test parameters.

Holland [23] performed both MRI and EBT examinations in a group of 16 patients (chronic pulmonary thromboembolism suspects) with a high probability ventilation perfusion scan. Pulmonary angiography served as the standard in all but four cases in which surgical thromboendarterectomy was performed. Twenty-four lesions were identified with pulmonary angiography in the 32 pulmonary arterial systems examined. EBT identified all but two of these chronic PE with a sensitivity of

92%, specificity of 100%, and accuracy of 94%. Both false negative findings were due to adherent chronic clot in the inferior aspect of the main pulmonary artery.

In their various reports Teigen et al. [21–23] found a sensitivity of 65% (95% confidence interval 42.8–82.6), with a specificity of 97% (85.5–99.9). This study included all patients referred for pulmonary angiography from March 1992 to March 1993 because of clinical suspicion of PE disease which 'may have been based' on results of ventilation-perfusion scanning and other non-invasive tests (such as lower extremity ultrasound, D-dimer assays, or even clinical suspicion). The experience in 60 patients was reported in their last report, and 38 of these patients had a ventilation perfusion scan (normal in one, high probability in 4 and intermediate probability in 33 patients).

Pulmonary angiography served as the reference test, which revealed a prevalence of PE in this patient group of 38% (23 of 60 cases). A total of 61 emboli were found, of which 26 were localised in the central vascular zones (area 1, 2, 3, 5, 8, 9, 11) and 35 in peripheral zones, including the segmental and subsegmental artery distribution.

When the central and peripheral vascular zones (n = 720) were analysed individually, there was no substantial difference in the diagnostic accuracy between EBT results and invasive pulmonary angiography with regard to clinically significant PE. In the 420 central vascular zones sensitivity (with 95 % confidence intervals) was reported to be 71 % (48.9–87.4) with a specificity of 98 % (95.7–98.9) and in the 300 peripheral zones these values were 79 % (61.6–91.0) and 98 % (95.5–99.4), respectively.

Findings at EBT and pulmonary angiography were discordant in nine patients. In one patient, the pulmonary angiogram was actually a false negative study (compared to the CT scan) because the area containing the evident luminal filling defect on EBT was not well depicted on the pulmonary angiogram due to patient motion artifact. In eight other patients, two of the pulmonary angiograms were actually false positive with the occlusion on the angiogram being due to a tumour in one patient and postradiation vascular changes in another patient, both of which were clarified by EBT. In two cases it seemed unlikely that the angiographic abnormalities explained the complaints of the patient.

In four patients with false negative EBT, all five of the emboli demonstrated by pulmonary angiography were very small and in subsegmental vessels. The authors, at that time, discussed the clinical relevance of missing these small emboli. In these four patients, the finding of small peripheral emboli on the angiogram did not lead to institution of anti-coagulation therapy and they were deemed to be clinically irrelevant.

Therefore, after revising their evaluation to reflect the explanations of false negative and false positive, it was estimated that the true sensitivity and specificity of EBT for PE may well approach 100 %.

Difficulties (pitfalls)

Indeterminate (uninterpretable) examinations occur infrequently and are mainly caused by technical problems such as extremely rapid respiratory rate, inability to obtain an accurate circulation time which can be associated with an examination in which there is poor opacification of the pulmonary arteries because of low cardiac output, large patient size, vascular distortion from the presence of tumour, or previous surgery on the heart and great vessels. Operator error can result in indeterminate examinations if the examination is not carried out with a timing close to that of the circulation time, which may be particularly important in

the upper lobe segments [40]. Occasionally patients experience a reaction to contrast material, which necessitates interruption or termination of the examination.

Potential sources of *false positive* EBT diagnosis of PE includes misinterpretation of a partial volume effect in an obliquely oriented vessel such as the lingula or the middle lobe artery and its branches. This source of error has been reduced with the conversion from thick slices (6 mm) to 3 mm slices. Partially opacified pulmonary veins can be confused with thrombosed arteries. Confusion with hilar or intersegmental lymph nodes and circumferential edema of the pulmonary artery wall that occurs with congestive heart failure may occur. Inadequate enhancement of vessels due to any cause may result in a false positive diagnosis. This can occur when there is decreased flow because of increased peripheral resistance.

Viewing the images on the workstation in an interactive mode and following each vessel dynamically through the scanned volume can prevent most of these errors. In this way, arteries emanate from the pulmonary hilum and veins flow to the left atrium, and it is possible to clearly differentiate structures such as lymph nodes from the more continuous course of these vessels.

False negative results may occur when vessels are obscured by surrounding parenchymal opacification such as consolidation or atelectasis, though patent arteries can often be seen to be opacified within atelectatic portions of the lung. Very small eccentric emboli or very small occluded vessels may be overlooked by the examiner. The ability of EBT to detect peripheral emboli has not been clearly established although results indicate that at least some of these emboli can be visualised in subsegmental branches either as intraluminal filling defects or as non-opacified vessels.

Considerations concerning differential diagnosis
With the EBT method, as with any computed tomography method, alternative diagnoses can be made on examinations for patients with possible PE. Coronary artery calcification as a sign of coronary atherosclerosis is visible. Thickened pericardium due to pericarditis or pericardial effusions are occasionally seen. Diseases of the aorta due to atheromatous disease such as aneurysm or dissection or penetrating ulcers with intramural hematoma can be discovered when scanning for PE. Also tumours of the heart, pulmonary arteries, pulmonary veins, or even bronchogenic tumours with constriction of the pulmonary arteries are occasionally found in patients being examined predominantly for possible PE.

Comparative value

EBT vs helical (or spiral) CT in the diagnosis of pulmonary embolism

No prospective studies have been reported comparing the diagnostic accuracy of EBT versus conventional fast (helical or spiral) CT in the diagnosis of PE. Advantages of EBT over conventional CT may be the shorter scan time of 100 or 200 msec (versus 1,000 msec with spiral CT) that can be expected to reduce motion artifact and motion unsharpness from cardiac motion and vascular pulsation, although this difference may only be of practical importance in the search for smaller emboli in peripheral vessels. It is expected that the results in EBT tomography and conventional CT will be similar with regard to the larger central vessels down to the segmental branches.

Although fast conventional CT may provide the ability to study time attenuation characteristics of lung parenchyma, it seems probable that if this were important, the more rapid image acquisition and the shorter exposure time and the ability to acquire multiple slices simultaneously would be an advantage of EBT in refining the diagnosis of the parenchymal effects of PE.

EBT vs MRI

Only one study compared EBT with MRI in the diagnosis of PE disease. In an abstract already referred to in this review, Holland [23] compared EBT with MRI using pulmonary angiography as reference test in 16 patients with a high probability ventilation-perfusion scan. MRI identified all clots in the main and right and left pulmonary arteries, including the 2 lesions missed by EBT. However, MRI failed to identify 1 clot in a 3rd generation vessel and did not identify any in the 4th generation branches obtaining a sensitivity of 79% and a specificity of 100%, with an accuracy of 84%, being slightly less than the values for EBT (92%, 100% and 94% respectively). The authors conclude that these preliminary results suggest that EBT is more accurate in diagnosing PE than MRI. However, advances in MR technology (as described in Chapter IV.8) will require further evaluation comparing these two techniques.

Examination speed and ease of patient monitoring currently favour the use of CT and detailed depiction of lung parenchyma and the mediastinum may provide for alternate diagnoses, as demonstrated in the series of Teigen [21–23]. Although MRI may not require the administration of intravenous contrast material, which could be considered as an advantage of MRI, current protocols as described in Chapter IV.8 have used contrast enhancement techniques to obtain more accurate images with MRI. With the use of venous saturation, MRI may be able to differentiate arteries from veins more easily than fast CT imaging. Finally, an advantage of MRI over EBT may be the option of combining MR angiography of the pulmonary vasculature with MR evaluation of the veins of the pelvis and legs in the same session for thromboembolic disease [41, 42]. However, if this were an important issue it would be possible to utilise either fast CT or conventional CT to inspect the pelvis and extremities as well for existence of intraluminal venous clots after the pulmonary arterial study had been completed.

Clinical value

The classical test parameters (sensitivity, specificity) neither completely inform about the clinical value of a test, to be expressed in terms of cost-effectiveness, nor provide information concerning the added value of a test with respect to already available information prior to implementation of the diagnostic test under consideration [40]. It is probably still too early to expect studies to be undertaken to provide more clinically relevant information with respect to the value of this new scanning technique in the diagnosis of PE, and because of this no data is available on this subject.

A recent cost-effectiveness analysis, performed by Van Erkel et al. [43], suggested that a diagnostic strategy which uses spiral CT will be more cost-effective than one that involves the use of pulmonary angiography, if the specificity of CT exceeds 92%, and that this protocol will have a lower associated mortality rate when the sensitivity of CT exceeds 85% [44].

Finally, what seems to be needed is a management study in which anticoagulant therapy is withheld in patients in whom scans are deemed to be negative. This would validate the accuracy and specificity of a negative CT scan for clinically relevant PE.

Discussion and future directions

There are several unresolved issues regarding the overall value of fast CT (EBT) for evaluation of patients suspected of having PE, and these controversies are being addressed in the current radiologic literature.

The issue of the detectability of small peripheral emboli is one of the major possible limitations on CT becoming the procedure of choice for evaluation of patients with clinically suspected PE. Moreover, the natural course and hence the clinical relevance of peripheral embolus is not clear.

The actual terminology used to describe the location of 'small peripheral pulmonary emboli' can be confusing. Terms such as 3rd order, 4th order, or 5th order branches, or, 3rd, 4th or 5th division branches are all used to describe 'small peripheral vessels.' Are these lobar, segmental and subsegmental locations? It would seem that the main pulmonary artery is the first, the right and left pulmonary arteries the second, the upper, lower, middle, and lingular the third, and their branches the segmental. Then branches of the segmental vessels, the subsegmentals, are really the 5th division or 5th order branches. It seems that the term 'small peripheral pulmonary embolus' is best applied to the emboli that are located in the branches beyond the segmental '4th division, 4th order' branches.

Up until recently, the pulmonary angiogram has been the unquestioned diagnostic standard for diagnosis or exclusion of PE in any location. But it has been recognised that pulmonary angiography can be false negative for PE in up to 9 % of patients [46]. Also, interobserver variability in regard to small peripheral pulmonary emboli is high [45, 46]. Nevertheless, negative pulmonary angiograms (including false negative studies and erroneously interpreted studies) have been deemed accurate in predicting a good patient outcome with no evidence of subsequent PE on follow-up [47–49]. Indeed, it is likely that many pulmonary angiograms have been interpreted as either positive or negative without the compulsion to name the actual vessel in which the (small) emboli were found.

Perhaps the insertion of CT into the pulmonary embolus diagnostic algorithm (formerly consisting of clinical suspicion, ventilation perfusion scintigraphy, lower extremity venous studies, and pulmonary angiography) will result in a need to identify the precise location and size of the PE. After all, CT is being asked to provide information which was not previously required because it was not always available with these other methods.

To further complicate the issue, it is even said that small peripheral pulmonary emboli are a common occurrence in asymptomatic humans and that one of the functions of the lung is to remove or filter these small pulmonary emboli [50]. It has been demonstrated that normal persons can have major perfusion defects on ventilation perfusion scans [51] that are indistinguishable from those caused by PE, but it was not proven that these defects were in fact due to PE in these normal volunteers.

So, if 'small peripheral emboli' occur, maybe even in normal persons, and if the established standard diagnostic procedure, pulmonary angiography, can fail to detect these with minimal long-term sequelae, perhaps the supposed inability of CT to detect these 'small peripheral pulmonary emboli' is not of great clinical importance.

Now, however, a review of the figures in this chapter shows clearly that many subsegmental emboli are visible and even emboli in the branches of subsegmental vessels, the sub-subsegmental vessels, are identifiable. They can be seen, but probably not all of them.

The issue of subsegmental vessel evaluation and the ability to detect PE in subsegmental vessels probably is more dependent on the size of the vessel than on the name of it. Actually, subsegmental vessels don't have proper names other than 'subsegmental'. Also, subsegmental vessels show considerable variation in size. Similarly, the branches of the segmental vessels are not all the same size. For instance, if the anterior segmental branches to the upper lobes are examined carefully, it is possible to see that they can be quite short, sometimes as short as 1 cm in length, before giving rise to a subsegmental branch. The first branch may be 1 mm or less in diameter and then the continuation of the segmental artery, in reality now a subsegmental branch, may be as large as 3 mm in diameter. In this situation the segmental branch gave rise to a 1 mm diameter branch and a 3 mm diameter branch.

Perhaps the best temporary resolution to the discussion is to reflect that some subsegmental pulmonary emboli can be seen and it may well be that the visibility depends upon the size of the vessel and on the size of the embolus within the vessel. If the subsegmental branch is big enough it can be evaluated for the presence or absence of filling defects. If it is quite small, and for instance completely obstructed, it may not be possible to accurately rule in or rule out a tiny occlusive embolus. This could be the case on either CT or pulmonary angiography.

Hence efforts to actually analyse all subsegmental branches in every study can be time-consuming and somewhat unrewarding. Perhaps the best course of action is to pay attention to any vessel that is large enough and opacified well enough to analyse for the presence or absence of embolus.

Another as yet unresolved question is the relative competence of spiral/helical CT versus EBT. It will not be possible to answer this question until a head to head comparison is done in a sufficient number of patients to be statistically significant. This can be carried out only in a setting that has both methods available for use, and these settings are limited in number. Also, the comparative accuracy would have to be judged by using either pulmonary angiography or clinical follow-up as a standard of reference.

There may be a theoretical advantage to EBT because of the shorter scan time and the short total examination time, but this may be relevant only in the situation where 'small peripheral pulmonary emboli' are deemed to be of clinical consequence.

Limitations of spiral/helical CT, voiced by those experienced with the techniques, include non-visualisation of subsegmental vessels, motion artifact or unsharpness in the segmental and subsegmental vessels, inability to scan the entire chest in a single breath-hold and artifacts due to dense contrast material in the superior vena cava. These factors seem not to be a problem with EBT, where a 24 cm volume (almost the entire chest) can be scanned in 15 seconds (a reasonable single breath-hold) from the top down with thin (3 mm) collimation and undiluted contrast material without motion artifact because of short exposure time per scan (100 or 200 msec).

References

1. Boyd DP, et al. Computed transmission tomography of the heart using scanning electron beam. In: Higgins CB (ed). CT of Heart and Great Vessels; experimental evaluation in the clinical application. Futura 1983

2. McCollough B. Technical design of Ultrafast Computed Tomography. Radiol Clin N Am 1994; 32: 521–536

3. Galvin J. Ultrafast Computed Tomography of the Chest. Radiol Clin N Am 1994; 32: 775–793

4. Stephen RE, Joles H, Keyes WD, et al. Cine CT technique for dynamic airway studies. Am J Roentgenol 1985; 145: 35–36

5. Frey EE, Smith WL, Grandgeorge S. Chronic airway obstruction in children; evaluation with cine-CT. Am J Roentgenol 1987; 148: 347–352

6. Frey EE, Sato Y, Smith WL. Cine CT of the mediastinum in pediatric patients. Radiology 1987; 154: 19–23

7. Goldberg HI, Gould RG, Feuerstein IM. Evaluation of Ultrafast CT Scanning of the adult abdomen. Invest Radiol 1989; 24: 537–543

8. D'Agincourt L. Ultrafast CT makes bid in chest, body imaging. Diagn Imaging 1992; 1–5

9. Kaufmann RB, Peyser PA, Sheedy PE, et al. Quantification of coronary artery calcium by Electron Beam Computed Tomography for determination of severity of angiographic coronary artery disease in younger patients. JACC 1995; 25: 626–632

10. Gumey JW. No fooling around: direct visualization of pulmonary embolism. Radiology 1993; 188: 618–619

11. Stern EH, Webb R, Gamsu G. Dynamic Quantitative Computed Tomograhy – a predictor of pulmonary function in obstructive lung diseases. Invest Radiol 1994; 29: 564–569

12. Murata K, Takahashi M, Mori M. Chest wall and mediastinal invasion by lung cancer: Evalution with a multisection expiratory dynamic CT. Radiology 1994; 191: 251–255

13. Cutrone JA, Georgiou D, Yospur LS, et al. Metastatic spread of cervical carcinoma to the right ventricle and pulmonary arteries: diagnosis by ultrafast computed tomography. Am J Card Imaging 1995; 9: 275–279

14. Groell R, Kugler C, Aschauer M, et al. Quantitative perfusion parameters of focal nodular hyperplasia and normal liver parenchyma as determined by electron beam tomography. Br J Radiol 1995; 68: 1185–1189

15. Geraghty JJ, Stanford W, Landas K, Galvin JR. Ultrafast Computed Tomography in experimental pulmonary embolism. Invest Radiol 1992; 27: 60–63

16. Stanford W, Reiners TJ, Thompson BH, Landas SK, Galvin JR. Contrast enhanced thin slice Ultrafast Computed Tomography for the detection of small pulmonary emboli: studies using autologous emboli in the pig. Invest Radiol 1994; 29: 184–187

17. Minor RL, Oren RM, Stanford W, Ferguson DW. Biventricular thrombi and pulmonary emboli complication idiopathic dilated cardiomyopathy; diagnosis with cardiac ultrafast CT. Am Heart J 1991; 122: 1477–1481

18. Rooholamin SA, Galvin JR, Stanford W. Ultrafast CT in the detection of cardiac tumors and intracardiac and proximal pulmonary thromboembolism. Radiology 1989; 173(P): 481

19. Jamali IN, McKay CR, Embrey RP, Galvin JR. Electron beam computed tomography: use in pulmonary embolectomy. Ann Thor Surg 1995; 59: 1577–1579

20. Teigen CL, Maus TP, Sheedy PF II, et al. Diagnosis of pulmonary embolism with fast CT. Radiology 1991; 181 (P): 338

21. Teigen CL, Maus TP, Sheedy PF II, et al. Pulmonary embolism: diagnosis with electron beam CT. Radiology 1993; 188: 839–845, with reaction Radiology 1994; 191: 288–289

22. Teigen CL, Maus TP, Sheedy PF II, et al. Pulmonary embolism: diagnosis with contrast-enhanced electron beam CT and comparison with pulmonary angiography. Radiology 1995; 194: 313–319

23. Holland GA, et al. Prospective comparison of pulmonary MRA and UFCT for the diagnosis of pulmonary thromboembolic disease. Radiology 1993; 189 (P): 234

24. Sheedy PF, Welch TJ, Stanson AW, Breen JF, Maus TP. Fast CT for pulmonary embolus. Sem Ultrasound, CT, MRI 1996; 17: 324–338

25. Hoffman EA, Tajik JK, Petersen G, et al. Perfusion deficit versus anatomic visualization in detection of pulmonary emboli via EBT: validation in swine. Proceedings SPIE 1995; 2433: 26–36

26. Kalender WA. Thin-section 3D spiral CT: is isotropic imaging possible. Radiology 1995; 197: 578–580

27. Watt A. Volume rendering. In: 3D computer graphics. Addison Wesley 1993, 2nd edition; Chapter 9

28. Galvin JR, Gingrich RD, Hoffman E, et al. Ultrafast Computed Tomography of the chest. Radiol Clin N Am 1994; 32: 775–793

29. Webb WR, Stern EJ, Kanth N, Gamsu G. Dynamic pulmonary CT: findings in healthy adult men. Radiology 1993; 186: 117–124

30. Galvin JR, Gingrich RD, Hoffman E, et al. Ultrafast Computed Tomography of the chest. Radiol Clin N Am 1994; 32: 791, fig 20

31. Tajik JK, et al. An automate method for relating regional pulmonary structure and function: Integration of dynamic multislice CT and thin-slice high-resolution CT. Biomedical Image Processing and Biomedical Visualization. Proceedings SPIE 1993; 1905: 339–350

32. Wu MT, Chang JM, Chiang AA, et al. Use of quantitative CT to predict postoperative lung function in patients with lung cancer. Radiology 1994; 191: 257–262

33. Hoffman EA, et al. Matching pulmonary structure and perfusion via combined dynamic multislice CT and thin slice high-resolution CT. Comput Med Imaging Graphics 1995; 19: 101–112

34. Hoffman EA, Tajik JK, Petersen G, et al. Perfusion deficit versus anatomic visualization in detection of pulmonary emboli via EBT: validation in swine. Proceedings SPIE 1995; 2433: 30, fig. 7

35. Goldin JG, Yoon HC, Greaser LE, Nishimura E, Aberle DE. Prospective detection of pulmonary artery embolism using CT angiography in a porcine model. Am J Roentgenol 1997; 168 (Suppl): 28

36. Greaves SM. Pictorial essay: pulmonary thromboembolism: spectrum of findings in CT. Am J Roentgenol 1995; 165: 1359–1363

37. Milne ENC, Pistolesi M. Reading the chest radiograph. A physiological approach. Mosby 1993

38. Remy-Jardin M, Remy J, Cauain O, Petyt L, Wannebroucq J, Beregi JP. Diagnosis of central pulmonary embolism with helical CT: role of 2D multiplanar reformation. Am J Roentgenol 1995; 165: 1131–1138

39. Moons C. Diagnostic research; theory and application. Dissertation Erasmus University 1996

40. Remy-Jardin M, Remy J, Wattinne L, Giraud F. Central pulmonary thromboembolism: diagnosis with spiral volumetric CT with single breath-hold technique; comparison with pulmonary angiography. Radiology 1992; 185: 381–387

41. Gefter WB, Gupta KB, Holland GA. MR, CT enhanced diagnosis of pulmonary emboli. Diagn Imaging 1993; 80–85

42. Gefter WB, Habatu, Holland GA, Gupta KB, Henscke, Palevsky. Pulmonary thromboembolism: recent developments in diagnosis with CT and MRI. Radiology 1995; 197: 561–574

43. Erkel AR van, Rossum AB van, Bloem JL, Kievit J, Pattynama PM. Spiral CT angiography for suspected pulmonary embolism; a cost-effectiveness analysis. Radiology 1996; 201: 29–36

44. Rossum AB, Pattynama PMT, Tjin a Ton ER, et al. Pulmonary embolism; validation of spiral CT angiography in 149 patients. Radiology 1996; 201: 467–470

45. Quinn MF, Lundell CJ, Klotz TA, et al. Reliability of selective pulmonary arteriography in the diagnosis of pulmonary embolism. Am J Radiol 1987; 149: 469–471

46. Van Beek EJR, Bakker AJ, Reekers JA. Interobserver variability of pulmonary angiography in patients with non-diagnostic lung scan results: conventional versus digital subtraction arteriography. Radiology 1996; 198: 721–724

47. Novelline RA, Baltarowich OH, Athanasoulis CA, et al. The clinical course of patients with suspected pulmonary embolism and a negative pulmonary arteriogram. Radiology 1978; 126: 561–567

48. Van Beek EJR, Reekers JA, Batchelor D, Brandjes DPM, Peeters FLM, Büller HR. Feasibility, safety and clinical utility of angiography in patients with suspected pulmonary embolism and non-diagnostic lung scan findings. Eur Radiol 1996; 6: 415–419

49. Stein PD, Athanasoulis C, Alavi A, et al. Complications and validity of pulmonary angiography in acute pulmonary embolism. Circulation 1992; 85: 462–468

50. Dorfman GS, Cronan JJ, Tupper TB, Messersmith RN, Denny DF, Lee CH. Occult pulmonary embolism: a common occurrence in deep venous thrombosis. Am J Roentgenol 1987; 148: 263–266

51. Tetalman MR, Hoffer PB, Heck LL, Kunzmann A, Gottschalk A. Perfusion lung scan in normal volunteers. Radiology 1973; 106: 593–594

IV.8 Magnetic resonance imaging and angiography of the pulmonary vascular system

P. A. Wielopolski, M. Oudkerk, P. M. A. van Ooijen

1. MRI and MRA in the assessment of the pulmonary vasculature

Since the introduction of MRI in the late seventies, the ongoing breakthroughs in this technique have resulted in a versatile modality that offers a strong potential for a multitude of evaluation and diagnostic capabilities. Many topics have been investigated, such as pulmonary embolism (PE) [1 – 8], pulmonary circulation, blood flow patterns and vessel distensibility [7, 9], lung parenchyma [10], clots [4, 5], deep venous thrombosis [11], hypertension [5, 7] flow quantification [7], congenital defects [12] chronic versus acute conditions [6] and dynamic imaging [4, 5, 13] have been evaluated with MRI. Patient follow-up procedures after elective surgery or anticoagulant treatment can be easily performed non-invasively and may be accomplished as often as required [3, 4].

Furthermore, fast MRA promises to be an alternative for the morphological assessment of the pulmonary vascular tree and the circulatory system with the recent development of state-of-the-art MR angiographic techniques and breath-hold scan times [14, 15]. The routine administration of contrast agents has been explored to further enhance the pulmonary vasculature and parenchymal signal [16 – 18]. The use of hyperpolarised gases for mapping lung ventilation is also possible and it is undergoing major research at this stage, waiting for its validation in routine clinical practice [19, 20].

High resolution MR pulmonary angiography (MRPA), like other MRI techniques applied to the thorax, requires special attention for the following issues:

▪ Imaging in the presence of respiratory and cardiac motion [21, 22]. Well-established MRI and MRA techniques used in routine studies of the brain, neck and peripheral vasculature have not been reliable in producing consistent image quality in the thorax and abdominal vessels.

▪ Signal loss from the large magnetic field inhomogeneities present in the thoracic region (extensive air/tissue interfaces). Susceptibility differences lead to irreversible dephasing of the MR signal, especially with gradient recalled echo (GRE) techniques using thick slices (> 7 mm) and echo times (TE) > 4 msec. The signal loss that can arise translates into signal voids in the pulmonary vasculature, especially in small distal vessels, that could be misinterpreted as vessel cut-offs and confuse the diagnosis in PE cases [23, 24].

▪ Limited signal-to-noise ratios (SNR). Poor SNR often requires longer imaging time (usually improved by averaging multiple acquisitions) and consequently image quality could once more be compromised by motion.

Two features in new MRI hardware combined have made it possible to improve the quality of two-dimensional (2D) and three-dimensional (3D) MRPA. The strength and speed of the gradient system and signal reception using phased-array coil technology has provided a several-fold improvement in data encoding speed and volume coverage.

The MR gradient system is the most influential component for imaging of the pulmonary vascular anatomy with good image quality and good coverage. Recent MRI systems have imaging gradients with stronger peak gradient amplitudes (> 20 mT/m) and faster rise times (80 – 170 mT/m/msec). This results in the following improvements:

▪ Markedly increased data collection speed by making shorter repeat times (TR) possible; hence fast MRA protocols and high resolution morphologic imaging can be performed in breath-hold imaging times, together with good flexibility for balancing acquisition speed, SNR and resolution per unit time.

250

- Flow artifacts in MRA can be reduced by using shorter echo times (TE) and field echo times (FE).
- Echo times in the sub-millisecond range may be used, suppressing the effects of magnetic field inhomogeneities in GRE techniques.
- The execution of gradient events outside the acquisition window can be improved, providing better data sampling efficiency with lower acquisition bandwidths (reduced receiver sampling rates) and increased SNR.

However, increased speed can diminish SNR in the final image by an increase in acquisition bandwidth (large acquisition bandwidths produce noisier images). Fortunately, recently introduced phased-array coil technology, which covers large fields-of-view (FOV, panoramic imaging), more than doubles SNR, obtainable with body coil acquisitions, the standard for thoracic examinations [25].

The breakthrough in MRPA has been possible with a combination of these two features with the application of contrast agents for the generation of increased SNR (see Sections 8, 9 and 11).

2. MR signal formation

Spin echo and gradient echo readouts

A receiver coil acquires the MR signal from transverse magnetisation generated after the longitudinal magnetisation component stored along the main magnetic field is perturbed by radio-frequency (RF) excitation. This transverse magnetisation component can be read either in the form of a spin echo (SE) or a gradient recalled echo.

In a simple SE readout, a 90° RF excitation converts all the longitudinal magnetisation available to transverse magnetisation and is immediately followed by a 180° RF refocusing pulse to produce a spin echo (Fig. 1a). A GRE readout can collect the MR signal after the application of the 90° RF excitation but it requires that a bipolar readout imaging gradient be applied to dephase and consequently rephase the transverse magnetisation to form an echo (Fig. 1b).

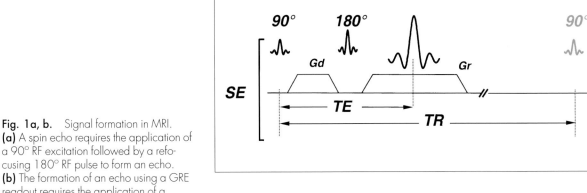

Fig. 1a, b. Signal formation in MRI.
(a) A spin echo requires the application of a 90° RF excitation followed by a refocusing 180° RF pulse to form an echo.
(b) The formation of an echo using a GRE readout requires the application of a dephasing gradient that is cancelled by a rephasing gradient to form an echo. The echo formed in SE readouts is insensitive to signal loss from magnetic field inhomogeneities and magnetic susceptibility changes with TE selected to coincide at twice the time interval between the 90°–180° RF pair, contrary in GRE readouts.
Gd = dephasing gradient;
Gr = rephasing gradient;
TR = repeat time;
TE = echo time;
α = flip angle/RF excitation angle.

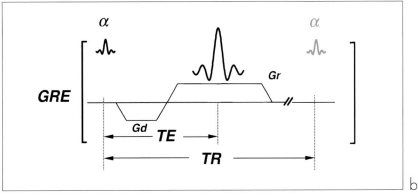

Sensitivity of spin echo and gradient recalled echo imaging to magnetic field inhomogeneities

Two-dimensional (2D) and three-dimensional (3D) acquisitions using SE techniques (and variants, see Section 4) are virtually insensitive to signal loss from field inhomogeneities (immunity to spin dephasing across a voxel, a volume element), losses that mainly arise from differences in the magnetic susceptibility between tissues . Imaging in the thorax and specifically lung parenchyma is especially problematic because of the extensive interfaces between water and air. The use of scans using SE readouts is optimal in this case. Gradient echo techniques do not share this immunity to field inhomogeneities and are regarded as less adequate for imaging the lung parenchyma.

Two-dimensional GRE techniques present greater sensitivity to signal loss (intravoxel dephasing) than their counterpart 3D GRE scans. Therefore, the latter are selected more often for imaging the pulmonary vasculature. The effect of field inhomogeneities in GRE is voxel dependent and results are improved with small voxel volumes. Thus, in addition to the use of the shortest TE possible and a 3D scan, data acquisition should proceed with the largest matrix size available and a large number of sections, all within SNR limits and scan time. These considerations minimise the intravoxel dephasing making GRE techniques compare more closely to SE techniques and provide a fast alternative to imaging in the thoracic region.

Signal manipulation and image contrast

In conventional SE imaging, proton-density, T1- and T2-weighted images are acquired by setting a specific repetition time (TR) and echo time (TE). Proton-density weighting may be acquired by using long TR and short TE. T2 weighting is adjusted by lengthening TE. Intermediate values of TR with short TE produce T1-weighted images.

The rigid $90°$-$180°$ combination in conventional SE readouts slows the longitudinal magnetisation recovery, restricting the maximum possible signal that may be requested for a particular TR. Imaging techniques using GRE readouts, on the other hand, can modify the RF excitation or flip angle ($\leq 90°$, partial flip angle imaging) to produce optimal signal strength for a specific tissue at a fixed TR value. The flexibility of GRE techniques to use partial flip angles provides proton-density, T1-, T2-, T2*- and T1/T2-weighted images with short TR settings that makes it more compatible for breath-hold imaging. Section 5 reviews some of the contrast generation strategies possible with GRE techniques.

It is important to note that recently introduced scans using SE readout variants, referred to as fast SE, make them competitive to GRE scans for fast imaging in the thorax with good signal-to-noise and resolution and single-shot imaging capabilities. Fast SE techniques make use of multiple refocusing $180°$ RF pulses after the initial $90°$ RF excitation and are discussed in more detail in Sections 4, 7 and 9.

3. MR data acquisition

The k-space matrix

The acquired MR signal is sorted into a matrix of discrete points that has been termed the k-space matrix (Fig. 2). K-space is defined as the spatial frequency domain and it contains the spatial frequencies that represent the number of sine wave cycles per unit length of an object. An inverse discrete fast Fourier transform (IFFT) is applied to this matrix to produce an anatomical image. The k-space matrix can be multidimensional, e. g., to resolve an object in three dimensions a 3D k-space matrix is collected and processed.

Relation between k-space and image signal and contrast

K-space contains information that provides all spatial frequencies acquired to form the complete image and not only a portion. However, the information in the central portion and that towards the edges of the k-space matrix defines completely different image features. The central portion of the k-space matrix (low spatial frequencies) relates to the contrast between tissues (Fig. 3a). Data points towards the edges of the k-space matrix (high spatial frequencies) characterise the smaller details and edge information in the image (Fig. 3b).

Thus, the knowledge of the contribution of each portion of the k-space matrix to the resulting image is important and has many practical implications

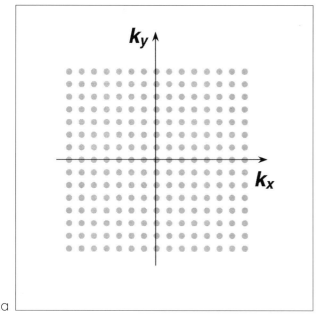

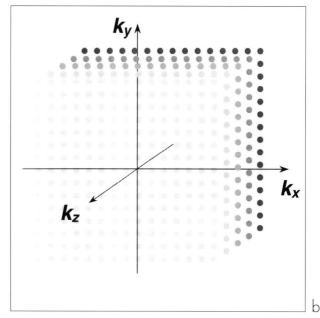

Fig. 2a, b. The k-space matrix denotes the spatial-frequency domain. The digitised MR signal is stored in this domain into a 2D **(a)** or a 3D **(b)** array of points to reconstruct a 2D or a 3D representation of the object after the application of an inverse fast Fourier transform (IFFT). The time interval between phase encoding steps (in-plane and along the section select phase encoding directions, k_y and k_z respectively) is usually associated to TR, the repetition time of the MRI experiment. In general, all points along the readout (frequency encoding) direction (k_x) are collected for each MR signal reception event.
k_x = frequency encoding direction; k_y = in-plane phase encoding direction; k_z = section select phase encoding direction.

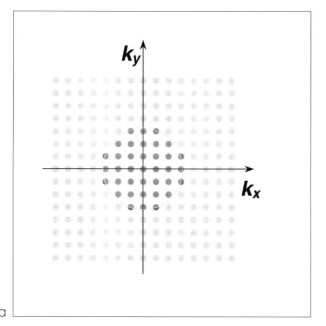

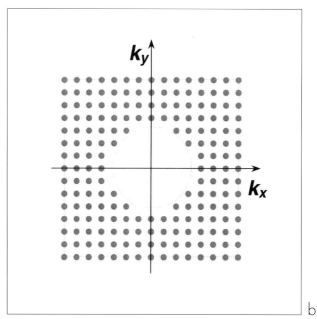

Fig. 3a, b. Each portion of k-space has different weightings in the image domain. **(a)** The centre of k-space (low spatial frequencies) mostly contains information about the resulting image contrast. **(b)** On the other hand, the edges of k-space are associated with edge information and, therefore, are linked to image resolution. Objects that are very small (on the order of a pixel or a voxel in 2D and 3D, respectively) contain energy that is spread over all k-space points.
k_x = frequency encoding direction; k_y = in-plane phase encoding direction

with respect to image contrast, SNR and resolution, especially in magnetisation-prepared GRE acquisitions (see Section 5) and acquisitions occur-ring during the transient T1 shortening induced in the blood pool with dynamic contrast injections as in contrast-enhanced MRPA (see Section 8).

2D and 3D imaging times

The time varying MR signal received is digitised to form a row of data (frequency encoding process, 1D encoding). In general, to resolve a 2D or 3D acquisition the MR signal must be repeatedly acquired and phase-encoded accordingly to form an image or a volume data set. Assuming that a single in-plane phase encoding step is acquired per TR, the time necessary to encode a 2D image is determined by

Equation 1

Acquisition time 2D $= (N_y TR)N_{acq}$

where N_y indicates the number of in-plane phase encoding steps and N_{acq} the number of signal averages performed. An extra phase encoding is required to resolve sections in a 3D acquisition. Defining the number of sections or 3D partitions as N_z, the acquisition time is given by

Equation 2

Acquisition time 3D $= (N_y TR)N_z N_{acq}$

The time to acquire a 3D data set amounts to that of a 2D acquisition weighted by the number of sections desired. Imaging time for 2D and 3D acquisitions is the same if the number of sections acquired is identical. 3D acquisitions present an additional advantage. If all imaging parameters are kept the same (TR, TE, flip angle) as in its counterpart 2D technique, the SNR of 3D acquisitions augments as the square root of the number of partitions collected.

Equations 1 and 2 only represent the imaging time in the very general case. Scan time for 2D and 3D can be shortened appropriately depending on specific phase encoding strategies (see below). Shortening scan time makes it possible to collect data using breath-holds and eliminate some of the detrimental effects that respiratory motion produces on 2D and 3D images.

Motion sensitivity of 2D and 3D imaging

3D acquisitions are most appealing for thoracic and pulmonary vascular imaging because of their SNR possibilities and reduced sensitivity to field inhomogeneities. However, 3D acquisitions present a serious drawback with respect to motion artifacts. Each section of a 2D acquisition is independent from the others acquired, while in 3D, sections are reconstructed after the data acquisition has been completed (slice-select phase encoding).

Thus, for 3D acquisitions the motion artifacts propagate across the entire data set while in 2D they will be constrained to the slices where motion occurred. Therefore, imaging planes and phase encoding directions must be carefully chosen to minimise ghosting artifacts over the lung parenchyma (see Section 8).

k-space ordering

Two basic ordering schemes are used most commonly during the filling of k-space: sequential and centric ordering. Additional k-space ordering schemes (e.g. spiral, elliptical ordering) that are important for conventional MRA and contrast-enhanced MRPA are discussed later.

Sequential ordering is standard in most MRI and MRA techniques used. Denoting N_y as the number of in-plane phase encoding lines chosen for scanning in a 2D imaging strategy, k-space is acquired from its most negative value of the phase-encoding table, $-N_y/2$, and linearly increases towards its most positive value, $N_y/2 - 1$ (Fig. 4a). This is equivalent to first filling the negative high spatial frequency information, traversing through the centre of k-space during the middle of the acquisition and ending up collecting the positive higher spatial frequencies. The centre of k-space may be acquired asymmetrically in some techniques to manipulate the image contrast more adequately (e. g., with partial Fourier scanning and contrast-enhanced MRPA; see Sections 3 and 8).

Centric ordering first encodes the centre of k-space before toggling back and forth between negative and positive phase encoding values to collect the number of N_y lines set (Fig. 4b). Thus, the first view acquired is 0, continuing to collect phase encoding lines 1, -1, 2, -2, and so forth until reaching the highest spatial frequencies (set at $N_y/2$). This scheme is used specifically to assure that image contrast, e. g., as set by a magnetisation preparation scheme (see Section 5), can be obtained in the reconstructed image virtually independent from sequence scanning parameters. This scheme has also been used for scans that commence data collected when a particular condition is reached and the contrast that develops should be encoded at that particular moment, as in "smart preparation" in contrast-enhanced MRPA (Section 8).

K-space segmentation is a concept that is associated with shorter scan times and corresponds to one of the many concepts that are used extensively in fast MRI, particularly for fast SE scans (see Section 4). In essence, k-space segmentation

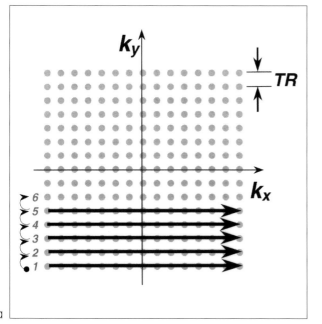 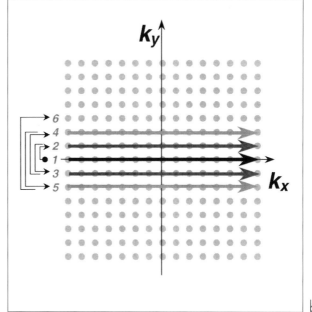

Fig. 4a, b. Sequential and centric phase-encoding schemes. **(a)** With a sequential phase-encoding order, the phase encoding table scans k-space linearly from its most negative value as defined by the maximum number of lines collected, N_y, to its most positive value. The centre of k-space is acquired during the middle of the scan. **(b)** During centric phase-encoding ordering, data is collected starting from the centre of k-space and the phase encoding table values toggle about this point to collect the positive and negative values of k-space one at a time. The arrows between k-space lines indicate the succession of the lines collected.
k_x = frequency encoding direction; k_y = in-plane phase encoding direction; TR = repetition time.

is a data collection strategy that is mainly used to fit in two particular situations:

- To share a contrast that is prepared among several lines of data collected. This is used to improve the quality of magnetisation-prepared GRE scans. It serves the purpose to eliminate the time required to repeat particular events, such a presaturation band or a pause between a string of RF excitations executed very rapidly, that would be applied for each phase encoding line.
- To collect more data that is to be synchronised with a specific physiological event, e.g., data collection during systolic or diastolic events, by lowering the time resolution of the dynamic event encoded but making it possible to collect breath-hold cine acquisitions by virtue of the time reduction involved.

The time-saving factor involved during k-space segmentation can only be envisioned with the above situations. When this is the case, this accounts for a reduction in scanning time that is proportional to the number of lines collected. K-space segmentation is usually performed in a sequential interleaved fashion (Fig. 5), that is, to collect lines as in the sequential ordering case (see above) but with

phase encoding jumps equal to the number of shots that must be performed to fill the number of phase encoding lines of the matrix size chosen. The sequential interleaved order reduces ghosting artifacts that can appear from the step-like changes in amplitude or phase in the raw data between the lines encoded by each echo.

This strategy has been used in 2D MRPA and 3D MRPA in scans that necessitate the elimination of signal from unwanted structures with a time-efficient scheme, such as the use of saturation bands to suppress venous or arterial components (see Section 7). K-space segmentation is also used to produce breath-hold scans that synchronise data collection with a specific phase of the cardiac cycle, e.g., to maximise contrast between an embolus and blood when blood inflow effects are at maximum during systole or minimise flow dephasing effects in diastole.

Shortening data collection time

Rectangular field-of-view (RecFOV) makes it possible to increase the resolution per unit time or maintain resolution with shorter scanning when an object does not fill the entire view along the in-plane phase encoding direction for a predefined FOV.

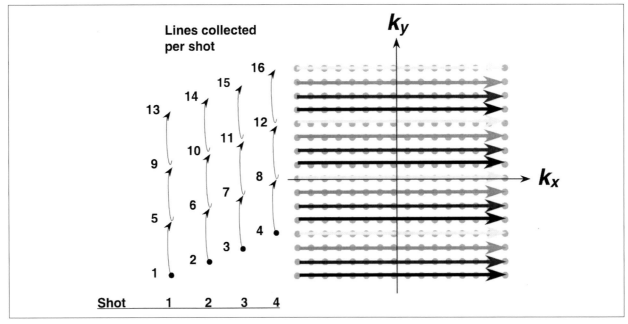

Fig. 5. With k-space segmentation a limited number of lines that share similar contrast characteristics are collected in rapid succession and placed in the raw data matrix. The pattern displayed is sequential interleaved. In this example, k-space is composed of a 16 × 16 matrix, and 4 shots collecting 4 k-space lines each has been chosen to encode the matrix. The lines are encoded in sequential order, e. g., 1, 5, 9, 13 for the first shot. If cardiac synchronisation is used, 4 heart cycles are required to fill the entire matrix. The curved arrows between k-space lines indicate the succession of the lines collected.
k_x = frequency encoding direction; k_y = in-plane phase encoding direction.

The decrease in imaging time possible is performed by scaling down the original number of in-plane phase encoding lines by the ratio between the extend of the object along the in-plane phase encoding direction and the predefined FOV. During scanning, the phase encoding gradients are amplified accordingly by this ratio while the image is compressed after the IFFT is performed to produce the correct aspect ratio.

For both 2D and 3D measurements, the acquisition time can nearly be halved by collecting half of the k-space data and use several post-processing algorithms to recover the complete resolution (Fig. 6). This has been known as partial Fourier imaging [26–28]. This is possible because of the conjugate symmetry of the Fourier transform that permits recreation of the k-space portion that was not acquired. Partial Fourier along the in-plane phase encoding direction (Fig. 6a) or along the frequency encoding direction (Fig. 6b) can be used effectively to decrease scan time without a loss in resolution. The first option is more widely known and used, consisting of decreasing the number of scanned k-space lines. Partial Fourier along the frequency encoding is particularly useful for shortening TR in MRPA scans by collecting only a partial number of points, therefore shortening the readout window and consequently TR. In this case the time saving will be greater with lower readout bandwidths.

Partial Fourier applied to GRE techniques with very short echo times (TE < 2 msec) can be attempted for MRPA without major artifacts (Figs. 6c and d). Phase cancellation from out-of-phase water-fat condition distorts the phase estimate but this is not a problem for imaging the pulmonary vasculature, as there is minimal contribution from fat signal in the lungs. Partial Fourier has a small drawback with respect to SNR, generating images that can be noisier by a factor of $\sqrt{2}$ (at most, half of the phase encoding steps are acquired as compared with full k-space coverage).

Several partial Fourier algorithms have also been devised that are more robust for reconstructing images generated with GRE techniques. The main difference between the available partial Fourier algorithms is the sensitivity of the reconstructed image to unwanted phase contributions that arise from magnetic field inhomogeneities and flowing blood [29]. Particularly, POCS (Projection onto convex sets) partial Fourier [30] improves MRPA, but has not yet been clinically implemented.

In general, the conventional data encoding process collects a rectangle or a rectangular volume of data points to form a 2D or a 3D k-space data set, respectively. However, isotropic resolution

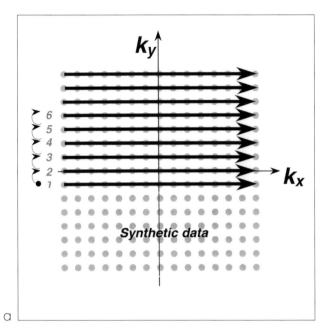

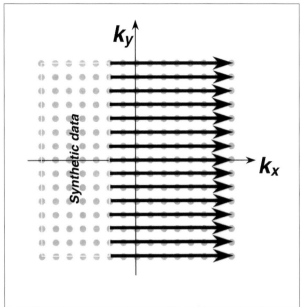

a

b

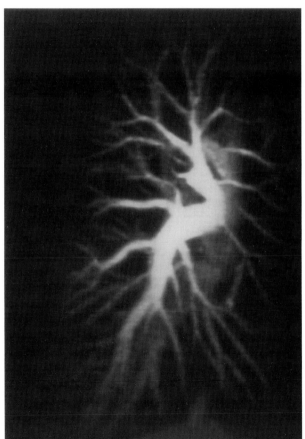

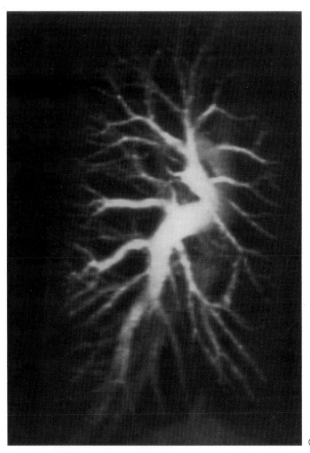

c

d

Fig. 6a–d. Partial Fourier acquisition of k-space. Ideally, only half of the k-space data is necessary to reconstruct an image without any loss in resolution. **(a)** Partial Fourier along the in-plane phase encoding direction. **(b)** Partial Fourier along the frequency encoding direction. Both strategies are useful to decrease imaging time, decreasing the number of lines and the TR used for imaging, respectively. **(c)** MIP image of a 3D MRPA scan collected with an echo asymmetric in the frequency encoding direction. **(d)** MIP image with the data processed with partial Fourier along the frequency encoding direction. Echo asymmetry was approximately 31 % (40 points rather than 128 points collected before the echo for a 256 point readout). The resolution enhancement is not as apparent on the MIP as compared to the original sections. There is an SNR penalty (maximum loss of $\sqrt{2}$) as well as fidelity in the reconstruction depending on the particular partial Fourier algorithm selected.

k_x = frequency encoding direction; k_y = in-plane phase encoding direction.

data sets for 2D images or 3D volumes are produced by collecting all data points to conform to the area of an ellipse or an ellipsoidal volume in the k-space domain, respectively, with the appropriate radius as required by the field-of-view (FOV) in each axis. For scans in which the FOV in all encoding directions and the number of data points collected is the same, the data conforms to a circle or a sphere in k-space for 2D and 3D imaging, respectively, with a diameter equal to the scanned imaging matrix.

The statement above suggests that the edges of k-space for a rectangular area or a rectangular volume of k-space data do not necessarily contribute actively in the resolution of the reconstructed images (unless the data is interpolated by zero filling to a higher matrix size, see below). Therefore, the time necessary to acquire the edges of k-space can be spared. The potential time savings are represented by the ratio between the area or volume to be encoded and that covered in the conventional case. For example, a cubic volume can be encoded using a cylinder or a sphere of k-space data (Fig. 7) to cut imaging time by approximately 21 % and 48 %, respectively.

Cylindrical acquisitions are straightforward to implement for 3D imaging and require a predetermined filling pattern that will only depend on the acquisition strategy used (e. g., normal or contrast-enhanced imaging). Although the time saving is greater if an ellipsoid is encoded, it is impossible to describe an adequate k-space trajectory with conventional signal readouts (remember that there is no inherent time saving with a conventional frequency encoding as it is possible to collect any arbitrary number of points). Therefore, special 3D k-space trajectories have been formulated that employ time-varying imaging gradients during data collection (stack of spirals, cones, etc.) [31].

The utilisation of interpolation to produce isotropic voxels (cubic volume elements), despite the size of the k-space data collected, has been advantageous for MRA to improve the overall display of vascular structures, especially for small vascular

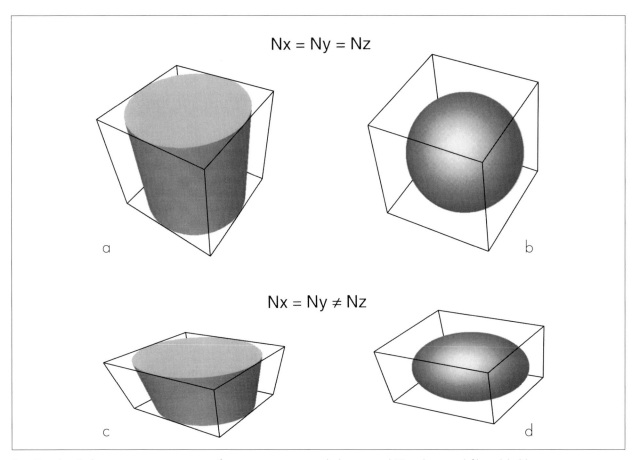

$Nx = Ny = Nz$

a

b

$Nx = Ny \neq Nz$

c

d

Fig. 7a – d. Reducing scan time is important for scanning patients with documented PE and essential if breath-hold imaging is performed. Time saving is practical for 3D imaging. Using a cylindrical coverage (**a**) or a sphere (**b**), scan time can be reduced by 21 % and 48 %, respectively, when compared to a cubic data set (time saving proportional to the ratio between the volumes scanned to that of a cube). **c**) and **d**) show the cases for 3D when the number of points along the k_z axis is different from k_x and k_y. There is no loss in resolution in either case. N_x, N_y and N_z define the number of points collected along each k-space direction.

branches. Interpolation can be performed in the image domain but it is more efficient and is more beneficial when it is performed using the raw data directly. The best interpolation possible is known as sinc interpolation. This is accomplished by placing the original raw data collected into a larger 2D or 3D matrix (reconstruction matrix) and zero-filling those k-space values that have not been collected (most commonly the outer edges of k-space) prior to image reconstruction using the IFFT. The improved vascular presentation is appreciated mostly in regions where the vessel would otherwise display a clear staircase pattern with the original reconstruction matrix (Fig. 8).

There is an additional advantage to interpolation by zero-filling, that is, it can compensate some of the signal loss that may arise from intravoxel phase cancellation (reducing the phase dispersion caused by flow dephasing or field inhomogeneities across a smaller reconstructed voxel) [32].

This property is clearly desirable for MRPA because it helps to reduce the dephasing occurring from magnetic field susceptibility differences.

Sinc interpolation is becoming increasingly popular for producing 3D image data sets with isotropic voxels without the need to increase the acquisition time, especially for breath-hold examinations. The reconstructed resolution will not be higher than that of the originally collected raw data. Nonetheless, when conventional encoding is performed (a cubic data set) the k-space values at the edges of the raw data can now help to improve the resolution. Interpolation requires additional memory to perform the computation and storage space for a larger data set.

The projection reconstruction technique has been proposed and recently reintroduced [33, 34] to mitigate susceptibility and flow artifacts by providing ultrashort TE (< 1 msec) required for a signal-loss-free MRA. Scanning time is longer than with

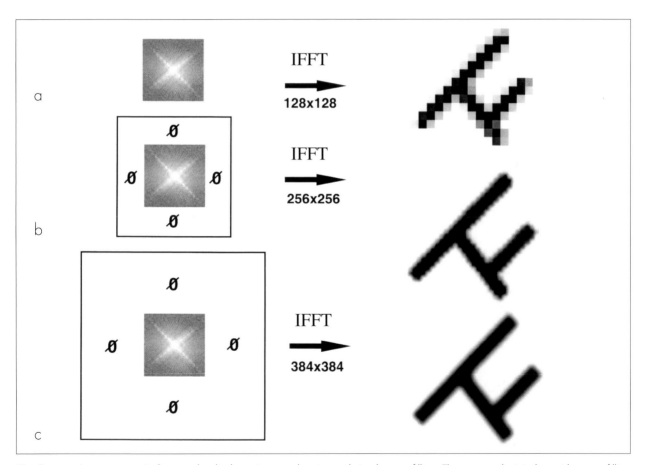

Fig. 8a–c. Improvements in the vascular display using raw data interpolation by zero filling. The process depicted considers zero filling of the raw data to a larger matrix and the application of an inverse Fourier transform to produce the interpolated image with smaller isotropic voxels. Using a raw data set of 128 × 128 points, a simulated structure is reconstructed showing a staircase pattern (a). After zero filling, the interpolation to a matrix size that is twice (256 × 256 points, (b) or trice (384 × 384 points, (c) the original size can produce a much better display of the structure without the necessity to increase scan time. By using this type of interpolation, the smaller voxels reconstructed can present less phase dispersion as well and therefore can regain some signal loss from phase effects that can prevail across the original voxel size.

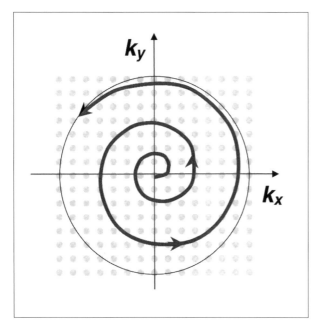

Fig. 9. Time saving is possible for 2D using a circular coverage of k-space, e. g. using a spiral k-space trajectory. The acquisition is approximately 27 % faster than that of standard spin warp encoding. The trajectory makes ultrashort TE imaging possible and it is inherently flow compensated. The gradients are oscillated in tandem to describe the trajectory.
k_x = frequency encoding direction;
k_y = in-plane phase encoding direction.

conventional spin warp imaging but new encoding and reconstruction strategies make possible higher resolution images with a substantially reduced imaging time [35].

Although spiral encoding has not yet been reported for MRPA, this k-space trajectory is becoming increasingly popular (Fig. 9) [36]. Spiral encoding describes a spiral trajectory through k-space using two gradients oscillated in tandem in the imaging plane. Spiral scanning is intrinsically flow compensated (centre of k-space is collected first) and reduces many of the blurring and displacement artifacts when visualising flowing blood. Additionally, the gradient moments of a spiral trajectory are small near the origin of k-space, smoothly varying and circularly symmetric over k-space. Rewinding is inherent in a spiral trajectory and does not require the extreme hardware requirements to achieve short TE. Acquisition is approximately 27 % faster than with standard spin warp encoding (time savings proportional to the area ratio between a square and a circle).

Both k-space encoding patterns are sensitive to static magnetic field inhomogeneities, which produces some blurring in the reconstructed image (increasing with longer readout windows).

4. Conventional and fast SE techniques

Conventional SE techniques acquire one line of data per TR. Even for a multi-echo SE scan, commonly performed to acquire images at different echo times during the same imaging session (e. g., proton-density and T2-weighted together), one single line of data is collected per image per TR. This can be a lengthy acquisition process when a long TR is required.

Fast SE (FSE) techniques have been conceived to reduce the scanning time without a significant loss in contrast (Fig. 10) [37, 38]. Fast SE features the same idea as in multi-echo SE scans but encodes the echoes generated in the same k-space matrix using the concept of k-space segmentation (see Section 3). The decrease in encoding time is specially noted for long T2-weighted scans using long TR.

Fast spin echo imaging originates from 2D RARE (Rapid Acquisition with Relaxation Enhancement) scans, a single shot imaging technique phase encoding a long train of echoes generated by multiple 180° RF refocusing pulses after the initial 90° RF excitation with a short echo train spacing (ETS)

[39]. In fast SE, the length of the echo train (ETL) has been reduced to an adequate number that balances acquisition time and filtering effects that can blur the image along the in-plane encoding direction (from signal decay in tissues with short T2).

FSE imaging shares the great advantage from conventional SE with respect to insensitivity to magnetic field inhomogeneities and presents, among other things, a better SNR profile than most GRE scans.

Although the initial application of RARE was geared to produce heavily T2-weighted images (CSF myelography and urography), the introduction of new imaging hardware and the addition of partial Fourier data collection and reconstruction (see Section 3) enables snapshot scans with good SNR and sub-second imaging times. This has made it possible to incorporate the use of HASTE (Half fourier Acquisition Single shot Turbo spin Echo) imaging (Fig. 11) [40]. HASTE has been used in many applications but its major asset is the short scanning time, making it possible to collect images in uncooperative patients and scan in the

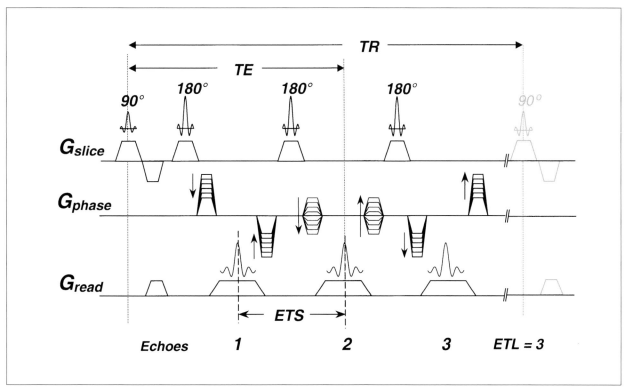

Fig. 10. Fast SE imaging. A 90° RF excitation pulse is followed by a string of 180° refocusing RF pulses that are closely spaced. One echo is generated for each 180° RF pulse applied. The separation between the 180° or the echoes is known as echo train spacing or ETS. The signal of the echo train generated decays with the T2 relaxation of the tissues imaged. The echoes are usually encoded in k-space using a sequential interleaved trajectory (see Fig. 5). The echo that coincides with the centre of k-space mainly determines the image contrast. In this example, 3 echoes are collected. The second echo weights the resulting image contrast. Scan time is 1/3 of that of a conventional SE readout. TR is defined as the total time necessary per shot.

N_y = number of in-plane phase encoding lines; $N_{shot} = N_y/ETL$ = number of shots; G_{read} = readout gradient; G_{phase} = in-plane phase encoding; G_{slice} = section select gradient; ETL = echo train length; ETS = echo train spacing.

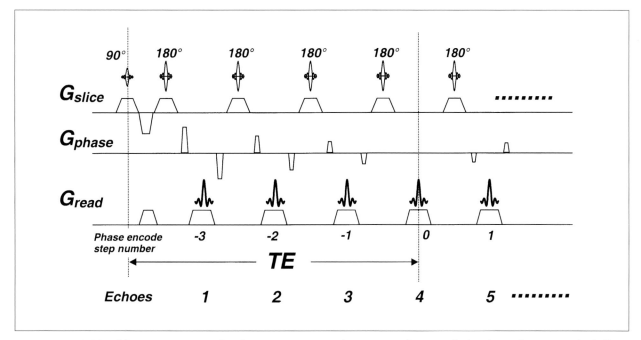

Fig. 11. HASTE (Half fourier Acquisition with Turbo SE) imaging. Partial Fourier encoding is applied to shorten the scan time by half. The contrast is defined by the echo that is made to coincide with the centre of k-space (the 4th echo in the diagram). The echo train length (ETL) is equal to the number of in-plane phase encoding steps, N_y. The TR is infinite because of the single shot nature of the scan.

G_{read} = readout gradient; G_{phase} = in-plane phase encoding; G_{slice} = section select gradient

thorax without the necessity of breath-holding. Because the image is collected under a long echo train decaying with T2, blurring along the in-plane phase encoding is generally observed for tissues with short T2 relaxation times. The amount of blurring is dictated by the T2 relaxation time of each tissue with respect to the length of the acquisition.

5. Gradient recalled echo imaging

GRE imaging offers a variety of tissue contrast possibilities that can be generated in the same imaging time without changing TR, opposite to what is generally possible with SE readouts. Proton-density, T1-, T2- and T1/T2-weighting is possible depending on the strength and state of the transverse and longitudinal magnetisation components for a particular T1 and T2 and a choice of TR and RF excitation angle.

There are two major distinctions between GRE sequences depending on the state of the longitudinal and transverse magnetisation. Steady-state incoherent (SSI) GRE techniques refer to those techniques in which only the longitudinal magnetisation is used during the acquisition. Techniques that combine both longitudinal and transverse magnetisation components to generate the signal are referred to as steady-state coherent (SSC) GRE techniques (see Section 10).

In SSI GRE techniques the signal contribution to the image formation comes exclusively from longitudinal magnetisation recovered between two successive RF excitations. The acronym FLASH (Fast Low Angle SHot) has been used extensively (other acronyms comprise RF-spoiled GRASS or SPGR, spoiled Gradient Recalled Acquisition in the Steady State (see Haacke et al. [41] for a summary of all abbreviations used by system manufacturers for most techniques clinically available). Figure 12 illustrates a typical 3D FLASH sequence diagram.

The signal intensity for SSI GRE techniques assumes no contribution from transverse magnetisation prior to each RF excitation to the signal formation, resulting in a very well known expression given by

Equation 3

$$S = \frac{M_o \sin\alpha (1 - E1) E2^*}{(1 - \cos\alpha E1)}$$

where α is the RF flip angle, $E1 = \exp(-TR/T1)$ and $E2^* = \exp(-TE/T2^*)$. This expression is important for setting the optimal imaging parameter corresponding to a specific T1 relaxation time.

For sufficiently small flip angles and short TR, the image contrast is predominantly proton-density weighted ($S \sim M_o \sin\alpha$); otherwise, T1 contrast can develop at larger flip angles. T2* weighting can

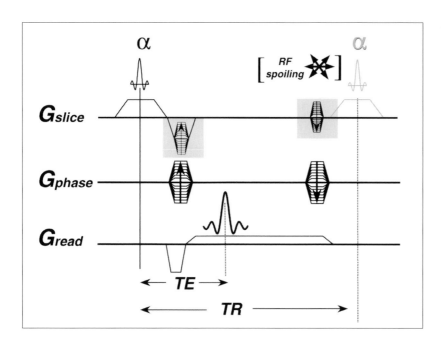

Fig. 12. Diagram of a 3D SSI GRE imaging technique primarily referred to as FLASH (Fast Low Angle SHot) imaging. The use of RF spoiling (changing the phase of the RF angle per phase encoding step in conjunction with rewinder phase encoding tables after reading the signal) is effective for producing signal that is weighted by only the longitudinal magnetisation component during steady-state conditions. FLASH is also known as RF-spoiled gradient recalled acquisition in the steady state (RF-spoiled GRASS).

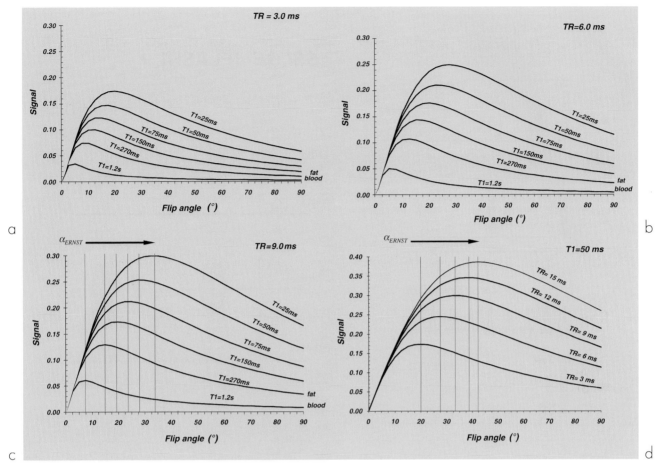

Fig. 13a–d. Signal intensity behaviour for SSI GRE techniques (FLASH imaging). Simulations performed for different values of TR for several T1 relaxation values as a function of flip angle **(a)** TR = 3.0 msec, **(b)** TR = 6.0 msec, **(c)** TR = 9.0 msec. Note in **(c)** the arrow indicating that the Ernst angle, the RF excitation that produces optimal SNR, increases as the T1 relaxation decreases at a fixed TR. In **(d)**, a fixed T1 of 50 illustrates that optimal SNR is met at increasing RF flip angles with longer TRs. T1 relaxation values considered were 25 msec, 50 msec, 75 msec, 150 msec, 270 msec and 1,200 msec. The longest values correspond to the T1 relaxation of fat and blood, respectively. Short T1 relaxation values have been chosen to illustrate the enhancement possible when using paramagnetic and superparamagnetic contrast agents to enhance the signal of blood.

only be generated by lengthening TE, making the image more sensitive to signal loss from susceptibility changes between air/tissue interfaces (or within a blood clot). Figure 13 illustrates the signal behaviour for various T1 relaxation values and TR. For SSI GRE imaging applied at a particular TR, the maximum signal can be obtained by choosing the RF excitation at the optimal angle, usually referred to as the Ernst angle or α_E (E tref) E. The Ernst angle is given by

Equation 4

$$\alpha_E = \cos^{-1}(E1)$$

At α_E (E tref), the signal will be

Equation 5

$$S\alpha_E = \sqrt{\frac{1 - E1}{1 + E1}}$$

Which is roughly proportional to $\sqrt{TR/2T1}$. For a fixed TR, the Ernst angle decreases as T1 increases and, vice versa, a decrease in T1 will increase the Ernst angle. Figure 13d illustrates the signal behaviour for a fixed T1 and a varying TR indicating that higher flip angles are necessary to obtain the optimal signal at longer TR. Maximum contrast between two tissues occurs at a different flip angle than the Ernst angle. All the above equations are necessary to calculate the optimal excitation for contrast-enhanced MRA scans.

Generally, GRE sequences for MRPA will refer to the application of SSI GRE techniques.

A magnetisation preparation (MP) period prior to a short TR SSI GRE sequence (a FLASH sequence), as depicted in Figure 14, can modify effectively the initial longitudinal magnetisation to produce an image with improved contrast with sub-second SSI GRE acquisitions. This technique has been known as turboFLASH imaging [42].

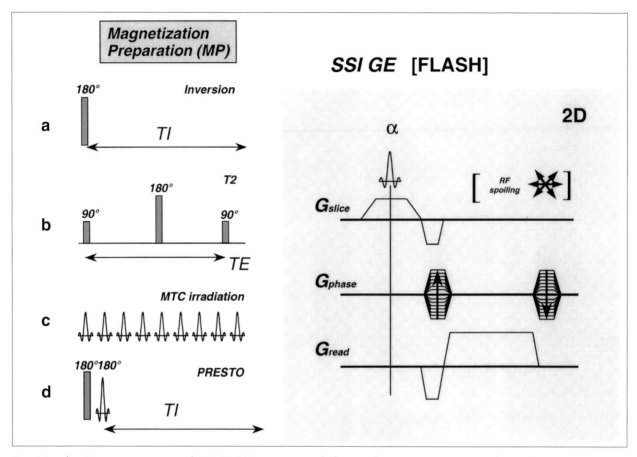

Fig. 14a–d. Magnetisation prepared (MP) SSI GRE acquisition with short TR. The MP stage may consist of a simple 180° pre-inversion pulse (inversion recovery) to provide strong T1-weighting **(a)**. A 90°x–180°y–90°x driven equilibrium pulse scheme produces T2-weighting **(b)**. A long train of RF pulses can be used to augment the magnetisation transfer contrast (MTC) and accentuate signal attenuation in tissues with higher density of bound water molecules **(c)**. A black blood preparation can be used. This executes a non-selective inversion over the entire imaging volume immediately followed by a selective inversion to restore full magnetisation in the imaging slice. For **(d)**, imaging is performed after a suitable delay time (inversion time of blood, TI = T1 · ln 2 ~800 msec) that permits the inflow of initially inverted blood into the imaging region and procures a null longitudinal magnetisation to render blood black. This MP is known as a PRESTO preparation and is used in a multitude of imaging scenarios to help eliminate the signal from blood while maintaining high SNR for stationary tissues.
FLASH = Fast Low Angle SHot; TE = echo time; TI = inversion time; G_{slice} = slice selection gradient; G_{phase} = phase encoding gradient; G_{read} = frequency encoding gradient; α = RF flip angle.

Increased T1 weighting is possible after the application of an inversion pulse (Fig. 14a). A T2 magnetisation preparation scheme or magnetisation transfer pulses can also be applied (Figs. 14b and c, respectively). A special preparation that has been increasingly used in later years for many techniques is referred to as a black blood preparation or PRESTO, illustrated in Figure 14d [43] (see also Section 9). The methodology of MP SSI GRE scans has been applied effectively for the detection of pulmonary emboli for 2D and 3D scans (see Section 9). Additionally, the T1 weighted turboFLASH sequence is generally used for timing the delivery of contrast material in contrast-enhanced MRPA scans

A transient behaviour develops, related to the approach to steady-state, between the prepared longitudinal magnetisation and the signal obtained during the application of the string of RF excitations that is used to form the signal. During this transient, the signal can be encoded. The equations that drive the signal evolution of different magnetization preparation SSI experiments is given by

Equation 6

$$M_o \sin\alpha [M_s + (M_t - M_s)r^{n-1}] \text{ for } n \geq 1$$

in which the term M_t is directly related to the state of the magnetisation after the application of the particular RF scheme that will encode the desired contrast (T1, T2, diffusion weighting, etc.). Equation 7 indicates some useful values for M_t,

Equation 7

$$M_t = 1 \tag{a}$$
$$M_t = (1 - 2E_{TI}) \tag{b}$$

$$M_t = \frac{M_s q(1 - r^{N-1}) + 1 - E_{TW}}{1 - qr^{N-1}} \qquad \text{(c)}$$

$$M_t = \frac{E_{Ti}[M_s q(r^{N-1} - 1) + E_{TW} - 2] + 1}{1 - E_{TI}qr^{N-1}} \qquad \text{(d)}$$

where $E1 = \exp(-TR/T1)$, $r = E1\cos\alpha$, $M_s = (1-E1)/(1-r)$, $E_{TI} = \exp(-TI/T1)$, $E_{TW} = \exp(-TW/T1)$ and $q = E_{TW}\cos\alpha$. Equation 7a demonstrates that the longitudinal magnetisation starts from Mo for a simple 2D SSI GRE scan that collects data during the approach to steady-state. Equation 7b is the typical signal received when the MP is an inversion pulse where TI is the inversion time to the start of data collection. Equation 7c and Equation 7d are general extensions to Equation 7a and Equation 7b in which the experiment is continuously repeated with an effective pause or a recovery interval TW. This is useful for a 2D scan exciting the same slice repeatedly or a 3D experiment.

The approach to steady-state produces different signal strengths during data encoding. This introduces a filter function that can affect the resolution and the appearance of each tissue depending on their size relative to the imaging field-of-view and the specific pattern utilised to fill k-space. The filter function is complex but may be regarded as a high pass filter that enhances sharp features such as edges and tissue boundaries. Edge enhancement is more prominent with an inversion pulse used for the magnetisation preparation, which is important for morphological imaging and for detection of pulmonary emboli.

6. MR properties of lung parenchyma, blood and blood clots

Three tissue MR parameters have been predominantly used to produce the differentiation between tissues: the proton density, the T1 relaxation time (rate of recovery of the longitudinal magnetisation) and the T2 relaxation time (rate of decay of the transverse magnetisation). Only the latter two can be exploited adequately to provide the necessary differentiation between blood and blood clots.

The water distribution and relaxation times of lung parenchyma are difficult to quantify due to the cyclic alteration of blood flow through the vessels, cardiac output, vascular permeability and changes in position and inflation during respiration. There is a large difference in the amount of blood present proportional to lung tissue and interstitial fluid in the least dependent areas when compared with that seen in the lower zones of the lung where the vasculature is distended with blood.

The composition of the lung is gravity-dependent, and this contributes to the complexity of the data interpretation. The various perfusion zones help create a continuous change in the lung composition from the least dependent to the most dependent areas. Thus the proton density and relaxation parameters are related to the proportion of blood in relation to air, lung tissue and interstitial fluid and differences should be expected depending on the measurement site. A more detailed description of the magnetic properties of lung parenchyma has been compiled by Cutillo [44].

The MR signal of blood is proportional to its proton density, which is similar to that of other tissues and constituents. The relaxation times in blood have been found to be a linear function of the hematocrit (H). This is a direct consequence of the fast exchange occurring between the intracellular and extracellular water due to the random passage of water molecules, particularly between the plasma and the red blood cells (RBCs) [45–47].

The relaxation rates of blood, R_{blood}, depend predominantly on the relaxation rates of the RBCs ($1/\tau_c$) and the plasma ($1/\tau_p$), weighted by the relative population of protons existing in each environment, fc and fp, respectively (see Table 1). Thus,

Equation 8

$$\begin{aligned} R_{blood} &= \frac{fc}{\tau_c} + \frac{fp}{\tau_p} \\ &= \frac{H}{\tau_c} + \frac{1-H}{\tau_p} \\ &= \frac{1}{\tau_c} + H\left(\frac{1}{\tau_c} + \frac{1}{\tau_p}\right) \end{aligned}$$

Paramagnetic relaxation effects are usually not seen in most tissues. Blood is an exception in that its properties are strongly coupled to the presence of hemoglobin (Hb) in the RBCs and its oxidation states. Thus, the relaxation in whole blood is similar to that of an Hb solution, despite the effects of

Table 1. Relaxation times for blood and plasma. T2 measurements performed with a Meiboom-Gill-Carr-Purcell sequence using an interpulse spacing of 3 msec.

Variable	T1 (msec)	T2 (msec)
Anticoagulant Plasma		
EDTA	1,754	455
Citrate	1,786	526
Heparin	1,563	455
Blood		
EDTA	1,124	181
Citrate	1,042	222
Heparin	1,064	182

EDTA = sodium ethylenediaminetetraacetate
citrate = sodium citrate (adapted from reference [45])

membrane exchanges and of plasma proteins [48, 49].

Hemoglobin binds free O_2 to form oxyhemoglobin (oxyHb) when the O_2 binds to the heme iron in its reduced ferrous state (Fe^{++}). Hemoglobin alternates between oxyhemoglobin and deoxyhemoglobin (deoxyHb) as the oxygen is exchanged between the RBCs in the lungs and capillaries.

When the blood is exposed to certain drugs, or oxidising agents in vitro or in vivo, the ferrous iron (Fe^{++}) of the molecule is converted into ferric iron (Fe^{+++}) forming methemoglobin (metHB). In the circulation, some oxidation of deoxyHb occurs transforming a portion of the deoxyHb into metHb. Nevertheless, an enzymatic system in the RBCs, the NADH-methemoglobin reductase (NADH is the reduced form of nicotinamide-adenine dinucleotide), converts the metHb into deoxyHb again.

Table 2. Relative change in the relaxation times of blood for different stages in the oxidation process.

Stages	T1	T2
Intact RBC with oxyHb	=	=
Intact RBC with deoxyHb	=	<<
Intact RBC with metHb	<<	<<
Free metHb	<<	>
Hemosiderin	=	<<

> indicates prolongation of relaxation time
<< indicates marked shortening
= indicates no change (from reference [171])

With continued oxidative denaturation, metHb is further reduced to derivatives known as hemichromes.

In blood, the paramagnetic properties are confined to the RBCs. DeoxyHb and metHb are paramagnetic because they contain unpaired electrons, while oxyHb is not, given that the heme iron electron spin is cancelled by the oxygen electron spin. Hemichromes do not have unpaired electrons like metHb does, so the molecule is not paramagnetic.

The paramagnetism of deoxyHb and metHb can affect the relaxation times in two ways. The first is seen in deoxyHb and metHb, and it manifests itself as shortening in the T2 relaxation time, a consequence of the presence of increased magnetic field inhomogeneities. This is caused by the concentration of Hb in RBCs which produces microscopic magnetic field inhomogeneities that increase the dephasing effects of diffusing molecules between the RBC interior and the extracellular plasma [46–49]. Even with the use of SE readouts, the effect is marked because water molecules diffuse to regions with very different magnetic field strengths within small distances between RF excitations that increases phase dispersion, even more when the field inhomogeneities are not static, as in this case.

The dependence of T2 has been investigated using a Meiboom-Gill-Carr-Purcell pulse sequence (Table 1). This has provided an estimate for the mean residence time of water inside the RBC of about 10 msec [46]. The T2 shortening and susceptibility effects (comprised under T2*) are better seen with GRE imaging techniques [50], producing major signal attenuation with increasing echo times, illustrating the magnitude of the field inhomogeneities present. The T2 relaxation enhancement increases as the square of the local field gradient and it has been demonstrated to be as much as 1.6 times stronger for intracellular metHb than for extracellular deoxyHb [49]. Biologic field gradients are caused by the heterogeneity in magnetic susceptibility and are directly proportional to the applied main magnetic field. The T2 relaxation of RBC lysates does not change with different magnetic field strengths because the susceptibility effects once present when RBCs were intact is eliminated.

On the other hand, the direct magnetic interaction between the water protons with unpaired electron spins reduces the T1 relaxation time, as in the case of metHb (distances between Hb and water molecules are well within 3 Å). This effect is not possible in deoxyHb because the water molecules cannot approach the heme iron closely enough to

Table 3. Appearance of hemorrhage at different stages of clot formation. Signals in T1- and T2-weighted scans as compared against white matter.

Stage	Time	Comp	Hemoglobin	T1	T2
Hyperacute	≤ 24 h	Intra	OxyHb	low	high
Acute	1 – 3 d	Intra	DeoxyHb	isointense	low
Subacute					
Early	3 + d	Intra	MetHb	high	low
Late	7 + d	Extra	MetHb	high	midly high
Chronic					
Center		Extra	Hemichromes	medium	medium
Rim	14 + d	Intra	Hemosiderin	low	low

Comp = composition/intracellular/extracellular (adapted from Reference [48])

make an important contribution to proton relaxation enhancement. Much of the T1 relaxation enhancement is also due to the electron spin relaxation time of metHb, which is closer to the Larmor frequencies used in MRI [48]. Table 2 summarises the changes in the relaxation times for the different stages of oxidation of blood as compared to intact blood.

The proportion of fibrin, platelets, RBCs and other components varies for each clot and over time as Hb progresses from its oxygenated state to deoxyHb, to metHb, and finally to hemisiderin. Acute intracerebral hemorrhage contains blood at varying stages of clot formation and retraction and the effects on the relaxation times are depicted in Table 3, showing the form of hemoglobin that prevails for each clot formation stage. The relaxation rates for blood and plasma before and after clotting are summarised in Table 4. These are the relaxation times that must be taken into account when defining the sensitivity of a specific MRI technique to clot detection within a vessel.

Improved contrast between blood and thrombi can be obtained by taking advantage of blood motion itself. Blood flow has been exploited extensively to form the basis of conventional time-of-flight (TOF) and phase-contrast MRA evaluations (see below). In essence, in TOF MRA techniques stationary tissue will remain with relatively low signal whenever the signal enhancement possible by flowing blood into the imaging section is high. In phase-contrast MRA, the phase that can be accumulated from moving blood (essentially the phase is made proportional to flow velocity) is the mechanism that provides contrast while stationary

signal will have a null contribution to the formation of the vascular image. This can be performed with both SE and GRE techniques but most MRA used today fall into the latter category. In both TOF and phase contrast techniques, the signal from thrombi can be low but the range of signal variability depending on the age of blood clots (variable T1 relaxation values, see above) will modulate the contrast possible with TOF MRA.

Other methodology has also been exploited, mostly with the use of techniques using SE readouts. Blood motion can provide negative contrast, that is, provide an image in which blood will have no signal while surrounding tissues will have higher signal intensities. These techniques fall under what has been referred to as black blood MRA (Section 9). Thrombi can be rendered bright against the darker signal from blood.

Table 4. Relaxation times for blood and plasma before and after clotting. T2 measurements performed with a Carr-Purcell-Meiboom-Gill sequence using an ETS spacing of 3 msec (adapted from reference [45]).

	T1 (msec)	T2 (msec)
Plasma		
Before clotting	1,639	500
Unretracted clot	1,724	500
Retracted clot	1,667	208
Blood		
Before clotting	1,250	182
Unretracted clot	1,205	172
Retracted clot	833	95

7. Conventional MRPA

Basic principles

Conventional MRA is defined as all MRA techniques that only exploit the effects of blood motion to sensitise the MR signal accordingly to provide vascular contrast. MRA techniques can use blood flow to produce higher signal than surrounding tissues through a time-of-flight (TOF) phenomena or induce motion dependent changes in the phase of the MR signal received (mainly sensitising the signal to blood velocity) [51]. Techniques using the latter effect are the basis of phase contrast MRA and flow quantification techniques [52].

The low proton density of the lung parenchyma surrounding the pulmonary vessels provides signal that is practically that of background noise. This fact alone provides superb contrast for identifying the pulmonary vessels using either SE or GRE techniques [53]. The fact that background signal is nearly non-existent is rather unique for this region of the body and can be exploited effectively. TOF MRA rather than phase contrast MRA protocols has been exploited because of this fact, as it is not necessary to suppress background tissue. Additionally, TOF MRA is faster, which reduces the detrimental effects of motion with large volume coverage and breath-hold imaging capabilities.

Vascular enhancement with TOF MRA is produced from the higher signal amplitude produced when fully magnetised blood enters the imaging slice or imaging volume that contains stationary tissues with a lower steady-state signal.

During data acquisition stationary tissue reaches a steady state value (saturation state, Equation 3). Fully magnetised blood may enter the imaging volume and replace or mix with previously excited blood, providing additional magnetisation that stationary tissues do not see. Blood saturation can occur, particularly in a 3D experiment as the spin travels through the imaging volume after experiencing many RF excitations, which drives its signal to its particular steady-state value (given also by Equation 3).

Many parameters influence the blood signal in conventional TOF MRA. The signal is a function of the longitudinal magnetisation of blood, its flow velocity, the relative vessel position with respect to the imaging volume and scanning parameters such as TR, RF excitation angle and the spatial dependence of the RF excitation profile.

Considering a plug-like flow profile for a vessel entering perpendicular to the imaging volume with a constant velocity V_f, the number of RF excitation pulses (NRF) that flowing blood experiences at location D downstream from the edge of the volume is

Equation 9

$$N_{RF} = \text{integer part of} \left(\frac{D}{V_f TR} \right)$$

The signal from blood along the vessel from the edge of the volume will evolve in a similar fashion as the approach to steady state for an SSI GRE sequence starting from fully magnetised blood. That is, the same temporal behaviour seen with the approach to steady state (see Section 5) can be observed spatially varying along the vessel from the entry point to the imaging volume. As seen from the edge of the volume, the signal from fully magnetised blood along the vessel due to inflow of freshly magnetised spins evolves toward equilibrium conditions following the same behaviour as the approach to equilibrium curve for FLASH in a stationary tissue. Equation 10 describes the signal behaviour along a vessel with constant plug flow perpendicular to the imaging volume for a standard TOF experiment for blood crossing an imaging volume with a constant RF excitation (usually not the case, see below),

Equation 10

$$S = M_o \sin\alpha \left[M_s + (1 - M_s)r^{n-1} \right]$$

where $E1 = \exp(-TR/T1)$, $r = E1 \cos\alpha$ and $Ms = (1 - E1)/(1 - r)$, α being the RF excitation angle. The signal at position D is calculated by setting $n = N_{RF}$ according to Equation 9. Note the resemblance between Equation 10 and that of the approach to equilibrium of a SSI GRE experiment as stated by Equation 6 with $M_i = 1$. This indicates that the temporal variation of the signal of blood as it receives an increasing number of excitations appears spatially imprinted along a vessel with blood flowing into the volume at a constant velocity.

Equation 9 indicated that the number of RF pulses experienced by flowing blood is preserved as long as the product $V_f TR$ is maintained constant, indicating that any combination that satisfies this condition will provide the same enhancement pattern along the vessel. For any blood flow velocity, the enhancement along the vessel will be more uniform at longer TR (complete refreshment/replacement). Likewise, blood entering at higher velocities with shorter TR will produce a similar effect if the product $V_f TR$ is the same. Nevertheless, the contrast between the flowing spins and surrounding stationary material will be greater in the latter case, which is desirable for better blood/blood clot contrast because surrounding tissue will saturate more at shorter TRs. The opposite situation arises when lower flow velocities and short TR are selected, resulting in a fast decay of the signal along the vessel, especially when a high flip angle is used. As the number of excitations experienced by blood within the imaging volume increases, the optimal signal enhancement approaches the optimal flip angle for SSI GRE imaging during steady-state conditions, expressed by the Ernst angle (see Equation 4).

The variation in flow velocities in the pulmonary arteries can be large between healthy patients suspected of PE and those that are afflicted by the condition. Therefore, it is necessary to know a priori the flow velocities in order to select an adequate flip angle, given that TR is usually maintained constant to maintain the same imaging time and resolution for all studies (using either breath-hold or free-breathing scans).

Vascular signal enhancement

Significant signal enhancement for blood can be obtained using a form of excitation-recovery scheme that has been termed as a syncopated excitation in early MRPA literature [53]. For a 3D SSI GRE scan, a syncopation is performed by disrupting the steady-state signal of tissue receiving multiple RF excitations (usually set to the number of sections encoded) by including a recovery period between in-plane phase encoding lines. For blood moving into a region of interest, the recovery time incorporated helps its magnetisation to be replenished faster and for a longer vessel stretch (through inflow) than that of surrounding tissues. Several k-space ordering schemes may be used to augment the signal from blood in this case, not readily possible with a steady-state approach.

Incorporating the wait period, denoted here as TW, after a finite number of RF excitations, N, before proceeding to encode another portion of k-space leads to a signal evolution that is characterised by

Equation 11

$$S(k,n) = M_o \sin\alpha \left[M_s(1 - r^{n-1}) + TR^n - 1 \right]$$

where

$$T = \frac{M_s q(1 - r^{N-1}) - E_{TW} + 1}{1 + qr^{N-1}}$$

with $E_{TW} = \exp(-TW/T1)$, $E1 = \exp(-TR/T1)$, $q = E_{TW}\cos\alpha$ and $r = E1\cos\alpha$. Equation 11 is derived by setting the magnetisation at a particular excitation during the RF string to be equivalent to the magnetisation at the corresponding excitation in the preceding RF string, so that a steady-state regime is forced. The index k is analogous to any of the in-plane phase-encoding steps and n relates to one of the RF excitations utilised to encode N sections. In practice, Equation 11 is only part of the contribution to the signal of flowing blood as it occurs that during the acquisition, inflow effects still modulate the signal in the blood vessel. The effects are clearly seen as TR becomes shorter, higher flip angles are used and a centric ordered acquisition of k-space is performed.

The signal for flowing blood at a constant velocity in a 3D SSI GRE scan using an ideal RF excitation (rectangular profile) obeys Equation 6. In practice, however, the slice excitation profiles are not ideal and do not excite portions of the volume with the same RF excitation angle. This situation is not desirable when a target image contrast is required within the entire imaging volume (e.g. T1-weighted imaging of the brain). Nonetheless, the non-ideal excitation profile is more interesting in the context of MRA, even more so for MRPA.

As blood enters the imaging volume it experiences an increasing number of excitations and, in the case of a non-ideal RF excitation profile, different flip angles along its path. Because saturation will always occur as blood experiences more RF pulses, a vessel will demonstrate this signal decay. Nonetheless, it is possible to devise an RF excitation profile that helps counteract this saturation effect, making it possible to maintain approximately the same signal for a specific length along the vessel path. The creation of an RF profile that satisfies such conditions has been investigated by several researchers, using RF excitation profiles with the acronyms TONE (Tilted Optimised N Excitation) [54] and VUSE (Variable-angle Uniform Signal Excitation) [55], the latter designed to take into account an average velocity for moving blood and resulting in statistically better enhancement for MRPA than the former. Figure 15 illustrates a diagram comparing both concepts against the ideal excitation profile. VUSE is the spatial analogue to the optimisation performed when using SSI sequences with a temporally incremental RF excitation angle tuned to a particular T1 relaxation time [56]. The end excitation angle at the edge of the volume (opposite to the inflow site) is set to 90° (within the limits of the RF amplifier when using short RF excitation pulses).

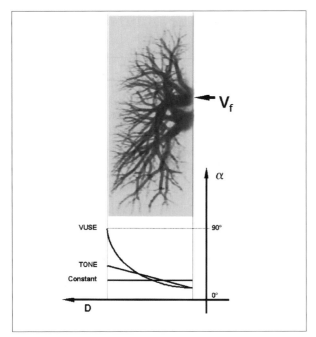

Fig. 15. Signal optimisation for conventional arterial MRPA using spatially varying RF excitation profiles. For freshly magnetised blood entering the right pulmonary tree in this example, the RF angle that blood sees as it travels into the imaged volume can be optimised to produce a homogeneous vascular enhancement from the entrance point towards higher order branches. Two profiles have been investigated. TONE (tilted optimised non-saturating excitation) creates a linearly varying RF flip angle along the imaging volume. VUSE (variable-angle uniform signal excitation), is the spatial equivalent to the approach to equilibrium signal given by Equation 6, and produces the best enhancement possible. Both TONE and VUSE profiles are optimised by estimating the inflow blood flow velocity into the pulmonary arterial tree. Constant flip angles produce an uneven enhancement when high flip angles are used, with lower flip angles SNR is not optimal but the enhancement is homogeneous. The VUSE profiles provide additional suppression of veins as the end flip angle towards the opposite edge of the volume approaches 90°.

Asymmetric echo readouts and RF excitations

To reduce the sensitivity to flow artifacts and susceptibility artifacts for MRPA, compact gradient waveforms with shorter echo and field echo (FE) times must be used. The parameter FE denotes the time that it takes to produce an echo along the readout direction from the instant the readout gradient is switched on. This has been accomplished by collecting the echo asymmetrically [57], setting the number of data points collected before the echo formation as a design parameter. In practice, MRA and MRPA sequences have been implemented with an echo asymmetry of 50% (e.g., echo centred at $^1/_4$ of the readout window) in conjunction with motion compensated gradient waveforms. The echo asymmetry is defined here as the percentage ratio between twice the number of

points sampled before the echo and the number of points collected along the frequency encoding direction. Slightly higher degrees of echo asymmetry have also been used to permit smaller FOV and shorter TR, necessary for good spatial coverage and resolution in breath-hold MRPA. When higher degrees of echo asymmetry are employed, resolution loss can be restored using partial Fourier reconstruction techniques or specialised processing such as CORE (Constrained Reconstruction) (Fig. 6) [26, 58].

Section selection and slice-select phase encoding are time-consuming processes with conventional spin warp encoding. For MRPA a substantial reduction in the section select refocusing is possible by using as well asymmetric RF pulses [59] without distorting the slice profiles significantly. This concept is similar to that of the asymmetric echo along the readout direction described above. This strategy makes it possible to refocus the excited spins faster and relaxes the gradient requirements needed for more compact gradient waveforms. These schemes also prove effective for producing a shorter TE.

MRPA techniques

Spin echo pulse sequences are typically associated with low signal from flowing blood. However, with the incorporation of gradient moment nulling techniques for flow and motion compensation, the pulmonary vasculature could be displayed hyperintense on SE images over the lung parenchyma (Fig. 16a). Short echo times and thick slices were selected to minimise the washout of blood spins, making sure that flowing blood is exposed to both the exciting and refocusing portion of the spin echo sequence. Cardiac triggering is used to collect the data during diastole, when the blood flow velocity in the pulmonary arteries is lowest. Drawbacks include restricted volume coverage, lengthy imaging times, and overlap of arterial and venous information. Images may also suffer considerably from respiratory ghosting artifacts from subcutaneous and intrathoracic fat and excessive blurring that can degrade the vessel information. This technique is disappointing for the detection of pulmonary emboli due to the lack of contrast between vessel and thrombus.

Snapshot imaging with fast SE scans (HASTE) has demonstrated bright signal from blood despite the long train of RF pulses applied and the fact that blood is moving during the entire acquisition (~200–400 msec). The technique exploits the long T2 relaxation time of blood compared to that

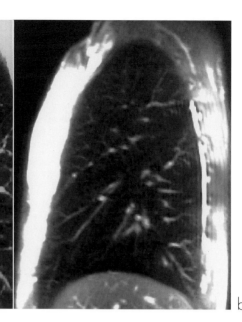

Fig. 16a, b. **(a)** Respiratory-gated/cardiac-triggered sagittal SE image showing superb resolution in the distal branches of the pulmonary arteries (arrow). Single-slice SE, TE = 22 ms, 192 × 256 matrix with FOV = 200 mm, 20.0-mm thick slice, N$_{acq}$ = 3, threshold = 50% and a single scan collected under open-gate conditions on expiration (acquisition time of 45 min). **(b)** Single-shot HASTE imaging can deliver similar vascular information virtually during free breathing with acquisition times of less than 300 msec. Single-slice HASTE, echo spacing = 4 msec, TE = 64 msec, 128 × 256 matrix with FOV = 200 × 350 mm, 6-mm thick slice.

a

b

of surrounding tissues. An example collected during free breathing is illustrated in Figure 16b. Signal from flowing blood is maintained by a principle known as even-echo rephasing. Even-echo rephasing occurs on every other 180° RF refocusing pulse and can be regarded as a form of flow compensation mechanism in this case (phase errors do not accumulate for flow moving at constant velocity). Relatively short echo times are used to ensure that blood signal remains high and to reduce the effects of wash-in and wash-out phenomena commonly presented in SE scans (black blood imaging). Blood maintains its signal while flowing in the plane of section and especially along the readout direction (along which even-echo rephasing occurs). Signal from vessels entering the imaging volume perpendicularly can appear but is likely only in cases of slow flow.

HASTE imaging can be regarded as a fast angiographic roadmap for the pulmonary vascular system (see STAR imaging with HASTE readouts below). The choice of a long effective echo time with HASTE techniques can prove adequate to distinguish dark emboli from brighter surrounding blood. Additionally, the short acquisition time does not require breath-holding. However, it is likely that images present flow voids in the pulmonary arteries, confusing the interpretation with the lack of signal from thrombi.

Miyazaki et al. [60] have produced a rough projection MRPA using a breath-hold double shot HASTE scan (SPEED, Swap Phase Encode Extended Data). Each scan is identical but the direction of the readout gradient is swapped with the in-plane phase encoding gradient. This strategy

tries to compensate for blood that does not remain bright in one shot that is available on the other. The resulting images are combined (using MIP) to obtain a projection-like MRPA with reduced signal voids. Images can be somewhat different in that geometric distortions (lower distortion with larger readout gradients) and phase-encoding aliasing effects can arise (requiring large field-of-views). 3D SPEED has also been implemented using multiple breath-holds (Fig. 17) to produce thinner sections that can be reformatted or use additional image post-processing. Eventually, 3D SPEED could be used for PE detection because of the long effective TE used (TE > 100 msec).

The diverse GRE MRPA techniques that have been investigated have mainly focused on the problem of PE detection. Time-of-flight (TOF) [61] rather than phase contrast [62] concepts have been exploited because of speed and no need for background suppression. Work using phase contrast MRA in the thorax has been described by Yuasa [63].

Two-dimensional TOF GRE techniques maximally use the natural enhancement possible from fully magnetised blood flowing into the imaging region [64, 65]. Despite facing both motion and magnetic susceptibility problems, Hatabu et al. [66] demonstrated high spatial resolution, single thin-slice images with 2D GRE scans illustrating peripheral pulmonary vessels with breath-hold acquisitions (6th and 7th order branches). However, long overall imaging time with large regions of interest and image misregistration from inconsistent breath-holding proved inadequate for 3D display.

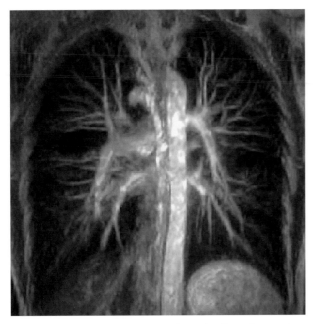

Fig. 17. 3D SPEED MRPA acquired on a healthy volunteer. A 40 mm volume was scanned coronally (20 sections, 2 mm thick), cardiac gated, selecting an effective TR equal to 4 cardiac periods, TEeff = 120 msec, 256 x 256, FOV = 380 x 380 mm and N_{acq} = 1. The HASTE readout (TE/ETS = 120/5 msec) was gated to diastole to minimise signal voids from flow-related dephasing. Images resulting from a MIP of 2 interleaved acquisitions with the in-plane phase encoding direction swapped with the frequency encoding direction. Intermittent breath-holds were performed for approximately 3 minutes. The arms were positioned above the head to eliminate in-plane phase encoding aliasing.

Many variations have been examined since to cover larger imaging volumes, most notably:

- Single thick slab projection (20–50 mm thick) (Fig. 18) [67],
- Sequential acquisition of thin slices (Fig. 19) [68],
- Thin slices acquired in an interleaved slice mode (Figs. 20 and 21) [69],
- Thin slice, sequential segmented k-space acquisitions [70, 71].

The choice of TR depends on the breath-hold length, directly influencing the number of slices and matrix size desired. Single thick slice imaging can use short to intermediate TR values (4–100 msec), depending mainly on breath-hold length. Sequential acquisitions use short TR (4–12 msec) while interleaved acquisitions use long TR (100–200 msec). Segmented acquisitions use in general short TR (4–12 msec). Echo times are short to counteract the effect of signal loss from magnetic susceptibility differences between water/air interfaces (TE < 3 msec, mainly using asymmetric echo positions in the sampling window). Readout bandwidth, flip angle and TR are usually chosen accordingly to provide appropriate SNR and a compromise with saturation or signal enhancement possible with fresh inflowing blood. Flow compensation is usually not employed to keep both TE and TR short.

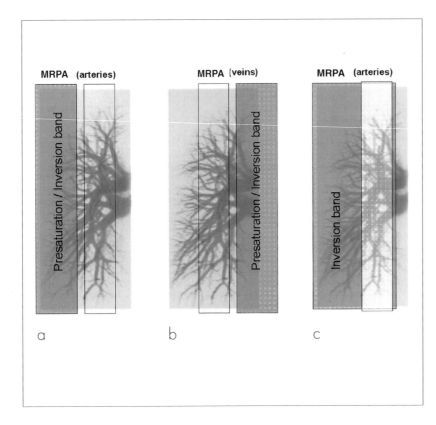

Fig. 18a–c. Single thick slab projection 2D MRPA set-up. An intermediate TR is chosen to reduce blood saturation. Without the application of a presaturation/inversion slab the image formed contains both arteries and veins (**a**). A venous-only MRPA can be acquired by placing the inversion/presaturation slab at the arterial input (**b**). Venous suppression can be performed as well by changing the position of the inversion/presaturation slab laterally (to a certain extent because all unwanted blood cannot be eliminated effectively). The inversion/presaturation slab can be applied once or for all RF excitations (**c**) The application of a single selective inversion over the volume with a delay time prior to acquisition to permit fresh arterial blood to enter the imaging slab can produce an arterial-only MRPA (venous blood is nulled out during the acquisition). This is advantageous for cardiac-triggered scans, the inversion applied prior to systole while the signal readout is performing during diastole. The signal is read using short TR and preferably the inversion/presaturation slab is positioned over the imaging volume during the QRS and imaging is performed in diastole using short TR.

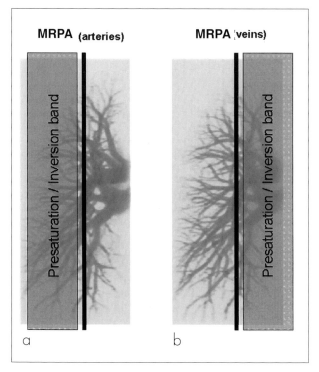

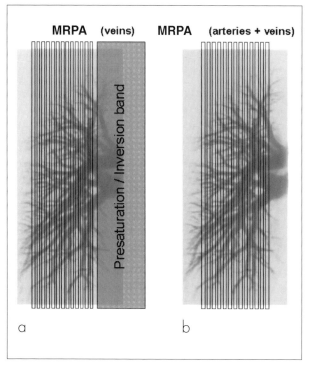

Fig. 19a, b. *Multi-slice sequential 2D MRPA set-up. Slices are acquired one after the other in rapid succession. Using short TR, a single slice can be encoded in less than a second. Arterial **(a)** or venous **(b)** MRPA are possible with the application of a travelling presaturation band on either side of the imaged slice, respectively. For an arterial-only MRPA, it is convenient to locate the central phase encoding steps of each slice to match with the peak arterial inflow.*

Fig. 20a, b. *Long TR, short TE multi-slice interleaved 2D MRPA. Breath-holds are possible by selecting a long TR (100-200 msec) to encode between 10 to 30 slices. **(a)** The application of a presaturation/inversion band over the heart permits the acquisition of a venous-only MRPA. **(b)** Differentiation between arteries and veins is produced exclusively by selecting the appropriate flip angle that permits higher SNR in the arteries. Slices should be scanned starting from the lateral wall towards the centre of the thorax (ascending and descending order).*

Cardiac synchronisation has been applied for sequential and segmented k-space acquisitions. This is performed either to synchronise the centre k-space lines (contrast) to a specific cardiac phase (e. g., to enhance inflow effects to differentiate arteries from veins or to create a cine loop) [65] or to reduce ghosting artifacts from cardiac motion and pulsatile blood flow. Interleaved acquisitions can support some form of cardiac synchronisation but these have not been reported for MRPA as they necessitate special acquisition data encoding to fill k-space depending on the TR and the number of slices chosen.

Inflow of freshly magnetised blood into the imaging region can provide arterial and venous differentiation depending on the technique and imaging parameters used, mainly through a suitable combination between TR and the flip angle applied. The incorporation of cardiac synchronisation to acquire the centre k-space lines during peak systole permits a higher degree of arterial and venous differentiation. However, the differentiation is clearly dependent on the difference between arterial and venous blood flow velocities.

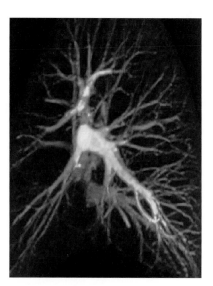

Fig. 21. *Maximum intensity projection (MIP) of a breath-hold multi-slice interleaved 2D MRPA acquisition in the right lung of a healthy subject. The acquisition encoded 26 sagittal slices (2.5 mm slice thickness) with TR/TE = 160/2.4 msec, $\alpha = 35°$, 150×512 matrix, FOV = 180×350 mm^2, 24 sec acquisition. Good differentiation between arteries and veins is possible with good arterial inflow to the imaged volume. Manual segmentation of the thorax was performed prior to MIP. Body phased-array coil detection.*

273

Selective imaging can be performed more effectively using presaturation or inversion slabs. This can be achieved in several ways depending on the imaging technique selected:

- For sequential acquisitions, travelling presaturation bands can be applied before the excitation of each slice [72, 73]. The presaturation band is applied on the side closer to the heart for arterial suppression (venous MRPA) or away from the heart to suppress veins (arterial MRPA).
- Using a presaturation or an inversion slab on either side of the imaging volume for thick slice projections or interleaved acquisitions (Figs. 18–20).
- Signal inversion prior to imaging fully magnetised blood flowing into the volume of interest [11, 74]. This technique should use cardiac triggering and apply the inversion slab prior to

systole. A suitable inflow delay is then used to synchronise the collection of the centre of k-space during diastole. K-space segmentation can be very effective in reducing imaging time for arterial or venous MRPA [75].

The application of 3D GRE techniques was proposed to better circumvent susceptibility effects and improve signal-to-noise ratios and resolution [76]. Moreover, 3D MRPA techniques can deliver isotropic data sets, enabling greater possibilities for morphological analysis and display of the pulmonary vasculature using multiplanar reformations (MPR), maximum intensity projections (MIP) and volume rendering. However, isotropic 3D data sets require extended imaging time, promoting vessel blurring and ghosting from respiratory motion. Free-breathing 3D MRPA techniques can prove to be attractive as they gain advantage over breath-hold techniques on uncooperative patients and

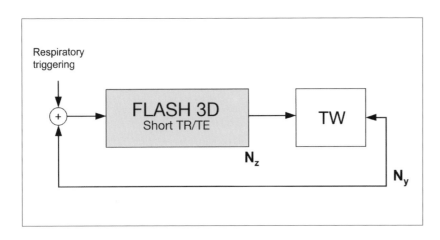

Fig. 22. Diagram of a syncopated 3D MRPA scan. After a string of RF excitations, in this case encoding all the slice select phase steps Nz, a wait time TW is included for inflow of fresh blood into the imaging volume. The process is repeated for all the in-plane phase encoding lines selected, Ny. Data is encoded using a FLASH 3D sequence with short TR/TE. Respiratory synchronisation can be included after each TW period to reduce image blurring.

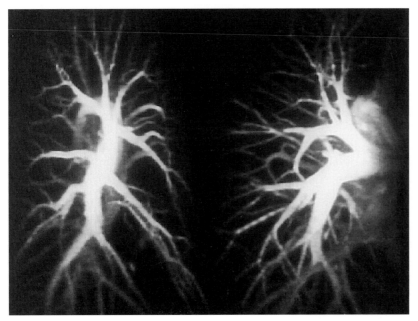

Fig. 23. Two MIP views of a free-breathing syncopated 3D MRPA in the right lung of a healthy subject. 128 coronal slices (1.5 mm slice thickness) were encoded with TR/TE = 8.2/2.8 msec, $\alpha = 12°$, TW = 500 msec, 64 × 256 matrix, FOV = 110 × 200 mm^2 and $N_{acq} = 8$. The thorax was segmented manually prior to MIP. Body Helmholtz coil reception. TW = wait time.

open the possibility for higher spatial resolution and coverage. At first, free-breathing 3D MRPA was met with enormous scepticism after unsuccessful conventional 3D MRA strategies in the abdomen. Breath-hold 3D MRPA was investigated by MacFall et al. [67], proving better visualisation of peripheral pulmonary segments than thick slice breath-hold 2D MRPA. Severe limitations in spatial resolution, coverage and signal-to-noise ratios were still present. The set-up for 3D MRPA is identical to that of the thick single slice technique (Fig. 18).

Image quality was significantly improved by Wielopolski et al. [76] with a free-breathing syncopated 3D GRE technique (Figs. 22 and 23). A recovery time (TW) was included between bursts of data collection to enhance the arterial flow entering a sagittal 3D volume (Fig. 24). Signal averaging was considered to suppress ghosting from respiration at the expense of vessel blurring that affected mostly pulmonary vessels close to the diaphragm. Two reports corroborated the improved results for 3D MRPA over 2D MRPA acquisitions [70, 73].

Acquisitions monitoring respiration with belts over the thoracic trunk [77, 78] and navigator echoes [74, 79] soon proved advantageous to improve vessel definition without substantial increases in scanning time [74, 80]. Wielopolski investigated the impact of respiratory triggered 3D MRPA using respiratory belts. This was met with varying degrees of improvement over the syncopated 3D MRPA technique (Fig. 25). The idea to directly monitor the diaphragmatic motion using navigator echoes (a pen-like excitation through the diaphragm) provided better correlation with pulmonary vessel motion than the indirect measurement performed with respiratory belts and, in principle, could yield better results [81].

Two measurement possibilities using navigator echoes may be considered, one accepting data in real-time mode (prospectively) [21, 74] or sorting data retrospectively collected over the entire respiratory cycle (oversampling) [82]. Wang et al. [74] investigated the first possibility. With additional electrocardiographic triggering and selective inversion over the region of interest, exclusive enhancement of the pulmonary arterial tree was possible using TOF effects with venous signal greatly suppressed. The overall quality of segmental arteries was significantly better than that of 3D MRPA collected with free breathing; comparison also reported in this study.

Retrospective navigator gated scans have not yet been reported for MRPA, perhaps because of the large amount of data necessary to produce the final image and the excessive scan time necessary to sample the entire respiratory period. Reports using this technique have only been assessed for imaging the coronary arteries [83], providing some insight into the effectiveness of the technique. Unfortunately, inconsistent results have been reported [84] which may tend to worsen in patients with suspected PE because these are often dyspneic and unable to cooperate during the scan.

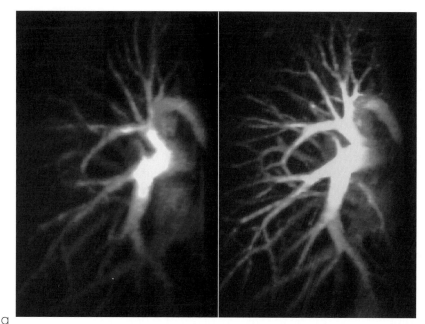

Fig. 24a, b. Effect of TW on signal enhancement in syncopated 3D MRPA. Imaging parameters were the same as in Figure 23 but comparing TW = 0 msec (**a**) with TW = 500 msec (**b**). The delay produces greater enhancement of the pulmonary arteries and better visualisation of high order branches. The signal enhancement in the pulmonary veins observed in (**b**) is produced only from longitudinal magnetisation recovery and not from inflow effects. The thorax was segmented manually prior to MIP. Body Helmholtz coil reception. TW = wait time.   a

b

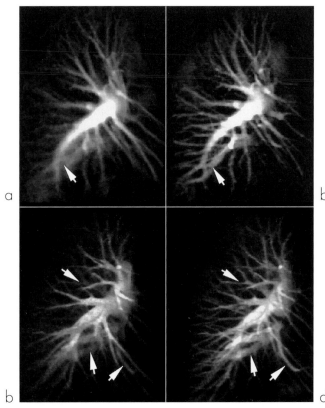

a

b

Fig. 25a – d. Comparison between free-breathing and respiratory triggered syncopated 3D MRPA on the right lung of two healthy subjects. Syncopated 3D MRPA technique with averaging (N_{acq} = 8) **(a, c)**. Respiratory triggered acquisition using respiratory belts (N_{acq} = 1) **(b, d)**. Respiratory triggering can reduce blurring at the base of the lung **(a, b)**. Nonetheless, this improvement may be minimal **(c, d)**. The arrowheads point at veins to illustrate the difference in signal enhancement between the two acquisition schemes, the respiratory triggered scan being more proton-density weighted because of the long effective TW between data acceptances (~2–4 sec). Imaging time was comparable for both acquisition modes (approximately 13 minutes). Imaging parameters as in Figure 23 but FOV = 110 x 260 mm². Volume rendering after manual segmentation of the thorax. Body coil reception.

Arterial-only or venous-only MRPA using subtraction techniques

Conventional MRPA techniques can be used to produce angiograms with good vessel selectivity, e. g., an arterial-only or venous-only MRPA using subtraction. Blood tagging can offer the required selectivity to view only selected portions of the pulmonary vascular tree. Two techniques that are of interest are described here.

To produce an arterial-only MRPA, a complex or a magnitude subtraction can be performed between two data sets that are identical except for the longitudinal magnetisation of inflowing arterial blood that has been previously tagged with a selective adiabatic inversion pulse (180° RF pulse) or a pre-

saturation pulse over the heart. Signal encoding can then be performed with any technique that is robust for imaging moving blood.

The concept has been investigated by several researchers and has received several acronyms such as STAR (Signal Targeting with Alternating Radiofrequency) and SIR (Selective Inversion Recovery) [85, 86]. The alternating inversion bands should have identical characteristics and be placed symmetrically about the centre of the imaging volume. This produces a cleaner subtraction as it suppresses any difference that may appear between the two data sets from magnetisation transfer effects.

Figure 26 illustrates an example collected over a large imaging volume using a single shot HASTE readout. HASTE is adequate for this application to demonstrate bright blood and the acquisition benefits from good magnetic field inhomogeneity insensitivity for projection imaging, thanks to the SE readout. With this single shot imaging scenario, the addition of cardiac triggering produces optimal inflow of the tagged blood into the pulmonary arteries (tagging performed prior to systole with the readout performed in mid-late diastole when blood flow and cardiac movements are small). To minimise subtraction errors from breath-holding, the two data sets should be collected in an interleaved fashion when averaging is used.

This tagging and subtraction methodology can be extended to a 3D imaging scenario to benefit from any imaging post-processing scheme that can aid in the evaluation (Fig. 27). Although interleaved data collection would minimise subtraction errors from unstable breath-holding (single shot case above), it is inefficient for a 3D scenario because it requires an inflow delay and a recovery time to assure that blood from one acquisition does not interfere with the other. Therefore, a sequential collection scheme, which collects one 3D volume first with the tag pulse on one side and the other later, permits continuous inflow of tagged blood into the volume. For an arterial-only MRPA, a subtraction is performed between the data set with the tagging pulse outside the thorax and that acquired with the tag over the heart. The venous-only MRPA is produced automatically with the data set acquired with the tagging pulse applied over the heart.

The venous MRPA data set will show bright signal where the signal void is generated on the arterial MRPA. Interaction between the three data sets that are obtained (arteries, veins and both) in conjunction with a multiplanar reconstruction platform can provide the confidence needed to determine whether the cut-off seen in the arterial MRPA is in effect an embolus by inspecting the location in the venous MRPA data set.

Arterial-only or venous-only MRPA scans can be generated using sequential 2D MRPA scans with travelling presaturation bands (Fig. 19). Blood tagging is based on the same time-of-flight principle but benefits from a greater efficiency in certain circumstances. Subtraction can produce a rapid display of the entire pulmonary arterial tree without the need for image post-processing because stationary tissues surrounding blood are automatically suppressed. Subtraction also offers similar results to contrast-enhanced MRPA scans for thrombus detection (see Section 8).

Unfortunately, all the subtraction techniques still depend on blood flow velocities and may not be reliable in all patients, especially for those with low cardiac output or slow flow (such as in pulmonary hypertension). Breath-holding is also very important in order to eliminate subtraction errors that may mimic filling defects or vessel cut-offs. If SNR permits, long inflow delays can be used for mapping lung perfusion without contrast agents.

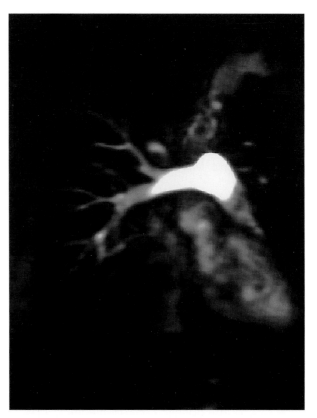

Fig. 26. Coronal oblique view of the right pulmonary arterial tree acquired with a breath-hold, subtraction-based cardiac-triggered HASTE incorporating an arterial blood tagging pulse. Tagging was performed using an inversion band over the heart prior to systole and an inflow delay of 400 msec was used to image the tagged blood during mid diastole. Readout per shot was 320 msec with a 20 mm slice thickness, ETS/TE = 4.4/36 msec, 128 x 256 matrix, FOV = 450 x 450 mm^2 and 3 signal averages performed to increase SNR (~20 sec breath-hold). Body phased-array coil acquisition. (Image courtesy of J. Gaa, Radiology, University Hospital Mannheim, Mannheim, Germany).

Fig. 27. Arterial and venous MRPA using subtraction between data sets collected with and without blood tagging pulses. The data set collected with a presaturation/inversion band over the arm, labelled **(a)**, produces a set containing both arteries and veins. Placing the presaturation/inversion band over the heart, labelled **(b)**, produces a set that should only contain signal from veins. Subtraction between **a** and **b** produces an arterial-only MRPA data set. To increase the effect of the presaturation/inversion band, the readout flip angle of the 3D GRE sequence must be small and a short TR should be employed (< 10° for TR < 5 msec). Low flip angle readouts produce results that are less dependent on blood inflow velocities and result in a more homogeneous display of the arterial pulmonary tree.

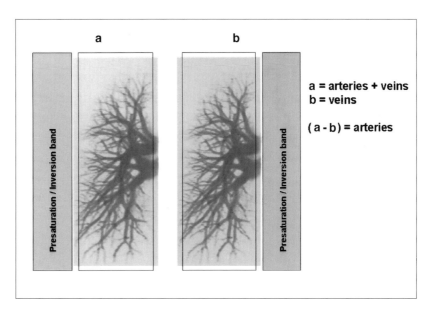

a = arteries + veins
b = veins

(a - b) = arteries

8. Contrast-Enhanced MRPA

The improvement in acquisition speed that is possible with faster MRI gradient hardware usually requires additional help to improve SNR and image contrast. Therefore, agents affecting the characteristic relaxation time of blood have been devised in recent years that have shown positive impact for fast MRPA and MRA in different regions in the body.

The T1 relaxation of blood can be shortened with the intravenous administration of paramagnetic contrast agents (gadolinium Gd^{3+} chelates) and ultra-small iron oxide particles (USPIOs). When present at the right concentration, the T1 relaxation time of blood can drop to values below 50 msec and produce results that are virtually flow independent for any MRA acquisitions (substantially shorter than the T1 relaxation time exhibited by fat, approximately 270 msec). The T2 relaxation time of blood also changes, remaining shorter than the T1 relaxation time.

The dynamic T1 shortening experienced in the presence of a paramagnetic contrast medium, $T1_{blood}(t)$, can be modelled in relation to the concentration of the contrast medium in time according to

Equation 12

$$\frac{1}{T1_{blood}(t)} = \frac{1}{T1_{blood}} + R1_{Gd} \cdot [Gd](t)$$

where at 1.5 T the relaxivity of pure blood, $T1_{blood}$, is approximately 1,200 msec and the relaxivity of Gd-DTPA, $R1_{Gd}$, approximately $4.5\,s^{-1}mmol^{-1}$. The concentration of Gd-DTPA, indicated by [Gd], depends on the dose and how it is being administered during image acquisition. There is a similar equation for the T2 relaxation of blood.

Contrast enhanced MRPA can be performed in two modalities, using acquisitions that take place during the transient T1 relaxation effects in blood after a bolus injection of a contrast agent or during steady-state conditions using intravascular contrast agents. Thus far, MRPA has only been performed during dynamic contrast injections in routine application.

Assuming a one-compartment model, the concentration of the contrast agent can be related to the rate of contrast injection and the cardiac output as illustrated by Equation 13 [87, 88]

Equation 13

$$[Gd] = \frac{(\text{rate of Gd injection in mol/sec})}{(\text{cardiac output in L/sec})}$$

where [Gd] denotes the steady-state concentration of Gd-DTPA that is expected when the injection time is long enough that no variations in concentration occur during the MRPA acquisition. The T1 relaxation induced in blood can be computed by combining Equation 12 and Equation 13. This yields T1 relaxation values for blood of 36 msec and 18 msec for 1 ml/sec and 2 ml/sec injections for a typical cardiac output of 5 L/min, respectively. Under realistic imaging conditions, these relaxation values are adequately supported by commercial imaging hardware for the resolution that is necessary for the evaluation of the MRPA for full lung coverage (approximately $5\,mm^3$ voxels). Injection rates greater than 4 ml/sec may not yield better MRPA quality. Shortening TR is only possible to a certain extent, given that the readout window directly affects the SNR and resolution possible for the available gradient amplifier. The RF excitation must be kept below the maximum output of the RF amplifier and RF exposure limits to the patient.

With the T1 relaxation times expected in blood after the administration of contrast, optimal imaging parameters can be computed using the signal for FLASH imaging (SSI GRE imaging, Equation 3). This assumes that the T1 relaxation is maintained constant during the entire scan time. The signal intensity plots illustrated in Figure 13 provide the characteristic signal behaviour for FLASH imaging for short TR scans, as currently implemented in advanced 3D MRPA protocols with the range of T1 relaxation times expected for contrast-enhanced scans.

Evaluation of the patient's breath-hold ability should be performed prior to every examination using a sagittal or a coronal imaging plane to generate images at a rate of 1 per second that demonstrate the diaphragmatic position. Patients who are short of breath will not be able to produce images with adequate resolution to effectively review arteries beyond 4th order branches of the pulmonary tree. Studies have shown that adequate resolution for evaluation is possible if breath-holds are held consistent at least for half of the scan time, preferably during the centre of the data acquisition (sequential scanning) [89]. A breath-hold time of less than 17 seconds has been appropriate

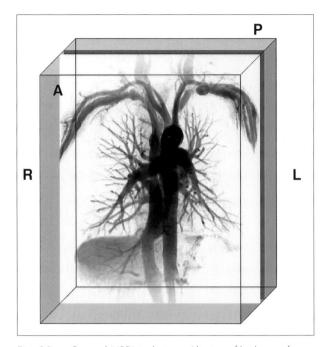

Fig. 28. Coronal MRPA technique. Aliasing of both arms frequently occurs into the imaging volume for a small FOV setting, therefore, resolution must be sacrificed to keep the imaging time short. The set-up is advantageous in that a single injection and a single breath-hold are performed.

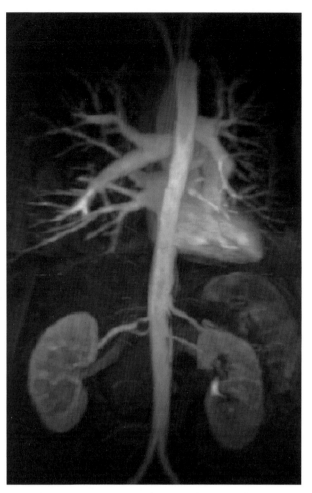

Fig. 29. MIP reconstruction of a coronally acquired contrast-enhanced 3D MRPA. Body phased-array coil detection using FLASH 3D, TR/TE/α = 3.65/1.6 msec/30°, 390 Hz/pixel acquisition bandwidth, 170 x 512 matrix, 390 Hz/pixel acquisition bandwidth, FOV = 420 x 420 mm^2, 100 sections of 1.25 mm reconstructed thickness, 26 sec acquisition. A contrast bolus of 30 ml (Gd-DTPA) was delivered via a power injector at 2 ml/sec followed by 20 ml of saline at 2 ml/sec.

for all patients with good outcomes for the assessment [90].

In most contrast-enhanced MRPA clinical studies breath-hold fast 3D GRE scans acquired during the first pass of a Gd-DTPA contrast bolus have been used [91–95].

Imaging protocols varied with respect to acquisition orientation (sagittal, transverse, coronal or double oblique volumes). Coronal and sagittal orientations are most often used for assessing PE. Coronal imaging is preferred if a single contrast injection is performed (Figs. 28 and 29). Breath-holds have ranged between 15 sec and 30 sec with imaging parameters tailored to obtain results that take into account the patient's breath-hold ability [96]. Coronal scanning with short breath-hold acquisitions may prove ineffective for PE de-

tection at sub-segmental level unless both lungs are entirely covered with appropriate spatial resolution (voxels < 5 mm^3). It is also important in coronal scanning that the in-plane phase encoding loop is scanned faster than the section select phase encoding loop. This can reduce ghosting from heart motion whenever all in-plane phase encoding lines are acquired in less than one cardiac cycle.

Shorter breath-holds with satisfactory spatial resolution necessitate that each lung be scanned separately (Fig. 30). For a sagittal set-up two contrast injections must be administered [97]. Several examples using this set-up are shown in Figure 31.

Contrast-enhanced 3D MRPA makes use of the shortest TR that it is possible by the MRI gradient hardware in order to generate the desired resolu-

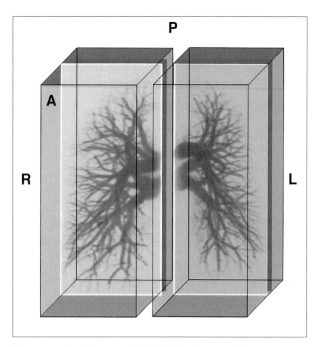

Fig. 30. Double sagittal slab MRPA technique. The technique focuses on one lung at a time to obtain good resolution within a reasonable short breath-hold interval that permits the evaluation of arterial branches down to sub-segmental level. The contrast dosage must be split in two to provide the vascular enhancement necessary for each vascular territory separately.

tion within a prescribed, short imaging time. Nonetheless, satisfactory SNR is the parameter that modulates the appropriate choice for TR and readout acquisition bandwidths that are employed for all MRPA protocols. Typical TR and TE values range between 3 to 6 msec and 1.0 to 3.5 msec, respectively, for fast MRI gradient hardware. Readout acquisition bandwidths have been set, in general, to less than 500 Hz/pixel.

The readout flip angle is chosen according to the expected concentration (T1 relaxation induced) of the contrast medium in blood during the scanning time and calculated according to the optimal flip angle formula for FLASH imaging (Ernst angle, Equation 4). Flip angles values that have been used have ranged between 15° to 60°. Higher flip angles for scans with longer TR or higher contrast concentration or both. The RF amplifier and

heat exposure limits on patients (specific absorption ratios, SAR) may limit the application of short RF excitations that are required for short TR sequences.

Contrast arrival time to the pulmonary vasculature and the pulmonary circulation time (transit time between arterial and venous phase) are very short, which makes it nearly impossible to obtain arterial-only MRPA data sets in all patients. An analysis over data generated in our institution using a dynamic 3D MRPA acquisition (3D MRPP) is described (see Sections 9 and 11).

Figure 32 illustrates the course of signal enhancement for different vascular compartments in the cardiothoracic circulatory system after a short bolus of contrast. From these curves, several parameters can be calculated. The time of arrival of contrast to the pulmonary arteries (PA), lung parenchyma (PP), pulmonary veins (PV) and descending aorta (Ao) can be seen. The transit time through the pulmonary circuit (τ) can be derived from the time difference between the PA and PV intensity curves. The bolus dispersion time (T_{bd}), that is, the associated expansion of the bolus shape during the time it remains in the pulmonary circulation, can be calculated. The enhancement speed recorded in the pulmonary artery (E_{rt}), has been set as the time elapsed from the start of enhancement and half the intensity is reached.

The transit time τ is very short, approximately 3.6 sec, and remains fairly constant in all patients. Similar values have been recorded by other investigators using dynamic contrast enhanced scans with high temporal resolution [98, 99]. It is also important to note that the bolus can spread considerably depending on the condition of the patient, with recorded values between 4.98 sec and 20.25 sec (mean 8.71). The speed of enhancement in the pulmonary artery, E_{rt}, has a large variation as well with a range of 0.5 sec to 5.2 sec (mean 2.10). The effect of these parameters on MRPA image quality has not been yet correlated adequately. In general, studies that have a short time of arrival to the PA with small E_{rt} and T_{bd} provide the best enhancement in the MRPA (Fig. 33).

Fig. 31a–f. Imaging examples for the double sagittal slab technique. Volume rendering was performed on the data of a healthy volunteer (a) and on patients referred for PE with abnormal V/Q scans but confirmed normal with conventional pulmonary angiograms (b–f). Two separate 17 sec breath-hold scans were performed using 20 ml of contrast (Gd-DTPA) per acquisition. A variable contrast injection rate was performed first with 5 ml at a flow rate of 1 ml/sec followed by 15 ml at 2 ml/sec and flushed by 20 ml of saline at 2 ml/sec. Contrast delivery was timed after a test bolus scan to produce optimal enhancement in the pulmonary arteries. Each sagittal slab contains 96 sections acquired with FLASH 3D, TR/TE = 3.65/1.6 msec, α = 25°, 390 Hz/pixel acquisition bandwidth, 106 x 512 matrix, FOV = 220 x 320 mm^2, 1.25 mm reconstructed slice thickness, 17 sec acquisition. Body phased-array coil detection. The thorax was segmented manually prior to volume rendering. Views reconstructed correspond to a RAO 25° projection.

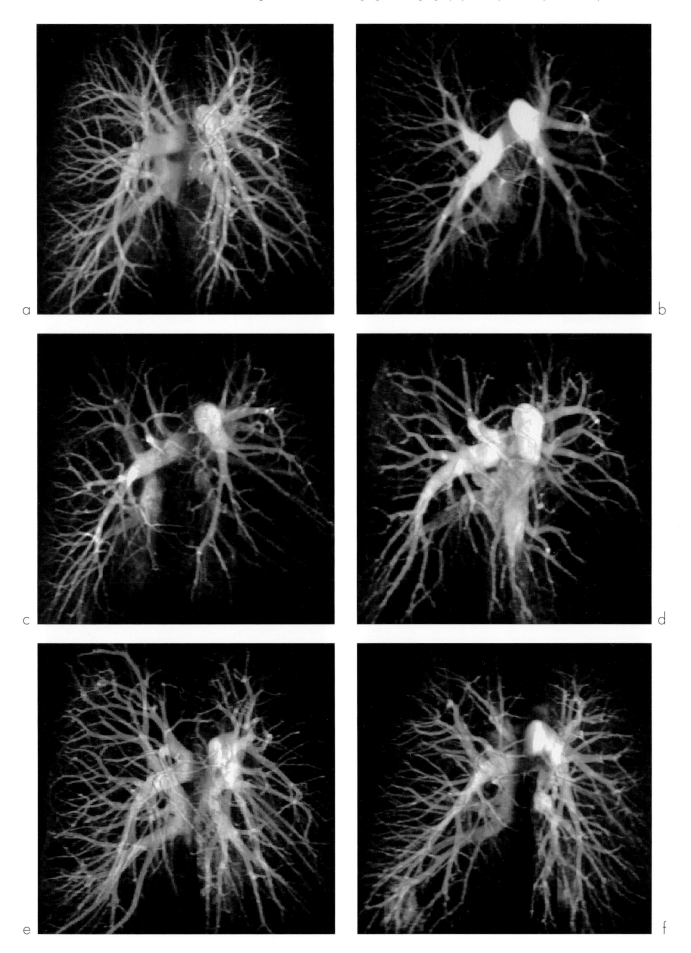

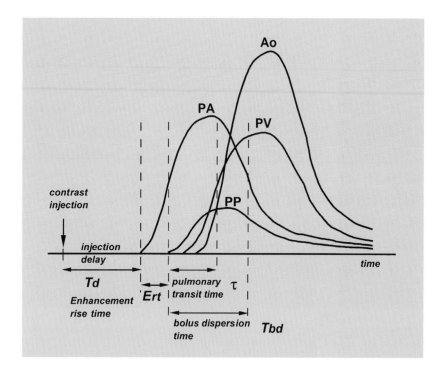

Fig. 32. Typical enhancement curves through the pulmonary artery (PA), pulmonary parenchyma (PP), pulmonary vein (PV) and aorta (Ao) after the injection of a short bolus of contrast. T_d indicates the time between the start of injection and the instant that enhancement in PA appears. The enhancement rise time, Ert, is defined between Td and half the maximum intensity at PA. The bolus dispersion time, T_{bd}, is calculated as the full width half maximum of the PA curve. The transit time through the pulmonary circuit, τ is the time interval between one half of the maximum enhancement recorded at PA and PV.

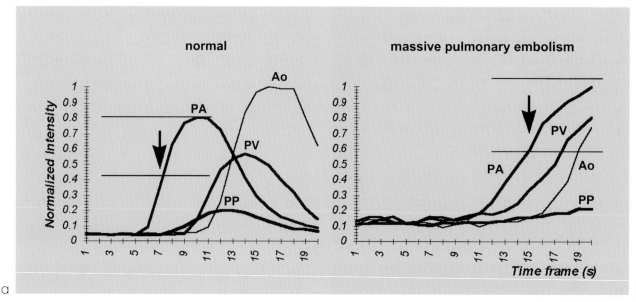

Fig. 33a, b. Representative signal intensity curves in the descending pulmonary artery (PA), pulmonary vein (PV), posterior pulmonary parenchyma (PP) and the descending aorta (Ao) **(a)** normal patient. Patient with large thrombi lodged in both descending pulmonary arteries **(b)**. The dynamic acquisition was performed with a time resolution of 1 sec after the injection of an 8 ml bolus of Gd-DTPA at a rate of 4 ml/sec and flushed with 20 ml of saline at a rate of 2 ml/sec.

The average arrival time to the pulmonary arteries after start of injection, denoted as T_d, is 4.9 seconds. The data illustrated in Table 5 summarises the analysis on 55 patients referred for PE in our institution (including 13 patients with the disease). Thus, if a contrast timing scan is obviated and a best guess technique is used, the contrast injection should be started approximately 5 seconds prior to the MRPA scan.

Contrast is generally administered through an intravenous catheter placed into the antecubital vein. A long bolus will extend the plateau during which the acquisition is to be performed. Excellent results for MRA and MRPA have been reported using a fixed dose of contrast of 40 ml (approximately a double dose of contrast). Single dose injections (approximately 20 ml) have also been reported to produce good results for either coronal

Fig. 34a – e. Possible contrast concentration curves that can appear in the pulmonary arteries following a bolus of contrast. **(a)** Single dose of contrast delivered over a shorter period than that of the MRPA acquisition produces constant signal enhancement during the entire scan time. **(b)** Double dose of contrast delivered during the same time as in **(a)** produces twice the signal enhancement. **(c)** Double dose of contrast delivered for a longer time than that in **(a)** and **(b)** still produces constant enhancement during the acquisition but part of the contrast is misused. **(d)** Double dose delivered during shorter time that **(a)** and **(b)** can produce more enhancement but over a smaller portion of k-space. The cases depicted in **(a – c)** produce equal k-space weighting and consequently no filtering artifacts in the reconstructed images. The case in **(d)** represents the case where considerations in the way k-space is encoded (see Figure 35) must be taken into account to minimize filtering artifacts during image encoding. **(e)** represents a variable infusion rate to shape the contrast curve during the acquisition. Differentiation between arteries and veins depends on the position where the center k-space is collected relative to the appearance of contrast in the arteries and veins respectively (refer to Table 5).

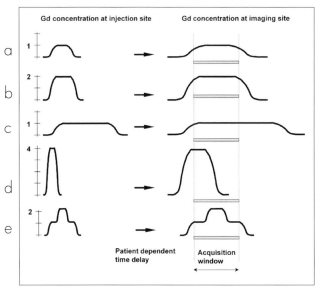

[100] or sagittal data collection strategies [101] when timing is optimal and sequence parameters are tuned accordingly (Fig. 34). Hany et al. [101] have determined that a double dose of contrast (0.2 mmol/kg) is optimal for any MRA examination (dose ranging between single dose and quadruple dose).

Injection flow rates are set to 2 ml/sec although variable rates have been reported to produce a greater enhancement during the collection of the central k-space lines whenever a limited amount of contrast agent is used [102]. A saline flush greater than 15 ml (2 ml/sec flow) must always follow the contrast injection [103].

Several cases for contrast enhancement curves that may appear in the pulmonary arteries after a contrast injection include

- A single dose of contrast delivered over a shorter period than that of the duration of the MRPA acquisition produces constant signal enhancement during the entire scan time (Fig. 34a)
- Double dose of contrast delivered during the same time producing twice the signal enhancement (Fig. 34b)
- Double dose of contrast delivered for a longer time producing a constant enhancement during the acquisition but part of the contrast is misused (Fig. 34c)
- Double dose delivered to provide more vascular enhancement but over a smaller portion of k-space (Fig. 34d)

Table 5. Circulation times from the injection site to and through the pulmonary vasculature quantified using a 3D dynamic contrast-enhanced scan with a time resolution of 1 sec.

Circulation parameters (55 patients, mean age = 50.2 years)	(sec)
Arrival time to PA	5.00
Arrival time to 1/2 intensity at PA	6.99
Arrival time to 1/2 intensity at PP	9.69
Arrival time to 1/2 intensity at PV	10.60
Arrival time to 1/2 intensity at Ao	13.08
Enhancement rise time (E_{rt})	2.10
Pulmonary transit time (t)	3.60
Bolus dispersion time (T_{bd})	8.71
Maximum E_{rt}	0.50
Minimum E_{rt}	5.20
Maximum T_{bd}	20.25
Minimum T_{bd}	4.98

Contrast injection was performed at the antecubital vein using a power injector delivering a short bolus of contrast with 8 ml at a rate of 4 ml/sec flushed with 20 ml of saline at a rate of 2 ml/sec. All values represent averages over data collected on 55 patients and measured at 2 different sites in each data set. Thirteen patients presented PE by conventional pulmonary angiography.

PA = descending pulmonary arteries
PV = pulmonary veins
PP = posterior pulmonary parenchyma
Ao = descending aorta

In Figures 34a-c, the signal is uniform for all k-space values and consequently no filtering artifacts (blurring or edge enhancement) will be present in the reconstructed images. Figure 34d represents the case where considerations in the way k-space is encoded. These are necessary to produce the least amount of filtering artifacts while achieving appropriate vascular contrast between pulmonary arteries and veins. Variable contrast delivery flow rates have been proposed (Fig. 34e), enabling contrast to appear for all k-space values but with a higher concentration during the collection of the center of k-space. Under real conditions, the contrast washout period can be elongated, providing a buffering effect. This varies depending on physiology and patient condition.

Precise differentiation between pulmonary arteries and veins depends on the concentration of the contrast agent in each compartment at the time the center of k-space is acquired. The time at which peak enhancement occurs in each vascular compartment is not fixed and can vary enormously in patients referred for MRPA. Four different strategies for contrast delivery and scanning are therefore possible:

- Best guess technique
- Test bolus technique
- Automated bolus detection (smart prep)
- MR fluoroscopy

From these, only the first two have been reported for MRPA. The best guess technique considers an educated guess to what the contrast arrival time may be between the injection site and the pulmonary arteries. This is difficult to determine from the patient condition alone because the arrival time can change substantially when emboli are present. In general, guessing yields sub-optimal results and provides a wide spectrum of enhancement patterns between the pulmonary arteries and

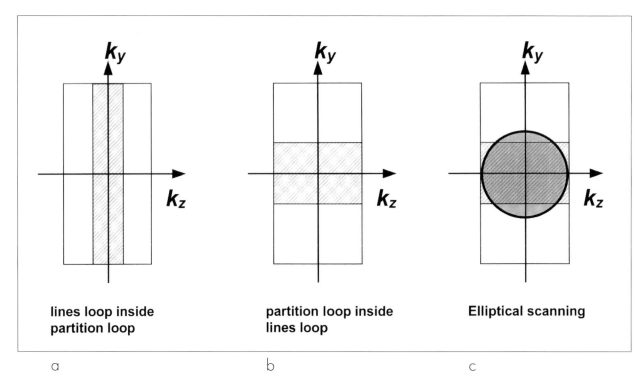

lines loop inside partition loop

partition loop inside lines loop

Elliptical scanning

a   b   c

Fig. 35a-c. Shape of the k-space area covered in the k_y-k_z plane by different encoding strategies for the same time interval during the center of k-space. **(a)** In-plane phase encoding steps acquired in the inner most loop, inside the section select phase encoding loop. **(b)** Reversed loop as in **(a)**, with the section select phase encoding in the inner most loop. **(c)** Elliptical encoding collecting both phase encoding steps with symmetrical weighting in both k_y and k_z. The three schemes differ substantially in the way filtering and ghosting artifacts appear along both phase encoding directions and the possible signal difference between arteries and veins (see text). When a short bolus of contrast generated roughly a gaussian contrast enhancement curve during the acquisition window defined by the shaded areas and with the peak signal during the center of k-space, the elliptical encoding scheme produces optimal weighing because of its symmetry in the k_y-k_z plane and the highest degree of suppression between arterial and venous structures with short transit times and artifact equilibration along both phase encoding directions. In the limit that contrast enhancement is the same for the entire k-space and the transit time between the arterial and venous phases is long, the schemes only differ in the ghosting pattern that blood pulsation, heart motion and breath-holding may create in the final images.

veins. The estimated contrast travel time should be taken as the average arrival time to the pulmonary artery as shown in Table 5, that is, approximately 5 seconds (from an injection in the antecubital vein).

A test bolus injection (using 1–3 ml contrast) is required in routine practice. A dynamic 2D T1-weighted scan with a time resolution of 1 s is usually employed to determine arrival time to the main pulmonary arteries. This involves additional scanning time and analysis of the contrast enhancement time course but results are more consistent and generally lead to optimal enhancement of the pulmonary arteries. However, it must be considered that the injection delay may change between the test scan and the MRPA.

In the event that sequential k-space encoding is used and the center of k-space is collected in the middle of the acquisition time, the timing of contrast prior to scanning can be calculated as [110]

Equation 14

$$Imaging\ Delay = Estimated\ Contrast\ Travel\ Time$$
$$+ \frac{Injection\ Time}{2}$$
$$- \frac{Imaging\ Time}{2}$$

Note that if the injection time is the same as the imaging time, the imaging delay is equal to the estimated contrast travel time. For the test bolus technique, the estimated contrast travel time is taken as the moment when contrast appears in the pulmonary artery.

Guessing or data analysis prior to scanning can be offset using real time monitoring of the arrival of contrast to the pulmonary arteries with an automated bolus detection scheme and trigger (smart prep) [107, 109] or an operator dependent scan trigger using MR fluoroscopy [108]. With „smart prep", the operator places a small measuring voxel in the main pulmonary artery to detect the signal changes induced by the passage of the contrast. The signal coming from the voxel is processed in real time and decisions are made after setting a suitable threshold over the background signal. Upon detection, the MRPA scan starts data collection automatically or the operator is alerted to start the scan manually. MR fluoroscopy collects instead an entire image in any desired plane to monitor the contrast arrival from which breath-hold and start of scan is instructed. MR fluoroscopy may be more reliable for MRPA as there is no need for positioning the „smart prep" measuring

voxel to detect the contrast and eliminates any failure to detection if the monitor voxel does not appear correctly positioned at all times because of breathing. Both schemes involve that operator delivers the instruction conveniently to the patient (which may be difficult in some cases). Centric or elliptical ordering of k-space should be used in these cases.

Temporally resolved 3D contrast-enhanced MRPA could be used to completely eliminate timing considerations (see Dynamic contrast-enhanced MRPA imaging). Nonetheless, temporally resolved data must have the appropriate spatial/time resolution and coverage to permit a precise evaluation of each arterial lumen.

For sequential encoding a variable flow rate can yield greater enhancement during the center of k-space. For a centric ordering scheme, encoding should start whenever contrast arrives at the pulmonary artery while the contrast is delivered at a constant flow rate. Most importantly is the speed at which the central portion of k-space is encoded (in the k_y-k_z plane) that determines the separation between arterial and venous enhancement and the filtering artifacts that occur along both phase encoding directions.

Scan choice is dependent on the size of the central k-space data that is related to the encoded matrix (k_y-k_z plane, number of sections and in-plane phase encoding steps chosen). There are two setups that can be envisioned: scanning the in-plane phase encoding steps inside the section select phase encoding loop or the other way around. Considering that the same number of points around the center of k-space is scanned, the resulting pattern for each one of these ordering schemes is illustrated in Figures 35a and 35b, respectively. The best representation of the contrast encoded and the milder filtering effects occur in the case of Figure 35b, performing the acquisition using the „faster" loop in the direction of the smaller amount of phase encoding steps. This ordering scheme should be used for either sagittal or coronal orientation setups. However, increased ghosting laterally can occur for coronal MRPA which may be unacceptable for a good evaluation and therefore, the reversed looping of Figure 35a is generally used.

Elliptical encoding provides the best compromise (Fig. 35c). Symmetrical weighting of the contrast enhancement curve in the k_y-k_z plane is possible with the same k-space area scanned as in Figure 35a and Figure 35b. Both phase encoding are played such that k-space is accessed from its center in a spiral fashion This scheme also produces the best venous suppression possible, minimum amount of filtering (equal weighting in both directions) and ghosting evenly distributed along both phase encoding directions.

Elliptical encoding can yield a higher degree of venous suppression and artifact reduction whenever the Ert time (enhancement rate) and the bolus dispersion time are short, as determined from a test bolus scan. However, for a short bolus of contrast, sequential encoding represents the best choice because the acquisition window can be twice as long in comparison to any centric ordering scheme.

Image artifacts in contrast-enhanced MRPA

Two types of artifacts can be distinguished: those that are derived from physiologic conditions (such as breath-holding and blood pulsation) and the ones that are coupled to the change in concentration of the contrast agent during data acquisition.

Poor breath-holding can produce inadequate results for high order branches but the resulting MRPA can still have diagnostic quality for the vessels with larger diameter (Fig. 36). The reason for this is that vessel display has a direct link to the speed that is used to acquire the centre k-space lines. Therefore, it is possible to affirm that the presence of thrombus can be confirmed with a good degree of confidence to the 3rd order branches with poor breath-holds. Even dyspneic patients who present with emboli in the larger vessels can be diagnosed with contrast-enhanced MRPA.

Ghosting can arise from blood pulsation during the acquisition (Fig. 37). The superimposition of ghosted vessels over others can produce signal voids (signal cancellation) that can be confused with a thrombus. Careful review along both phase encoding directions with multiplanar reformatting can indicate the presence of such an artifact. Ghosting is mainly present because the acquisition is not synchronised with the cardiac motion.

Ghosting artifacts can arise from two different origins, one related exclusively to variations in the signal intensity of blood during the acquisition and the other associated to changes in the phase of the signal. Both effects are intensified with high signal produced by the contrast-enhanced blood. Since MRPA sequences do not use flow compensation to achieve speed, there will be some variation in the phase of the signal from blood pulsation.

Artifacts related to contrast agents depend on the concentration of the contrast agent during the course of the acquisition. These artifacts tend to disappear since the concentration during the entire acquisition remains constant. Therefore, there will be no special weighting associated for each portion of k-space scanned.

Contrast agents induce a T2 and T2* shortening in blood which can result in unwanted signal loss. The TE of the MRPA acquisition is chosen such that it is several-fold shorter than the T2* relaxation of the contrast-enhanced blood. However, the contrast concentration can be so high that the T2* shortening is comparable to TE, resulting in a signal intensity drop in the vessel. This can be noted in the majority of cases in the subclavian vein

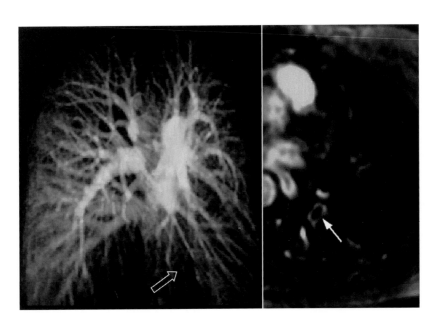

Fig. 36. Images corrupted with blurring from poor breath-holding. Vessels towards the periphery are completely blurred and the scan may be considered non-diagnostic. In this case, an embolus appearing in the right descending pulmonary artery can be seen clearly with MPR despite blurring (arrow), providing a positive result for the detection of PE. The block arrow points at a region with a clear lack of vascular enhancement.

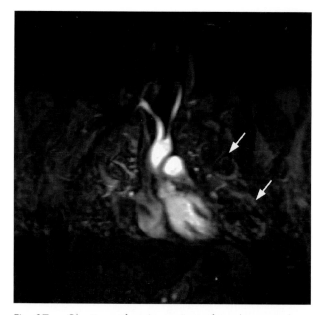

Fig. 37. Ghosting artifacts (arrows) arise from changes in the phase of the MR signal due to blood pulsation and heart motion. The pulsation artifacts can be accentuated further when the signal intensity of blood changes during the acquisition from changes in the T1 relaxation. The artifacts can propagate over the vasculature and can create local enhancement or signal voids.

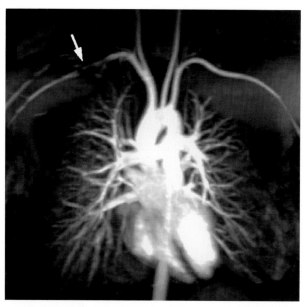

Fig. 38. Susceptibility signal loss caused by the passage of contrast. Signal loss is appreciated in the subclavian vein for an increase in the local concentration of contrast agent (arrows) despite the short TE utilised for scanning (TE = 1.6 ms). The local change in magnetic susceptibility affects nearby tissues and vessels and can be better appreciated in the raw images. The radius of action for such artifacts is highly dependent on the concentration of contrast during the acquisition of the centre of k-space and the TE of the contrast-enhanced MRPA acquisition.

(Fig. 38), which is close to the point where the contrast agent is injected. The local dephasing that is produced can affect the signal of surrounding tissues and other vessels as well. This void can be misinterpreted as a possible stenosis or thrombus and can be better appreciated on the original sections of the MRPA.

Good contrast timing is required to form an arterial MRPA only data set. To achieve good vessel selectivity with short circulation times between arteries and veins there should always be a sharp peak T1 relaxation shortening occurring at different positions in k-space. The T1 relaxation shortening occurs during a brief period of the acquisition and has a Gaussian-like shape over a small portion of k-space. When the Gaussian curve (maximum T1 relaxation shortening) occurs during the collection of the edges of k-space, ringing and edge enhancement are produced in the image of the vessel (Fig. 39). This edge-enhancement produces a darkening of the vessel centre that may be confused with an embolus if the signal characteristics of the MRPA scan are not known for the chosen imaging parameters. Blurring (or vessel smoothing) occurs when the maximum T1 relaxa-

tion occurs only during the centre of k-space, creating an effect that is similar to a low pass filter.

Saturation can occur, which manifests itself as a local or global signal intensity decrease, when a stenosis or a thrombus restricting blood flow is present. Mixing of contrast-enhanced blood with normal blood can be slower and therefore a longer T1 relaxation time will occur when compared to other vessels where contrast may be more concentrated. Saturation occurs more often with the use of a short contrast bolus. It indicates that the flip angle chosen is too high for the concentration of contrast expected. Luckily, in cases of saturation, the blood T1 relaxation values have remained shorter than that of surrounding thrombus. This is nicely demonstrated in Figure 54 along the descending pulmonary artery of a patient with a large embolus.

High venous signal is a by-product of wrong contrast timing, indicating that the centre of k-space was acquired after most of the contrast had already passed through the pulmonary arterial system. Artifacts in the arteries are not likely to appear because there is always some residual contrast during the entire length of the scan that pro-

287

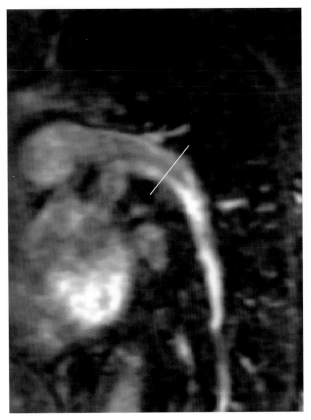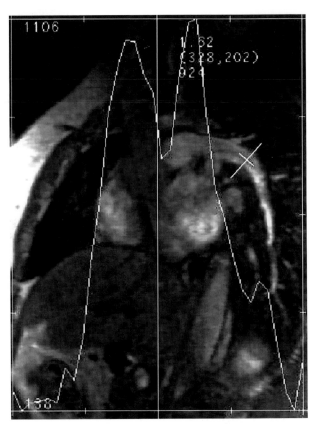

Fig. 39a, b. Signal profile across the left descending pulmonary artery indicative of ringing artifacts in the vessel from inadequate signal distribution across k-space. A one-sided signal enhancement of the high k-space data occurred to produce a mild high pass filter effect on the data reflected as an enhancement of the vessel edges. The dip in the signal intensity in the centre of the vessel can be confused with a thrombus.

vides T1 relaxation enhancement for the arteries. Figure 54d illustrates the results of a hand injection without the correct timing demonstrating much higher intensity in the pulmonary veins.

Intravascular contrast agents

Dynamic injections provide one single chance to obtain fast breath-hold MRPA with good image quality. To overcome this constraint and enhance the limited resolution and SNR possible with ultra-fast breath-hold acquisitions, a variety of intravascular contrast agents have been investigated that produce similar steady-state T1 relaxation effects in blood as gadolinium complexes during dynamic injections. The time that these new contrast agents remain in blood varies, depending on the size of the molecule and its excretion metabolism, ranging between 20 minutes to several hours. Studies already performed on animals have produced a continuous several-fold enhancement of

pulmonary vessels and pulmonary parenchyma [111–113].

When the contrast agent is confined to the blood compartment, a steady-state condition for the T1 and T2 relaxation values is achieved. The time dependence can be eliminated from Equation 12, making the design independent of all considerations of k-space scanning exposed earlier.

Intravascular contrast agents are undergoing clinical trials at present, but may soon become available for general use. A Gd complex binding reversibly to albumin with a high T1 relaxivity profile (MS-325) holds promise in many respects (steady-state and dynamic imaging) [114, 115]. Ultra-small particle superparamagnetic iron oxides (USPIOs, e. g. CLARISCAN*, NC100150, Nycomed Amersham) have also been evaluated in parallel [80].

Using NC100150 enables imaging of the pulmonary vasculature with continous breathing due to the longer presence of the contrast agent in the blood which enables the use of navigator echoes for respiratory triggering. This is of importance in the investigation of pulmonary embolism where the patients can have problems to hold their breath long enough to get sufficient image quality. It also enables longer acquisition times for higher resolution and cardiac triggering, which improves the image quality further by avoiding motion arte-

facts from the heart. Due to the prolonged imaging window NC100150 further enables dual imaging of pulmonary embolism and detection of the source of the emboli.

Both contrast agent types equally enhance arteries and veins during the steady-state phase (Fig. 40).

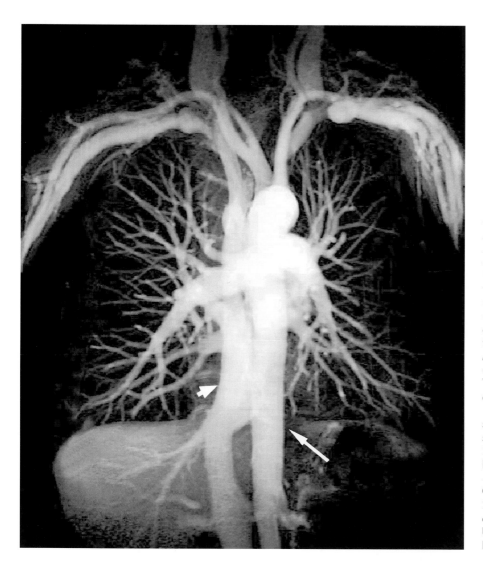

Fig. 40. Pulmonary vascular imaging in a patient with suspected PE using the intravascular contrast NC100150 (Nycomed Amersham) acquired during the steady-state phase. Veins and arteries appear uniformly enhanced, as can be noted between the inferior vena cava (arrowhead), usually appearing unenhanced during a dynamic acquisition using Gd-DTPA injections, and the aorta (arrow). MRPA performed with 3D FLASH using
TR/TE = 4.5/1.7 msec,
$\alpha = 30°$, 390 Hz/pixel,
108 mm coronal slab with scanned/reconstructed sections = 36/72,
200 x 512 matrix,
FOV = 450 x 450 mm^2,
32 sec breath-hold.
Contrast dosage was
2 mg Fe/Kg. (Raw slices courtesy of Dr. André Duerinckx, UCLA Veterans Hospital, Los Angeles, USA).

9. Clinical evaluation of MRPA for pulmonary embolism

Few studies report on the use of MRPA for the detection of PE. Earlier reports mainly focus on the utility of conventional TOF 2D GRE scans. A single clinical report has been presented with contrast-enhanced 2D GRE. Although an increasing number of studies allude to the application of contrast-enhanced 3D scans for MRPA because of its robustness and easy interpretation, only a single clinical study has been published. The result of the literature survey is summarised in Table 6. The imaging parameters show the difference between imaging protocols, especially for contrast-enhanced MRPA where resolution, coverage and breath-hold time can vary substantially.

Conventional MRPA

Schiebler et al. [116] evaluated 18 patients prospectively with 2D sequential MRPA (TR/TE/α = (6.8–9.8)/2.2/20°, 128×256 matrix, breath-hold, 2 averages, sagittal) in conjunction with cardiac-gated SE and cine 2D GRE with spatial modulation of magnetisation (SPAMM). The overall sensitivity for the detection of acute pulmonary emboli was 85 % (42 % for chronic emboli). Confirmation was performed with conventional angiography on 8 patients, 5 with radionuclide ventilation/perfusion (V/Q) scan, and 6 had direct surgical intervention.

Table 6. Sensitivity and specificity values for MRPA techniques used for the detection of acute and chronic PE.

Reference	MRPA technique	Data collection Mode	Number Patients	Sensitivity %	Specificity %
CONVENTIONAL TOF TECHNIQUES					
2D studies					
Grist et al. [117][a]	2D sequential TOF GRE	breath-hold	20	92/100	62
Schiebler et al. [116][b]	2D sequential TOF GRE	breath-hold	18	85/42	–
Sostman et al [118][c]	2D sequential TOF GRE	free breathing averaging	25	71	97
CONTRAST-ENHANCED TECHNIQUES					
2D studies					
Loubeyre et al. [119][d]	Magnetization-prepared 2D sequential CE GRE	multiplanar free breathing dynamic	23	70	100
Bergin et al. [121][e]	2D interleaved CE GRE	breath-hold	55	36/72	65/59
3D studies					
Meaney et al. [94][f]	3D CE GRE	breath-hold coronal slab single injection	30	87	97
Oudkerk et al. [90][g]	3D multi-slab CE GRE	breath-hold double sagittal slabs double injection	82	83	97

[a] sensitivity from 2 different readers

[b] acute versus chronic emboli

[c] sensitivity for expert readers

[d] MR evaluation only on proximal pulmonary branches

[e] sensitivity and specificity for central and segmental vessels, respectively

[f] analysis excluding 3 patients with unreadable scans

[g] new numbers were not yet reported, study shows a reader learning curve

TOF = time-of-flight, GRE = gradient recalled echo imaging, 2D = two-dimensional, 3D = three-dimensional, CE = contrast-enhanced.

A study by Grist et al. [117] reported on the accuracy of a similar breath-hold 2D sequential MRPA set-up (TR/TE/α = (6.8 – 12)/(2.2 – 3.4)/20 – 30°, 128 × 256 matrix, breath-hold, 4 averages, sagittal). A sensitivity of 92 % – 100 % and specificity of 62 % was reached in 20 patients evaluated prospectively (16 with angiographic correlation, 4 with known PE).

Sostman et al. [118] investigated a free-breathing 2D sequential GRE scan (TR/TE/α = 12/(1.8 – 2.8)/30°, 256x256 matrix, 8 averages, sagittal) in 25 patients. Several levels of expertise were discussed, reporting sensitivities ranging between 43 % and 92 % and specificities between 67 % and 100 %. In the expert group, a mean sensitivity of 73 % and specificity of 97 % was obtained. Study confirmation was performed using a decision tree involving conventional angiography and radionuclide V/Q scans.

Initial comparison between conventional and contrast-enhanced MRPA

One single study by Rubin et al. [69] using Gd-DTPA (gadopentetate dimeglumine) compared breath-hold 2D sequential, cardiac compensated 2D interleaved and 3D GRE MRPA, reporting worst image quality for the 2D sequential case.

Another report using dynamic imaging during Gd-DTPA injection was reported by Loubeyre et al. [119]. The group envisioned a multi-slice setup using 2D sequential magnetisation-prepared (MP) GRE scans for the assessment of the proximal pulmonary arteries, selecting a set of three imaging planes with thick slices (20 mm) to encase the main pulmonary artery and the proximal pulmonary branches. One set was acquired every 1.5 sec, collecting data repeatedly during quiet breathing for approximately one minute.

2D contrast-enhanced MRPA studies

Using the multiplanar MRPA setup described above using a thick-section magnetisation prepared 2D GRE scan (TR/TE/α = 6.5/3.0 (msec)/12°, inversion time to null blood = 300 msec, 128 × 128 matrix, free breathing) [120], Loubeyre et al. [119] imaged 23 consecutive patients with suspected PE. A comparison with pulmonary angiography yielded a sensitivity of 70 % and a specificity of 100 % only for proximal pulmonary emboli (segmental emboli were completely missed).

More recently, Bergin et al. [121] investigated the accuracy of a 2D interleaved acquisition (TR/TE/ α = 113/4.3 (msec)/70°, 128 × 256 matrix, breath-hold) combined with spiral contrast-enhanced CT angiography in 26 patients with chronic thrombolytic disease. After angiographic and surgical confirmation, MRPA provided a sensitivity of 36 % and specificity of 65 % for thrombus detection in central vessels and higher values for segmental vessels, reaching a sensitivity of 72 % and specificity of 59 %. The poor figures may be attributed to the thickness of the slices utilised (10 mm).

3D contrast-enhanced MRPA studies

The report by Isoda et al. [91] may be considered the first clinical experience with breath-hold contrast-enhanced 3D MRPA. The group investigated 13 patients (9 with lung cancer, 1 metastatic lung tumour, 2 pulmonary sequestrations, 1 suspicious PE) with a contrast-enhanced 3D GRE scan (TR/TE/α = 12/5 (ms)/20°, 16 slices, 100 × 128 matrix, breath-hold 19 sec, coronal, test bolus injection). Correlation with conventional angiography revealed a sensitivity of 80 %, specificity of 95 % and an accuracy of 94.5 % for the detection of segmental artery stenosis or occlusion.

More recent investigations with breath-hold contrast-enhanced 3D MRPA using higher spatial resolution protocols have reported the routine visualisation of 5th to 7th order branches and have provided data sets that can be reformatted to assess any vessel obstruction caused by emboli with increased accuracy. Meaney et al. [94] investigated 30 consecutive patients prospectively (TR/TE/α = 6.5/1.8 (ms) /40° – 45°, 32 slices, 128 × 256 matrix, breath-hold 27 sec, coronal, fixed injection delay 7 – 10 sec, dose 0.3 mmol/kg Gd-DTPA). Readings by three independent radiologists provided sensitivities of 100 %, 87 % and 75 % (mean 87.3 %) and specificities of 95 %, 100 % and 95 % (mean 96.6 %), respectively, when compared with conventional angiography. The overall score by consensus agrees on 100 % sensitivity and a specificity of 95 %, however, without including data from 3 patients with unreadable MRPAs.

Wielopolski et al. [102] reported the implementation of a double sagittal protocol to cover both lungs completely with high spatial resolution (TR/TE/α = 3.65/1.6 (msec)/25°, 44 slices-96 reconstructed, 106 × 512 matrix, breath-hold 17 sec, 2 sagittal slabs, test bolus injection, dose 20 ml Gd-DTPA per lung) (Figs. 41 – 44). A preliminary evaluation by Oudkerk et al. [90] performed in 82 patients using this protocol provided a sensitivity of

291

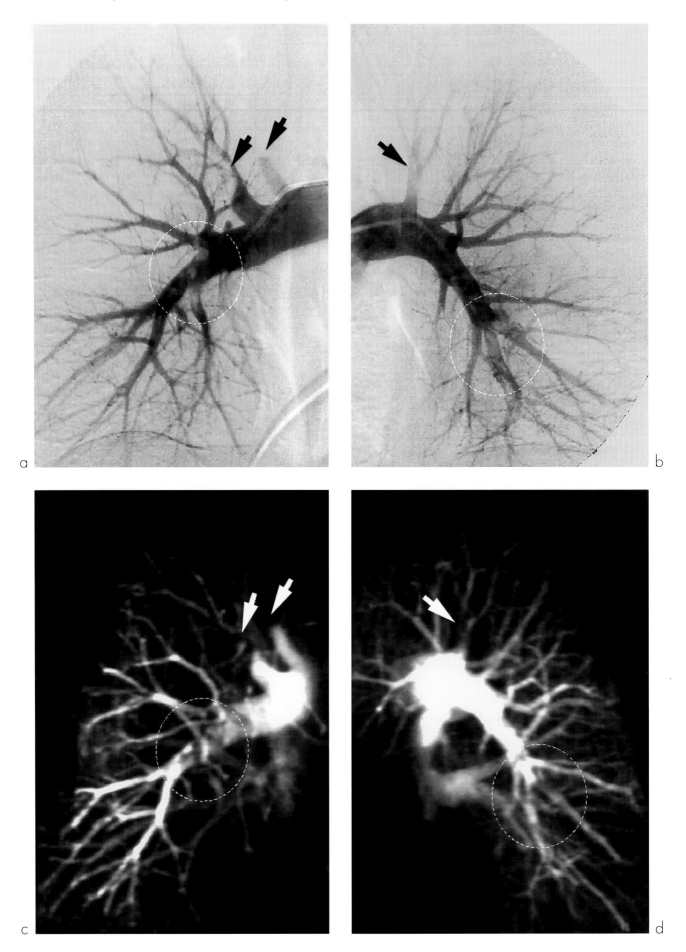

Fig. 41a–g. Initial and follow-up examinations of a patient with PE with multiple emboli lodged in both right and left pulmonary arteries. Right **(a)** and left **(b)** coronal oblique digital subtraction angiograms (RAO and LAO 25° views) acquired within one hour after the MRPA. Volume rendering of the right **(c)** and left **(d)** pulmonary arterial trees from a contrast-enhanced 3D MRPA acquisition. **(e)** Multiplanar reformations along first to third order branches of the arterial tree in both lungs demonstrate the location of many of the thrombi seen in **(a)–(d)**. The follow-up examination after 3 months of thrombolitic therapy shows complete clearance of all thrombi in both right **(f)** and left **(g)** pulmonary arterial systems. Comparison between first and follow-up examinations reveals in the latter reduced vessel diameters in both pulmonary arterial systems. Volume rendering was performed with a transparency setting similar to that of an X-ray projection to make the MRPA compare more closely to the digital subtraction angiogram. Arrow and arrowheads point at the location of thrombi in **(a)** through **(e)**. Circular dashed region illustrates a region with major opacification defects. A double sagittal slab contrast-enhanced 3D MRPA protocol was performed with acquisition parameters such as in Figure 31.

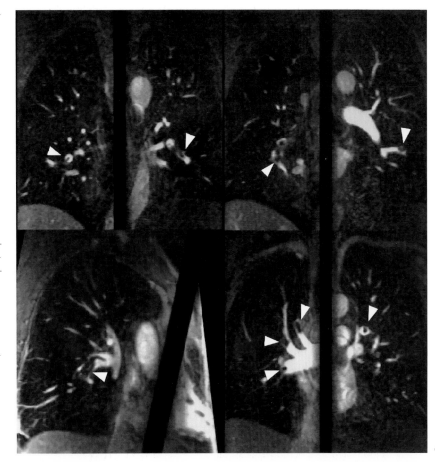

e

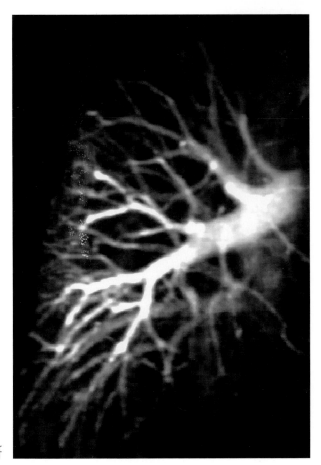

f

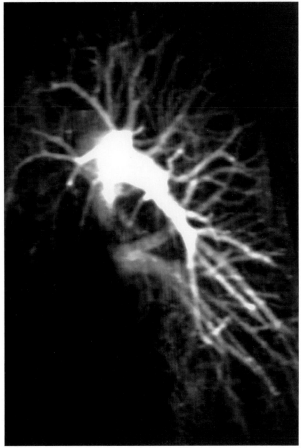

g

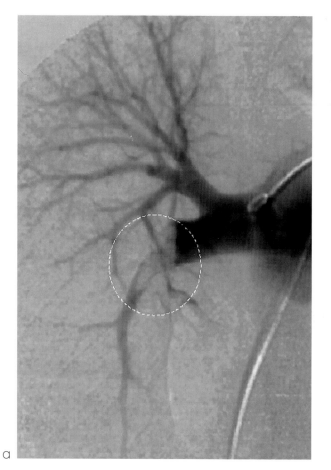

a

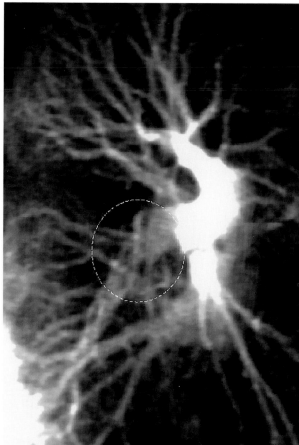

b

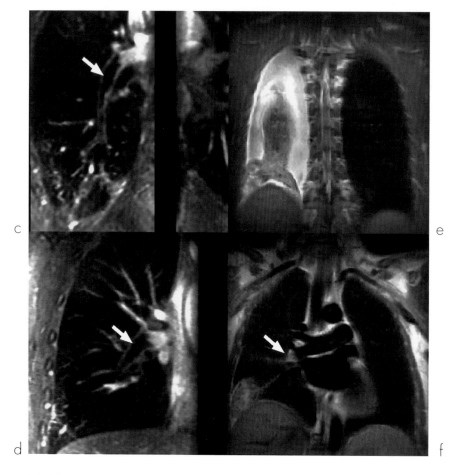

c

d

e

f

Fig. 42a–f. Patient with a massive thrombus in the right descending pulmonary artery. The conventional pulmonary angiogram **(a)** compares closely to the projection obtained with contrast-enhanced 3D MRPA **(b)**. Circular dashed regions demonstrate the location of the embolus. **(c)** and **(d)** depict two perpendicular MPR images along the massive embolus. Black blood HASTE illustrates a large pleural effusion in the posterior right lung, by-product of the massive embolus **(e)**. Arrow and arrowheads point at the location of the thrombus. A double sagittal slab contrast-enhanced 3D MRPA protocol was performed with acquisition parameters as in Figure 31. The black block HASTE was collected with a 5 mm thickness, ETS/TE = 4/32 msec, 780 Hz/pixel readout, 5 mm slice thickness, 192 × 256 matrix, FOV = 330 × 330 mm^2. The thrombus can also be appreciated in this setting (arrows) **(f)**.

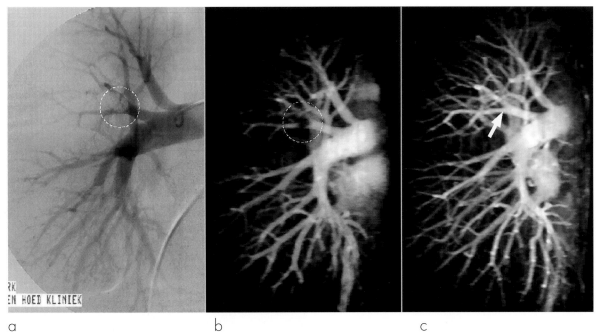

a   b   c

Fig. 43a–c.   Initial and follow-up MRPA examinations of a patient with a small embolus lodged in the anterior segmental artery of the right upper lobe. **(a)** Conventional pulmonary angiography. **(b)** Initial contrast-enhanced 3D MRPA demonstrates the signal void associated with the embolus. Circular dashed region encircles the location of the embolus in **(a)** and **(b)**. **(c)** The follow-up contrast-enhanced MRPA examination demonstrates complete clearance of the embolus (arrow) after 3 months following anticoagulant therapy. A double sagittal slab contrast-enhanced 3D MRPA protocol was performed with acquisition parameters as in Figure 31. **(b)** used half the dosage of contrast as compared to **(c)**.

83 % and specificity of 97 %, respectively. Conventional angiography was performed in all patients after and within one hour of the MRPA examination. Sensitivity was hampered by the learning curve of the radiologist involved in the evaluation. Lung perfusion defects can appear in many circumstances (Fig. 45) but PE can only be diagnosed if the thrombus occluding the lumen is visualised after inspection with MPR (Fig. 46). Another indication that may show during review is a pulmonary branch with lower signal intensity than others. This sign seldom appears but has been seen with emboli blocking a branch almost entirely, producing a lower concentration of the contrast agent in the vessel with reduced blood flow. This is similar to inadequate bolus timing. Pulmonary perfusion with sufficient temporal resolution (one image per second) has documented regional differences of contrast arrival.

Dynamic contrast-enhanced MRPA imaging

Time-resolved acquisitions for MRPA have been investigated with 2D projection MRA [122, 123] and 3D MRA [124, 125]. The time-resolved acquisition concept using fast 2D GRE sequence (FLASH, RF spoiled GRASS) after contrast injection is not new. Many reports exist using the technique to map perfusion in several organs. This technique has been used by Loubeyre et al. for diagnosing PE [119].

The more recent reports of Hennig et al. [122] (Fig. 47) and Wang et al. [123] (Fig. 48) have employed thicker slices to produce a projection MRPA with higher spatial and time resolution using the shorter TR/TE possible with newer imaging gradient hardware. Wang et al. use a complex subtraction that proves more beneficial for imaging the lung as it overcomes phase cancellation in voxels containing stationary and flowing material and removes some of the residual background phase associated with magnetic susceptibility.

Departing from 2D dynamic MRPA concepts, the 3D time-resolved volumetric imaging concept of Korosec et al. [126] (3D TRICKS, 3D Time-Resolved Imaging of Contrast Kinetics) has also been applied for dynamic MRPA. This was demon-

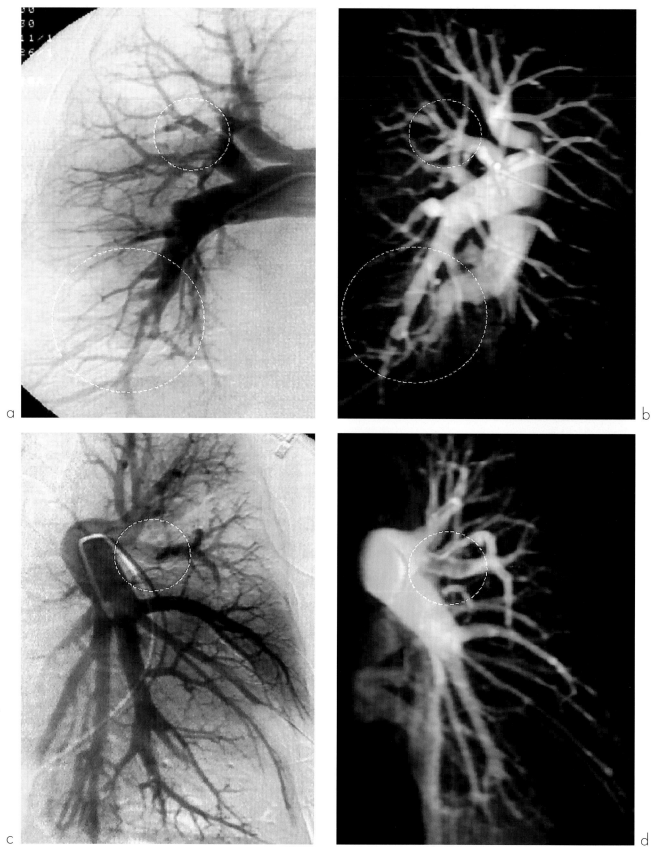

Fig. 44a–d. Initial contrast-enhanced 3D MRPA on a patient with multiple emboli lodged in both lungs. Dashed circular regions on the conventional RAO 25° right pulmonary angiogram show the signal voids associated with the emboli. **(b)** Volume rendering of the 3D contrast-enhanced MRPA demonstrates similar vascular anatomy. Opacity settings were not adequate to clearly show the voids (overprojection). A nice correlation is possible on the left lung between the conventional pulmonary angiogram **(c)** and the volume-rendered MRPA acquisition **(d)**. A double sagittal slab contrast-enhanced 3D MRPA protocol was performed with acquisition parameters as in Figure 31.

Fig. 45. Perfusion defect detected in the posterior section of the left lower lobe in the patient. The perfusion defect was not associated with the presence of a blocking thrombus, confirmed after assessing the pulmonary artery feeding the associated segment using multiplanar reformation. Perfusion defects are better appreciated with increased enhancement of the lung parenchyma.

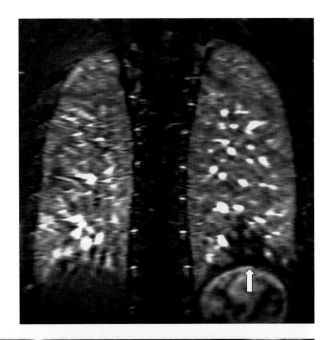

Fig. 46a, b. Thrombus and perfusion defect detected in a patient with suspected PE. **(a)** Multiplanar reformation demonstrates the location of a large embolus centrally located in the descending right pulmonary artery and the associated sub-segmental perfusion defect towards the posterior section of the lung parenchyma (encircled regions). **(b)** The follow-up examination after 3 months of thrombolitic therapy demonstrates complete thrombus clearance with complete restoration of perfusion towards the previously compromised region. Contrast injected manually using a 7 sec delay to image acquisition.

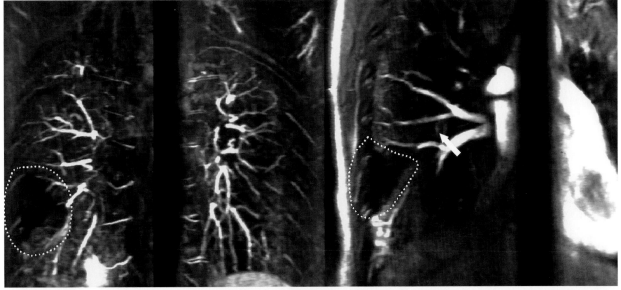

a

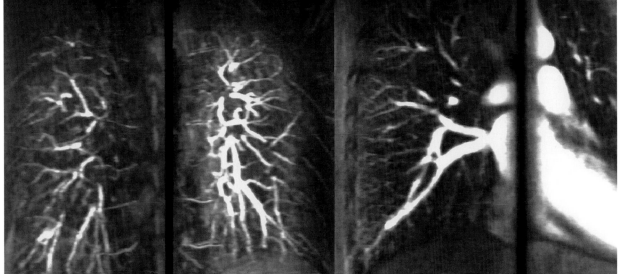

b

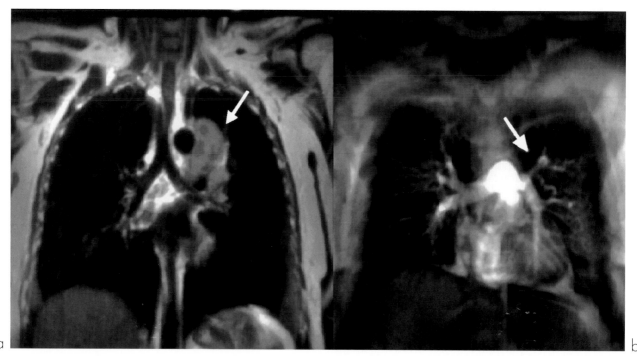

a   b

Fig. 47a, b. Malignant obstruction. 51 year old male with bronchogenic carcinoma in the left upper lobe **(a)** producing pulmonary arterial stenosis **(b)**. Time-resolved magnitude projection MRPA using a thick slice 2D FLASH sequence with dynamic contrast injection and a temporal resolution of 1 sec. The acquisition used a TR/TE = 3.4/1.6 msec, $\alpha = 35°$, 256 × 256 matrix, FOV = 380 × 380 mm^2. 0.1 mmol/Kg of Gd-DTPA was injected (20 ml) at a flow rate of 6 ml/sec (flushed with 20 ml of saline). Image accompanied by a morphological slice collected with a HASTE acquisition. Body phased-array coil acquisition. (Image courtesy of J. Laubenberger, Freiburg University, Freiburg, Germany).

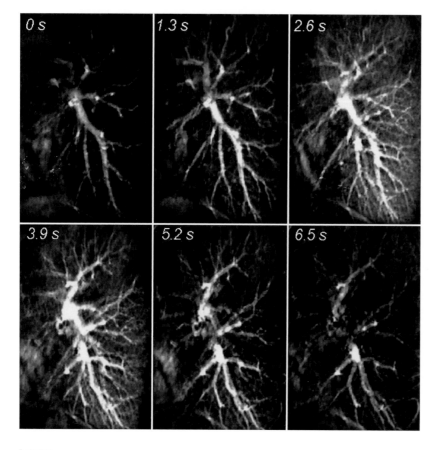

Fig. 48. Complex subtraction, breath-hold, time-resolved 2D sagittal projection MRPA on the right lung of a healthy subject. Frames where acquired with a time resolution of 1.3 sec after a hand injection of 0.1 mmol/Kg Gd-DTPA injection (flushed with 20 ml of saline). The acquisition used a TR/TE = 10/2.5 msec, $\alpha = 45°$, 128 × 256 matrix, FOV = 380 × 380 mm^2 and a slab thickness of 50 mm. A pre-contrast arrival image was used as mask for the complex subtraction to demonstrate only the contrast-enhancing vessels and parenchyma. Body phased-array coil acquisition. Relative time of each frame is identified (in seconds). (Image courtesy of Y. Wang, Diagnostic Radiology, Mayo Clinic, Rochester, USA).

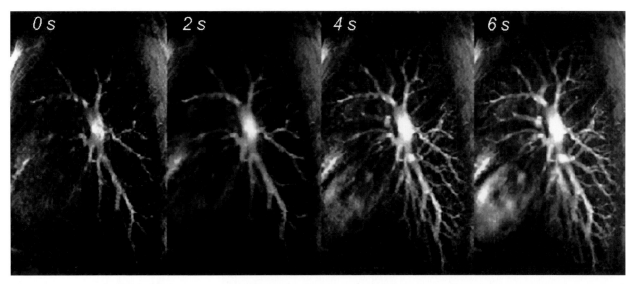

Fig. 49. Time-resolved MIP of a dynamic contrast-enhanced acquisition in the right lung of a healthy volunteer using a cardiac-triggered 3D TRICKS acquisition. The frames displayed were produced with a temporal resolution of 2 sec per volume while view sharing used a temporal aperture of 8 seconds. The time resolution was good enough to demonstrate the pulmonary arteries prior to the enhancement of parenchyma and pulmonary veins. A 256 × 256 partial Fourier matrix was selected with TR/TE = 25/4.9 msec, α = 25°, FOV = 240 × 180 mm². The lung was covered with 8 sagittal sections (12 mm thick). 36 ml of Gd-DTPA was injected at a rate of 1.6 ml/sec, followed by 20 ml of saline. Relative time of each frame is shown (in seconds). Body phased-array coil acquisition. (Image courtesy of D. Peters, Department of Radiology, Madison University, Wisconsin, USA).

strated by Peters et al. [124] using 3D TRICKS in conjunction with cardiac triggering, observing the passage of contrast through the pulmonary vasculature with good temporal resolution (2 sec) to observe the selective enhancement of arteries and veins with good spatial resolution (Fig. 49). To maintain both good spatial and good temporal resolution, k-space filling is performed in a segmented fashion (k-space segmentation using blocks of contiguous data) and k-space data is shared between the volumes encoded. Depending on the set-up, the centre of k-space can be updated at reasonable time resolution while high k-space lines are shared between several data sets using time interpolation with a sliding acquisition window that updates these values at lower speed. Using this methodology, good temporal and spatial resolution can be obtained with low readout bandwidths and using MRI scanners with slower imaging gradients. Wielopolski et al. [102] applied a similar k-space sharing concept to a 3D scan making use of a faster gradient hardware. The implementation was based on an ultrashort FLASH TR/TE sequence (TR/TE = 1.7/0.8 msec) covering the entire thorax with a time resolution of 1 volume per second with a short sliding window

of 1.5 sec. This was intended to produce both a low resolution MRPA (with 2.6 × 2.6 × 9 mm³ voxel sizes) and volumetric perfusion imaging of the entire lung parenchyma (Fig. 50).

Volumetric acquisitions with multi-shot echo-planar imaging (EPI)

MRPA can be attempted in a fraction of the time of standard without sparing resolution with 3D GRE MRPA incorporating segmented echo planar imaging (EPI) readouts [127]. The sampling density of segmented EPI is unparalleled, with sampling rates greater than 1 msec/per line and an ample reduction in radio-frequency power deposition. Heid et al. [128] have demonstrated this for whole-body MRA with acceptable image quality. A representative sequence diagram of a 3D segmented EPI acquisition is illustrated in Figure 51.

Coverage and resolution can be maintained for different breath-hold lengths because of the signal encoding speed, requiring only that TR, the number of echoes encoded per RF excitation and the readout bandwidth be balanced appropriately. A smaller number of echoes per excitation make pos-

299

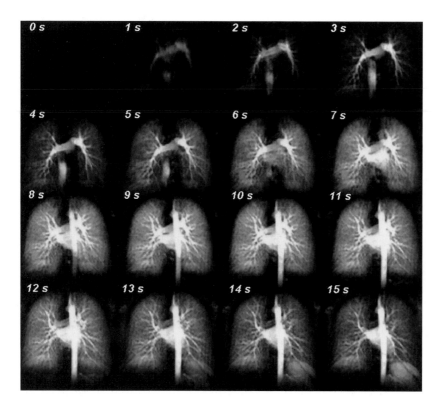

Fig. 50. Volumetric lung perfusion scan collected in a patient with suspected PE using an ultrafast 3D GRE acquisition after administering a bolus of 8 ml of Gd-DTPA delivered at a flow rate of 4 ml/sec. A coronal maximum intensity projection was performed over a 64 mm volume in the posterior section of the lung. Twenty coronal sections were acquired per volume-frame at a rate of 1 volume-frame/sec. Frames 1 through 16 (from 20 acquired, 400 images) are displayed in collage form. The relative time sequence is indicated in seconds. The 3D FLASH acquisition used a TR/TE = 1.7 msec/0.90 msec, $\alpha = 12°$, 9 mm slice thickness and FOV = 330 × 330 mm^2. Body phased-array coil acquisition.

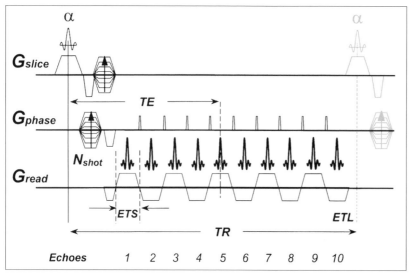

Fig. 51 3D multi-shot EPI sequence diagram. For each rf excitation, 10 echoes are collected (ETL = 10). Segmentation is performed along the in-plane phase encoding direction.
α = rf excitation angle;
G_{read} = readout gradient;
G_{phase} = in-plane phase encoding;
G_{slice} = section select gradient;
ETL = echo train length;
ETS = echo train spacing.

sible shorter TRs, and vice versa, a larger number of echoes will require longer TRs. The issues of blood saturation are identical to those discussed for conventional 3D TOF MRA, and susceptibility effects for the longer echoes of the echo train must be carefully measured to reduce signal losses and issues related to chemical shift interference and flow artifacts [129, 130].

Figure 52 illustrates a contrast-enhanced MRPA acquisition using 3D multi-shot EPI acquisition covering the entire thoracic volume, acquired in one single breath-hold (16 sec) with isotropic resolution and with one contrast injection. Signal loss from magnetic susceptibility dephasing between vessels and air in the lungs can be maintained small by keeping a short effective TE (asymmetric encoding along the in-plane phase encoding direction). This makes it possible to visualise the pulmonary vasculature out to the lung periphery (within SNR limits of the receiver coil used). Additional time savings can be incorporated using partial Fourier scanning that can be robust with very short TE (< 2 msec) and the number of echoes encoded per RF excitation, ETL, is small (< 6).

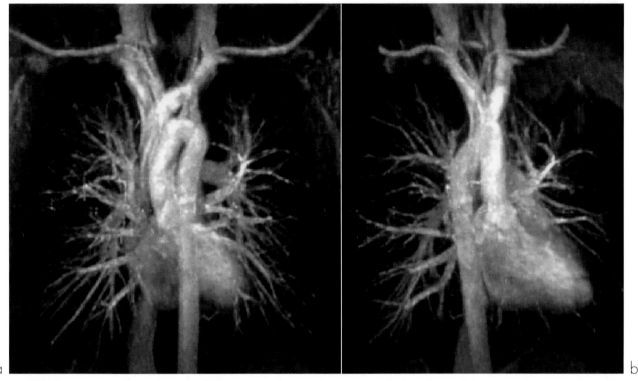

a   b

Fig. 52a, b. Contrast-enhanced 3D MRPA acquired with 3D multi-shot EPI on a healthy subject. A non-selective RF excitation was realized and encoding was performed over the entire thorax in a coronal plane with a matrix size of $110 \times 180 \times 256$ with a FOV of $200 \times 280 \times 320 \, \text{mm}^3$. Five echoes were encoded (ETL = 5) with TR/TE = 4.92/2.30 msec, $\alpha = 35°$. Fat suppression pulses were not applied. Signal reception performed with a body phased-array coil. A single injection of 0.1 mmol/Kg of Gd-DTPA was used. **(a)** left anterior oblique MIP projection and **(b)** right anterior oblique projection (Images courtesy of Oliver Heid, Siemens AG, Erlangen, Germany).

Comparison between breath-hold conventional and contrast-enhanced MRPA for the detection of thrombi

Thrombi are best detected with sequential and segmented k-space 2D MRPA techniques because of the high contrast that can develop between the signal from saturated blood clot and that of blood freshly entering into the thin imaging slice. Although sensitivity for thrombus detection increases with higher flip angles, high blood flow velocities are necessary; angles to avoid blood saturation effects that may obscure thrombi (e. g., a pulmonary vessel running in the plane of section).

In contrast-enhanced MRPA, blood signal can be optimised for any TR and contrast dosage. 2D interleaved MRPA scans can be used but 3D MRPA can offer better SNR and contrast between blood and clot.

Figures 53 and 54 present two cases of patients who received a preliminary examination that tested positive for PE and had a follow-up examination after anticoagulant therapy. A low flip angle, breath-hold 3D MRPA was compared to a contrast-enhanced 3D MRPA acquisition covering the same region of interest (sagittal slab) in the right lung of each patient. The pulmonary embolus that could be easily seen on the contrast-enhanced 3D MRPA in both cases (Figs. 53c and g, Fig. 54c) could not be appreciated on the conventional scan (Figs. 53b and f, Fig. 54b) because of small signal differences between blood and blood clot as a result of the lower flip angle acquisition. Figure 54 also illustrates the saturation effects that are possible when the concentration of Gd-DTPA is lower in the almost completely blocked pulmonary descending artery. The emboli can still be appreciated while the proton density weighted conventional 3D MRPA scan has lower signal for the embolus and can be appreciated if the location is known. The pulmonary angiograms (Figs. 53a and e, Fig. 54a) corroborate the initial findings on the initial contrast-enhanced 3D MRPA scan while the follow-up examinations illustrate the effectiveness of the anticoagulant therapy (Figs. 53d and h, Fig. 54e).

Contrast-enhanced MRPA can improve the display of pulmonary vessels in patients with congenital heart disease [131], atelectasis (Fig. 55), arteriovenous malformations [132, 133], scimitar syn-

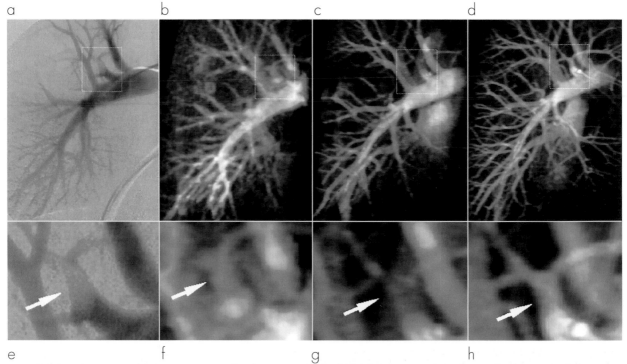

a   b   c   d

e   f   g   h

Fig. 53a–h. Comparison between conventional and contrast-enhanced 3D MRPA on a patient with a small pulmonary embolus in the middle right pulmonary artery. **(a)** Conventional pulmonary angiogram. **(b)**. The magnified views of **(e–h)** correspond to the rectangular view (white dashed square) in **(a–d)** with arrows pointing at the vessel containing the small thrombus. Note that in conventional MRPA the contrast between thrombus and blood does not permit good differentiation **(f)**, better seen on the contrast-enhanced scan **(g)**. **(d)** and **(h)** illustrate the 3D MRPA acquisition after anticoagulant therapy (3 months after first examination) with complete clearance of the blood clot. For the conventional 3D MRPA scan, a sagittal acquisition was performed using FLASH 3D with TR/TE = 3.5/1.4msec, α = 5°, 110 mm, 44 sections (2.5 mm), 96 × 256 matrix, FOV = 220 × 340 mm^2, 15 sec breath-hold. Volume rendering was used for **(b–d)** after manual segmentation of the thorax. Same patient illustrated in the comparison of Figure 43. Contrast-enhanced 3D MRPA parameters as in Figure 31.

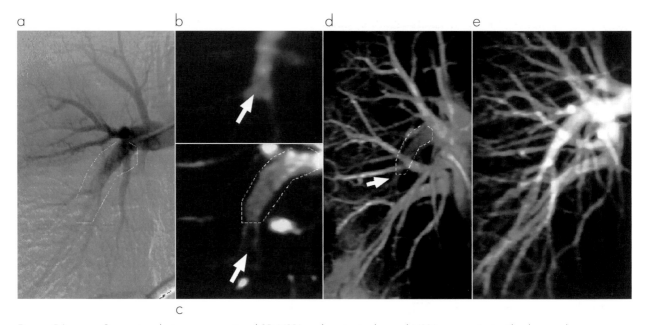

a   b   d   e

c

Figure 54a–e. Comparison between conventional 3D MRPA and contrast-enhanced MRPA on a patient with a large pulmonary embolus lodged in the right descending pulmonary artery. **(a)** Conventional pulmonary angiogram. The irregular dashed region indicates the right descending pulmonary artery. **(b)** Illustrates an MPR view from the conventional 3D MRPA along the vessel with no clear depiction of the thrombus (arrow). The contrast-enhanced 3D MRPA acquisition clearly demonstrates better contrast, making it possible to discern the thrombus from blood (arrow). Note that blood saturation is obvious along the vessel from inadequate bolus timing (no test bolus scan performed). The higher intensity closer to the heart is attributed to a slightly higher contrast concentration and additional TOF enhancement effects from inflowing blood directly from the heart to the sagittal imaged slab. Imaging parameters for the contrast-enhanced MRPA as in Figure 31. Imaging parameters for the conventional MRPA as in Figure 53. For **(d, e)** volume rendering was used after manual segmentation of the thorax. Same patient as shown in Figure 46.

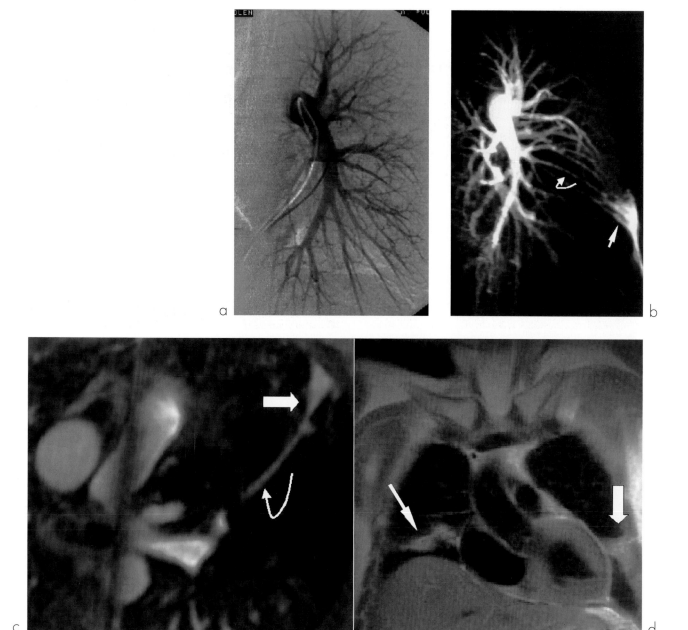

Fig. 55a – d. MRPA in the left lung of a patient suspected of PE demonstrates the signal enhancement produced in atelectasis. The conventional pulmonary angiogram **(a)** does not show such enhancement, clearly visible in the MRPA data set rendered along the same view **(b)**. An MPR reformation along the feeding vessel to the collapsed lung (block arrow) is demonstrated **(c)**. The morphological section collected with a free-breathing single-shot PRESTO HASTE **(d)** illustrates another region with atelectasis, including the one illustrated in the example indicated by the block arrow. Imaging parameters as in Figure 31.

drome [134], thoracic malignancies and vascular compression [135, 136] (Figs. 56 and 57) pulmonary hypertension (Fig. 58) [137].

In pulmonary hypertension, increased pulmonary arterial pressure and pulmonary vascular resistance produces a typical pattern of dilated central pulmonary arteries, tortuous vessels and a pruned appearance of peripheral pulmonary vascular segments (Fig. 58). This process can appear in chronic PE as well. To assess the severity of the vascular disease, a functional evaluation must be performed with conventional techniques and should be considered alternative to any MRPA technique utilised in the study. In the case of hypertension, this can be estimated using a 2D cine GRE scan by documenting the loss of normal systolic distension and diastolic collapse [7] Velocity-encoded cine MRI can also illustrate the lower peak systolic flow velocities with increased retrograde flow as compared to healthy individuals [138].

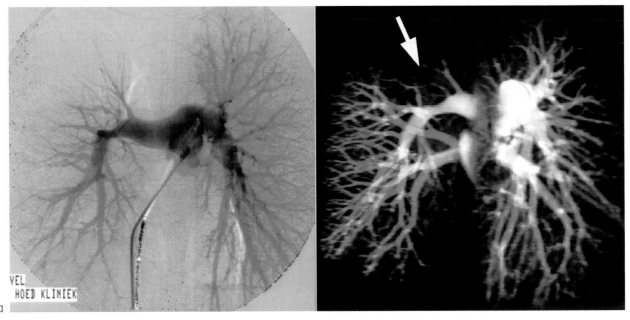

Fig. 56a, b. Patient with a cervix carcinoma presented with a perfusion defect in the right upper lobe on the perfusion radionuclide scan. **(a)** Digital subtraction angiogram corresponds nicely to the volume-rendered results of the 3D MRPA acquisition **(b)**. The arrow point to the narrowing provoked by the growing mass. The non-enhancing mass was completely suppressed on the MRPA examination, illustrating an important feature of contrast-enhanced MRPA for showing only vascular information, not possible with spinal or electron beam CT. The morphological examination confirmed the presence of a mass pressing over the right pulmonary artery. Imaging parameters as in Figure 31.

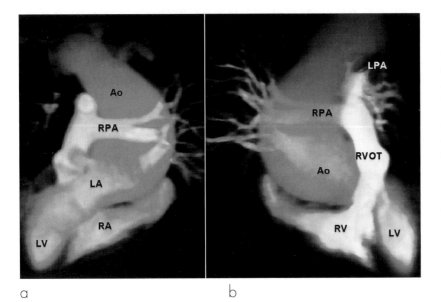

Fig. 57a, b. Two volume-rendered views of the main pulmonary arteries showing also an aortic aneurysm. Note that the timing was chosen for imaging the pulmonary arteries and therefore the aortic aneurysm and aorta appear with lower signal intensity. Data acquisition using a single sagittal slab positioned over the heart. **(a)** posterior volume-rendered projection and **(b)** anterior volume-rendered projection.

Ao = Aorta; RPA = right pulmonary artery; LPA = left pulmonary artery; LA = left atrium; RA = right atrium; LV = left ventricle; RV = right ventricle. Imaging parameters as in Figure 31 but using a single sagittal slab and contrast injection.

Black blood imaging

Many procedures have been used to eliminate blood signal in the so-called "black blood" techniques to display vascular information when high contrast against surrounding background is possible. However, the significance of black blood techniques is not clear for the display of the pulmonary vascular anatomy because lung parenchyma has low signal. Additionally, airways also present no signal and can be confused with vascular structures. Nonetheless, black blood techniques can be useful for the detection of intravascular abnormalities and PE.

With T1- and T2-weighted SE sequences (Fig. 59), anatomic views of the central pulmonary arteries and veins have been obtained with excellent contrast between vessel walls and dark blood [139]. Emboli lodged in vessels can be detected despite their varying signal intensities with age, making SE-based imaging techniques interesting for the diagnosis of PE [140–143].

A study by Erdman et al. [144] used a multi-phase cardiac gated SE technique in 86 patients on a

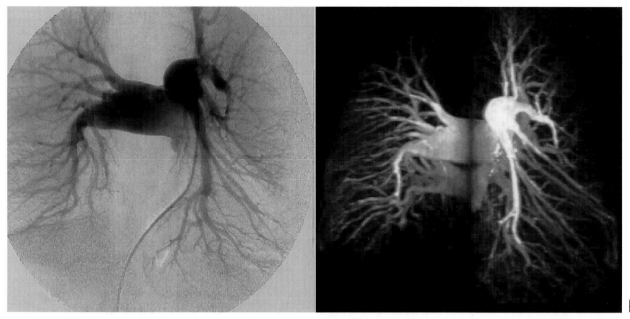

a   b

Fig. 58a, b. Patient with pulmonary hypertension. **(a)** Digital subtraction angiogram illustrates the larger main and central pulmonary artery diameters consistent with the disease. **(b)** Corresponding volume-rendered results from the double slab 3D MRPA acquisition. Imaging parameters as in Figure 31.

prospective and blinded interpretation. In 36 patients with angiographic correlation, the technique provided a sensitivity of 90% and specificity of 77% for the detection of large and medium-sized pulmonary emboli.

Hatabu et al. [145] used cardiac-triggered SPAMM SE (SPAtial Modulation of Magnetisation) to reduce the ambiguity between slow-flowing blood and thrombus. The technique imprinted a grid pattern prior to systole and evaluated its dynamics during the entire cardiac cycle, positively detecting thrombi whenever the pattern remained unchanged within the vessel lumen. The evaluation in 12 patients with chronic pulmonary hypertension yielded an accuracy of 96% for distinguishing persistent slow flow signal from clot.

Degradation from respiratory motion and slow blood flow have been reduced significantly with the introduction of breath-hold 2D fast SE scans [146], making possible high quality, improved spatial resolution morphological imaging of the pulmonary vasculature using cardiac triggering (Fig. 60). The single-shot variant referred to as HASTE (*Half Fourier Acquisition Single-shot Turbo SE*) imaging [147] (Fig. 11) can produce fine morphological views of the lung and the pulmonary vessel lumen and vessel wall, virtually motion artifact free even when acquired during free breathing and without cardiac triggering (Fig. 61). Breath-hold and cardiac triggering can be incor-

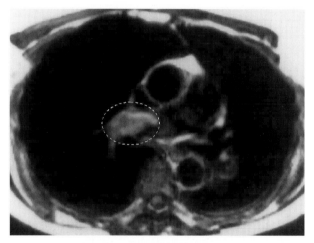

Fig. 59. SE technique with dephasing gradients along the slice select direction provides excellent vessel wall/blood contrast that allows easy visualisation of the pulmonary emboli. A central pulmonary embolus (encircled) appears as a region of higher signal intensity within the vessel as compared with surrounding tissues. Clot exhibits a shorter T1 than muscle, and consequently, a lower T1 than blood. A multi-slice SE scan was used with an effective TR = 700 msec and TE = 22 msec, slice thickness of 8 mm, 192 × 256 matrix with FOV = 400 mm, and 3 acquisitions. Body coil reception.

porated to produce anatomical views that can be used to inspect the vessels in the plane of section, e. g., along the main pulmonary arteries (Fig. 62).

305

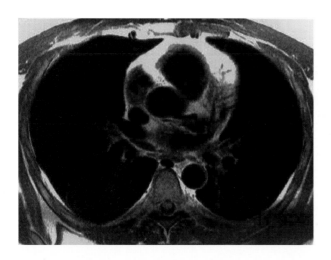

Fig. 60. Single slice, breath-hold T2-weighted fast SE scan. A black blood preparation is used to better suppress the signal from blood. Acquisition was performed in the transverse plane on every other heartbeat for 20 heartbeats, using a 5 mm slice, ETS/TE = 7.12/57 msec, 260 Hz/pixel readout, 150 × 512 matrix, FOV = 260 × 420 mm². A 110 msec acquisition window was used per trigger. Body phased-array coil acquisition.

a   b   c

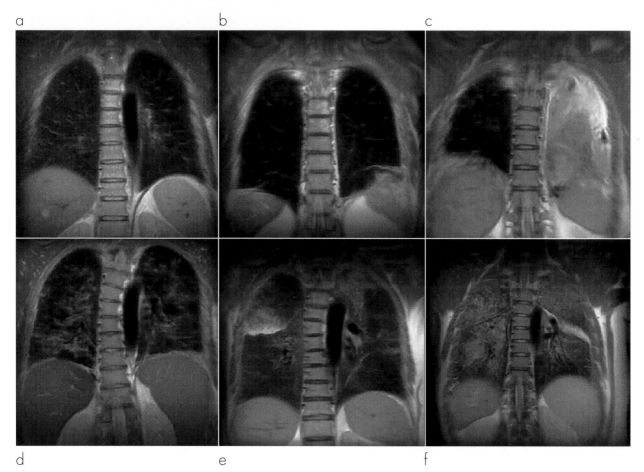

d   e   f

Fig. 61a–f. Examples of black blood HASTE used for a quick free-breathing scout collecting 30 slices over the entire thorax. Six selected cases are displayed from patients that were referred for suspected PE. Image selection was based only on the appearance of the lung parenchyma in each case. Little can be said about the state of the lung parenchyma (CT examination was not available to determine the different patterns observed). The black blood HASTE acquired each slice in 416 ms without cardiac gating, ETS/TE = 4/32 msec, 780 Hz/pixel readout, 5 mm slice thickness, 192 × 256 matrix, FOV = 330 × 330 mm². Body phased-array coil acquisition.

The incorporation of a black blood preparation [148] in both fast SE and HASTE has contributed to reducing the appearance of intraluminal signal from slow moving blood, improving the detection of pulmonary thrombi (Fig. 63).

Because the T1 of blood clots can be shorter than that of blood, a T1-weighted scan covering the entire thorax can be used to attempt their detection. Ultrafast T1-weighted acquisitions, as illustrated in the comparison of Figure 64, can demonstrate clearly the short T1 component of thrombi but can-

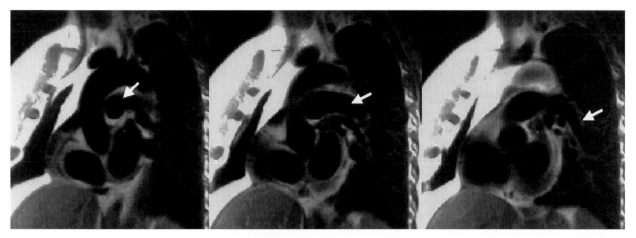

Fig. 62. Breath-hold, cardiac-triggered black blood HASTE along the left pulmonary artery (arrows). Breath-hold was performed to obtain complete registration. Acquisition parameters as in Figure 61.

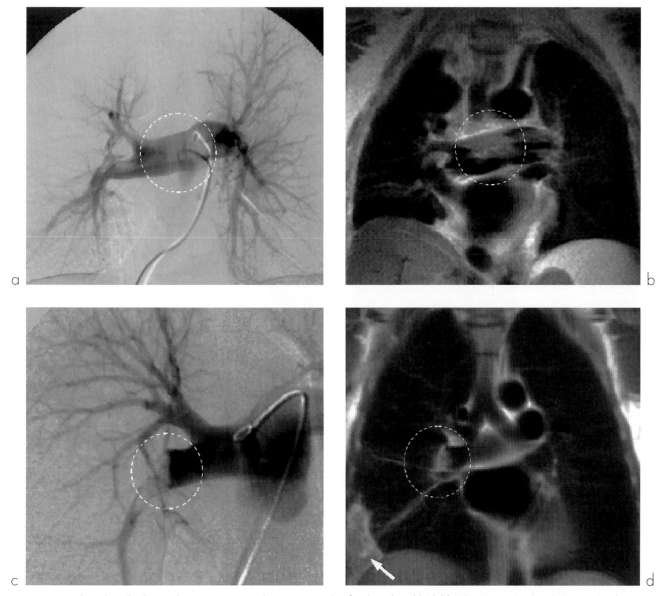

Fig. 63a–d. Thrombi detected in two patients with proven PE with a free-breathing black blood HASTE scan. **(a, c)** Conventional pulmonary angiograms. On the black blood HASTE scans, arrows point at thrombi located centrally **(b)** and at the origin of the right descending pulmonary artery **(d)**, respectively. Arrow in **(d)** points at a pleural effusion. Acquisition parameters for black blood HASTE as in Figure 61.

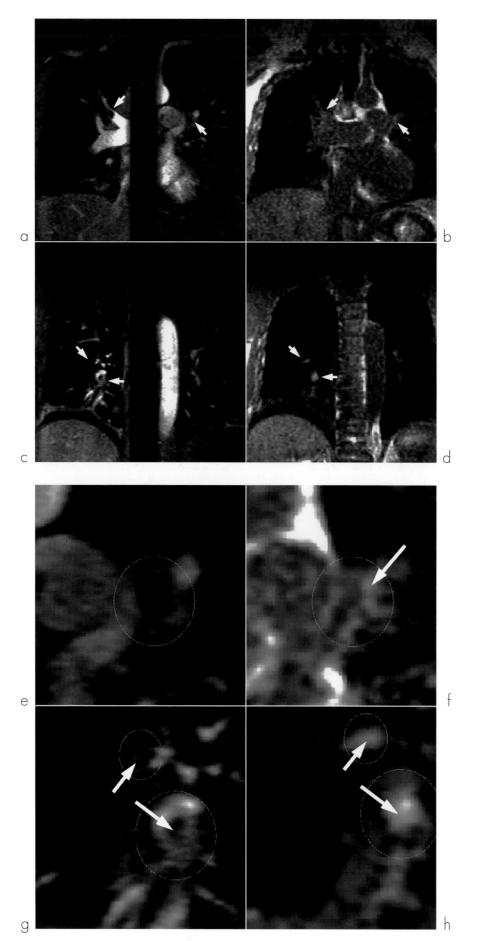

Fig. 64a–h. Possible blood clot detectability using ultrafast breath-hold 3D T1-weighted FLASH scanning both lungs in a single breath-hold prior to MRPA. A comparison with a contrast-enhanced MRPA scan with high sensitivity to clot detectability **(a, c)** is used as a guide to detect the signal from clot on the ultrafast T1-weighted scan **(b, d)**. The arrowheads in the coronal sections point at the location of the emboli. **(e–h)** illustrate magnified views from emboli in **(a–d)**, demonstrating enough sensitivity to view the emboli in the right lower lung base but not for the thrombus lodged in the bifurcation of the main left descending pulmonary artery. Timing for the contrast injection for the contrast-enhanced scan (double sagittal slab protocol) was not adequate to produce high SNR for the pulmonary arteries in this case. The SNR of the T1-weighted scan is not adequate to differentiate clotted blood with characteristics similar to those of surrounding blood. The imaging parameters for the ultrafast FLASH scan were
TR/TE = 1.8/0.9 msec,
$\alpha = 9°$ Hz/pixel readout,
128 x 256 matrix,
FOV = 330 x 460 mm,
80 sections 2.5 mm thick.
The double sagittal slab contrast-enhanced 3D MRPA protocol was performed as indicated in Figure 31. Both scans covered the entire pulmonary vasculature.

not provide the required sensitivity to view other parts of the blood clot (T1 closer to that of blood) because of poor SNR, even with the use of phased-array coil reception. The acquisition of a 3D volume makes it possible to investigate the entire vascular tree with multiplanar reformation.

Magnetisation-prepared gradient recalled echo imaging

Magnetisation-prepared GRE acquisitions can detect thrombi using a non-selective inversion pulse prior to a short TR GRE readout module, as proposed by Wielopolski et al. [149], using a 3D acquisition scheme to enhance resolution and signal-to-noise ratios and provide 3D multiplanar refor-

mation capabilities for arterial lumen inspection. The technique proved sensitive for the detection of some thrombi, as it provided a positive high contrast against suppressed blood. Recently, Moody et al. [150] have revisited this concept using a single-shot 2D MP GRE approach in patients with proven pulmonary emboli, concluding positively on the sensitivity of the approach.

The choice on the inversion time makes this black blood imaging possible. Nonetheless, it is possible to suppress the signal from thrombi instead by using a short inversion time to make the signal from surrounding blood bright. A comparison for different inversion times is illustrated in Figure 65. The use of a T2 or magnetisation transfer preparation can produce a similar effect by suppressing the signal from thrombus (shorter T2 than blood

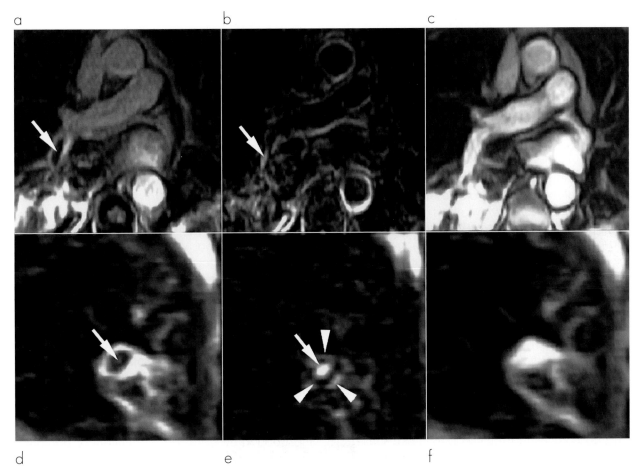

Fig. 65a–f. Pulmonary embolus in the right descending pulmonary artery may be depicted with different signal intensities depending on the imaging parameters chosen for a single-shot magnetisation-prepared (MP) 2D GRE scan. In this case, an inversion pulse and a delay are used as magnetisation preparation prior to image acquisition. **(a)** Inversion time tuned to suppress the signal from blood demonstrates a bright clot (arrow). Small arrowheads in **(c)** point to unsuppressed signal from the vessel wall and high-spatial frequency artifacts from remnant signal from blood. **(b)** Without an inversion pulse, a proton-density weighted image is generated with no discernible contrast between thrombus and blood. **(c)** Choice of a short inversion time suppresses the signal from the embolus (arrow) while moderate signal is maintained for surrounding blood. **(d–f)** correspond to views perpendicular to the ones shown in **(a–c)**. The 2D MP GRE acquisition used a TR/TE/α = 3.5 msec/1.6 msec/10°, 8 mm slice thickness and a 3.3 x 3.0 mm^2 in-plane resolution. Body phased-array coil acquisition.

and higher magnetisation transfer coefficient) while maintaining high signal for blood.

The inversion-based MP GRE technique can be problematic for the detection of clot in small vessels for three reasons:

- vessel walls are not suppressed and signal remains in peripheral small vessels because of partial volume effects
- a long string of low flip angle RF pulses (typically 80–128) after a single magnetisation preparation can suppress blood signal only in the larger vessels (poor suppression of high spatial frequencies during signal encoding typically forming the signal of small vessels). The remnant signal in the vessel wall can be observed in Figure 65 [151].

- Signal-to-noise for MP GRE approaches is usually low because of the low RF excitation readout used to maintain the prepared contrast.

Advantages to the 2D and 3D MP GRE techniques include blood-flow independent results, a drawback often found with non-contrast-enhanced MRA techniques (conventional TOF MRA) for obtaining high blood signal with slow flow.

Both SE and fast MP GRE approaches have a limited scope for PE detection and may only identify intraluminal abnormalities up to 4th order branches reliably. The incorporation of negative contrast agents to suppress blood signal (shortening T2 and T2* dramatically) can prove useful for rapid thrombus imaging [152].

10. Display and evaluation of MRPA

The evaluation of vascular data sets of patients with suspected PE can be a difficult task because of the extent and complexity of the pulmonary vascular tree. Furthermore, the evaluation can be hampered with data sets that are not free from artifacts (blurring in non-cooperative patients or ghosting from blood pulsation) or present poor vascular enhancement (poor inflow effect in conventional TOF MRA or wrong timing for contrast-enhanced scans). Several image post-processing tools can be used, among which multiplanar reformation (MPR), maximum intensity projections (MIP) and volume rendering are widely available options in standard 3D workstations. A suitable combination of these image post-processing tools permits the evaluation of all branches for the eventual detection of thrombi in PE.

Other image presentation and post-processing techniques for MRA have been reviewed in detail by Siebert et al. [153] but they have not been analysed for MRPA. It is important to note that 3D image post-processing routines only make sense for an improved evaluation and display of the MRPA data when SNR, contrast and resolution are adequate.

Multiplanar reformation (MPR)

Multiplanar reformation is an excellent tool for the evaluation that is simple to use and effective for intraluminal vessel inspection. MPR permits the refor-

mation of double oblique planes along any particular vessel path, making it possible to localise intraluminal defects directly. Three planes are most often visualised at once, e. g. the target orientation along a vessel and two adjunct perpendicular views. It is common to produce a reformatted image with a thicker slice than that set by the voxel dimensions. This helps to visualise longer vessel sections (in cases with vessel tortuousity) without hiding intraluminal defects completely through partial volume effects.

Multiplanar reformations can be time-consuming, as it is necessary to inspect every arterial branch separately. Thrombus visualisation is also highly dependent on its location within a vessel. Cases that are fairly easy to document conform to those where thrombi are completely surrounded by bright blood (Fig. 66a). Experience is binding for the detection of thrombi lying against a vessel wall (partial narrowing or constriction) (Figs. 66b and c) or when complete vessel cut-off occurs (requiring good knowledge of the pulmonary anatomy) (Fig. 66d). The latter two can be problematic because a thrombus can be easily missed when the signal is similar to that of the darker lung parenchyma (especially with contrast-enhanced scans using a high contrast dosage at high flip angles). In any case, the review is significantly facilitated when using an MPR platform that is highly interactive, fast and provides adequate localisation freedom.

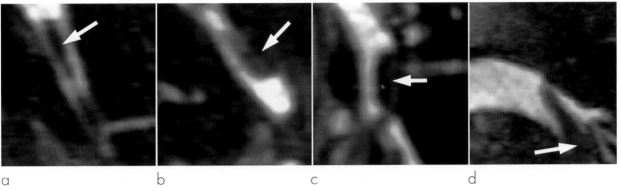

Fig. 66a–d.   Four examples from patients with documented PE illustrating the possible location of thrombi after multiplanar reformation of the corresponding 3D contrast-enhanced MRPA. **(a)** Embolus located centrally in the vessel lumen. **(b, c)** Emboli lodged against the vessel wall producing a partial occlusion (stenosis). **(d)** Embolus totally occludes the left pulmonary descending artery. All arrows point at the location of the blood clot, confirmed with conventional pulmonary angiography.

Maximum intensity projection (MIP) and volume rendering

The most commonly used and widely available technique for vascular visualisation is MIP. The concept behind MIP is straightforward. The MIP algorithm projects rays through voxels of a volume data set and forms an image that has the signal intensity of those voxels that contain the highest intensity values encountered along the casting ray. Another technique that provides a higher degree of control over the display of the MRPA is volume rendering. Volume rendering assigns to voxels particular properties such as opacity, colour and shininess (among others that are definable). These properties are later selectively added to form the rendered image along a specific view. With volume rendering a voxel can be made completely opaque whenever the opacity value assigned is one or, otherwise, completely transparent if the opacity value is set to zero. Intermediate opacity values make it possible to distinguish overlapping vessels or to enhance features that may be hidden within a vessel, e.g. a thrombus. The volume rendering process is more computationally expensive than MIP and requires faster processing hardware for interactive display. These techniques are illustrated in Figure 67.

To demonstrate the main difference between MIP and volume rendering, simulated vessels (software generated) are used that contain different thrombi shapes in similar locations as demonstrated in pulmonary arteries of patients with proven PE. The simulated vessels are constructed from the different cross sections illustrated in Figure 68. The vessel lumen has been assigned a value of 100% with emboli and background at 20% and zero, respectively. Two cases account for the signal of an intact

vessel or a completely occluded one (Figs. 68a and e). Three cases are of interest for the visualisation:

- A cylindrical embolus completely contained and in the centre of the vessel lumen (Fig. 68b)
- A small cylindrical embolus placed near to the vessel wall (Fig. 68c)
- An irregular embolus obstructing half of the vessel lumen (Fig. 68d).

As noted in Figures 69 to 71, MIP has major drawbacks compared to volume rendering techniques. Completely intraluminal defects or small emboli relative to the vessel lumen will not be displayed in a MIP image. It is clear that the only instance where MIP demonstrates the unequivocal presence of an embolus will be when this is larger than one half of the vessel lumen and with the condition that a large area is attached to the lumen wall. If this is the case, part of the casting rays will pass through the embolus without touching the lumen with higher signal intensity (see Figure 71 with viewing angles at 60° and 120°). Volume rendering, on the contrary, can show any intraluminal defect independent of size and location of the thrombi. Because the properties of the voxels can be changed at will, the embolus can be extracted from the histogram of intensities and its brightness and opacity enhanced so that it appears brighter than the vessel lumen itself.

Unfortunately, the single vessel display does not correspond to reality because features and other vessels do not overlap in the reconstruction, especially when vessel information is abundant, as in the case of MRPA. Practically, finding thrombi will be a more realistic task towards the peripheral pulmonary vasculature, where vessel overlap is less likely to occur. There is another situation where

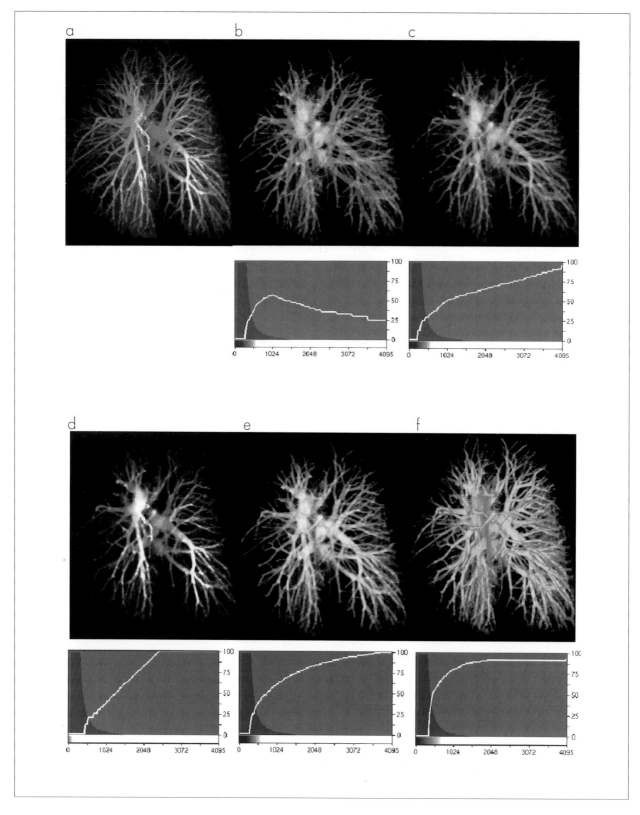

Fig. 67a–f. Appearance of MIP and several settings of voxel opacity during volume rendering. **(a)** MIP. **(b)** Opacity setting corresponding to an image similar to a x-ray projection, showing clear overlap between vessels (all vessel intensities are equalised). **(c, d)** An increase in the opacity value for voxels with higher intensity in the histogram produces more contrast between vessels with higher and lower intensity levels. **(e)** An increase in the curvature of the opacity control (close to assigning equal opacity levels for all intensity values) produces highly contrasted vessels, as in surface rendering, another known type of 3D display setting **(f)**. All the graphs demonstrate the histogram of intensity values of the vascular data set (ranging from 0 to 4095). The opacity curve is controlled using the white tracing in the histogram, making it possible to assign the opacity level selectively for each intensity value of the histogram. This comparison was produced from the MRPA data set collected after anticoagulant therapy in the patient demonstrated in Figure 81.

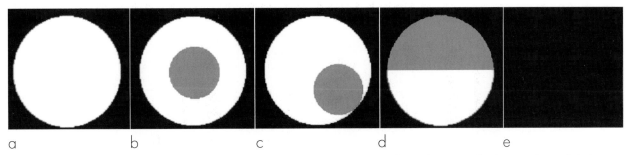

Fig. 68a–e. Cross section of several vessels used to compare the resulting images formed by MIP and volume rendering. **(a)** Plain vessel. **(b)** Embolus completely embedded within the vessel lumen. **(c)** Small embolus closer to the vessel wall. **(d)** Embolus attached to the vessel wall obstructing one half of the vessel lumen. **(e)** Vessel completely occluded. The signal intensity for the vessel was set to 100 % while emboli and background are approximately 20 % and zero, respectively. The cases illustrated correspond to the possible variations that have been found in patients with proven PE (see Fig. 66).

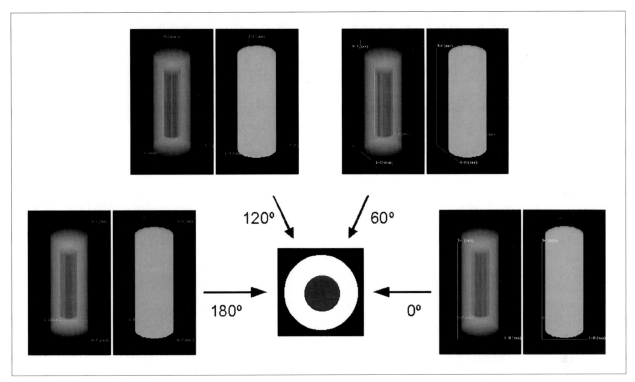

Fig. 69. Comparison between MIP and volume rendering for an embolus completely embedded and centred within the vessel lumen. Projections from all angles demonstrate the same images given the symmetry of the set-up. Images to the left and right of each comparison correspond to volume rendering and MIP, respectively. The embolus can be appreciated with the opacity setting used for volume rendering while it is completely masked with MIP.

MIP can fail completely. Such is the case when the reconstructed vessel cannot rotate on its axis, e. g., a horizontal vessel viewed in a coronal rotation where the casting rays always pass through the bright vessel and the embolus.

MIP presents some additional serious drawbacks. Because one single value is recorded along the casting ray, MIP cannot provide depth information that results in a loss in the spatial position of individual vessels along the casting ray. MIP obscures features that have lower intensity (as illustrated in Figs. 69 and 71), as is the case of intraluminal pul-

monary emboli (Fig. 72). A partial solution to these two issues has been the cine viewing of the processed images at different angles. Another solution has been "sliding" thin slab MIPs through the entire vascular data set. A "sliding" MIP can provide enough vascular coverage to ease the integration of all the vascular information as it is played in the cine loop while it provides a better chance for the detection of intraluminal emboli. More peripheral emboli are easy to detect with both volume rendering and MIP (Fig. 73).

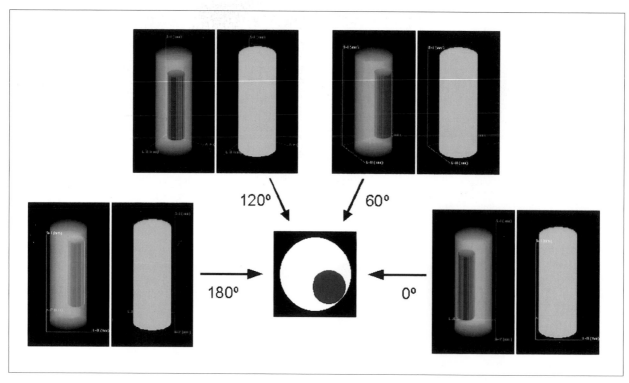

Fig. 70. Comparison between MIP and volume rendering for a small diameter embolus completely embedded within the vessel but close to the vessel wall. Images to the left and right of each comparison correspond to volume rendering and MIP, respectively. The embolus can be appreciated with the opacity setting used for volume rendering while it is still completely masked with MIP. Note that the intensity of the embolus for the rendered projections at 0° and 180° differ to illustrate the shorter distance between the observer and the embolus for the former.

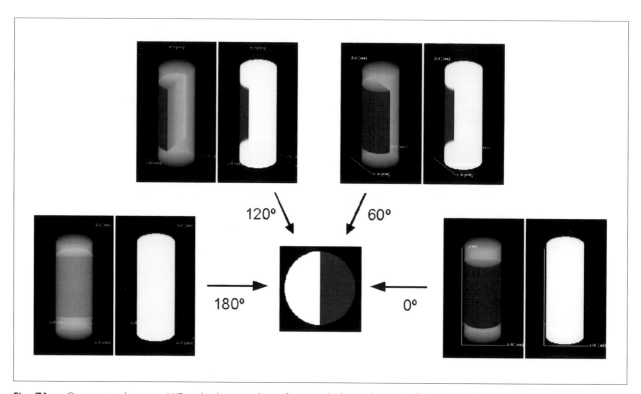

Fig. 71. Comparison between MIP and volume rendering for an embolus occluding half of the vessel lumen. This is the only case where MIP can demonstrate the presence of an embolus. In order to appreciate the embolus, several projections must be reconstructed and played in a cine loop to illustrate the defect. Note that the size of the signal void is smaller than the size of the embolus because information is masked. Images to the left and right of each comparison correspond to volume rendering and MIP, respectively. The embolus can be appreciated with the opacity setting used for volume rendering while it is completely masked with MIP.

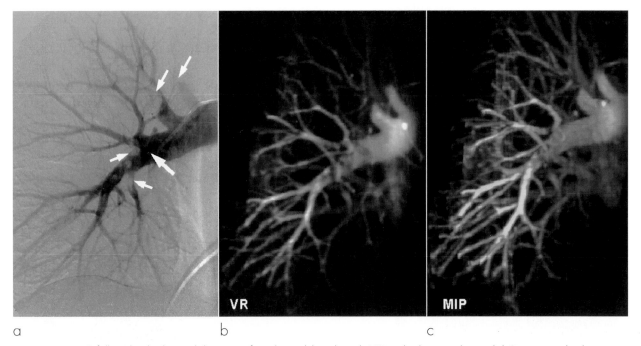

a   b   c

Fig. 72a–c.   Pitfalls in the display and detection of intraluminal thrombi with MIP and volume rendering. **(a)** Conventional pulmonary angiography. **(b)** Volume rendering with an X-ray projection setting. **(c)** MIP. MIP masks the location of a large intraluminal thrombus in the right descending pulmonary artery (large arrow) from overprojection from surrounding brighter blood.

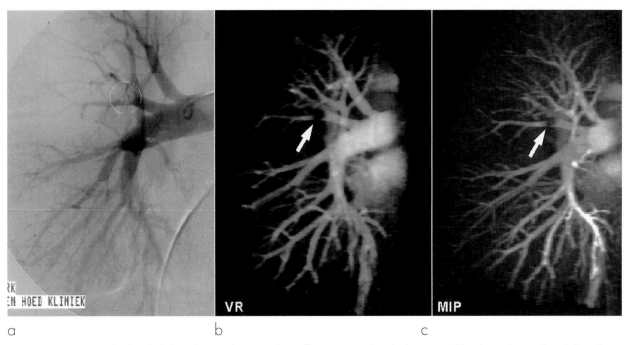

a   b   c

Fig. 73a–c.   More distal emboli that often produce vessel cut-offs at segmental and sub-segmental levels are depicted similarly with both reconstruction types. **(a)** Conventional pulmonary angiography. **(b)** Volume rendering with an X-ray projection setting. **(c)** MIP.

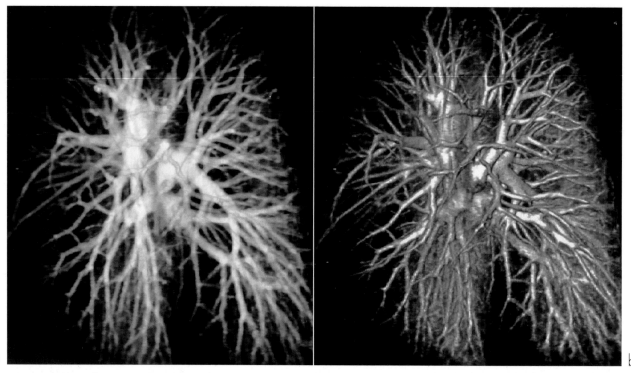

a   b

Fig. 74a–d. Differences in depth and vessel geometry perception using volume rendering without and with lighting applied. **(a, c)** Volume rendering with an opacity setting to create an x-ray like projection provides no depth perception but permits a clear view of overlapping vessels. **(b, d)** The application of lighting on the vessel surface automatically produces high contrast in the image, adding depth cues that make it clear to appreciate the spatial relationships between vessels. Lighting is usually applied using a point light source that can be directed from a view different from that of the observer. The light is reflected according to the normal surface computed during the rendering process (surface primitives) and the shining properties assigned through the opacity control (rough or smooth surface).

Unfortunately, cine viewing is not always available to a clinician during review, because this requires a graphics workstation that can perform this kind of viewing user-friendly and at an acceptable speed. New 3D printing methodology using volumetric multiplexed transmission holography can provide 3D reviewing on a single sheath of holographic film, making it also more transportable [154].

Optimal visualisation can also be difficult because of the signal variability between data sets. Contrast enhancement differences will always be present between arteries and veins but also from the existence of atelectasis, pneumonia, hemorrhage, pleural effusion and tumours that can overlap during the formation of suitable images that provide a global visualisation of the entire vascular structure. A targeted reconstruction or structure segmentation is therefore appropriate.

Surface shading display

Lighting is another feature that can be exploited in conjunction with volume rendering to improve the visualisation of spatial relationships between the pulmonary vessels and provide additional depth cues (Fig. 74). Lighting is performed by directing a light source (that can be assigned from any point in space) over the surface representation of the vessel tree that is computed during rendering and recording into an image the resulting light reflected. The quality of the reflection is dependent on the opacity settings used, producing a more diffuse or a polished appearance of the vascular surface. Lighting necessitates additional computation, as it is necessary to calculate the surface primitives and their surface normals to determine the direction in which the light will be reflected (signal intensity with respect to the view from the observer).

Combining multiplanar reformation and vascular visualisation

Multiplanar reformation can also be combined with volume rendering (or MIP) with the incorporation of "clipping" planes in the 3D vascular volume to demonstrate any pulmonary vessel branch in relation to its surroundings. Clipping planes are double oblique planes that cut into the volume to

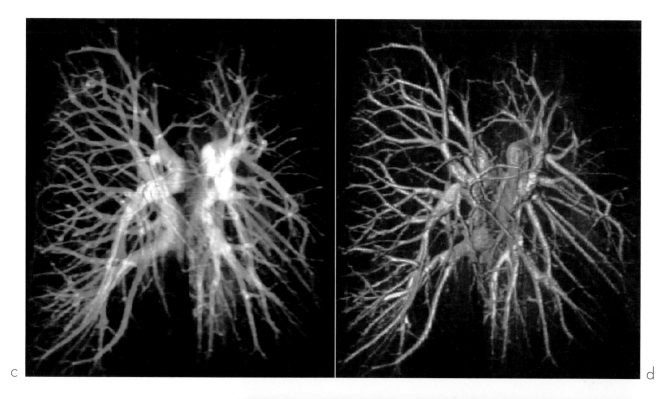

c

d

Fig. 75a, b. Multiplanar reformation by means of a double oblique clipping plane during active volume rendering to observe a long thrombus lodged in both the right descending **(a)** and right ascending **(b)** pulmonary arteries. The vascular information reconstructed corresponds to that on the other side of the clipping plane. The white frames surrounding the vascular region represent the clipping planes used.

a

b

stop the rendering process at the surface defined by the plane. In this way, a thrombus lodged inside a pulmonary vessel can be accompanied with all the surrounding vascular information for improved visualisation (Fig. 75).

The observer viewing angle can be adjusted with the clipping plane held constant to permit other views of the vascular territory. The number of clipping planes that can be applied is virtually unlimited (but software dependent). Clipping planes can also be used to eliminate interference from unwanted structures during the volume rendering process.

Automatic segmentation of the thoracic wall using MR sequence properties

Segmentation of the thoracic wall must be performed to demonstrate the complete pulmonary vascular tree. Manual segmentation can be difficult without the appropriate imaging workstation. An option exists that uses the inherent motion properties of SSC GRE scans to provide a semi-automatic form of segmentation of the thorax.

SSC GRE techniques use both longitudinal and transverse magnetisation components to form the image, producing a signal that is roughly independent of TR, whenever the TR selected is much shorter than the T2 relaxation. The signal strength of SSC GRE techniques demands that the transverse magnetisation is available for many RF excitations so that it contributes to the signal formation. Motion, as is the case of flowing blood, can destroy this delicate requirement and create signal fluctuations in the image of an otherwise homogeneous

tissue. Therefore, quasi-static tissue in the thorax can appear in the reconstructed images while flowing blood is completely eliminated. This provides a means to produce a binary mask that has only the signal from the thoracic wall and that can be used to set to zero all voxels that belong to the thorax in the MRPA acquisition (Fig. 76) [155].

This procedure can produce a mask that is reasonable for automatic processing of the right pulmonary vasculature, as illustrated in Figure 77. Because liver moves during the acquisition with respiratory motion, it cannot be masked out because its signal is dephased during the sensitive SSC GRE acquisition (the mask and MRPA data used for Figure 77 were acquired during free-breathing). Because of this motion sensitivity, it is more problematic to produce a clean display of the left pulmonary tree. The heart moves and it is nearly impossible to produce a binary mask that would eliminate it from the MRPA data prior to data reformation and display.

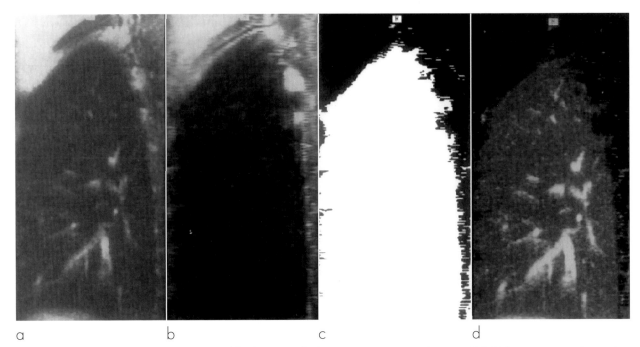

a   b   c   d

Fig. 76a–d. Semi-automatic segmentation of the thoracic wall. The sensitivity to motion of certain SSC GRE sequences can be used to create images that do not contain vessel information that can be used to produce a binary mask to eliminate the thorax. **(a)** illustrates a coronal slice acquired with a free-breathing syncopated 3D SSI GRE approach. **(b)** demonstrates the corresponding level acquired with a motion sensitive SSC GRE scan. **(c)** Binary mask image. **(d)** Binary mask multiplied by the MRPA data removes the unwanted thorax. The heart and the liver move and may not appear in the motion-sensitive acquisition and cannot be eliminated from the MRPA scan using the mask but can by other means.

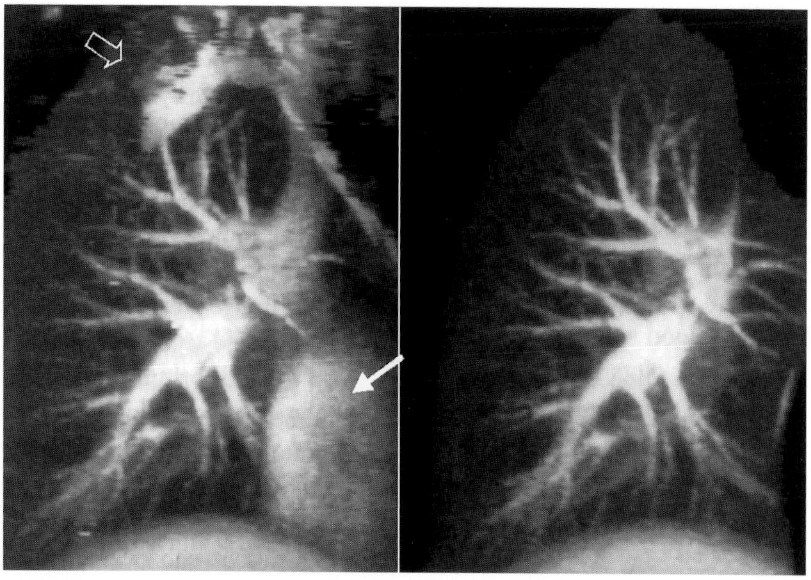

Fig. 77a, b. MIP generated from the same data set as in Figure 76 after using the computed mask from a flow sensitive SSC GRE sequence to eliminate the entire thoracic wall. **(a)** Automatic segmentation. **(b)** Manual segmentation. Note that because the heart and liver move more during the SSC GRE acquisition they do not provide signal that could be used in the mask and therefore remain. Note that the signal from the superior vena cava and subclavian artery and vein (arrows) do not appear in the mask and therefore are shown in **(a)**.

a   b

11. MR lung perfusion and ventilation

Lung parenchymal perfusion (MRPP) has been investigated with several techniques using intravascular contrast agents [156, 157], arterial spin tagging [85, 158] and dynamic imaging of the passage of a concentrated bolus of contrast material [102, 159–161]. Intravascular contrast agents used in a feasibility study using a PE model [157] positively characterised the perfusion deficit produced but has been not yet entered clinical trials, nor has the concept been pursued with current developments. Arterial spin tagging, an interesting concept using subtraction between images acquired with and without tagged blood, has been attempted using long inflow delays. The tagging approach does not require contrast agents but has poor SNR and requires patient cooperation (see Fig. 26).

Dynamic imaging with fast 2D or 3D GRE imaging has proven robust and can be readily applied for clinical practice. Dynamic perfusion in a pig model with induced PE illustrated wedge perfusion defects detected after complete occlusion of a pulmonary descending artery [159]. The imaging strategy has been employed on patients with proven pulmonary emboli with similar results [159–162]. Unlike in radionuclide perfusion scans, pulmonary vessels are readily demonstrated in conjunction with parenchymal perfusion and could be assessed simultaneously (low resolution MRPA).

With the acquisition speed possible with fast gradient hardware, the entire lung perfusion can be mapped virtually during quiet breathing after contrast injection using a 3D ultrashort TR/TE GRE scan with a time resolution of 1 volume per second (volume of 20 slices) [162] (Figure 78, 79).

The 3D data collection permits the review of the enhancing parenchyma and pulmonary vessels in any desired orientation (Fig. 80). With image subtraction from a baseline volume, only vessels and the enhancing parenchyma are appreciated. Investigation in patients with proven PE demonstrates the lack of perfusion in the areas that are affected by thrombi (Fig. 81). Perfusion MR with contrast agents has also been investigated clinically to quantify perfusion after lung transplantation [161].

The addition of MR pulmonary ventilation (MRPV) would provide a complete set-up for the diagnosis of PE as the entire examination might be performed in one single setting in combination with perfusion and MRPA. Animal work was first attempted using aerosolised Gd [156], but it has not been attempted on humans. Inhalation of hyperpolarised noble gases such as He [163, 164] and Xe [165] has been presented recently with exceptional image quality, tomographic imaging and the same functionality as radionuclide ventilation scans. Noble gas hyperpolarisation has been pos-

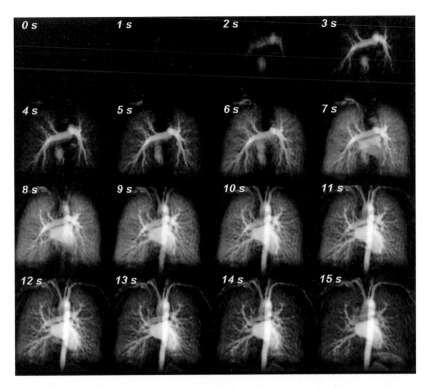

Fig. 78. Normal MRPP collected on a patient with suspected PE. A MIP of the posterior section of the lungs (64 mm) is illustrated. Data was acquired with a 3D TurboFLASH sequence using TR/TE/TI/α = 1.75/0.9/0 msec, 9°. Twenty sections were acquired per volume-frame at a rate of 1 volume-frame/sec after the injection of a short bolus of 8 ml of Gd-DTPA at a rate of 4 ml/sec and flushed with 20 ml of saline at 2 ml/sec. Frames 1 (f1) through 16 (f16) are displayed in a collage form. The collage display enhances the integration of all the perfusion information. The displayed data was formed after subtraction from a non contrast-enhanced frame. Resolution per volume is 84 x 128 x 20 with a FOV of 320 x 320 mm^2. The MRPP data shown corresponds to the patient illustrated in Figure 31 f.

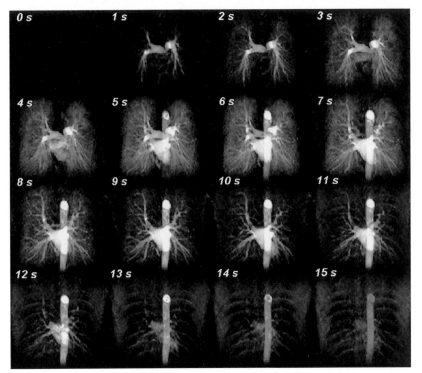

Fig. 79. Normal MRPP collected on a patient with suspected PE. A 64 mm MIP of the posterior section of the lungs is presented. Imaging parameters as in Figure 78. Note the faster passage of contrast through the pulmonary vasculature as compared to the patient of Figure 78 for the timing of the bolus of contrast. MRPP data from the same patient as in Figure 31e.

sible after laser optical pumping followed by electron-nuclear polarisation transfer, leading to a large increase in the nuclear spin polarisation available to several orders of magnitude (10^5) compared to that of water protons at thermal equilibrium. Extensive work is now being conducted to study lung disease [164, 166]. An excellent re-

view has been published by Kauczor et al. on this topic [167].

Hyperpolarised gases are expensive to produce. On the other hand, ventilation-like scans have been attempted using molecular oxygen [168, 169]. Oxygen has a weak paramagnetic effect that can be detected with imaging sequences sen-

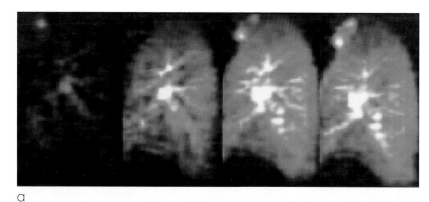

a

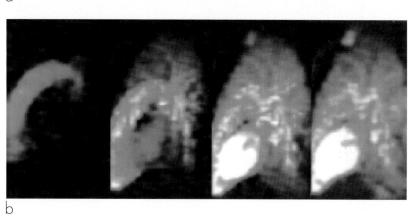

b

Fig. 80a, b. Sagittal multiplanar reformats from a coronally acquired 3D MRPP data set as illustrated in Figure 78 and Figure 79. The time succession of the contrast-enhancing parenchyma is seen from left to right with a 4-second time difference between frames. The reconstructed slice thickness is 25 mm. A normal perfusion pattern in both lungs is observed in this case. Volume rendering rather then MIP is used for display to equalise the signal intensity in the entire lung parenchyma and eliminate intensity signal decay towards the centre of the imaged volume from non-uniform signal reception using a body phased-array coil. Acquisition parameters as in Figure 78. **(a)** Right lung, **(b)** left lung

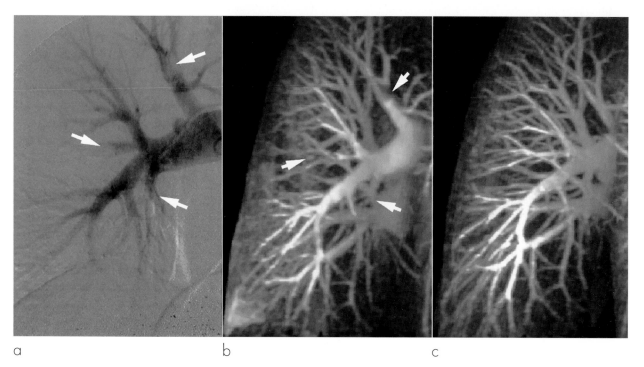

a   b   c

Fig. 81a–e. First and follow-up examinations of a combined MRPA and MRPP protocol on a patient with confirmed PE by conventional pulmonary angiography. **(a)** Conventional pulmonary angiography. The arrows indicate the location of several thrombi. **(b)** MIP view corresponding to the conventional pulmonary angiogram can demonstrate clearly the emboli illustrated in (a). **(c)** MIP of the follow-up examination shows complete clearance. **(d)** A 20 mm MIP in the posterior wall of the lung illustrates multiple perfusion defects in both lungs (arrows). **(e)** MRPP examination after 2 months of thromboembolytic therapy: all perfusion defects are dissolved. A double sagittal slab contrast-enhanced 3D MRPA protocol was performed with acquisition parameters as in Figure 31. Two emboli were present in the left pulmonary vasculature, seen in both the MRPA and conventional pulmonary angiogram.

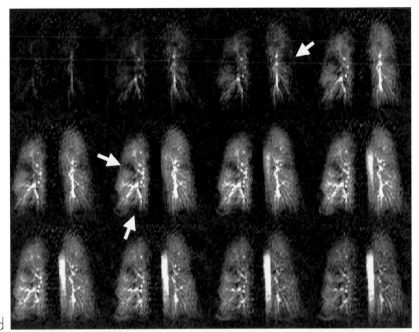

d

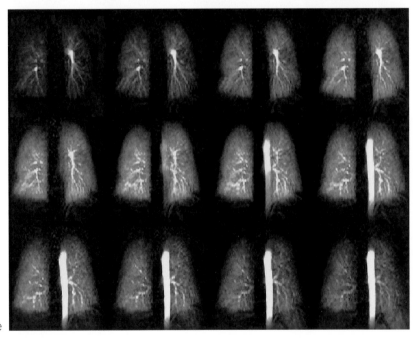

e

sitive to T1 relaxation. Results have been encouraging, especially considering that oxygen is readily available and can be applied safely to patients. Additionally, oxygen lung ventilation scanning can be performed in conjunction with perfusion and MRPA without any changes in the MRI hardware. That has been proven especially effective in patients with proven PE (Fig. 82) [170]. Oxygen MRPV provides poor SNR in comparison to scans using hyperpolarised gases (reason for the low resolution image in Figure 82) and the enhancement is not only confined to the air spaces, as oxygen diffuses rapidly into the pulmonary vasculature during inhalation.

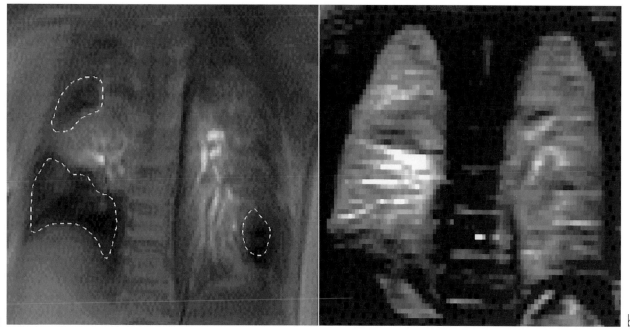

Fig. 82a, b.   Perfusion and ventilation mismatch in a patient with proven PE. **(a)** One frame of the MRPP using a 15 mm thick slice acquired with time-resolved 2D turboFLASH imaging with a temporal resolution of 1 frame/sec after contrast administration (20 ml of Gd-DTPA). Dashed contours encircle regions with perfusion defects. **(b)** Oxygen MRPV scan demonstrates a uniform enhancement of the lung parenchyma. PE was confirmed on the contrast-enhanced MRPA scan. The parameters of turboFLASH were TR/TE/TI = 3.4/1.6/600 msec, α = 12°, 128 × 128 matrix, FOV = 380 × 380 mm^2. The oxygen MRPV scan was produced after the subtraction of two data sets acquired during breathing of normal air and air with 100% oxygen saturation at 10 l/min. A T1 weighted inversion recovery, short TE HASTE scan was used with ETS/TE = 4/20 msec. Body phased-array coil acquisition. (Image courtesy of Q. Chen, New England Medical Center, Boston, USA).

12. Conclusions

Magnetic resonance imaging offers good flexibility for the non-invasive morphological and functional assessment of the pulmonary vasculature. Numerous MRI and MRA techniques are under investigation for use in patients with suspected PE.

The resurgence of thoracic MRI has been triggered by the improvements in image quality with the introduction of MRI scanners with stronger imaging gradients, faster data acquisition capabilities and improved signal reception with the incorporation of phased-array coil technology. Magnetic resonance pulmonary angiography has considerable potential in this context.

Although contrast-enhanced MRPA may have a good future for the diagnosis of difficult conditions, it is still under development and improvements are constantly marking new scenarios for their applicability in clinical trials. Several points must be kept in mind. The availability of high-end MRI scanners does not surpass that of CT units. Even when the optimal MRPA procedure is avail-able, scanning time is still longer than CT angiography, there are difficulties in monitoring patients conveniently with life-support devices and image quality can degenerate in many patients who cannot breath-hold adequately or are uncooperative. Finally, diagnostic experience is required to make the assessment in difficult cases if using MRPA alone.

The administration of contrast agents that enhance the signal from blood has broadened the scope of MR pulmonary angiography. MR pulmonary angiography is considered to be competitive to contrast-enhanced spiral computed tomography (CT) and electron-beam CT (EBCT) angiography. High quality and fast morphological imaging of the thorax has also developed in parallel that can now help corroborate the cause of vascular abnormalities, and functional data demonstrating lung ventilation and perfusion can address a wider range of vascular and airway diseases. MRPP and MRPV have the potential to replace lung scintigraphy.

References

1. Alderson PO, Martin EC. PE: Diagnosis with multiple imaging modalities. Radiology 1987; 164: 297–312

2. Kelley MA, Carson JL, Palevsky HI, Schwartz JS. Diagnosing PE: New facts and strategies. Ann Intern Med 1991; 1 T4: 300–306

3. Moore EH, Gamsu G, Webb WR, Stulbarg MS. Pulmonary embolus: Detection and follow up using magnetic resonance. Radiology 1984, 153: 471–472

4. Gamsu G, Hirji M, Moore EH, Webb WR, Brito A. Experimental pulmonary emboli detected using magnetic resonance. Radiology 1984; 153: 467–470

5. White RD, Winkler ML, Higgins CB. MR imaging of pulmonary arterial hypertension and pulmonary emboli. Am J Roentgenol 1987; 149: 15–21

6. Posteraro RH, Sostman HD, Spritzer CE, Herfkens RJ. Cine-gradient refocused MR imaging of central pulmonary emboli. Am J Roentgenol 1989; 152: 465–468

7. Bogren HG, Klipstein RH, Mohiaddin RH, et al. Pulmonary artery distensibility and blood flow patterns: A magnetic resonance study of normal subjects and of patients with pulmonary artery hypertension. Am Heart J 1989; 118: 990–999

8. Moser KM. Pulmonary vascular physiology and pathophysiology. In: Weir EK, Reeves JT (eds). Lung Biology in Health and Disease (V 38, chapter Pulmonary Vascular Obstruction due to Embolism and Thrombosis. Marcel Dekker, Inc., New York, 1989.

9. Mohiaddin RH, Paz R, Theodonopoulos S, et al. Anatomic and flow MR imaging of pulmonary arteries in patients following single lung transplantation. Radiology 1990; 177 (Suppl.): 139

10. Thakur ML, Vinitski S, Mitchell DG, et al. MR imaging of pulmonary parenchyma and emboli by paramagnetic and superparamagnetic contrast agents. Magnetic Resonance Imaging 1990, 8: 625–630

11. Spritzer CE, Sostman HD, Wilkes DC, Coleman RE. Deep venous thrombosis. Experience with gradient-echo MR imaging in 66 patients. Radiology 1990; 177: 235–241

12. Gomes AS, Lois JF, Williams RG. Pulmonary arteries: MR imaging in patients with congenital obstruction of the right ventricular outflow track. Radiology 1990; 174: 51–57

13. Gefter WB, Hatabu H, Dinsmore BJ, et al. Pulmonary vascular cine MR imaging: A noninvasive approach to dynamic imaging of the pulmonary circulation. Radiology 1990; 176: 761–770

14. Kauczor HU. Contrast-enhanced magnetic resonance angiography of the pulmonary vasculature. A review. Invest Radiol 1998; 33(9): 606–617

15. Bongartz G, Boos M, Scheffler K, Steinbrich W. Pulmonary circulation. Eur Radiol 1998; 8(5): 698–706

16. Hatabu H. MR pulmonary angiography and perfusion imaging: recent advances. Semin Ultrasound CT MR 1997; 18(5): 349–361

17. Hatabu H, Gaa J, Kim D, Li W, Prasad PV, Edelman RR. Pulmonary perfusion: qualitative assessment with dynamic contrast-enhanced MRI using ultra-short TE and inversion recovery turbo FLASH.. Magn Reson Med 1996; 36(4): 503–508

18. Amundsen T, Kvaerness J, Jones RA, et al. PE: detection with MR perfusion imaging of lung – a feasibility study. Radiology 1997; 203(1): 181–185

19. Kauczor H, Surkau R, Roberts T. MRI using hyperpolarized noble gases. Eur Radiol 1998; 8(5): 820–827

20. Johnson GA, Cates G, Chen XJ, et al. Dynamics of magnetization in hyperpolarized gas MRI of the lung. Magn Reson Med 1997; 38(1): 66–71

21. Axel L, Summers RM, Kressel HY. Respiratory effects in two-dimensional Fourier transform MR imaging. Radiology 1986; 160: 795–801

22. Lewis CE, Prato FS, Drost DJ, Nicholson RL. Comparison of respiratory triggering and gating techniques for the removal of respiratory artifacts in MR imaging. Radiology 1986; 160(3): 803–810

23. Morris AH, Blatter DD, Case TA, et al. A new nuclear magnetic resonance property of lung. J Appl Physiology 1985; 58: 759–762

24. Bergin CJ, Glover GH, Pauly JM. Lung parenchyma: magnetic susceptibility in MR imaging. Radiology 1991; 180: 845–848

25. Hayes CE, Roemer PB. Volume imaging with MR phased arrays. Magn Reson Med 1990; 16: 181–191

26. Liang ZP, Boada FE, Constable RT, Haacke EM, Pauterbur PC, Smith MR. Constrained reconstruction methods in MR imaging. Rev Magn Reson Med 1992; 4: 67–185

27. McGibney G, Smith MR, Nichols ST, Crawley A. Quantitative evaluation of several partial Fourier reconstruction algorithms used in MRI. Magn Reson Med 1993; 30(1): 51–59

28. Haacke EM Lindskog ED, Lin W. Partial-Fourier imaging. A fast, iterative, POCS technique capable of local phase recovery. J Magn Reson 1991; 92: 126–144

29. Haacke EM, Masaryk TJ, Wielopolski PA, et al. Optimizing blood vessel contrast in fast three-dimensional MRI. Magn Reson Med 1990; 14(2): 202–221

30. Cuppen JJ, Groen JP, Konijn J. Magnetic resonance fast Fourier imaging. Med Phys 1986; 13(2): 248–253

31. Irarrazabal P, Nishimura DG. Fast three dimensional magnetic resonance imaging. Magn Reson Med 1995; 33(5): 656–662

32. Parker DL, Du YP, Davis WL. The voxel sensitivity function in Fourier transform imaging: applications to magnetic resonance angiography. Magn Reson Med 1995; 33(2): 156–162

33. Bergin CJ, Noll DC, Pauly JM, Glover GH, Macovski A. MR imaging of lung parenchyma: a solution to susceptibility. Radiology 1992; 183: 673

34. Bergin CJ, Pauly JM, Macovski A. Lung parenchyma: projection reconstruction MR imaging. Radiology 1991; 179: 777

35. Peters DC, Mistretta CA, Korosec FR, et al Using projection reconstruction with a limited number of projection to increase image resolution or acquisition speed. Proceedingsbook Intern Soc Magn Reson Med (ISMRM) 1998; 1: 182

36. Meyer C, Hu B, Nishimura D, Macovski A. Fast spiral coronary artery imaging. Magn Reson Med 1992; 28: 202–213

37. Melki PS, Jolesz FA, Mulkern RV. Partial RF echo planar imaging with the FAISE method. I. Magn Reson Med 1992; 26: 328–341

38. Melki PS, Jolesz FA, Mulkern RV. Partial RF echo-planar imaging with the FAISE method. II. Magn Reson Med 1992; 26: 342–354

39. Hennig J, Nauerth A, Friedburg H. RARE imaging: a fast imaging method for clinical MR. Magn Reson Med 1986; 3: 823–833

40. Stehling MK, Holzknecht NG, Laub G, Bohm D, von Smekal A, Reiser M. Single-shot T1- and T2-weighted magnetic resonance imaging of the heart with black blood: preliminary experience. MAGMA 1996; 4(3–4): 231–240

41. Haacke EM, Frahm J. A guide to understanding key aspects of fast gradient-echo imaging. J Magn Reson Imaging 1991; 1(6): 621–624

42. Haase A, Matthaei D, Bartkowski E, Duhmke E, Leibfritz D. Inversion recovery snapshot FLASH MR imaging. J Comp Assist Tomogr 1989, 13: 1036–1040

43. Edelman RR, Chien D, Kim. Fast selective black blood MR imaging. Radiology 1991; 181(3): 655–660

44. Cutillo AG. Application of magnetic resonance to the study of the lung. Futura Publishing Company 1996, Armonk, NY, USA

45. Blackmore CG, Francis CW, Bryant RG, Brenner B, Marder VJ. Magnetic resonance imaging of blood and clots in vitro. Invest Radiol 1990; 25: 1316–1324

46. Bryant RG, Marill K, Blackmore C, Francis C. Magnetic relaxation in blood and blood clots. Magn Reson Med 1990; 13: 133–144

47. Fullerton GD. Magnetic Resonance Imaging, Vol. I. Mosby Year Book, Inc., second edition, 1992.

48. Brooks RA, DiChiro G. Magnetic resonance imaging of stationary blood: A review. Med Phys 1987; 14(6): 903–913

49. Gomori JM, Grossman RI, Yu-Ip C, Asakura T. NMR relaxation times of blood: Dependence on field strength, oxidation state, and cell integrity. J Comp Assist Tomogr 1987; 11(4): 684–690

50. Edelman RR, Johnson K, Buxton R, et al. MR of hemorrhage: A new approach. Am J Neuroradiol 1986; 7: 751

51. Graves MJ. Magnetic resonance angiography. Br J Radiol 1997; 70: 6–28

52. Dumoulin CL. Phase contrast MR angiography techniques. Magn Reson Imaging Clin N Am 1995; 3(3): 399–411

53. Wielopolski PA.. Pulmonary arteriography. Magn Reson Imaging Clinics N Am 1993; 1: 295–313

54. Nagele T, Klose U, Grodd W, Nusslin F, Voigt KJ. Nonlinear excitation profiles for three-dimensional inflow MR angiography. Magn Reson Imaging 1995; 5(4): 416–420

55. Friedli JL, Paschal CB. Evaluation of variable-angle uniform signal excitation, tilted optimized nonsaturating excitation, and flat radio-frequency pulses in free-breathing non-contrast-enhanced pulmonary MR angiography. Radiology 1997; 202(3): 863–867

56. Stehling MK. Improved signal in "snapshot" FLASH by variable flip angles. Magn Reson Imaging 1992; 10(1): 165–167

57. Nishimura DG, Jackson JI, Pauly JM. On the nature and reduction of the displacement artifact in flow images. Magn Reson Med 1991; 22: 481–492

58. Haacke EM, Liang ZP, Izen SH. Constrained reconstruction: a superresolution, optimal signal-to-noise alternative to the Fourier transform in magnetic resonance imaging. Med Phys 1989; 16(3): 388–397

59. Nishimura DG, Macovski A, Jackson JI, Hu RS, Stevick CA, Axel L. Magnetic resonance by selective inversion recovery using a compact gradient echo sequence. Magn Reson Med 1988, 8: 96–103

60. Miyazaki M, Ichinose N, Sugiura S, Kassai Y, Kanazawa H, Machida Y. A novel MR angiography technique: SPEED acquisition using half-Fourier RARE. J Magn Reson Imaging 1998; 8(2): 505–507

61. Keller P. Time-of-flight magnetic resonance angiography. Neuroimag Clin N Am 1992; 4: 639–656

62. Dumoulin CI, Hart HR Jr. Magnetic resonance angiography. Radiology 1986; 161: 717–720

63. Yuasa Y. Phase-contrast magnetic resonance angiography in the abdomen and thorax. Magn Reson Imaging Clin N Am 1993; 1: 327–338

64. Keller PJ, Drayer BP, Fram EK, Williams KD, Dumoulin CL, Souza SP. MR angiography via 2D acquisitions but yielding a 3D display: A work in progress. Radiology 1989; 173: 527–532

65. Foo THF, MacFAll J, Hayes C, Sostman H, Slayman B. Pulmonary vasculature: Single breath-hold MR imaging with phased-array coils. Radiology 1992; 183: 473–477

66. Hatabu H, Gefter WB, Kressel HY, Axel L, Lenkinski RE. Pulmonary vasculature: High resolution MR imaging. Work in progress. Radiology 1989; 171: 391–395

67. MacFall JR, Foo TKF, Sostman HD. Thick section, single breath-hold MR pulmonary angiography. Invest Radiol 1992; 27: 318–322

68. Hatabu H, Gefter WB, Listerud J, et al. Pulmonary MR angiography utilizing phased-array surface coils. J Comput Assist Tomogr 1992; 16: 410–417

69. Rubin GD, Herfkens RJ, Pelc NJ, et al. Single breath-hold pulmonary magnetic resonance angiography, optimization and comparison of three imaging strategies. Invest Radiol 1994; 29: 766–772

70. Laissy JP, Assayag P, Henry-Feugeas MC, et al. Pulmonary time-of-flight MR angiography at 1.0 T: comparison between 2D and 3D tone acquisitions. Magn Reson Imaging 1995; 13: 949–957

71. Seelos KC, von Smekal A, Steinborn M, Gieseke J, Kaas P, Urban J, Redel DA, Reiser M. MR angiography of the heart and thoracic blood vessels. Use of rapid ECG-triggered techniques with multiplanar reconstruction capability. Radiologe 1994 Aug; 34(8): 454–461

325

72. Foo TKF, MacFall JR, Sostman HD, Hayes CE. Single-breath-hold venous or arterial flow-suppressed MR imaging with phased-array coils. J Magn Reson Imaging 193; 3: 611–616

73. Isoda H, Masui T, Hasegawa S, et al. Pulmonary MR angiography: a comparison of 2D and 3D time-of-flight. J Comput Assist Tomogr 1994, 18(3): 402–407

74. Wang Y, Rossman PJ, Grimm RC, Wilman AH, Riederer SJ, Ehman RL. 3D MR angiography of pulmonary arteries using real-time navigator gating and magnetization preparation. Magn Reson Med 1996; 36: 579–587

75. Foo TK, MacFall JR, Sostman HD, Hayes CE. Single-breath-hold venous or arterial flow-suppressed pulmonary vascular MR imaging with phased-array coils. J Magn Reson Imaging 1993; 3(4): 611–616

76. Wielopolski PA, Haacke EM, Adler LP. Three-dimensional MR imaging of the pulmonary vasculature: Preliminary experience. Radiology 1992; 183: 465–472

77. Ehman RL, McNamara MT, Pallack M, Hricak H, Higgins CB. Magnetic resonance imaging with respiratory gating: techniques and advantages. Am J Roentgenol 1984; 143: 1175–1182

78. Bailes DR, Gilderdale DJ, Bydder GM, Collins AG, Firmin DN. Respiratory ordered phase encoding (ROPE): a method of reducing respiratory motion artifacts in MR imaging. J Comput Assist Tomogr 1985; 9: 835–838

79. Sachs TS, Meyer CH, Hu BS, Kohli J, Nishimura DG, Macovski A. Real-time motion detection in spiral MRI using navigators. Magn Reson Med 1994; 32: 639–645

80. Ahlstrom H, Johansson L, Ragnarsson A. Pulmonary MRA during continuous breathing using a blood pool agent and navigator echo. Proceedingsbook Int Soc Magn Reson Med (ISMRM) 1998; Vol. I: 170

81. Liu Y, Riederer SJ, Rossman PJ, Grimm RC, Debbins JP, Ehman RL. A monitoring, feedback and triggering system for reproducible breath-hold MR imaging. Magn Reson Med 1993; 30: 507–511

82. Hofman MB, Paschal CB, Li D, Haacke EM, van Rossum AC, Sprenger M. MRI of coronary arteries: 2D breath-hold vs 3D respiratory-gated acquisition. J Comput Assist Tomogr 1995; 19(1): 56–62

83. Post JC, van Rossum AC, Hofman MB, Valk J, Visser CA. Three-dimensional respiratory-gated MR angiography of coronary arteries: comparison with conventional coronary angiography. Am J Roentgenol 1996; 166(6): 1399–1404

84. Stehling MK, Balci C, Reiser M. Navigator echo coronary MRA: controversial results. Proceedingsbook Int Soc Magn Reson Med (ISMRM) 1997; Vol. I: 911

85. Edelman RR, Siewert B, Adamis M, Gaa J, Laub G, Wielopolski P. Signal targeting with alternating radio-frequency (STAR) sequences: application to MR angiography. Magn Reson Med 1994; 31(2): 233–238

86. Wang SJ, Hu BS, Macovski A, Nishimura DG. Coronary angiography using fast selective inversion recovery. Magn Reson Med 1991; 18(2): 417–423

87. Prince MR. Body MR angiography with gadolinium contrast agents. Magn Reson Imaging Clin N Am 1996; 4(1): 11–24

88. Maki JH, Chenevert TL, Prince MR. Three-dimensional contrast-enhanced MR angiography. Top Magn Reson Imaging 1996; 8(6): 322–344

89. Maki JH, Chenevert TL, Prince MR. The effects of incomplete breath-holding on 3D MR image quality. J Magn Reson Imaging 1997; 7(6): 1132–1139

90. Oudkerk M, de Bruin HG, Wielopolski PA, Hicks SG, Obdeijn AIM, Berghout A. PE detection using contrast-enhanced, breath-hold 3D magnetic resonance angiography. In: Oudkerk M, Edelman RR (eds). High-power gradient MR imaging. Advances in MRI II. Blackwell Science Publishers, Berlin 1997: 78–86

91. Isoda H, Ushimi T, Masui T, et al. Clinical evaluation of pulmonary 3D time-of-flight MRA with breath-holding using contrast media. J Comput Assist Tomogr 1995; 19(6): 911–919

92. Wielopolski P, Hicks S, Obdeijn AIM, Oudkerk M. PE Detection using Contrast-Enhanced, Breath-hold 3D Magnetic Resonance Angiography: Preliminary Experience. Proceedingsbook Int Soc Magn Reson Med 1996; Vol. II: 705

93. Steiner P, McKinnon GC, Romanowski B, Goehde SC, Hany T, Debatin JF. Contrast-enhanced, ultrafast 3D pulmonary MR angiography in a single breath-hold: initial assessment of imaging performance. J Magn Reson Imaging 1997; 7(1): 177–182

94. Meaney JF, Weg JG, Chenevert TL, Stafford-Johnson D, Hamilton BH, Prince MR. Diagnosis of PE with magnetic resonance angiography. N Engl J Med 1997; 336(20): 1422–427

95. Leung DA, Debatin JF. Three-dimensional contrast-enhanced magnetic resonance angiography of the thoracic vasculature. Eur Radiol 1997; 7: 981–989

96. Gay SB, Sistrom CL, Holder CA, Suratt PM. Breath-holding capability of adults: implications for spiral computed tomography, fast-acquisition magnetic resonance imaging, and angiography. Invest Radiol 1994; 29: 848–851

97. Wielopolski PA, Oudkerk M, Hicks SG, Berghout A. Breath-hold 3D MR pulmonary angiography after contrast material administration in patients with pulmonary embolim: correlation with conventional pulmonary angiography. Radiology 1996; 201 (Suppl): 202

98. Hatabu H, Gaa J, Kim D, Li W, Prasad PV, Edelman RR. Pulmonary perfusion: qualitative assessment with dynamic contrast-enhanced MRI using ultra-short TE and inversion recovery turbo FLASH. Magn Reson Med 1996; 36(4): 503–508

99. Wang Y, Johnston DL, Breen JF, et al. Dynamic MR digital subtraction angiography using contrast enhancement, fast data acquisition, and complex subtraction. Magn Reson Med 1996; 36(4): 551–556

100. Bongartz G, Boos M, Scheffler K, Steinbrich W. Pulmonary circulation. Eur Radiol 1998; 8(5): 698–706

101. Hany TF, Schmidt M, Davis CP, Gohde SC, Debatin JF. Diagnostic impact of four postprocessing techniques in evaluating contrast-enhanced three-dimensional MR angiography. Am J Roentgenol 1998; 170(4): 907–912

102. Wielopolski PA, Hicks SG, Bruin HG de, Oudkerk M. Breath-hold three-dimensional lung perfusion imaging and pulmonary angiography after contrast administration. In: Oudkerk M, Edelman RR. High-power gradient MR-imaging. Advances in MRI II. Blackwell Science 1997, Berlin: 71–77

103. Schoenberg SO, Knopp MV, Prince MR, Londy F, Knopp MA. Arterial-phase three-dimensional gadolinium magnetic resonance angiography of the renal arteries. Strategies for timing and contrast media injection: original investigation. Invest Radiol 1998; 33(9): 506–514

104. Earls JP, Rofsky NM, DeCorato DR, Krinsky GA, Weinreb JC. Breath-hold single-dose gadolinium-enhanced three dimensional MR aortography: usefulness of a timing examination and MR power injector. Radiology 1996; 167(4): 981–987

105. Maki JH, Prince MR, Londy FJ, Chenevert TL. The effects of time varying intravascular singla intensity and k-space acquisition order on three-dimensional MR angiography image quality. J Magn Reson Imaging 1996; 6: 642–651

106. Maki JH, Chenevert TL, Prince MR. The effects of incomplete breath-holding on 3D MR image quality. J Magn Reson Imaging 1997; 7(6): 1132–1139

107. Foo TK, Saranathan M, Prince MR, Chenevert TL. Automated detection of bolus arrival and initiation of data acquisition in fast, three-dimensional, gadolinium-enhanced MR angiography. Radiology 1997; 203(1): 275–280

108. Wilman AH, Riederer SJ, Huston III J, Wald JT, Debbins JP. Arterial phase carotid and vertebral artery imaging in 3D contrast-enhanced MR angiography by combining fluoroscopic triggering with an elliptical centric acquisition order. Magn Reson Med 1998; 40: 24–35

109. Ho VB, Foo TK. Optimization of gadolinium-enhanced magnetic resonance angiography using an automated bolus-detection algorithm (MR SmartPrep). Original investigation. Invest Radiol 1998; 33(9): 515–523

110. Maki JH, Prince, Chenevert TC. Optimizing three-dimensional gadolinium-enhanced magnetic resonance angiography. Original investigation. Invest Radiol 1998; 33(9): 528–537

111. Bàck JC, Kaufmann F, Felix R. Comparison of gadolinium-DTPA and macromolecular gadolinium-DTPA polylysine for contrast-enhanced pulmonary time-of-flight magnetic resonance angiography. Invest Radiol 1996; 31(10): 652–657

112. Frank H, Weissleder R, Bogdanov AA Jr, Brady TJ. Detection of pulmonary emboli by using MR angiography with MPEG-PL-GdDTPA: an experimental study in rabbits. Am J Roentgenol 1994; 162(5): 1041–1046

113. Li KC, Pelc LR, Napel SA, et al. MRI of PE using Gd-DTPA-polyethylene glycol polymer enhanced 3D fast gradient echo technique in a canine model. Magn Reson Imaging 1997; 15(5): 543–550

114. Lauffer RB, Parmelee DJ, Dunham SU, et al. MS-325: albumin-targeted contrast agent for MR angiography. Radiology 1998; 207(2): 529–538

115. Grist TM, Korosec FR, Peters DC, et al. Steady-state and dynamic MR angiography with MS-325: initial experience in humans. Radiology 1998; 207(2): 539–544

116. Schiebler ML, Holland GA, Hatabu H, et al. Suspected PE: prospective evaluation with pulmonary MR angiography. Radiology 1993; 189(1): 125–131

117. Grist TM, Sostman HD, MacFall JR, et al. Pulmonary angiography with MR imaging: preliminary clinical experience. Radiology 1993; 189(2): 523–530

118. Sostman HD, Layish DT, Tapson VF, et al. Prospective comparison of helical CT and MR imaging in clinically suspected acute PE. J Magn Reson Imaging 1996; 6(2): 275–281

119. Loubeyre P, Revel D, Douek P, et al. Dynamic contrast-enhanced MR angiography of PE: comparison with pulmonary angiography. Am J Roentgenol 1994; 162(5): 1035–1039

120. Revel D, Loubeyre P, Delignette A, Douek P, Amiel M. Contrast-enhanced magnetic resonance tomoangiography: a new imaging technique for studying thoracic great vessels. Magn Reson Imaging 1993; 11(8): 1101–1105

121. Bergin CJ, Sirlin CB, Hauschildt JP, et al. Chronic thromboembolism: diagnosis with helical CT and MR imaging with angiographic and surgical correlation. Radiology 1997; 204: 695–702

122. Hennig J, Scheffler K, Laubenberger J, Strecker R. Time-resolved projection angiography after bolus injection of contrast agents. Magn Reson Med 1997, 37(3): 341–345

123. Wang Y, Johnston DL, Breen JF, et al. Dynamic MR digital subtraction angiography using contrast enhancement, fast data acquisition, and complex subtraction. Magn Reson Med 1996; 36(4): 551–556

124. Peters DC, Korosec FR, Frayne R, Grist TM, Mistretta CA. Cardiac-gated contrast-enhanced time-resolved 3D imaging of the pulmonary arteries. Proceedings-book Int Soc Magn Reson Med (ISMRM) 1997; 3: 1859

125. Frayne R, Grist TM, Korosec FR, et al. MR angiography with three-dimensional MR digital subtraction angiography. Top Magn Reson Imaging 1996; 8(6): 366–388

126. Korosec FR, Frayne R, Grist TM, Mistretta CA. Time-resolved contrast-enhanced 3D MR angiography. Magn Reson Med 1996; 36(3): 345–351

127. Wielopolski PA, Simonetti OP, Duerk JC. Echo-planar imaging angiography. In: Schmitt F, Stehling MK, Turner R (eds). Echo-planar imaging: theory, technique and application. Springer-Verlag, Berlin, 1998: 8: 291–296

128. Heid O, Marr S, Vock P. Ultrafast. Gd-enhanced 3D segmented EPI MR angiography of the complete abdomen. Eur Radiol 1997; 7 (suppl): 431

129. Wielopolski PA, Simonetti O, Duerk J. Echo-Planar Imaging Angiography. In: Schmitt F, Stehling MK, Turner R (eds). Echo Planar Imaging. Springer Verlag, Berlin 1998: Chapter 5

130. Luk Pat GT, Meyer CH, Pauly JM, Nishimura DG. Reducing flow artifacts in echo-planar imaging. Magn Reson Med 1997; 37(3): 436–447

131. Hartnell GG, Cohen MC, Meier RA, Finn JP. Magnetic resonance angiography demonstration of congenital heart disease in adults. Clin Radiol 1996;51(12):851–857

132. Vrachliotis TG, Bis KG, Kirsch MJ, Shetty AN. Contrast-enhanced MRA in pre-embolization assessment of a pulmonary arteriovenous malformation. J Magn Reson Imaging1997; 7(2): 434–436

133. Berthezene Y, Howarth NR, Revel D. Pulmonary arteriovenous fistula: detection with magnetic resonance angiography. Eur Radiol 1998; 8: 1403–1404

134. Vrachliotis TG, Bis KG, Shetty AN, Simonetti O, Madrazo. Hypogenetic lung syndrome: functional and anatomic evaluation with magnetic resonance imaging and magnetic resonance angiography. J Magn Reson Imaging 1996; 6(5): 798–800

135. Low RN, Sigeti JS, Thomas Song SY, Shimakawa A. Dynamic contrast-enhanced breath-hold MR imaging of thoracic malignancy using cardiac compensation. J Magn Reson Imaging 1996; 6: 625–631

136. Marcilly MC, Howarth NR, Berthezene Y. Bronchial carcinoid tumor: demonstration by dynamic inversion recovery turbo-flash MR imaging. Eur Radiol 1998; 8: 1400–1402

137. Bergin CJ, Hauschildt J, Rios G, Belezzuoli EV, Huynh T, Channick RN. Accuracy of MR angiography compared with radionuclide scanning in identifying the cause of pulmonary arterial hypertension. Am J Roentgenol 1997; 168(6): 1549–1555

138. Kondo C, Caputo GR, Masui T, et al. Pulmonary hypertension: pulmonary flow quantification and flow profile analysis with velocity-encoded cine MR imaging. Radiology 1992; 183: 751–758

139. Gamsu G, Webb WR, Sheldon P, et al. Nuclear magnetic resonance imaging of the thorax. Radiology 1983; 147: 473–480

140. Thickmann D, Kressel HY, Axel L. Demonstration of pulmonary embolus by magnetic resonance imaging. Am J Roentgenol 1984; 142: 921–922

141. Gamsu G, Hirji M, Moore EH, Webb WR, Brito A. Experimental pulmonary emboli detected by magnetic resonance imaging. Radiology 1984; 153: 467–470

142. Pope CF, Sostman D, Carbo P, Gore JC, Holcomb. The detection of pulmonary emboli by magnetic resonance imaging. Invest Radiol 1986; 22: 937–947

143. Fisher MR, Higgins CB. Central thrombi in pulmonary arterial hypertension detected by MR imaging. Radiology 1986; 158(1): 223–226

144. Erdman WA, Peshock RM, Redman HC, et al. PE: comparison of MR images with radionuclide and angiographic studies. Radiology 1994; 190(2): 499–508

145. Hatabu H, Gefter WB, Axel L, et al. MR imaging with spatial modulation of magnetization in the evaluation of chronic central pulmonary thromboemboli. Radiology 1994; 190: 791–796

146. Olson EM, Bergin CJ, King MA. Fast SE MRI of the chest: parameter optimization and comparison with conventional SE imaging. J Comput Assist Tomogr 1995; 19(2): 167–175

147. Gaa J, Fischer H, Laub G, Georgi M. Breath-hold MR imaging of focal liver lesions: comparison of fast and ultrasound techniques. Eur Radiol 1996; 6(6): 838–843

148. Edelman RR, Chien D, Kim D. Fast selective black blood MR imaging. Radiology 1991; 181(3): 655–660

149. Wielopolski PA, Haacke EM, Adler LP. Evaluation of the pulmonary vasculature with three-dimensional magnetic resonance techniques. MAGMA 1993; 1: 21–34

150. Moody AR, Liddicoat A, Krarup K. Magnetic resonance pulmonary angiography and direct imaging of embolus for the detection of pulmonary emboli. Invest Radiol 1997; 32(8): 431–440

151. Wielopolski PA, Haacke Em, Adler LP. Three-dimensional MR imaging of the pulmonary vascular system. In: Cutillo AG (ed). Application of Magnetic Resonance to the Study of the Lung. Futura Publishing Company, Armonk NY, USA, 1996: 11:341 343; 11:364–365

152. Thakur ML, Vinitski S, Mitchell DG, et al. MR imaging of pulmonary parenchyma and emboli by paramagnetic and superparamagnetic contrast agents. Magn Reson Imaging 1990; 8: 625–630

153. Siebert JE, Rosenbaum. Image presentation and postprocessing. In: Potchen EJ, Haacke EM, Siebert JE, Gottschalk A (eds). Magnetic resonance angiography, concepts and applications. Mosby-Year Book, Inc. St Louis, USA, 1993: Chapter 11, 220–245

154. Vannan MA, Cao QL, Pandian NG, Sugeng L, Schwartz SL, Dalton MN. Volumetric multiplexed transmission holography of the heart with echocardiographic data. J Am Soc Echocardiogr 1995; 8(5 Pt 1): 567–575

155. Wielopolski PA, Haacke EM, Adler LP. Three-dimensional pulmonary vascular imaging. In: Potchen EJ, Haacke EM, Siebert JE, Gottschalk A (eds). Magnetic resonance angiography, concepts and applications. Mosby-Year Book, Inc. St Louis, USA, 1993: Chapter 12, 246–277

156. Berthezone Y, Vexler V, Clement O, Muhler A, Moseley ME, Brasch RC. Contrast-enhanced MR imaging of the lung: assessments of ventilation and perfusion. Radiology 1992; 183(3): 667–672

157. Berthezone Y, Vexler V, Price DC, et al. Magnetic resonance imaging detection of an experimental pulmonary perfusion deficit using a macromolecular contrast agent. Polylysine-gadolinium-DTPA40. Invest Radiol 1992; 27(5): 346–351

158. Chen Q, Siewert B, Bly BM, Warach S, Edelman RR. STAR-HASTE: perfusion imaging without magnetic susceptibility artifact. Magn Reson Med 1997; 38: 404–408

159. Hatabu H, Gaa J, Kim D, Prasad PV, Edelman RR. Pulmonary perfusion: quantitative assessment with dynamic contrast-enhanced MRI using ultra-short TE and inversion recovery Turbo Flash. Magn Reson Med 1996; 36: 503–508

160. Amundsen T, Kvaerness J, Jones RA, et al. PE: detection with MR perfusion imaging of lung-a feasibility study. Radiology 1997; 203: 181–185

161. Berthezone Y, Croisille P, Bertocchi M, Houzard C, Bendib K, Revel D. Lung perfusion demonstrated by contrast-enhanced dynamic magnetic resonance imaging. Application to unilateral lung transplantation. Invest Radiol 1997; 32(6): 351–356

162. Wielopolski P, Hicks S, de Bruin H, Oudkerk M. Localizing pulmonary emboli: combining breath-hold three-dimensional lung perfusion imaging and 512 matrix pulmonary angiography after contrast administration. Proceedingsbook Int Soc Magn Reson 1997, Vol I: 130

163. Bachert P, Schad LR, Bock M, et al. Nuclear magnetic resonance imaging of airways in humans with use of hyperpolarized 3He. Magn Reson Med 1996; 36(2): 192–196

164. Kauczor HU, Ebert M, Kreitner KF, et al. Imaging of the lungs using 3He MRI: preliminary clinical experience in 18 patients with and without lung disease. J Magn Reson Imaging 1997; 7(3): 538–543

165. Mugler JP 3rd, Driehuys B, Brookeman JR, et al. MR imaging and spectroscopy using hyperpolarized 129Xe gas: preliminary human results. Magn Reson Med 1997; 37(6): 809–815

166. Kauczor HU, Hofmann D, Kreitner KF, et al. Normal and abnormal pulmonary ventilation: visualization at hyperpolarized He-3 MR imaging. Radiology 1996; 201(2): 564–568

167. Kauczor HU, Surkau R, Roberts T. MRI using hyperpolarized noble gases. Eur Radiol 1998; 8: 820–827

168. Edelman RR, Hatabu H, Tadamura E, Li W, Prasad PV. Noninvasive assessment of regional ventilation in the human lung using oxygen-enhanced magnetic resonance imaging. Nat Med 1996; 2(11): 1236–1239

169. Penzkofer H, Loffler R, Peller M, et al. Multisection ventilation imaging of the human lung after breathing of 100% oxygen. Proceedingsbook Int Soc Magn Reson Med (ISMRM) 1998; Vol. I: 454

170. Chen Q, David V, Levin D, et al. Ventilation-perfusion MRI of PE. Proceedingsbook Int Soc Magn Reson Med (ISMRM) 1998; Vol. I: 453

171. Gomori JM, Grossman RI, Goldberg HI, Zimmerman RA, Bilaniuk LT. Intracranial hematomas: Imaging by high-field MR. Radiology 1985; 157: 87–93

Chapter V
Vena Cava Filter Devices

V. Vena cava filter devices – types, effectiveness, indications, complications

J. A. Reekers, H. Harmsen, Y. L. Hoogeveen, R. W. Günther

History of management of venous thromboembolism

Surgical interruption

In 1784 John Hunter performed the first femoral vein ligation in managing deep venous thrombosis (DVT) of the lower limb and subsequent pulmonary embolism (PE) [1]. A century later, in 1893, Bottini [2] successfully performed ligation of the inferior vena cava (IVC). In 1960 Barrit and Jordan established anticoagulation therapy for venous thromboembolism with heparin, when they published the results of the only controlled trial of heparin treatment versus placebo in patients with PE [3]. In 1969, Coon et al. reviewed the effectiveness of heparin in preventing recurrent fatal PE in 639 patients presenting with a single pulmonary embolus. In only six patients (1 %) did fatal recurrent PE occur when treated with heparin [4]. At the time of the publication of these studies on heparin, IVC ligation was favoured above femoral vein ligation because of the high rate of fatal recurrent PE (5–8 %) with the latter technique [5]. However, IVC ligation was also associated with a recurrent PE rate of 6 %, of which 2 % fatal, and an operative mortality of 14 % [5]. Following reports of a chronic venous insufficiency rate as high as 33 % in patients with ligation therapy, plication of the IVC gained preference above ligation [6]. External clips with more facile administration than plication were developed to accomplish the same effect on the IVC [7]. Nevertheless, clipping and plication techniques still had a recurrent PE rate of 4 %, of which 1.7 % fatal, an operative mortality rate as high as 12 % and a high incidence of chronic venous insufficiency (67–69 %) [5, 7]. These reported complication rates led to further investigations to determine other means of preventing venous thromboembolism.

Development of intraluminal devices

Intraluminal devices were subsequently developed and were placed into the IVC by surgical cutdown of the internal jugular vein, without the need for laparotomy or general anesthesia, to achieve lower insertion mortality rates. In 1970, the Mobin-Uddin umbrella filter (MU) was introduced [8]. The original small design (23 mm) had a high incidence of (sometimes even lethal) migration [9, 10]. A larger model (28 mm) had a high risk (60–70 %) of total caval occlusion [11, 12, 13]. The Kimray-Greenfield stainless steel filter (KG) was introduced in 1973 and with its special conical design achieved a caval patency rate of up to 98 % [14].

The next step in the development of the filters was a new method of introduction of the intraluminal devices into the IVC: the transcutaneous placement of vena cava filters. The Kimray-Greenfield filter was originally designed for surgical insertion. However, in 1984, the percutaneous insertion by means of a 28 French introducer sheath via the internal jugular vein [15] and subsequently by the femoral vein [16], were reported. Although this new technique made filter placement substantially easier, Alexander et al. reported a higher incidence of morbidity (such as PE, caval thrombosis, renal dysfunction, venous gangrene, insertion site thrombosis, filter misplacement, and bleeding) when filters were inserted percutaneously compared to surgical filter placement (8 % and 25 %, respectively) [17]. Moreover, femoral insertion of the Kimray-Greenfield filter was accompanied by a high incidence of insertion site thrombosis (19–41 %) [18, 19], partly due to the large size of the introducer sheath (29.5F) and the necessity of dilating the insertion site and the subsequent prolonged compression for hemostasis. Solutions were found in the development of filters that could be loaded through much smaller introducer sheaths, like the Bird's Nest filter (14F) [20], Simon Nitinol filter (9F) [21], LGM-Venatech (12F) [22] and the Titanium Greenfield filter (14F) [23]. With these smaller introducer sheaths, the incidence of insertion site venous thrombosis decreased for the Titanium Greenfield filter to 2–8% [7, 24, 25] while for the Bird's Nest, Simon Nitinol and Günther filters this incidence fell to 0% [26].

Filter types

The different filter types (past and present) can be divided into 3 groups: (1) permanent filters, (2) permanent filters with optional retrievability, and (3) temporary filters.

1. Permanent filters (Fig. 1)

Mobin-Uddin umbrella (MU) (1967)
The MU filter consisted of a domed, perforated disk with whale bones, resembling those in an umbrella, made of stainless steel covered with a silastic layer. It was inserted surgically by cutdown of the jugular vein precluding general anesthesia. The original small 23 mm design was associated with a high incidence of, sometimes even lethal, migration [9, 10]. A subsequent larger 28 mm model was associated with a high risk of total caval occlusion (60–70%), resulting in lower extremity venous stasis [13, 27, 28]. It was therefore withdrawn from the market.

Kimray-Greenfield stainless steel filter (KG) (1973)
Known as simply 'the Greenfield', this conical shaped stainless steel filter comprises six struts with distal hooks for attachment to the caval wall. An advantage of this filter type is a caval patency rate of up to 98% due to the conical design so that 70% to 80% of the basket can be filled with

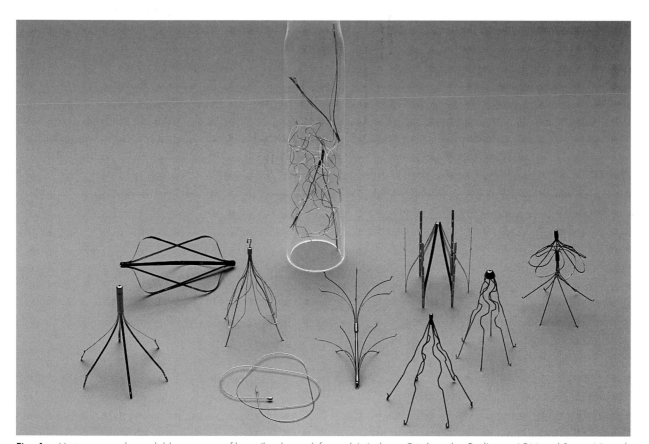

Fig. 1. Various currently available vena cava filters, (back row, left to right): Antheor, Günther tulip, Bird's nest, LGM and Simon Nitonol. Front row, left to right: Keeper, Dil, FCP, Greenfield titanium and Greenfield steel.

333

thrombus without a reduced blood flow. Besides demonstrating retention of trapped thrombi in the presence of continuous flow, the hooks on this filter are intended to ensure fixation to the venous wall [9, 11, 14, 29, 30]. The KG filter was initially inserted surgically. In 1984, the percutaneous insertion by means of an introducer sheath (24F) via the jugular vein or femoral vein was reported [15, 16].

Titanium Greenfield filter (TGF) (1987)

The flexibility of titanium allowed for introducer sheath size reduction from 28F to 14F outer diameter (OD) so that it could be inserted transcutaneously with a marked reduction in insertion site thrombosis, ranging from 2% to 8% [7, 24, 25]. A high incidence of caval wall penetration [31] and migration due to the higher flexibility of this titanium model, necessitated redesign of the filter and alteration of the strut hook angle to 80° (Titanium Greenfield filter with modified hook (TGF-MH)) [23]. These modifications resulted in enhanced attachment to the caval wall, with lower migration rates [7], and reported reduced caval penetration rates [31].

Bird's Nest filter (BNF) (1982)

Four stainless steel wires form a criss-cross web with a length of approximately 7 cm when positioned in the inferior caval vein. Four securing hook struts connected to this web anchor the filter to the caval wall: two struts form a proximal pointing V-shape and the other two a distal pointing V-shape [20]. The problem of migration encountered with the first smaller model (8F) [32] was overcome by redesigning the struts. This resulted in the definitive 11F model, which can be inserted through a 14F OD introducer sheath. The Bird's Nest filter is the first filter of choice for oversized caval veins up to 40 mm [33, 34]. A high incidence of caval thrombosis recently reported with this device was postulated to be the result of filter prolapse beyond the proximal struts and was considered to be operator dependent [35].

Simon Nitinol filter (SNF) (1977)

Composed of a nickel and titanium alloy, this device is shapeable under cold conditions (4°C–10°C) and regains its preformed shape when warmed to body temperature. The filter consists of a cone-shaped disk, formed from wires in overlapping loops, with six hooked legs [21, 36]. The introducer sheath size measures only 9F OD, making it suitable for antecubital vein insertion [36]. It has been questioned whether the material or the design could be thrombogenic because of

the high rate (19.6%) of short-term vena caval thrombosis [7, 37]. Furthermore, a recent report on long-term follow-up (> 180 days) in 22 patients implanted with a SNF revealed substantial leg fracture in 7 [38].

LGM-Vena Tech filter (VTF) (1986)

Made of phynox, this filter is similar in shape to the Greenfield filter but is additionally fitted with six stabilising struts. Pre-packaged in a 10F carrier, the VTF is inserted through a 12F OD introducer sheath via the jugular vein or femoral vein with the use of a guidewire [22, 39]. The device is restricted to IVC diameters of 28 mm or less. The stabilising struts are intended to prevent tilting and asymmetric placement of the filter; nonetheless, both tilting and migration have been reported [12, 35, 37, 40, 41]. The incidence of tilting is hypothesised as being related to the method of filter deployment and operator experience [12, 37]. The filter has no ferromagnetic properties and causes no artifacts or motion on magnetic resonance imaging (MRI) [42].

Keeper (Filcard) filter (KF) (1989)

The conical Keeper filter differs from the Greenfield filter in that double instead of single anchoring hooks are located on each of its six struts for attachment to the caval wall. The material used is phynox and is MRI compatible. A 12F introducer sheath is used for insertion by the jugular or femoral route. Although the KF is commercially available, only limited clinical data is available [43].

OPCETRA filter (OPCETRA) (1992)

The design of this filter is the result of a mathematical approach towards optimal central trapping, minimal flow resistance and optimal stability. This phynox filter consists of 5 long struts that form a cone for clot trapping and five short struts opposite that form a small cone intended to reduce tilting. Curved hooks are located alternately on the inside and outside of the long struts for attachment and stabilisation of the filter. It can only be inserted by the jugular vein through a 12F OD introducer sheath, with use of a guide wire [44].

Cardial filter (CAR) (1987)

This cone-shaped stainless steel device differs from other designs in that, besides six struts with anchoring hooks, there are two slightly longer struts for stabilisation of the filter. It can be introduced through a 10F introducer sheath via the jugular or femoral route. Its efficacy in vitro has been reported to be superior to Greenfield and LGM filters [45, 46].

Vascor filter (VAS) (1991)

The VAS is a cone-shaped stainless steel filter with six struts equipped with anchoring hooks at the ends and three longer struts, which assist in centring of the filter in the IVC. The filter can be introduced surgically or transcutaneously through a 7F introducer sheath via the brachial or jugular vein but not via the femoral approach [47]. With an in vitro efficacy similar to the Cardial filter [46], preliminary clinical experience has shown no recurrent PE, a 96% patency rate and no proximal migration [47].

Anthéor filter (ANT) (1990)

This self-centring design with a double helix basket has the possibility to be applied as a permanent or as a temporary filter. The permanent filter has hooks for caval wall fixation. The material used is phynox with an optional carbon coating intended to optimise hemocompatability and to postpone fibrinous reaction of the caval wall where there is contact with the filter. The filter can be introduced by the femoral, jugular or brachial vein [48] despite the rigidity of the filter [45]. Recently this device was withdrawn from the market, possibly due to the design of the single hooks and filter migration.

The Cordis TrapEase PVCF

This is a nitinol self-expandable, symmetrical double-basket shaped filter. The filter is cut from a single 2 mm tube. It is introduced through a long 6 Fr sheath. In-vitro tests have demonstrated a very good filtering capacity. A first clinical trial has been successfully performed. The next generation of this filter will also have the option of being retrievable.

Permanent filters with optional retrievability

Amplatz filter (AMP) (1984)

Cone shaped, this filter consists of stainless steel loops that end in eight struts with terminal hooks for attachment to the caval wall. A hook is attached to the caudal end of the filter for retrieval or repositioning [49]. The filter fits within a 14F sheath and can be placed via either a jugular or a femoral approach. Retrieval is only possible via the femoral vein due to the caudal position of the hook [50]. In the limited clinical data available [51, 52] this filter showed a relatively high rate of caval thrombosis (17.5% and 23%, respectively), with disconcerting occurrences of propagation

above the filter (6%). The high clot trapping rate or filter geometry was given as possible causes [51]. Filter retrievability was demonstrated 16 days after placement [52].

Günther basket filter (GBF) (1987)

The GBF filter consists of an onion-shaped basket formed by a helix of stainless steel wires with a cone on top ending in several struts with hooks for attachment. There are three planes of filtration. A hook is located centrally at both the apex and bot-

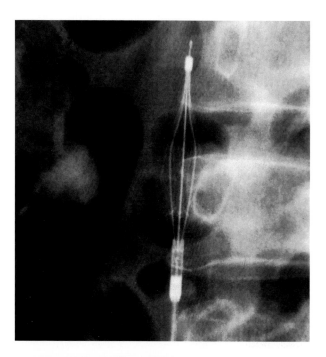

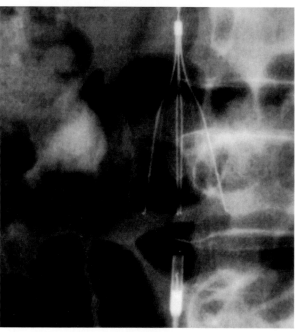

Fig. 2. Example of Günther tulip filter deployment. Note apical hook, which may be used for retrieval.

tom end so that retrieval is possible. Insertion is by the femoral or jugular route with the use of a 12F OD introducer sheath [53, 54]. The filter was removed from the market because of mechanical instability, such as disintegration of the basket and strut fracture [55, 56].

Günther Tulip filter (TF) (1992) (Fig. 2)

This half-basket filter is composed of stainless steel. The inverted tulip-shape is formed by four wires with four extended legs ending in hooks for attachment to the caval wall. At the apex a hook is present for retrieval. The filter can be inserted via the jugular or femoral vein using an 8.5F introducer sheath. The filter can be retrieved via the jugular approach through an 11F retrieval system. An in vivo study showed that 10 of 11 placed filters could be retrieved after 14 days by a jugular approach. One was attached so firmly to the caval wall that retrieval was not possible [57]. Clinically, Kunisch et al. [58] reported successful retrieval in 44 patients (mean implantation time of 6.1 ± 4.1 days), with a maximum of 14 days. Neuerburg et al. [59] reported the results of a multicentre study in which a total of 86 filters were implanted. The two filters intended for use as temporary implants were successfully removed after 6 and 11 days, respectively. In this patient series there was one fatal recurrent PE and 2 non-fatal events, 5 complete and 3 partial caval occlusions, and 3 caudal migrations of the filters.

FCP 2002 filter (FCP) (1988)

The FCP, which is made of phynox, consists of six struts forming a cone. Another six struts form an identical cone above the first thus forming a two tiered filter. The struts all end in little hooks for attachment. At the apex of the filter a little ring allows temporary wire attachment so that the filter can be retrieved by simply pulling this wire. Retrieval is possible up to 10 days after placement, during which time the 9F OD introducer sheath must remain in situ [60]. The latter can be a source of infection, as was reported by Textor et al. in 2 of 5 cases [61]. The design necessitates separate filters for jugular vein and femoral vein insertion [45, 62].

DIL filter (DIL) (1988)

The material used for this – no longer commercially available – unique filter design was a chromium-cobalt-stainless steel alloy. It consisted of a coiled memory wire which regained its pre-shaped form after introduction into the vena cava via the femoral, jugular or cubital vein using a 7F OD introducer sheath. Upon placement, the filter expanded to its preformed shape thereby flattening the vena cava (internal clip mechanism). The filter is retrievable as long as there is contact with the delivery sheath up to 8 days post-implantation. There were four different sizes of the DIL filter available for vena cava sizes varying from 1.9 to 2.8 cm [63]. It was necessary to measure the vena cava to ensure implantation of the correct filter size because a filter deployment defect could result in migration, penetration of the caval wall or caval thrombosis [64].

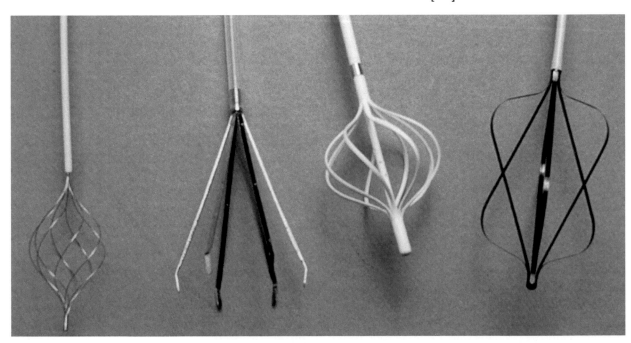

Fig. 3. Various currently used temporary vena cava filters *(left to right)*: Günther basket, LGT, Prolyser and Antheor.

Temporary filters (Fig. 3)

Anthéor temporary filter (ANTT)

As with the permanent version, this self-centring filter consists of a double helix. The phynox material is provided with a carbon coating, which is standard in the temporary model, to optimise hemocompatibility and to postpone fibrinous reaction of the caval wall where there is contact with the filter. The temporary device is without hooks but is kept in place by a catheter that is introduced through a 9.5 or 10.5 F introducer sheath depending on the filter diameter of 31 or 36 mm, respectively. To retrieve the filter, it is easily pulled back into the sheath which can be flushed. The filter can be introduced by the femoral, jugular or brachial vein [65] despite the filter's rigidity [45].

Prolyser filter (PRO)

The filter design consists of two flexible FEP tubes fused at the distal end. The outer tube is vertically cut so that eight strips are present around the central tube. When the inner tube is pulled back slightly, these strips form a basket with a variable diameter of 15–35 mm. At the distal end of the catheter, the inner tube culminates in an end-hole while inner tube side holes are located in the basket, allowing contrast injection and the administration of drugs at the basket site. The distal end-hole allows for a continuous saline drip infusion during the period of implantation. The filter can be inserted through an 8.5F introducer sheath via the femoral, jugular or brachial vein. A guide wire can be used. To retrieve the filter, the outer tube is pulled back resulting in folding of the basket and the whole system can be withdrawn from the vein. Because cardiac pulsations cause minimal movement between the filter and the vessel wall it is thought that this results in a delay of fibrous reaction and endothelisation of the filter and thus extends the period of retrievability [65, 66].

Tempo filter (LGT)

The Tempo filter, made of phynox, is cone-shaped consisting of eight legs attached to a shock-absorbing tethering catheter, which is anchored subcutaneously. The filter is placed percutaneously from the right internal jugular vein approach via a 12F introducer sheath. The legs contact the wall of the vena cava at two levels and centre the device in the vessel [67]. As there are no retaining hooks present on the filter legs, the filter is held in place by a tethering catheter, which is anchored subcutaneously at the puncture site, thereby reducing the risk of insertion site infection.

Cook filter (COOK)/Günther temporary filter (GüTmp)

This temporary filter consists of an unfolding basket, comprising ten 0.4 mm stainless steel wires, attached to a metal wire, which is introduced through a 6.5F introducer sheath via the femoral or jugular route. The basket is 4.5 cm long and has a diameter of maximal 30 mm. It is retrieved by pulling the wire and the collapsing basket back into the delivery sheath [65, 68].

Some experimental temporary filters

Dibie-Musset (DM) retrievable filter

The DM filter was designed on the same principles as the DIL filter, with the difference that this filter consists of a double stranded Nitinol thermic memory wire forming a double spiral when percutaneously inserted into the IVC via a 7F delivery catheter and released [69]. The intention of this coiled filter is to flatten the vena cava, thereby acting as an internal vena cava clip, while the double spiral forms a barrier for clots in the caval vein. The filter has a cobra-head loop, which allows for filter retrieval through a 9F retrieval system up to 15 days post-implantation [70].

Spring filter (SPR)

The SPR consists of a single 0.46 mm thick Nitinol wire that forms a loose flat spring at one end by coiling of the wire. The diameter varies in relation to the number of coils at the top of the wire. The principle of this filter is similar to that of the DIL filter and DM filter. It is introduced through a 7F introducer sheath and can be retrieved by pulling back the wire into the delivery sheath, thereby uncoiling the spring [71].

Retrievable Nitinol Filter (RNF)

Consisting of a single Nitinol wire with a 0.46 mm diameter, the RNF functions on the same principle as the Spring filter. It forms a conical spiral consisting of eight turns with decreasing diameter towards the top of the filter with a larger stabilising curve at the top. The filter is inserted and retrieved through a 5.5F delivery sheath, which is introduced through an introducer sheath [72].

Irie Retrievable IVC filter (Irie)

This experimental filter is intended for retrievability even after a prolonged period in the caval vein of up to four weeks [73]. It consists of two stainless steel conical units with a hook on each apex, placed with the limbs towards each other. The proximal unit is formed by six and the distal unit by four struts, of which two carry anchors for caval wall attachment. The limbs are bent internally so that they run parallel to the caval wall to prevent perforation. Both units are attached by a small spring that snaps when the filter is removed by pulling both hooks. In this way the filter can be retrieved, even after neointimal formation and incorporation of the caval wall has occurred, apparently without significant trauma to the wall [74]. Although the filter can be placed via the femoral or jugular vein, it must be retrieved via both sides simultaneously by trapping the hooks with snares: the proximal unit via the jugular and the distal unit via the femoral vein.

The Embolus Trap (ET)

This is a vena cava filter device made of Nitinol consisting of a central column from which two layers of three loops originate. At the loops anchoring hooks are present for fixation to the caval wall [75].

Effectiveness of vena caval filters

Becker and colleagues [76] combined the results of 13 consecutive series of patients with PE who were treated with stainless steel Greenfield filters. They also described an overall frequency of 2.4 % of recurrent PE (26 of 1094 of which 21 objectively proven) and a frequency of 0.7 % recurrent fatal PE (8 of 1094). Ballew et al. [77] reviewed 11 series of patients with PE treated with newer filter types and described an overall frequency of 2.9 % of recurrent PE (42 of 1428) and a frequency of 0.8 % recurrent fatal PE (12 of 1428). Table 1 shows percentages of recurrent and fatal PE for each filter type. In none of these studies was there any question of systematic screening for recurrent PE after filter placement, so that its true incidence is presumably much higher. The incidence of fatal recurrent PE is less likely to be biased and so these can be better used to evaluate the effectiveness of vena caval filters. Since no placebo controlled trials have been carried out, the mortality rate has to be compared to the estimated mortality of thromboembolism without treatment. A problem with this is that there are almost no data available describing the natural course of untreated thromboembolism. Only five studies [2, 3, 78, 79, 80] are known (including only one placebo controlled study [3]), in which an estimation is made of the mortality rate in untreated thromboembolism. All these studies date from before the introduction of pulmonary angiography and ventilation-perfusion scan in the seventies. Consequently, the described groups are probably not representative for the present population diagnosed with thromboembolism. In these studies, mortality rates of approximately 30 % are described (38 % in the placebo controlled study, of which 26 % autopsy confirmed cases [3]). A comparison of these data with the data on mortality in thromboembolic patients treated with a vena caval device (0.7 % and 0.8 % versus ± 30 %) strongly suggests that caval devices prevent fatal recurrent PE, despite the above-mentioned objections and the fact that objective scientific evidence is not available.

Table 1.

	Recurrent PE (in %)	Fatal PE (in %)
MU [9, 10, 27, 30]	4.6	2.9
KG [19, 75, 81, 82, 83, 84]	2.4	0.7
TGF [25, 41, 77]	5.0	1.6
TGF-MH [24, 35, 41, 85, 86]	2.5	1.1
BNF [35, 41, 81]	3.2	2.1
SNF [34, 36, 41, 81, 87]	2.9	1.0
VTF [22, 35, 40, 41, 88]	2.7	0.4
GBF [53, 55, 56]	5.8	0

Indications for vena cava filter placement

There are a few widely accepted absolute (a) indications for caval interruption in patients with venous thromboembolism and several relative (b) indications on which there is no general consensus or acceptance.

a) Absolute indications

- PE when there is a contraindication for anticoagulant therapy.
- Failure of adequate anticoagulation in preventing (recurrent) PE. If anticoagulation is not adequate and PE occurs, there is no strict indication for filter insertion. Furthermore, one must take into consideration the definition of recurrent PE, which should be defined as a major embolic event that has a close connection with the first embolic event and is proven by imaging modalities. If e. g. the second embolic event occurs after an interval of 6 weeks, there is no indication of filter insertion if anticoagulation is possible.
- Bleeding complications on anticoagulation.
- Prophylaxis in high-risk patients (e. g. cor pulmonale; occlusion of > 50% of pulmonary vasculature) with free-floating thrombus (i. e. patient described in Fig. 5).
- Prophylaxis of recurrent PE after successful pulmonary embolectomy [89].
- Patients with confirmed DVT and the presence of cardial or pulmonary arteriovenous shunt presenting paradoxical (arterial) embolism.

b) Relative indications

- Patients with small cardiopulmonary reserve who might not survive even a small PE [85, 90, 91].
- Patients with venographically proven presence of proximal large free-floating thrombus [37, 85].
- Prophylaxis of PE in the multiple trauma population with documented DVT in the past and the potential for a bedridden post-operative state [92].
- Prophylaxis of PE in cancer patients with DVT as an alternative to anticoagulation to decrease the risk of hemorrhage [93].
- Prophylaxis of PE in the orthopedic surgery population at high risk of PE.

- Prophylaxis of PE with vascular embolisation of arteriovenous malformations [94].
- Failure of a previously placed device [85, 95].

The indications for temporary caval interruption still need to be established. Temporary filters are frequently inserted prophylactically during short term fibrinolysis [96]. Furthermore, consideration is also given to temporary implantation as prophylaxis prior to surgery when there is a risk of displacement of thrombi and after PE, during pregnancy, and short-term contraindication to anticoagulation.

On the subject of contraindications to filter placement, a megacava should be considered a relative contraindication for most filters except the Bird's Nest filter. Megacavae may be observed in up to 5% of all cases [97]. It is therefore mandatory to perform cavography prior to filter implantation to ascertain the size and permeability of the IVC to exclude the possibility of caval anomalies and to localise the renal veins.

Many different groups of patients can be recognised differing in risk for developing DVT and subsequent PE. Therefore, 'tailor-made' prophylaxis/therapy of venous thromboembolism would be the best way to manage these different groups of patients. One must consider for each individual patient whether or not to use a filter, and if so, whether a temporary or permanent filter should be implanted and what type of filter could best be applied in the specific individual circumstances. Because of the absence of long term sequelae with the temporary devices, such a filter is preferred above a permanent filter in those cases where a filter is indicated for only a short period of time.

J. A. Reekers, H. Harmsen, Y. L. Hoogeveen, R. W. Günther

Filter placement

Approach for filter insertion (Fig. 4)

The sites of preference for filter insertion are the right jugular and the right femoral veins. These are relatively straightforward routes to the placement location. If these are not possible, the following alternatives are the left femoral vein and finally the left jugular vein. The latter is the most difficult approach. A transbrachial approach has been described in isolated cases and requires a very flexible introducer set, preferably with the smallest available dimensions (F-size).

Filter position (Fig. 5)

The position of the filter in the IVC is ideally at the L3/L4 level or if the source of the embolic event is in the upper extremities, in the SVC. In some cases it may be necessary to position the filter in the hepatic portion of the IVC, e. g. during pregnancy or if the IVC thrombus extends up to the renal veins. In these latter cases and for placement in the SVC, one should consider the filter type most suitable, preferably a short filter, e. g. Greenfield, Günther Tulip or the LGM-Vena Tech.

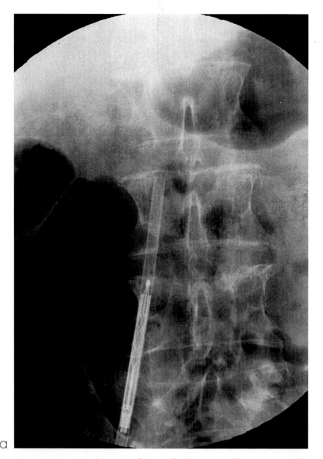
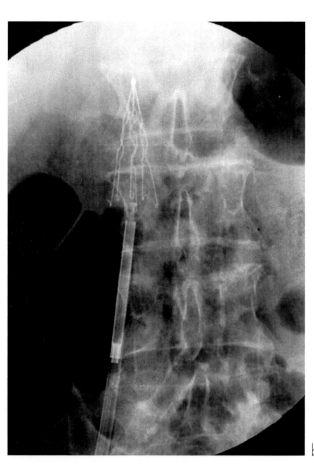

a   b

Fig. 4a, b. Deployment of Greenfield titanium filter using right femoral vein approach **(a)**. Note regular strut interval with central position of the apex which should be at the level of the renal veins **(b)**.

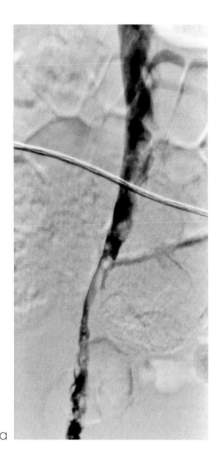

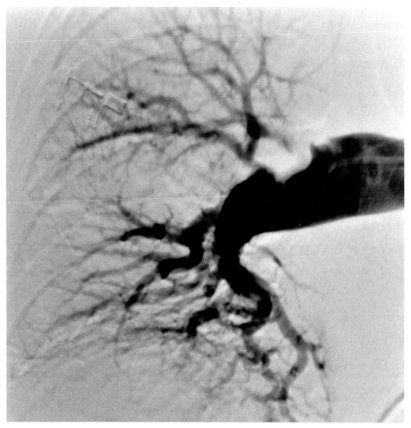

a

b

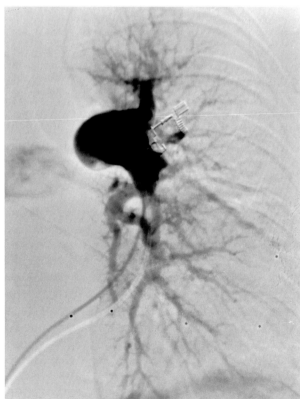

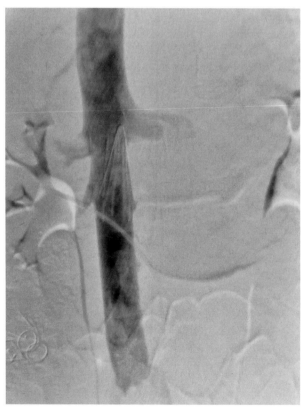

c

d

Fig. 5a–d. Young woman with known pulmonary hypertension. Anticoagulation was withdrawn for a surgical procedure and the patient developed acute respiratory and circulating distress. Catheterisation of the right femoral vein revealed extensive thrombus extending into the caval vein **(a)**. Pulmonary angiography showed adherent thrombus to right upper lobe with lower lobe atelectasis **(b)**. The left lung revealed extensive new embolism **(c)** when compared to previous angiogram (Fig. 4, chapter IV.5). A permanent LGM filter was successfully inserted **(d)** and the patient later underwent surgical thromboendarterectomy.

J. A. Reekers, H. Harmsen, Y. L. Hoogeveen, R. W. Günther

Patient groups in which filter placement could be effective

The trauma population

Due to immobilisation with subsequent venous stasis, vessel wall injuries and tissue damage with release of large amounts of thromboplastin, multiple trauma patients are at high risk for venous thromboembolism. Although confirmatory data are not available, it is estimated that incidence of DVT in patients with multi system trauma is on the order of 20%. However, different studies present ranges from 20% to 90% [98]. In general, treatment with anticoagulants is the therapy of first choice, but in this trauma patient population anticoagulants are frequently contraindicated and pneumatic compression is usually not possible because of fractures.

Brathwaite et al. [99] carried out a retrospective study in 70 trauma ICU patients of whom 36 where treated with anticoagulant therapy and 34 with a vena cava filter. In the group treated with anticoagulants there were 13 (36%) complications (recurrent PE, bleeding, heparin-induced thrombocytopenia) that demanded termination of anticoagulation. Coincidentally, these complications were related to an age over 55. In the group treated with vena caval filters there were no complications recognised. They stated that VCF should be placed in ICU trauma patients aged over 55. In the case of selected trauma patients at high risk for development of DVT and PE, several prospective studies show a significant decrease in incidence of PE and fatal PE when placement of a VCF is compared to standard prophylactic measures such as anticoagulants and external pneumatic compression [100, 101, 102, 103]. The authors indicate a preference for insertion of a VCF in these selected high risk trauma patients above standard prophylactic measures.

Orthopedic surgery

In all patients undergoing orthopedic surgery, the risk of venous thromboembolism is high, with the risk for DVT in hip and knee reconstruction surgery from 45% to 70%. Risk for PE after hip surgery is as high as 20% [104] with a fatal PE rate of 1% to 3% [104, 105, 106]. Low dose heparin is not very beneficial in orthopedic surgery [104] but LMW-heparin can reduce the incidence of proximal DVT and PE substantially [105, 107]. Despite standard prophylaxis, 10% to 30% of patients undergoing total hip arthroplasty (THA) will develop DVT and are thus at risk for PE [108]. However, the use of therapeutic anticoagulation can compromise the wound healing and increase the risk of wound infection [109].

Vaughn et al. performed pre-operative prophylactic filter placement in 44 patients undergoing THA or total knee arthroplasty (TKA). No fatal PE occurred in this group. In a second group of 24 patients, a VCF was placed post-operative when venous thromboembolism occurred. In this group there was one fatal PE, which was probably due to a filter site thrombosis, with massive PE confirmed at autopsy in both left and right lungs [109].

When performing a transoesophageal echocardiography after cuff deflation used for TKA during 3–15 minutes, Parmet et al. [110] observed echogenic material in the right side of the heart. One patient with a VCF had very little echogenic material as seen on ultrasonography. Whether this material is thrombus or not is unknown, but 2 cases of massive PE with subsequent cardiac arrest after cuff deflation have been described [111]. In at least one of the two patients there was no DVT prior to operation. The incidence of PE after cuff deflation is unknown and warrants further investigation.

Acetabular fracture surgery

Elderly patients with surgery for acetabular fracture form a distinct subset, being at extremely high risk of developing DVT and fatal PE (40% and 4%, respectively) [104]. Webb et al. [112] performed a prospective study in which 52 patients with acetabular fractures were divided into two groups: group one, with higher risk for DVT and PE, received a VCF as well as standard prophylaxis, while group two, with lower risk for DVT and PE, received only standard prophylaxis. In the higher risk group with VCF no clinical PE were identified but in the lower risk group, with only standard prophylaxis, there were two clinical cases of PE (7%) of which one was fatal. The researchers concluded that VCF placement is effective in preventing (fatal) PE in patients with acetabular fracture.

Neurosurgery

Patients undergoing neurosurgery are at high risk for DVT (9–50%) and fatal PE (1.5–3%) [104] due to prolonged surgery, paralysis, their frequently advanced age and underlying malignancies. In the case of stroke, the risk of DVT may be as high as 75% in the paralysed leg. Anticoagulants are contraindicated in patients with intracranial or spinal lesions because even minor bleeding can have calamitous consequences. Swann et al. [92] reviewed neurosurgical patients with symptomatic venous thromboembolism and compared subgroups treated with different therapeutic measures like VCF, anticoagulants or simply observation. Anticoagulation therapy had a 29% complication rate and a 15% mortality rate. Conversely, VCF placement prevented clinical PE in all cases. This led the authors to conclude that VCF placement in the neurosurgical patient with symptomatic DVT prevents PE and may be safer than anticoagulation therapy.

Wilson et al. [113] studied the efficacy of prophylactic VCF placement in patients with traumatic spinal cord injuries and paraplegia or quadriplegia and compared this with a historical control group. They advocated the prophylactic use of a VCF as the only effective long-term prophylaxis for PE in the patient with a spinal cord injury. Especially in these patients a long term prophylaxis for PE is required as most of the embolic events occur long after the traumatic event (range, 9–5993 d; median 79 d). Jarrel et al. [114] also concluded that the use of a VCF is effective for these patients but only in the presence of existing venous thromboembolism and in those in whom heparin treatment failed or was inadequate.

DVT during pregnancy

Although DVT during pregnancy is infrequent, PE is an important cause of maternal mortality. AbuRahma et al. [115] found retrospectively that pregnant patients with proximal DVT who were treated with a VCF and subcutaneous heparin tended to do better than patients with DVT treated with intravenous heparin and subcutaneous heparin. However, the group was too small to draw conclusions thereby warranting further research. Narayan et al. [116] reported the use of VCF in addition to standard full

anticoagulation in four pregnant women with proximal DVT and concluded that the use of these devices should be considered as a complementary prophylaxis for PE in pregnant women with DVT.

Cancer patients

Cancer and venous thromboembolism are associated (see also Chapter I). The incidence of PE in cancer patients varies from 6% to 35% depending on the type of tumour [108]. Anticoagulation therapy with heparin followed by oral warfarin is still the primary method of treatment; warfarin, however, has been shown to be less effective when compared to heparin [117]. However, in cancer patients there is a high complication rate of recurrent PE and major bleeding of 8% to 19% and 25% to 32%, respectively [118, 119]. Thrombocytopenia is often seen in this group of patients. The use of LMW-heparin instead of standard heparin shows a decrease of 50% in bleeding complications and mortality in cancer patients [117]. A number of papers describe the use of a VCF in cancer patients with venous thromboembolism and appeal for its use as the primary therapy because of the high rates of complications (recurrent PE and bleeding) with anticoagulant therapy [118, 119, 120]. Sarasin and Eckman [121] reviewed the literature and compared the use of a filter with anticoagulant therapy in cancer patients with venous thromboembolism. They concluded that the VCF was the primary choice of prophylaxis for PE because of bleeding complications in anticoagulant therapy and the related high costs when compared to filter placement. Prophylactic use, i.e. without signs of venous thromboembolism, of a VCF had no effect and anticoagulant prophylaxis had a negative effect on life expectancy [121]. Some authors question the use of a VCF in patients with an aggressive metastatic cancer, arguing that the quality and prolongation of life are not affected by filter placement [122, 123].

All the relative indications for permanent caval interruption are questioned by various authors for several reasons including effectiveness of VCF, costs, VCF associated morbidity and mortality. Furthermore, the lack of controlled randomised prospective studies must be counterbalanced before expansion of indications is justified.

J. A. Reekers, H. Harmsen, Y. L. Hoogeveen, R. W. Günther

Complications of vena cava filters

Fatal complications

In their review of 3,256 patients, Ballew et al. [77] reported only 4 deaths due to caval filters. These involved one case of cardiac arrest after filter placement [97], a case of filter misplacement into the heart [124], one embolisation of a Bird's Nest filter into the pulmonary artery [32] and one case of accidental puncture of the right carotid artery during placement of a filter [40]. Another death occurred as a probable result of septicemia from an infected filter [88].

Complications during insertion

Complications which can occur during insertion are:

1. Insertion site hematoma
2. Air embolism
3. Wound infection
4. Misplacement of the filter including:
   - asymmetry or entwining of the struts of the device. Especially reported of the titanium Greenfield filter (incidence up to 71 % [86])
   - tilting; tilting of the Venatech/L.G.M.filter is observed in up to 16 % of the placements [22]
   - improper anatomical placement of the filter; this includes placement in the heart [32], renal vein [12, 95], spermatic vein [95], iliac

vein [9, 10], lumbar vein [85] and suprarenal caval vein [85, 125]

5. Pneumothorax during internal jugular vein insertion
6. Vocal cord paralysis also due to internal jugular vein insertion
7. PE due to freed thrombus as a result of catheter manipulation

Insertion site thrombosis

Insertion site venous thrombosis is an important complication as this poses an additional risk for PE. When introduction is via the femoral route, the filter device protects against PE from insertion site thrombus, whereas this protection will be absent when the jugular route is chosen.

Incidence of insertion site thrombosis a few days after filter placement is high in cases of femoral insertion of the Greenfield filter (19–41 %) [18, 19] as well as for the Simon Nitinol filter with small introducer sheath (27.8 %) [36]. However, studies show that this incidence is considerably lower in the months following filter placement (2–8 %) [24, 25, 76] for the Greenfield filter as well as for the newer devices with small introducer sheaths (0–2 %) [26, 76]. The clinical significance of the initial high incidence of insertion site thrombosis is not known. Few patients develop clinical symptoms; nonetheless one could be advised to choose the femoral above the jugular route so that protec-

Table 2.

	Distal migration (in %)	Proximal migration (in %)	Wall penetration (in %)	Caval Thrombosis (in %)
MU [9, 10, 27, 30]	2.8	0.8	0.0	60–70
KG [19, 76, 81, 82, 83, 84]	38.9	3.5	17.6	6.3
TGF [25, 41, 77]	21.0	0.0	29.0	0.0
TGF-MH [24, 35, 41, 85, 86]	8.5	2.0	3.0	3.5
BNF [104, 106, 109]	0.0	0.0	6.2	17.5
SNF [34, 36, 41, 81, 87]	8.3	0.0	7.3	15.0
VTF [22, 35, 40, 41, 88]	6.9	1.3	0.5	13.4
GBF [53, 55, 56]	48.8	2.4	15.7	8.6

tion is always afforded against PE by the implanted device.

Caval obstruction and venous insufficiency of lower extremities

Short-term follow-up suggests that caval obstruction is not always clinically manifested. Short-term venous insufficiency of the lower limbs was determined on clinical symptoms in 5.3 % of the Greenfield filter series [76] and in 8.2 % of the newer filter series [77], while radiographic examination for vena cava obstruction showed an incidence of 6.3 % in Greenfield series [76] and in 11 % with newer filter series [77] (Table 2). Crochet et al. [40] report the data of long-term follow-up indicating more common venous insufficiency increasing from 37 % after two years, 42 % after four years up to 58.8 % six years after filter placement, although no correlation between IVC occlusion and trophic disease of the lower limbs has been established. It is difficult to estimate the contribution of filter placement in the manifestation of venous insufficiency of lower limbs because patients with DVT treated only with anticoagulants also exhibit an increasing incidence of insufficiency of up to 30 % to 45 % after 6 years [81]. Occurrence of sequelae after anticoagulation therapy compared to VCF placement for venous thromboembolism are in the same frequency range for chronic leg pain, swelling of the leg, skin changes with or without ulceration and recurrent thrombophlebitis [126]. The Mobin-Uddin (60–70 %), Bird's Nest (17.5 %), Amplatz (17.5 %) and Simon Nitinol filter (15 %) show a high incidence of short term caval thrombosis [76]. Filter occlusion may be due to a thrombogenic design or the result of successful clot trapping by the filter.

Caval penetration

Penetration of the caval wall is not uncommon. In series on routine radiographic surveillance for caval wall penetration a 17.6 % overall incidence of penetration was reported for the Greenfield filter [127] and a 9.1 % incidence of caval wall perforation on newer filter designs, especially the Titanium Greenfield filter (29 %) [77] (Table 2). These penetrations are probably caused by the sharp anchoring hooks in the designs for prevention of migration of the filter. Other designs and a redesign of the hooks in the TGF (leading to the MH-TGF) presented only 2 cases of penetration in three studies involving 168 patients [41, 85, 86]. Although the incidence is high, penetration only very rarely leads to clinical symptoms or fatal complications [77, 128].

Filter migration

Filter migration is a complication of concern because of the potentially fatal consequences (Table 2). The risks include migration to a location or position where the device no longer protects against PE or embolisation of the filter itself into the heart or pulmonary artery. Although theoretically these risks are real, in practice few clinical fatalities have been reported with filters other than the 23mm Mobin-Uddin umbrella. This latter filter demonstrated immediate proximal migration/embolisation of 0.8 %, of which 0.6 % fatal [10]. Filter migration occurs most often distally, i.e. in the opposite direction of blood flow. To recognise distal or proximal migration abdominal radiographs should be made. Migration is demonstrated when the filter moved more than 5 mm distal or proximal compared to earlier radiographs. Moving distances less than 5 mm can be due to differences in patient breathing, positioning and parallax of the roentgenogram beam [76].

Experience with temporary filters

Temporary devices are preferred above permanent filters in those cases where a filter is required for only a short period because of the anticipated absence of long term sequelae. With the majority of currently available temporary filters and retrievable (without tether) devices, removal must be before incorporation into the vessel wall occurs, which is after approximately 10 days. Only limited data is currently available concerning effectiveness and complications of temporary vena cava filters in vivo. Zwaan et al. [64] inserted three different types of temporary vena cava filters in 49 patients: 12 Cook filters, 11 Angiocor filters and 26 Antheor filters. Insertion took place in 7 patients via the femoral and in 42 patients via the brachial or jugular vein. All of these devices would appear to be highly effective since no PE occurred after filter insertion. Although complications such as filter migration, embolisation, caval wall perforation and caval thrombosis where not seen with the use of these temporary devices, a number of other complications occurred more often. These complications included (1) insertion site thrombosis (2 subclavian thromboses in 42 placements), (2) one catheter infection, (3) one dislocation of the catheter, (4) one air embolism, (5) one fracture of basket struts, and (6) 4 hematomas due to a combination of lysis therapy and filter placement. Retrieval of the filters succeeded in all patients. In these patients 4 filters captured thrombus, precipitating the problem on how to manage the filter with captured thrombus. When half of the volume of the basket is filled with thrombus it can still be retracted into the sheath (n = 2 patients). In 2 other patients in whom the filter basket was totally filled, the chosen retrieval strategy was to first perform 3 days of aggressive thrombolysis treatment with streptokinase.

Kuszyk et al. [66] performed animal experiments using the subcutaneously anchored Tempofilter. Their in vivo animal data demonstrated incorporation of filter legs into the caval wall by 3 weeks [66]. Clinical evaluation data on 66 patients (88.3% with duration of implantation longer than 21 days) with this filter [unpublished data cited in ref.66], reports successful retrieval in all 55 patients in whom this was attempted up to 6 weeks after placement. Complications with this filter included migration of more than 12 cm (3 patients), caval thrombosis (2 patients), externalisation of the fixation olive (3 patients) and perifilter thrombosis (9 patients). A recent article by Vos et al. [129] in which 11 Günther temporary filters were clinically evaluated in 10 patients reported successful and complication-free removal of 10 filters (implantation time, 7–10 days; mean 10 days). One filter had to be removed and replaced by a permanent filter due to patient manipulation of the filter; one patient developed sepsis, another an insertion site infection. Clinically no recurrent PE developed during the implantation period or within 7 months after filter removal. These authors concluded the Günther filter to be safe for short-term protection against PE. However, extra data must be awaited before recommendations can be made concerning indications, safety and effectiveness of temporary devices in general.

Randomised studies

Recently, a randomised clinical trial was published which compared the insertion of a cava filter versus no filter in 400 patients with proximal DVT who also received anticoagulant therapy [130]. PE was proven at baseline by angiography or lung scintigraphy in approximately 50% of these patients. The initial end points of the study showed significantly more recurrent PE within 12 days of inclusion in those without a filter (4.8% vs 1.1%, p = 0.02). During a period of follow-up of 2 years twice as many recurrent pulmonary emboli were seen in those who did not receive a vena cava filter (6.3% vs 3.4%), but this difference was not statistically significant. On the other hand, significantly more recurrent DVT developed in patients randomised to receive a vena cava filter (20.8% vs 11.6%, p = 0.02). Both short and long term mortality and bleeding complications were similar in both groups.

This study clearly shows that there are short-term benefits of vena cava filters in patients with proximal DVT. However, these benefits are counter-balanced by recurrent DVT that occurs in the longer term. Hence, it should be clear that at present the placement of a permanent vena cava filter should be severely restricted to those in whom other options are not feasible. Although not tested in this study, the use of retrievable or temporary cava filters may offer a better balance with the benefits during the first days, but without the complications in the long run.

Conclusion

Since the first percutaneous implantation of an inferior vena cava filter, a long list of permanent devices has evolved. The actual list of the most commonly used filters is, on the other hand, substantially shorter: in time the filters have themselves been filtered upon exposure of their safety, effectiveness, handling or ease of use, and complication rates record. As in the current arsenal of filters no one filter can be labelled as the 'ideal filter', each presenting with its own advantages and disadvantages, filter selection by a physician will be based on the published data in the literature, the filters handling and performance in the operator's own clinical setting, and the local patient population. The absolute indications for permanent filter placement are well delineated and generally accepted; the relative indications balance between the question whether caval interruption is at all required or whether temporary interruption should be used prophylactically in selected patients or patient groups. There is currently no consensus on the indications for temporary interruption, and also no substantial clinical data available upon which this can based. In the meantime, the list of devices with optional retrievability and temporary application is growing. A number of these devices are still in the developmental and experimental stages; others are being applied clinically on an increasing scale. However, the indications for their use and clinical benefit compared to current therapy have not yet been established. These must therefore be determined in well-controlled prospective randomised trials.

References

1. Hunter J. Observations on inflammation of internal coat of veins. Trans Soc Improvement Med Chir Knowledge 1793; 1: 18

2. Bottini, and Cited by: Dale WA. Ligation of the inferior vena cava for thromboembolism. Surgery 1958; 43: 22–44

3. Barrit DW, Jordan SC. Anticoagulant drugs in the treatment of pulmonary embolism: a controlled trial. Lancet 1960; 1: 1309–1312

4. Coon WW, Willis PW, Symons MJ. Assessment of anticoagulant treatment of venous thromboembolism. Ann Surg 1969; 170: 559–568

5. Bernstein EF. The place of venous interruption in the treatment of pulmonary thromboembolism. In: Moser KM, Stein M (eds). Pulmonary Thromboembolism. Mosby-Yearbook, St. Louis, 1973: 312–323

6. Piccone VA, Vida E, Yarnoz M, Glass BS, LeVeen HH. The late results of caval ligation. Surgery 1970; 68: 980–998

7. Greenfield LJ. Evolution of venous interruption for pulmonary thromboembolism. Arch Surg 1992; 127: 622–626

8. Mobin–Uddin K, McLean R, Jude JR. A new catheter technique of interruption of inferior vena cava for prevention of pulmonary embolism. Am Surg 1969; 35: 889–894

9. Cimochowski GE, Evans RH, Zarins CK, Lu CT, DeMeester TR. Greenfield filter versus Mobin-Uddin umbrella: the continuing quest for the ideal method of vena caval interruption. J Thorac Cardiovasc Surg 1980; 79: 358–365

10. Mobin-Uddin K, Utley JR, Bryant LR. The inferior vena cava umbrella filter. Prog Cardiovasc Dis 1975; 18: 391–399

11. Wingerd M, Bernhard VM, Maddison F, Towne JB. Comparison of caval filters in the management of venous thrombo-embolism. Arch Surg 1978; 113: 1264–1271

12. Grassi CJ. Inferior vena caval filters: analysis of five currently available devices [Review]. Am J Roentgenol 1991; 156: 813–821

13. Rao G. Long-term experience with the Mobin-Uddin umbrella. Int Surg 1980; 64: 223–230

14. Greenfield LJ, McCurdy JR, Brown PP, Elkins RC. A new intracaval filter permitting continued flow and resolution of emboli. Surgery 1973; 73: 599–606

15. Tadavarthy SM, Castadena-Zuniga W, Salamonowitz E, et al. Kimray-Greenfield filter: percutaneous introduction. Radiology 1984; 151: 525–526

16. Denny DF, Cronon JJ, Dorfman GS, Esplin C. Percutaneous Kimray-Green-field filter placement by femoral vein puncture. Am J Roentgenol 1985; 145: 827–829

17. Alexander JJ, Yuhas JP, Piotrowski JJ. Is the increasing use of prophylactic percutaneous IVC filters justified? Am J Surg 1994; 168: 102–106

18. Mewissen MW, Erickson SJ, Foley WD, Lipchik EO, Olson DL, McCann KM. Thrombosis at venous insertion sites after inferior vena caval filter placement. Radiology 1989; 173: 155–157

19. Kantor A, Glanz S, Gordon DH, Sclafani SJ. Percutaneous insertion of the Kimray-Greenfield filter: incidence of femoral vein thrombosis. Am J Roentgenol 1987; 149: 1065–1066

20. Roehm JOF, Gianturco C, Barth MH, Wright KC. Percutaneous transcatheter filter for the inferior vena cava: a new device for treatment of patients with pulmonary embolism. Radiology 1984; 150: 255–257

21. Simon M, Kaplow R, Salzman E, Freiman D. A vena cava filter using thermal shape memory alloy: experimental aspects. Radiology 1977; 125: 87–94

22. Ricco JB, Crochet DP, Sebilotte P, et al. Percutaneous transvenous caval interruption with the "LGM" filter: Early results of a multicenter trial. Ann Vasc Surg 1988; 2: 242–247

23. Greenfield LJ, Cho KJ, Tauscher JR. Evolution of hook design for fixation of the titanium Greenfield filter. J Vasc Surg 1990; 9: 345–353

24. Greenfield LJ, Proctor MC, Cho KJ, Cutler BS, Ferris EJ, McFarland D, Sobel M, Tisnado J. Extended evaluation of the titanium Greenfield vena caval filter [published erratum appears in J Vasc Surg 1995; 21 (1): 162]. J Vasc Surg 1994; 20: 458–464

25. Greenfield LJ, Cho KJ, Tauscher JR. Limitations of percutaneous insertion of Greenfield filters. J Cardiovasc Surg 1990; 31: 344–350

26. Ammann ME, Eibenberger K, Winkelbauer F, Walter RM, Dorffner R, Hormann M, Grabenwoger F. Thromboserate nach Kavafilterimplantation. Langzeitergebnisse. Ultraschall Med 1994; 15: 95–98

27. Wingerd M, Bernhard VM, Maddison F, Towne JB. Comparison of caval filters in the management of venous thromboembolism. Arch Surgery 1978; 113: 1264–1271

28. Grassi CJ. Inferior vena caval filters: analysis of five currently available devices [Review]. Am J Roentgenol 1991; 156: 813–821

29. Greenfield LJ, Michna BA. Twelve-year clinical experience with the Greenfield vena caval filter. Surgery 1988; 104: 706–712

30. Gomez GA, Cutler BS, Wheeler HB. Transvenous interruption of the inferior vena cava. Surgery 1983; 93: 612–619

31. Greenfield LJ, Cho KJ, Pais SO, et al. Preliminary clinical experience with the titanium Greenfield vena caval filter. Arch Surg 1989; 124: 657–659

32. Roehm JOF, Johnsrude IS, Barth MH, Gianturco C. The Bird's Nest inferior vena caval filter: Progress Report. Radiology 1988; 168: 745–749

33. Reed RA, Teitelbaum GP, Taylor FC, Pentecost MJ, Roehm JO. Use of the Bird's Nest filter in oversized inferior venae cavae. J Vasc Interv Radiol 1991; 2: 447–450

34. Korbin CD, Reed RA, Taylor FC, Pentecost MJ, Teitelbaum GP. Comparison of filters in an oversized vena caval phantom: intracaval placement of a bird's nest filter versus biiliac placement of Greenfield, Vena Tech-LGM, and Simon nitinol filters. J Vasc Interv Radiol 1992; 3: 559–564

35. Mohan CR, Hoballah JJ, Sharp WJ, Kresowik TF, Lu CT, Corson JD. Comparative efficacy and complications of vena caval filters. J Vasc Surg 1995; 21: 235–245

36. Simon M, Athanasoulis CA, Kim D, Steinberg FL, Porter DH, Byse BH, Geller S, Orron DE, Waltman AC. Simon nitinol inferior vena cava filter: initial clinical experience. Work in progress. Radiology 1989; 172: 99–103

37. Dorfman GS. Percutaneous inferior vena caval filters. Radiology 1990; 174: 987–992

38. Thomas DL, McFarland DR, Price MB, Ferris EJ. Fractures of Simon-Nitinol IVC filters: follow-up experience. J Vasc Interv Radiol; suppl. 8 (1): 197 (Abstract)

39. Cull DL, Wheeler JR, Gregory RT, Synder SO Jr, Gayle RG, Parent FN. The Vena Tech filter: evaluation of a new inferior vena cava interruption device. J Cardiovasc Surg 1991; 32: 691–696

40. Crochet DP, Stora O, Ferry D, Grossetete R, Leurent B, Brunel P, Nguyen JM. Vena Tech-LGM filter: long-term results of a prospective study. Radiology 1993; 188: 857–860

41. Ferris EJ, McCowan TC, Carver DK, McFarland DR. Percutaneous inferior vena caval filters: follow-up of seven designs in 320 patients [see comments]. Radiology 1993; 188: 851–856

42. Kiproff PM. Magnetic resonance characteristics of the LGM vena cava filter: technical note. Cardiovasc Intervent Radiol 1991; 14: 254–255

43. Lang M, Solovei G, Alame A, Deliere T, Segbaya P, Poitrineau O, Le Helloco A, Garnier LF, Rifai A, Delcour C, Barral F, Rousseau H. Evaluation du nouveau filtre cave percutane definitif Filcard (DF06). Abstract. RIPCV 3, Congres International, Toulouse, France, March 1993

44. Kraimps JL, De La Faye D, Drouineau J, Bensignor E, Barbier J. Optimal central trapping (OPCETRA) vena caval filter: results of experimental studies. J Vasc Interv Radiol 1992; 3: 697–701

45. Neuerburg J, Günther RW. Developments in inferior vena cava filters: A European viewpoint. Sem Interv Radiol 1994; 11: 349–357

46. Jausseran JM, Rubondy P, Caburol G, Ferdani M, Lablanne B, Chabert B. Blanc d'essai in vitro des filtres ombrelles caves. Phlebogie 1993; 46: 429–440

47. Rudondy P, Ferdani M, Reggi M, Jausseran JM. Interruption of the inferior vena cava using the Vascor filter: preliminary series of 51 cases. Cardiovasc Surg 1994; 2: 344–349

48. Zwaan M, Kagel C, Marienhoff N, Weiss HD, Grimm W, Eberhard I, Schwieder G. Erste Erfahrungen mit temporaren Vena-cava-Filtern. Fortschr Röntgenstr 1995; 163: 171–176

49. Lund G, Rysavy JA, Salomonowitz E. A new vena caval filter for percutaneous placement and retrieval: experimental study. Radiology 1984; 152: 369–372

50. Darcy MD, Hunter DW, Lund GB, Cardella JF. Amplatz Retrievable vena cava filter. Sem Interv Radiol 1986; 8 (3): 214–219

51. Epstein DH, Darcy MD, Hunter DW, Coleman CC, Tadavarthy SM, Murray PD, Castaneda-Zuniga WR, Amplatz K. Experience with the Amplatz retrievable vena cava filter. Radiology 1989; 172: 105–110

52. McCowan TC, Ferris EJ, Carver DK. Amplatz vena caval filter: Clinical experience in 30 patients. Am J Roentgenol 1990; 155: 177–181

53. Bull PG, Mendel H, Schlegl A. Gunther vena caval filter: clinical appraisal. J Vasc Interv Radiol 1992; 3: 395–399

54. Fobbe F, Dietzel M, Korth R, Felsenberg D, Bender S, Hamed M, Laass C, Sorensen R. Gunther vena caval filter: Results of long-term follow-up. Am J Roentgenol 1988; 151: 1031–1034

55. Perry JN, Wells IP. A long term follow-up of Gunther vena caval filters. Clin Radiol 1993; 48: 35–37

56. Becker CD, Hoogewoud HM, Felder P, Gal I, Ruijs PA, Triller J. Long-term follow-up of the Gunther basket inferior vena cava filter: does mechanical instability cause complications? Cardiovasc Intervent Radiol 1994; 17: 247–251

57. Neuerburg J, Gunther RW, Rassmussen E, Vorwerk D, Tonn K, Handt S, Kupper W, Hansen JV. New retrievable percutaneous vena cava filter: experimental in vitro and in vivo evaluation. Cardiovasc Intervent Radiol 1993; 16: 224–229

58. Kunisch M, Rauber K, Bachmann G, Rau WS. Temporary cava filter: Effective prophylaxis of pulmonary embolism in venous thromboses in the region of the pelvic vascular system and of the vena cava inferior? Fortschr Röntgenstr 1995; 163 (6): 523–526

59. Neuerburg JM, Günther RW, Vorwerk D, Donderlinger RF, Jäger H, Lackner KJ, Schild HH, Plant GR, Joffre FG, Schneider PA, Janssen JHA. Results of a multicentre study of the retrievable Tulip vena cava filter: early clinical experience. Cardiovasc Intervent Radiol 1997; 20: 10–16

60. Pietri J, Abet D. L'interruption partielle de la veine cave inférieure: premiers résultats d'un filtre endocave à double stage. J Mal Vasc 1988; 13: 288–289

61. Textor HJ, Strunk H, Schild HH. Temporary vena cava filter: critical comments. Fortschr Röntgenstr 1996; 165 (4): 371–374

62. Jackisch C, Schwenkhagen A, Budde T, Louwen F, Meschede D, Schober O, Holzgreve W, Schneider HP. Interventionelle Therapie der Vena cava inferior Thrombose in der Schwangerschaft-Einsatz eines neuartigen temporaren Vena-cava-Filters. Zentralbl Gynakol 1995; 117: 181–189

63. Dibie A, Lahille M, Palau R, Joussen JM, et al. Dil vena cava filter. A new percutaneous device. Experimental results. Circulation 1988; 78: 271

64. Nagele M, Konig C, Gorich C, Steudel A. DIL-Vena-Cava-Filter: Erfahrungen und Verlaufskontrollen bei 15 Patienten. Zentralbl Radiol 1994; 150: 242

65. Zwaan M, Kagel C, Marienhoff N, Weiss HD, Grimm W, Eberhard I, Schwieder G. Erste Erfahrungen mit temporaren Vena-cava-Filtern. Fortschr Röntgenstr 1995; 163: 171–176

66. Chavan A, Gulba D, Schaefer C, Daniel W, Galanski M. The Filcard temporary, removable vena cava filter: use in local thrombolytic therapy. Z Kardiol 1993; 82, Suppl 2: 191–193

67. Kuszyk BS, Venbrux AC, Samphilipo MA, Magee CA, Olson JL, Osterman FA. Subcutaneously tethered temporary filter: Pathologic effects in swine. J Vasc Interv Radiol 1995; 6: 895–902

68. Millward SF, Bormanis J, Burbridge BE, Markman SJ, Peterson RA. Preliminary clinical experience with the Gunther temporary inferior vena cava filter. J Vasc Interv Radiol 1994; 5: 863–868

69. Dibie A, Kareco T, Musset D, Dufaux J, Counord JL, Laborde F, Flaud P. Evaluation in vitro du filtre cave Dibie-Musset. Arch Mal Coeur 1994; 87: 115–122

70. Dibie A, Musset D, Maitre S, Parent F. DM Inferior Vena Cava Filter: Preliminary Clinical Results. Circulation 1996; 94 (suppl): J300

71. Xian ZY, Roy S, Hosaka J, Kuroki K, Kvernebo K, Enge I, Laerum F. In vitro evaluation of a new temporary venous filter: the spring filter. Cardiovasc Intervent Radiol 1995; 18: 315–320

72. Nakagawa N, Cragg AH, Smith TP, Castaneda F, Barnhart WH, De Jong SC. A retrievable nitinol vena cava filter: experimental and initial clinical results. J Vasc Interv Radiol 1994; 5: 507–512

73. Irie T, Yamauchi T, Makita K, Kusano S. Retrievable IVC filter: preliminary in vitro and in vivo evaluation. J Vasc Interv Radiol 1995; 6: 449–454

74. Vesely TM, Krysl J, Smit SR, Killon D, Hicks ME. Preliminary investigation of the Irie inferior vena cava filter. J Vasc Interv Radiol 1996; 7: 529–535

75. Mobin-Uddin K, Pleasant R, Mobin-Uddin O, Ahmad KA. Evolution of a new device for the prevention of pulmonary embolism. Am J Surg 1994; 168: 330–334

76. Becker DM, Philbrick JT, Selby JB. Inferior vena cava filters. Indications, safety, effectiveness [Review]. Arch Intern Med 1992; 152: 1985–1994

77. Ballew KA, Philbrick JT, Becker DM. Vena Cava Filter Devices. Clinics in Chest Medicine 1995; 16, 2: 295–305

78. Morrell MT, Truelove SC, Barr A. Pulmonary embolism. Br Med J 1963; 2: 830–835

79. Hermann RE, Davis JH, Holden WD. Pulmonary embolism: A clinical and pathologic study with emphasis on the effect of prophylactic therapy with anticoagulants. Am J Surg 1961; 102: 19–28

80. Zilliacus H. On specific treatment of thrombosis and pulmonary embolism with anticoagulants, with particular reference to postthrombotic sequelae: results of five years' treatment of thrombosis and pulmonary embolism at series of Swedish hospitals during years 1940–1945. Acta Med Scand 1946 (suppl) 171: 1–221

81. Browse NL, Clemenson G, Lea Thomas M. Is the postphlebitic leg always postphlebitic? Relation between phlebographic appearances of deep-vein thrombosis and late sequelae. Br Med J 1980; 281: 1167–1170

82. Berland LL, Maddison FE, Bernhard VM. Radiologic follow-up of vena cava filter devices. Am J Roentgenol 1980; 134: 1047–1052

83. Messmer JM, Greenfield LJ. Greenfield caval filters: long-term radiographic follow-up study. Radiology 1985; 156: 613–618

84. Rose BS, Simon DC, Hess ML, Van Aman ME. Percutaneous transfemoral placement of the Kimray-Greenfield vena cava filter. Radiology 1987; 165: 373–376

85. Greenfield LJ, Cho K, Proctor M, et al. Results of a multicenterstudy of the modified hook-titanium Greenfield filter. J Vasc Surg 1991; 14: 253–257

86. Sweeney TJ, Van Aman ME. Deployment problems with the titanium Greenfield filter [see comments]. J Vasc Interv Radiol 1993; 4: 691–694

87. McCowan TC, Ferris EJ, Carver DK, Molpus WM. Complications of the nitinol vena caval filter. J Vasc Interv Radiol 1992; 3: 401–408

88. Millward SF, Peterson RA, Moher D, Lewandowski BJ, Burbridge BE, Formoso A. LGM (Vena Tech) vena caval filter: experience at a single institution. J Vasc Interv Radiol 1994; 5: 351–356

89. Bauer EP, Laske A, Von Segesser LK, Carrel T, Turina MI. Early and late results after surgery for massive pulmonary embolism. Thorac Cardiovasc Surg 1991; 39: 353–356

90. Golueke PJ, Garrett WV, Thompson JE, Smith BL, Talkington CM. Interruption of the vena cava by means of the Greenfield filter: Expanding the indications. Surgery 1988; 103: 111–117

91. Rohrer MJ, Scheidler MG, Wheeler HB, Cutler BS. Extended indications for placement of an inferior vena cava filter [see comments]. J Vasc Surg 1989; 10: 44–49

92. Swann KW, Black PM, Baker MF. Management of symptomatic deep venous thrombosis and pulmonary embolism on a neurosurgical service. J Neurosurg 1986; 64: 563–567

93. Cohen JR, Grella L, Citron M. Greenfield filter instead of heparin as primary treatment for deep venous thrombosis or pulmonary embolism in patients with cancer. Cancer 1992; 70: 1993–1996

94. Thery C, Asseman P, Becquart J, Bauchart JJ, Jabinet JL, Marache P. Filtre cave temporaire permettant le diagnostic et la fibrinolyse chez les patients suspects d'embolie pulmonaire massive. Arch Mal Coeur Vaiss 1991; 84: 525–530

95. Jäger HR, Jackson JE, Allison DJ. Delayed pulmonary embolism after therapeutic vascular embolization of an arteriovenous malformation; Treatment with a venous filter. J Interv Rad 1993; 7: 153–156

96. Epstein DH, Darcy MD, Hunter DW, Coleman CC, Tadavarthy SM, Murray PD, Castaneda-Zuniga WR, Amplatz K. Experience with the Amplatz retrievable vena cava filter. Radiology 1989; 172: 105–110

97. Zolfaghari D, Johnson B, Weireter LJ, Britt LD. Expanded use of inferior vena cava filters in the trauma population [Review]. Surg Annu 1995; 27: 99–105

98. Pais SO, Tobin KD, Austin CB, Queral L. Percutaneous insertion of the Greenfield inferior vena cava filter: Experience with ninety-six patients. J Vasc Surg 1988; 8: 460–464

99. Brathwaite CE, Mure AJ, O'Malley KF, Spence RK, Ross SE. Complications of anticoagulation for pulmonary embolism in low risk trauma patients. Chest 1993; 104: 718–720

100. Webb LX, Rush PT, Fuller SB, Meredith JW. Greenfield filter prophylaxis of pulmonary embolism in patients undergoing surgery for acetabular fracture. J Orthop Trauma 1992; 6: 139–145

101. Khansarinia S, Dennis JW, Veldenz HC, Butcher JL, Hartland L. Prophylactic Greenfield filter placement in selected high-risk trauma patients. J Vasc Surg 1995; 22: 231–235

102. Rogers FB, Shackford SR, Ricci MA, Wilson JT, Parsons S. Routine prophylactic vena cava filter insertion in severely injured trauma patients decreases the incidence of pulmonary embolism [see comments]. J Am Coll Surg 1995; 180: 641–647

103. Leach TA, Pastena JA, Swan KG, Tikellis JI, Blackwood JM, Odom JW. Surgical prophylaxis for pulmonary embolism. Am Surg 1994; 60: 292–295

104. Consensus Conference: Prevention of Venous Thrombosis and Pulmonary Embolism. JAMA 1986; 256, no. 6: 744–749

105. Nicolaides AN, Arcelus J, Belcaro G, Bergqvist D, Borris LC, Buller HR, Caprini JA, Christopoulos D, Clarke-Pearson D, Clement D, et al. Prevention of venous thrombo-embolism. European Consensus Statement, 1–5 November 1991, developed at Oakley Court Hotel, Windsor, UK [editorial]. [Review]. International Angiology 1992; 11: 151–159

106. Paiement GD, Desautels C. Deep vein thrombosis: prophylaxis, diagnosis, and treatment-lessons from orthopedic studies [Review]. Clinical Cardiology 1990; 13: VI19–VI22

107. Eriksson BI, Kalebo P, Anthymyr BA, Wadenvik H, Tengborn L, Risberg B. Prevention of deep-vein thrombosis and pulmonary embolism after total hip replacement. Comparison of low-molecular-weight heparin and unfractionated heparin. J Bone Joint Surg 1991; 73: 484–493

108. Van Beek EJR, Büller HR, Ten Cate JW. Epidemiology of venous thromboembolism. In: Tooke JE, Lowe GO (eds). Textbook of Vascular Medicine. Arnold, London 1994: 15–50.

109. Vaughn BK, Knezevich S, Lombardi AV Jr, Mallory TH. Use of the Greenfield filter to prevent fatal pulmonary embolism associated with total hip and knee arthroplasty. J Bone Joint Surg 1989; 71: 1542–1548

110. Parmet JL, Berman AT, Horrow JC, Harding S, Rosenberg H. Thromboembolism coincident with tourniquet deflation during total knee arthroplasty [see comments]. Lancet 1993; 341: 1057–1058

111. McGrath BJ, Hsia J, Epstein B. Massive Pulmonary Embolism Following Tourniquet Deflation. Anesth 1991; 74: 618–620

112. Webb LX, Rush PT, Fuller SB, Meredith JW. Greenfield filter prophylaxis of pulmonary embolism in patients undergoing surgery for acetabular fracture. J Orthop Trauma 1992; 6: 139–145

113. Wilson JT, Rogers FB, Wald SL, Shackford SR, Ricci MA. Prophylactic vena cava filter insertion in patients with traumatic spinal cord injury: preliminary results. Neurosurgery 1994; 35: 234–239

114. Jarrell BE, Posuniak E, Roberts J, Osterholm J, Cotler J, Ditunno J. A New Method Of Management Using The Kim-Ray Greenfield Filter For Deep Venous Thrombosis And Pulmonary Embolism In Spinal Cord Injury. Surg Gynecol Obstet 1983; 157: 316–320

115. AbuRahma AF, Bastug DF, Tiley EH, Killmer SM, Boland JP. Management of deep vein thrombosis of the lower extremity in pregnancy. W V Med J 1993; 89: 445–447

116. Narayan H, Cullimore J, Krarup K, Thurston H, Macvicar J, Bolia A. Experience with the Cardial inferior vena cava filter as prophylaxis against pulmonary embolism in pregnant women with extensive deep venous thrombosis [published erratum appears in Br J Obstet Gynaecol 1992; 99 (9): 726]. Br J Obstet Gynaecol 1992; 99: 637–640

117. Naschitz JE, Yeshurun D, Lev LM. Thromboembolism in cancer. Changing trends [Review]. Cancer 1993; 71: 1384–1390

118. Whitney BA, Kerstein MD. Thrombocytopenia and cancer: use of the Kimray-Greenfield filter to prevent thromboembolism. South Med J 1987; 80: 1246–1248

119. Cohen JR, Grella L, Citron M. Greenfield filter instead of heparin as primary treatment for deep venous thrombosis or pulmonary embolism in patients with cancer. Cancer 1992; 70: 1993–1996

120. Calligaro KD, Bergen WS, Haut MJ, Savarese RP, DeLaurentis DA. Thromboembolic complications in patients with advanced cancer: anticoagulation versus Greenfield filter placement. Ann Vasc Surg 1991; 5: 186–189

121. Sarasin FP, Eckman MH. Management and prevention of thromboembolic events in patients with cancer-related hypercoagulable states: a risky business. J Gen Intern Med 1993; 8: 476–486

122. Rosen MP, Porter DH, Kim D. Reassessment of vena caval filter use in patients with cancer. J Vasc Interv Radiol 1994; 5: 501–506

123. Walsh DB, Downing S, Nauta R, Gomes MN. Metastatic Cancer: A relative contraindication to vena cava filter placement. Cancer 1987; 59: 161–163

124. Scurr JH, Jarrett PE, Wastell C. The treatment of recurrent pulmonary embolism: experience with the Kimray Greenfield vena cava filter. Ann Royal Coll Surg Engl 1983; 65: 233–234

125. Brenner DW, Brenner CJ, Scott J, Wehberg K, Granger JP, Schellhammer PF. Suprarenal Greenfield filter placement to prevent pulmonary embolus in patients with vena caval tumor thrombi. J Urol 1992; 147: 19–23

126. Fink JA, Jones BT. The Greenfield filter as the primary means of therapy in venous thromboembolic disease. Surg Gynecol Obstet 1991; 172: 253–256

127. Messmer JM, Greenfield LJ. Greenfield caval filters: long-term radiographic follow-up study. Radiology 1985; 156: 613–618

128. Bergqvist D. The role of vena caval interruption in patients with venous thromboembolism [Review]. Prog Cardiovasc Dis 1994; 37: 25–37

129. Vos LD, Tielbeek AV, Bom EP, Gooszen HC, Vroegindeweij D. The Günther temporary inferior vena cava filter for short-term protection against pumonary embolism. Cardiovasc Intervent Radiol 1997; 20: 91–97

130. Decousus H, Leizorovicz A, Parent F, et al. A clinical trial of vena caval filters in the prevention of pulmonary embolism in patients with proximal deep vein thrombosis. N Engl J Med 1998; 338: 409–415

Chapter VI
Conservative and Surgical Treatment

VI.1 The initial and long-term treatment of venous thromboembolic diseases

A. G. M. van den Belt, M. H. Prins, A. W. A. Lensing, J. Hirsh

Introduction

Although deep vein thrombosis (DVT) and pulmonary embolism (PE) were previously regarded as separate clinical entities, there is good evidence that they are expressions of a single disease process, namely, venous thromboembolism [1, 2]. The incidence of symptomatic venous thromboembolism in the general population is approximately 0.1 % per year. Anticoagulant therapy is the treatment of choice for most patients with venous thromboembolism [3]. A placebo-controlled randomised trial demonstrated that a regimen of intravenous heparin plus oral anticoagulants is more effective in preventing recurrent venous thromboembolism than oral anticoagulants alone [4]. Thus, to prevent thrombus extension, pulmonary embolisation, and recurrences, it is standard practice to treat patients with adjusted-dose, intravenous unfractionated heparin (UFH) for 5 to 10 days combined with oral anticoagulants for a period of at least 3 months. The dosage of oral anticoagulants is adjusted to prolong the prothrombin time to an International Normalised Ratio (INR) of 2.0 to 3.0. In patients with symptomatic DVT, UFH can also be administered by the subcutaneous route [5]. UFH treatment requires daily monitoring of the activated partial thromboplastin time (APTT) to adjust the dose to maintain the anticoagulant effect within a defined therapeutic range (i. e. APTT at least 1.5 times control). Laboratory monitoring is necessary because the anticoagulant response to heparin is highly variable over time between patients as well as in an individual patient [6, 7].

Low molecular weight heparins (LMWHs) are a relatively new group of anticoagulants. Compared with UFH, LMWHs have a longer plasma half-life and a better, almost complete bio-availability following subcutaneous injection, less inter- and intra-individual variability in anticoagulant response to fixed, body weight adjusted doses, and a more favourable antithrombotic to hemorrhagic ratio in animal models [8, 9]. As a result of these properties, a predictable anticoagulant effect can be achieved allowing once or twice daily subcutaneous administration of these compounds without dose adjustments and monitoring procedures as required for UFH. Nowadays, LMWHs are used instead of UFH for various indications. LMWHs have been extensively evaluated for the prevention of venous thromboembolism and have been shown to be safe and effective [10]. There is accumulating evidence from randomised clinical trials that these new anticoagulants are at least as effective and safe as UFH for the treatment of acute DVT. Only recently, the first clinical trials comparing LMWH with UFH in patients with PE have been published.

The optimal treatment duration with oral anticoagulants after an acute venous thromboembolic event is still unknown. Several subgroups of patients seem to benefit from prolonged anticoagulation. However, the ability of prolonged anticoagulant treatment to prevent venous thromboembolic complications should be balanced in the various subgroups against the potential for increased hemorrhagic complications. Recently, studies have become available on the long-term clinical course of patients with DVT who were treated according to current practice. In these studies, a high cumulative incidence of recurrent venous thromboembolism was found over the years following the acute thrombotic episode. In addition, studies have become available which compared short-term with long-term anticoagulant regimens. These recent studies challenge the appropriateness of the currently recommended duration of anticoagulant treatment.

In this chapter, at first a systematic review is provided on the effectiveness and safety of fixed-dose body weight adjusted subcutaneous LMWH compared to adjusted-dose UFH for the initial treatment of patients with acute DVT or PE. Secondly, studies evaluating the long-term risk for recurrent venous thromboembolic complications in patients with DVT and the optimal duration of anticoagulant therapy are reviewed.

Table 1. Randomised clinical trials: low molecular weight heparin versus unfractionated heparin for the treatment of venous thromboembolism.

Source, year	LMWH (alls.c.), dosage frequency	Dose: Anti-Xa units (per injection)	UFH route	UFH dose adjustment aPTT	UFH Bolus	OAC initiation/target INR	Duration initial treatment	Follow-up
Faivre et al. 1987 [26]	CY 222 *, twice daily	155 U/kg	s.c.	x2.0 to 3.0	+	not defined	10 days	§
Duroux et al. 1991 [29]	nadroparin, twice daily	+/-90 U/kg	i.v.	x1.5 to 2.0	−	not defined	10 days	§
Hull et al. 1992 [30]	tinzaparin, once daily	175 U/kg	i.v.	x1.5 to 2.0	+	day 2 / 2.0 to 3.0	6 days provided that INR was > 2.0	3 months
Prandoni et al. 1992 [32]	nadroparin, twice daily	+/-90 U/kg	i.v.	x1.5 to 2.0	+	day 7 / 2.0 to 3.0	at least 10 days; cessation if INR > 2.0	6 months
Lopaciuk et al. 1992 [33]	nadroparin, twice daily	92 U/kg	s.c.	x1.5 to 2.5	+	day 7 / 2.0 to 3.0	10 days	3 months
Simonneau et al. 1993 [34]	enoxaparin, twice daily	+/-100 U/kg	i.v.	x1.5 to 2.5	not reported	day 10 / 2.0 to 3.0	10 days	3 months
Lindmarker et al. 1994 [35]	dalteparin, once daily	200 U/kg	i.v.	x1.5 to 3.0	+	day on which venography was done / 2.0 to 3.0	at least 5 days; cessation if INR between 2.0 and 3.0 for 2 consecutive days	6 months
Luomanmäki et al. 1994	dalteparin, once daily	200 U/kg	i.v.	x1.5 to 3.0	not defined	during initial treatment/ not defined in abstract	5–10 days until therapeutic effect of OAC	§§
Levine et al. 1996 [37]	enoxaparin, twice daily	+/-100 U/kg	i.v.	60 to 85 sec	+	day 2 / 2.0 to 3.0	at least 5 days; cessation if INR was > 2.0 on two consecutive days	3 months
Koopman et al. 1996 [38]	nadroparin, twice daily	+/-100 U/kg	i.v.	x1.5 to 2.0	+	day 1 / 2.0 to 3.0	at least 5 days; cessation if INR > 2 in two measurement 24 hrs apart	6 months
Fiessinger et al. 1996 [39]	dalteparin, once daily	200 U/kg	i.v.	x1.5 to 3.0	+	day 1 or 2 / 2.0 to 3.0	5–10 days; cessation if INR between 2.0 and 3.0 on 2 consecutive days	§
Columbus Investigators 1997 [40]	reviparin, twice daily	+/-85 U/kg	i.v.	60 to 85 sec or x1.5 to 2.5	+	day 1 or 2 / 2.0 to 3.0	at least 5 days; cessation if INR > 2.0 on 2 consecutive days	12 weeks
Simonneau et al. 1997 [41]	tinziparin, once daily	175 U/kg	i.v.	x2.0 to 3.0	+	between day 1 and 3 / 2.0 to 3.0	at least 5 days; cessation if INR > 2.0 on 2 measurements 24 hrs apart	90 days

All trials: outcome assessment by investigators unaware of treatment allocation; OAC = oral anticoagulant therapy; § = no prospective follow-up; §§ = not clear whether prospective follow-up was done; * = intravenous bolus injection CY 222.

355

A. G. M. van den Belt, M. H. Prins, A. W. A. Lensing, J. Hirsh

Initial treatment of venous thromboembolism

This section summarises a systematic review, produced for the Cochrane Review Group on Peripheral Vascular Diseases, which is periodically updated and published in the Cochrane Library [11]. We have aimed to identify all randomised controlled clinical trials which compared LMWHs with UFH in the treatment of venous thromboembolism by electronic searching of Medline and Embase and by hand-searching relevant journals. In addition, studies were searched through personal communication with colleagues and pharmaceutical companies. The identified publications were reviewed independently by three reviewers (AGMB, MHP, AWAL) and assessed for inclusion based on predetermined criteria. Disagreements were resolved by consensus. The inclusion criteria were: 1) truly randomised in a way that precluded prior knowledge of the next treatment allocation (e. g. alternation would not suffice); 2) a comparison of adjusted-dose UFH versus fixed-dose subcutaneous LMWH; 3) an unconfounded comparison, such that one group differed from another only in the initial anticoagulant regimen; 4) inclusion of patients with confirmed venous thromboembolic disease (i. e., documented by venography or ultrasound in patients with suspected DVT and a perfusion ventilation lung scanning or pulmonary angiography in patients with PE) before randomisation; 5) prospective long-term follow-up to document the incidence of recurrent venous thromboembolic complications using objective diagnostic tests as well as mortality; and 6) independent assessment of suspected study outcomes by reviewers who were unaware of treatment assignment. Studies were excluded if they were duplicate reports or preliminary reports of data later presented in full, or were dose-ranging studies using other doses of LMWH than currently in use. In addition, studies which used intravenous or adjusted-dose LMWH, and those that used fixed-dose UFH were also excluded. Heparinoids were not considered for this analysis.

General information on the route of administration, the intensity of (low molecular weight) heparin and oral anticoagulant therapy, and the number of patients in the experimental treatment and control group having one of the predefined clinical outcomes were noted. Clinical outcomes were a) symptomatic recurrent venous thromboembolic complications during long-term (at least 3 months) follow-up; b) major hemorrhage during the initial treatment with (low molecular weight) heparin; and 3) death from any cause, specified for patients with and without cancer. In addition, if pre-

and post-heparin venograms were performed, the venographic outcome was classified as either improved or not improved (unchanged or deteriorated).

The following criteria were accepted for the diagnosis of recurrent DVT: a new constant intraluminal filling defect not present on the last available venogram; or if the venogram was not diagnostic, either an abnormal ^{125}I-fibrinogen leg scan, or an abnormal impedance plethysmogram or ultrasound result that had been normal before the suspected recurrent episode [12]. The following criteria were accepted for the diagnosis of PE: a segmental defect on the perfusion lung scan unmatched on the ventilation scan or chest roentgenogram, an abnormal pulmonary angiography, or a PE at autopsy. Hemorrhages were classified as major if they were intracranial, retroperitoneal, if they necessitated transfusion of packed red cells, if they led to interruption of antithrombotic treatment, or if they were fatal.

Analysis

The incidence of each of the clinical outcome measures and the changes in thrombus size between pre- and post-treatment venograms were used to calculate an odds ratio separately for each trial. These odds ratios were then combined across studies, giving due weight to the number of events in each of the two treatment groups in each separate study using the Mantel-Haenszel procedure, which assumes a fixed treatment effect [13, 14]. These analyses were performed both for the individual LMWH preparations and for all LMWH preparations combined. These analyses were performed for DVT and PE combined, as well as for PE alone. The statistical advisability of combining the trials was addressed with a test of homogeneity, which considers whether differences in treatment effect over individual trials are consistent with natural variation around a constant effect [14].

Description of studies

A total of 26 potentially eligible trials were considered for data extraction. Of these, 13 articles were excluded for the following reasons: dosage of UFH was not adjusted (n = 3) [15–17]; dose-ranging study (n = 1) [18], LMWH dosage was adjusted (n = 2) [19, 20], intravenous administration of LMWH (n = 2) [21, 22], results from patients treated for venous thrombosis of the upper limb and for PE could not be distinguished from those of patients with leg-vein thrombosis and because outcome was incompletely evaluated (n = 2) [23, 24], abstract with incomplete data which was later published in full (n = 2) [25, 26], duplicate report (n = 1) [27]. The remaining 13 studies which were included in the systematic review were published between 1988 and the end of 1997 [28–41]. Characteristics of the treatment regimens used in these trials are presented in Table 1. In all studies, patients received either LMWH or UFH for at least 5 days. The maximum length of (LMW) heparin was 10 days. Oral anticoagulation with a coumarin derivate was initiated within a range of day 1 to 10 after initiation of the (LMW) heparin. The majority of studies initiated oral anticoagulants within 24 to 48 hours of presentation. In all but one of the included studies [30], treatment allocation was not blinded due to the difference in route of administration between LMWH and UFH. All included studies compared fixed-dose, body weight adjusted, subcutaneous LMWH once [30, 35, 36, 39, 41] or twice daily [28, 29, 32–34, 37, 38, 40], with intravenous [29–32, 34–41], or subcu-

taneous [28, 33] UFH with daily dose adjustments within a specified target activated partial thromboplastin time range. Six brands of LMWH were used (nadroparin, tinzaparin, enoxaparin, reviparin, dalteparin, and CY 222). Heterogeneity was not found in any of the pooled analyses.

Recurrent venous thromboembolism

Nine studies evaluated the occurrence of symptomatic recurrent venous thromboembolism during long-term follow-up (3 to 6 months) in patients presenting with DVT or PE (Fig. 1). None of the individual trials proved statistically significant differences in the occurrence of recurrent symptomatic thromboembolic complications, nor did the analyses of the individual LMWHs. Compared with UFH, the reduction in the risk of recurrent venous thromboembolism at the end of follow-up with nadroparin, tinzaparin and enoxaparin varied from 35 to 46%. The analysis of the pooled results of all studies revealed a reduction in venous thromboembolic complications at the end of follow-up in favour of LMWH (OR 0.75; 95% CI, 0.55 to

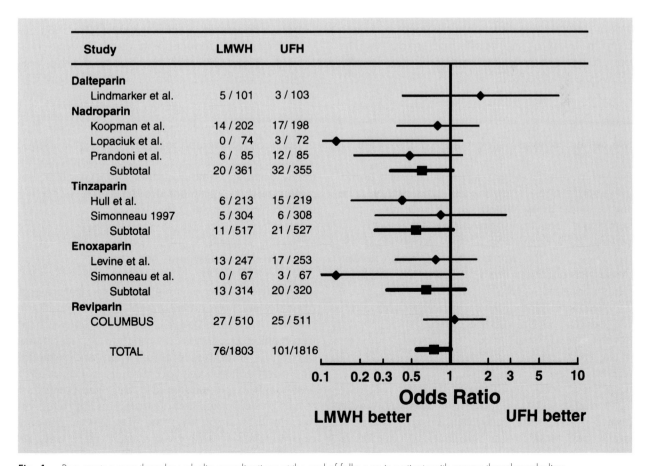

Fig. 1. Recurrent venous thromboembolic complications at the end of follow-up in patients with venous thromboembolism.

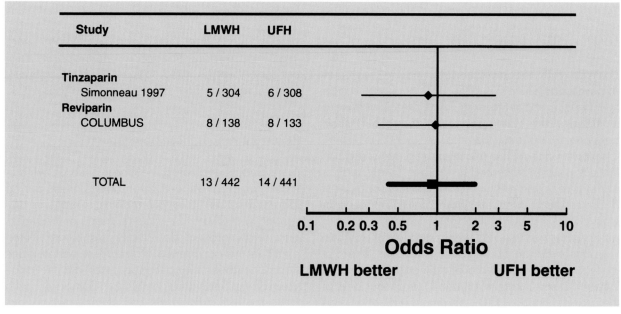

Study	LMWH	UFH
Tinzaparin		
Simonneau 1997	5 / 304	6 / 308
Reviparin		
COLUMBUS	8 / 138	8 / 133
TOTAL	13 / 442	14 / 441

Fig. 2. Recurrent venous thromboembolic complications in patients with PE.

1.01; p = 0.06). A total of 76 (4.2%) of the 1803 patients allocated to LMWH had venous thrombotic complications versus 101 (5.6%) of the 1816 patients allocated to UFH. The analysis of the individual LMWH preparations revealed a strong trend in favour of nadroparin and tinzaparin. The pooled odds ratio for the studies in patients with PE was 0.91 (95% CI, 0.42 to 1.97; p = 0.81) (Fig. 2).

Major hemorrhage during the initial treatment

All included trials evaluated the occurrence of major hemorrhage during the initial treatment. In a single study using tinzaparin [30], a statistically significant reduction in favour of LMWH was observed (OR 0.19; 95% CI, 0.06 to 0.59; p < 0.01). In the pooled results, major hemorrhage was observed in 23 (1.1%) of the 2158 patients allocated to LMWH versus 43 (2%) of the 2196 patients who received UFH (OR 0.55; 95% CI, 0.34 to 0.89; p = 0.02).

Mortality

Nine studies evaluated mortality during follow-up (Fig. 3). In a single study [30, 31], a statistically significant reduction in mortality in favour of LMWH was observed. Of the 1803 LMWH treated patients included in all studies, 94 (5.2%) died

versus 125 (6.9%) of the 1816 patients in the UFH group, for an odds ratio of 0.74 (95% CI, 0.57 to 0.98; p = 0.03). In six studies, mortality was specified for patients with and without malignant disease. In a single study [32], a statistically significant reduction in death in favour of LMWH in patients with malignant disease was found. Overall, 446 patients with malignant disease were included in these six studies. Of the 221 patients treated with LMWH, 31 (14%) died during follow-up, whereas 54 (24%) of the 225 unfractionated treated patients died (OR 0.53; 95% CI, 0.33 to 0.85; p < 0.01). Overall mortality in patients without cancer did not differ between the two treatment groups (OR 0.97; 95% CI, 0.61 to 1.56; p = 0.91).

Venographic assessment

In 7 studies, venograms were obtained before and after (LMW) heparin treatment in 1010 patients and were adjudicated by reviewers unaware of treatment allocation. A statistically significant reduction in thrombus size between pre-treatment and post-treatment venograms in favour of LMWH was found in two studies [32, 33]. The combined results of the studies demonstrated an improved venogram in 314 (62%) of the 506 LMWH patients and in 265 (53%) of the 504 UFH patients (p < 0.01).

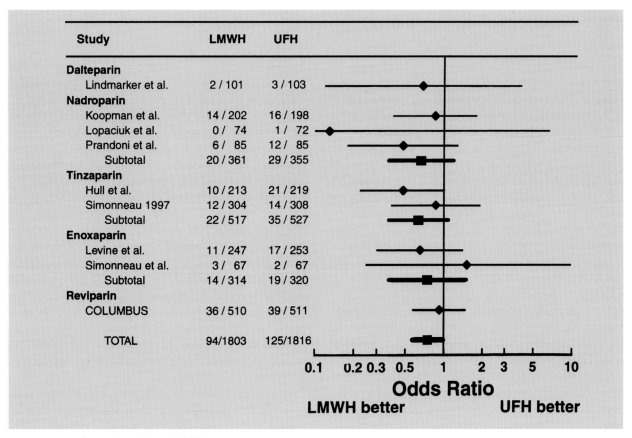

Study	LMWH	UFH
Dalteparin		
Lindmarker et al.	2 / 101	3 / 103
Nadroparin		
Koopman et al.	14 / 202	16 / 198
Lopaciuk et al.	0 / 74	1 / 72
Prandoni et al.	6 / 85	12 / 85
Subtotal	20 / 361	29 / 355
Tinzaparin		
Hull et al.	10 / 213	21 / 219
Simonneau 1997	12 / 304	14 / 308
Subtotal	22 / 517	35 / 527
Enoxaparin		
Levine et al.	11 / 247	17 / 253
Simonneau et al.	3 / 67	2 / 67
Subtotal	14 / 314	19 / 320
Reviparin		
COLUMBUS	36 / 510	39 / 511
TOTAL	94/1803	125/1816

Odds Ratio

LMWH better   UFH better

Fig. 3. Overall mortality at the end of follow-up.

The long-term risk of recurrent venous thromboembolism

A total of five studies were identified which addressed the long-term risk for recurrent venous thromboembolic events [42–46]. In a large follow-up study in 355 patients with a first episode of DVT who were treated for a period of three months [42], a cumulative incidence of recurrent venous thromboembolic complications was observed of 17.5% after two years. This incidence further increased to 25% at five years and 30% at 8 years of follow-up. The high risk for continuing venous thromboembolic complications following a first episode of DVT was consistent with the results of another study in which 454 patients with venous thromboembolism were treated with anticoagulants for a period of six months [43]. In this study, the cumulative incidence gradually increased to 9.5% at two years. Both studies demonstrated a decline in the risk of recurrence over time. Venous thromboembolic complications occurred in almost one of every four patients with a first episode of DVT after 12 years of follow-up of 58 patients [44]. In 1983, it was demonstrated that the rate of venous thromboembolic complications among 89 patients with recurrent DVT who were treated for three months was approximately 20% after an average follow-up of 20 months [45]. In a recent study, subsequent venous thromboembolic complications in 111 patients with recurrent venous thromboembolism, who were treated for six months, occurred in 21% during 4 years of follow-up [46]. From these studies and others [47, 48], four groups of patients can be identified who have a particularly poor prognosis for recurrent venous thromboembolism: those with idiopathic venous thromboembolism, those who are carriers of genetic mutations that predispose to venous thromboembolism such as antithrombin, protein C or S deficiency and the factor V Arg^{506}_Gln mutation [47], those with cancer [48], and those patients with anticardiolipin antibodies [49]. The prognosis is considerably better in patients who develop their first episode of venous thrombosis after surgery and who do not have continuing risk factors for recurrent venous thromboembolism [42].

Duration of anticoagulant therapy for deep vein thrombosis

Three clinical trials have been completed recently and have provided challenging information on the optimal duration of treatment for patients with a first episode of proximal DVT. Anticoagulant treatment regimens, which were compared, were 4 weeks versus 3 months in patients with DVT or PE [50], and 6 weeks versus 6 months [43] in patients with a first episode of venous thromboembolism. Another study in patients with a first episode of DVT used impedance plethysmography for the decision to discontinue treatment [51]. All patients with an abnormal IPG at 4 weeks were treated for 3 months, whereas patients with a normal IPG were randomised to continued treatment (3 months) or no treatment.

In the first study [49], recurrent venous thromboembolism during 1 year follow-up occurred in 14 (4%) of the 354 patients treated for 3 months as compared with 28 (7.8%) of the 358 patients treated for 4 weeks only (p < 0.04). In both treatment arms, recurrent venous thromboembolism occurred infrequently in patients with a postoperative thrombotic event. A similar statistically significant reduction in venous thromboembolic complications was found during 2 years of follow-up in a study comparing 6 weeks with 6 months of anticoagulant therapy [43]. Of the 443 patients allocated to the short-term treatment group, 80 (18.1%) developed a thrombotic complication compared with 43 (9.5%) of the 454 patients allocated to the long-term treatment group. In the third follow-up study [51], IPG at four weeks was used to direct the duration of treatment of patients with a first episode of DVT. All 192 patients with a persistently abnormal IPG were treated for 3 months and recurrent venous thromboembolism within a

period of one year occurred in 19 (9.9%). Of the 214 patients with a normalised IPG at four weeks, 105 were allocated to placebo and 109 were allocated to continue oral anticoagulants for another two months. During the 8 weeks following randomisation, 9 (8.6%) patients allocated to placebo and 1 (0.9%) of the oral anticoagulant treated patients developed a thrombotic complication, for a statistically significant difference (p < 0.01). At the end of the 11 months follow-up period, 12 (11.5%) of the 104 patients allocated to placebo and 7 (6.8%) of the 103 oral anticoagulant treated patients developed a thrombotic complication (not statistically significant). Of all 301 patients who received 3 months of oral anticoagulants (in the randomised trial or in the cohort study) 26 patients developed a venous thromboembolic complication. Interestingly, all these complications occurred in those patients with continuing risk factors for venous thrombosis.

The optimal duration of anticoagulant therapy was investigated in patients with a second episode of venous thrombosis [46]. Of the 227 patients, 111 were allocated to 6 months of anticoagulant treatment, and 116 were allocated to receive indefinite treatment. During 4 years of follow-up, recurrent venous thromboembolism occurred in 21% of the patients in the 6-month group versus 3% of the patients in the indefinite treatment group, for a statistically significant difference. Major hemorrhage occurred in 3 (2.7%) of the 111 patients in the 6-months group versus 10 (8.6%) of the 116 patients of the indefinite treatment group. Two of the bleeding episodes in the indefinite group were fatal.

Conclusion and treatment recommendations

Initial treatment

The systematic review on the therapeutic use of LMWH is based on a pooling of data from studies that have a high methodological quality and clinical similarity. Over 4,000 patients with a first venous thromboembolic event were included. This pooled analysis demonstrated that fixed-dose, body weight adjusted subcutaneous LMWHs are at least as effective as intravenous adjusted-dose UFH for the initial treatment of DVT and PE. Further-

more, the pooled analysis demonstrated a statistically significant reduction in the occurrence of clinically important hemorrhagic complications in favour of LMWH. An interesting finding was the statistically significant reduction in mortality with LMWH treatment, which was almost entirely due to an important imbalance in cancer deaths.

The use of LMWHs has multiple advantages as compared with UFH for the treatment of venous thromboembolic disease. The predictable pharmacokinetics of LMWHs do not only in theory obviate the need for laboratory monitoring and dose adjustments but indeed led in practice to favourable results without such monitoring. As a result of the specific features of LMWHs, these compounds are attractive to use in an out-of-hospital setting for the treatment of DVT. Comparable efficacy and safety profiles were found for outpatient treatment with LMWH and UFH treatment in hospital in two studies in patients with DVT [37, 38]. Both studies showed that out-of-hospital treatment was feasible for the majority of patients allocated to LMWH for a reduction in total hospital days of approximately 70 percent. Outpatient management was associated with a substantial cost reduction compared to inpatient treatment with UFH [52].

Compared to UFH treatment, equivalent efficacy and no relevant clinical differences in safety outcomes was demonstrated for the individual LMWHs enoxaparin, nadroparin, reviparin and tinzaparin. The majority of the patients included in the review had a DVT. Therefore, we conclude that the use of the aforementioned LMWHs is justified for the treatment of DVT. Further evaluation of dalteparin is desirable because a clinically relevant benefit in favour of UFH can not be excluded.

The comparison of LMWH (reviparin and tinzaparin) with UFH in patients with PE demonstrated equivalence regarding efficacy and safety. To further define the relative efficacy and safety of LMWHs and UFH in this specific subgroup of patients, it would be desirable to perform more clinical trials. Patients with PE and refractory hypotension do not qualify for LMWH treatment. In these patients thrombolysis is the regimen of choice.

All future LMWHs should be evaluated carefully before being introduced for the treatment of venous thromboembolism.

Long-term treatment

Patients with an episode of venous thromboembolism are usually treated with oral anticoagulants for a period of three months. Shorter courses of treatment have been associated with a statistically sig-

nificant and clinically important increase in the frequency of thromboembolic complications. Furthermore, a high recurrence rate was observed in long-term follow-up studies where patients received anticoagulant therapy for 3 months and in patients treated with oral anticoagulants for 6 weeks during the period between 6 weeks and 6 months following the first thrombotic episode. A trend towards a lower incidence of recurrent venous thromboembolism in patients with postoperative venous thrombosis and with reversible risk factors was reported in several studies.

Based on these results, it seems to be justified to recommend a treatment course of 6 months for patients with a first proximal DVT or PE without a reversible risk factor. For patients with specific conditions such as malignant disease or an inherited coagulation disorder, an even longer period might be indicated. However, supportive data are not yet available. Until unambiguous data is available on the incidence of recurrent thrombosis for patients with a postoperative venous thrombosis and a reversible risk factor, we recommend oral anticoagulant treatment for a period of 3 months for these patients. Because of the differences observed between subgroups of patients, new studies comparing different extended courses of anticoagulants should focus on the assessment of subgroup specific, long-term incidences of recurrent venous thromboembolism and on major hemorrhage.

In patients with a second episode of venous thromboembolism, treatment should probably be continued for at least 1 year, because cessation of therapy at 3 to 6 months is associated with a subsequent high rate of recurrent venous thromboembolic complications. Indefinite treatment may be indicated in patients with several recurrent thrombotic episodes. At present, long-term anticoagulant therapy remains a clinical judgement in the individual patient.

References

1. Huisman MV, Büller HR, Ten Cate JW, Van Royen EA, Vreeken J, Kersten MJ, Bakx R. Unexpected high prevalence of silent pulmonary embolism in patients with deep venous thrombosis. Chest 1989; 95: 498–502

2. Hull RD, Hirsh J, Carter CJ, Jay RM, Dodd PE, Ockelford PA, Coates G, Gill GJ, Turpie AG, Doyle DJ, Büller HR, Raskob GE. Pulmonary angiography, ventilation lung scanning, and venography for clinically suspected pulmonary embolism with abnormal perfusion lung scan. Ann Intern Med 1983; 98: 891–899

3. Hirsh J. Heparin. N Engl J Med 1991; 324: 1565–1574

4. Brandjes DPM, Heijboer H, Büller HR, De Rijk M, Jagt H, Ten Cate JW. Acenocoumarol and heparin compared with acenocoumarol alone in the initial treatment of proximal–vein thrombosis. N Engl J Med 1992; 327: 1485–1489

5. Hommes DW, Bura A, Mazzolai L, Büller HR, Ten Cate JW. Subcutaneous heparin compared with continuous intravenous heparin administration in the initial treatment of deep vein thrombosis. A meta-analysis. Ann Intern Med 1992; 116: 279–284

6. Basu D, Gallus A, Hirsh J, Cade J. A prospective study of the value of monitoring heparin treatment with the activated partial thromboplastin time. New Engl J Med 1972; 287: 325–327

7. Young E, Prins MH, Levine MN, Hirsh J. Heparin binding to plasma proteins. An important mechanism for heparin resistance. Thromb Haemostas 1992; 67: 639–643

8. Hirsh J. From unfractionated heparins to low molecular weight heparins. Acta Chir Scand. 1990; 556 (Suppl): 42–50

9. Hirsh J, Levine MN. Low molecular weight heparin. Blood 1992; 79: 1–17

10. Nurmohamed MT, Rosendaal FR, Büller HR, Dekker E, Hommes DW, Vandenbroucke JP, Briët E. Low-molecular-weight heparin versus standard heparin in general and orthopaedic surgery: a meta-analysis. Lancet 1992; 340: 152–156

11. Van den Belt AGM, Prins MH, Lensing AWA, Castro AA, et al. Fixed dose subcutaneous low molecular weight heparins versus adjusted dose unfractionated heparin in the treatment of venous thromboembolism. The Cochrane Library 1998

12. Büller HR, Lensing AWA, Hirsh J, Ten Cate JW. Deep venous thrombosis: new noninvasive tests. Thromb Haemostas 1991; 66: 133–139

13. Mantel N, Haenszel W. Statistical aspects of the analysis of data from retrospective studies of disease. J Nat Cancer Inst 1959; 22: 719–748

14. Collins R, Gray R, Godwin J, Peto R. Avoidance of large biases and large random errors in the assessment of moderate treatment effects: the need for systematic overviews. Stat Med 1987; 6: 245–250

15. Notarbartolo A, Salanitri G, Davi G, Averna M, Barbagallo C, Catalano I. Low molecular weight heparin in the short and long-term treatment of deep vein thrombosis in diabetic subjects. Med Prax 1988; 9: 393–405

16. Zanghi M, Morici V, Costanzo M, Astuto L, Salanitri G. Deep vein thrombosis of the legs: new therapy by means of low molecular weight heparins. J Intern Med Res 1988; 16: 474–484

17. Tedoldi A, Botticella F, Maloberti MR. Antithrombophilic effect of low molecular weight heparins in patients with deep vein thrombosis. Clin Trials Meta-analysis 1993; 28: 215–225

18. Handeland GF, Abildgaard U, Holm HA, Arnesen KE. Dose adjusted heparin treatment of deep venous thrombosis: a comparison of unfractionated and low molecular weight heparin. Eur J Clin Pharmacol 1990; 39: 107–112

19. Bratt G, Aberg W, Johansson M, Tornebohm E, Granqvist S, Lockner D. Two daily subcutaneous injections of Fragmin as compared with intravenous standard heparin in the treatment of deep venous thrombosis. Thromb Haemost 1990; 64: 506–510

20. Holm HA, Ly B, Handeland GF, et al. Subcutaneous heparin treatment of deep vein thrombosis: a comparison of unfractionated and low molecular weight heparin. Haemostasis 1986; 16 (Suppl): 30–37

21. Bratt G, Tornebohm E, Granqvist S, Aberg W, Lockner D. A comparison between low molecular weight heparin Kabi 2165 and standard heparin in the intravenous treatment of deep vein thrombosis. Thromb Haemost 1985; 85: 813

22. Vogel G, Machulik M. Efficacy and safety of a low molecular weight heparin (LMW-heparin Sandoz) in patients with deep vein thrombosis. Thromb Haemost 1987; 58 (Suppl): 427

23. Albada J, Nieuwenhuis HK, Sixma JJ. Treatment of acute venous thromboembolism with low molecular weight heparin (Fragmin). Circulation 1989; 80: 935–940

24. Harenberg J, Huck K, Bratsch H, et al. Therapeutic application of subcutaneous low-molecular-weight heparin in acute venous thrombosis. Haemostasis 1990; 20: 205–219

25. Fiessinger JN, Fernandez ML, Gatterer E, Ohlsson CG. Fragmin once daily versus continuous infusion heparin in the treatment of DVT: a European multicentre trial. Haemostasis 1994; 24 (Suppl 1): 44

26. Faivre R, Neuhart E, Kieffer Y, Toulemonde F, Bassand JP, Maurat JP. Subcutaneous administration of a low molecular weight heparin (CY 222) compared with subcutaneous administration of standard heparin in patients with acute deep vein thrombosis. Thromb Haemost 1987; 58 (Suppl): 120

27. Lockner D, Bratt G, Tornebohm E, Aberg W, Granqvist S. Intravenous and subcutaneous administration of Fragmin in deep venous thrombosis. Haemostasis 1986; 16 (Suppl): 25–29

28. Faivre R, Neuhart Y, Kieffer Y, Apfel F, Magnin D, Didier D, Toulemonde F, Bassand JP, Maurat JP. Un nouveau traitement des thromboses veineuses profondes: les fractions d'héparine de bas poids moléculaire. Etude randomisée. Presse Méd 1988; 17: 197–200

29. Duroux P. A Collaborative European Multicentre Study: a randomized trial of subcutaneous low molecular weight heparin (CY216) compared with intravenous unfractionated heparin in the treatment of deep vein thrombosis. Thromb Haemost 1991; 65: 251–256

30. Hull RD, Raskob GE, Pineo GF, et al. Subcutaneous low-molecular-weight heparin compared with continuous intravenous heparin in the treatment of proximal-vein thrombosis. N Engl J Med 1992; 326: 975–982

31. Green D, Hull RD, Brant R, Pineo GF. Lower mortality in cancer patients treated with low-molecular-weight versus standard heparin. Lancet 1992; 339: 1476

32. Prandoni P, Lensing AWA, Büller HR, et al. Comparison of subcutaneous low-molecular-weight heparin with intravenous standard heparin in proximal deep-vein thrombosis. Lancet 1992; 339: 441–445

33. Lopaciuk S, Meissner AJ, Filipecki S, et al. Subcutaneous low molecular weight heparin versus subcutaneous unfractionated heparin in the treatment of deep vein thrombosis: a Polish multicenter trial. Thromb Haemost 1992; 68: 14–18

34. Simonneau G, Charbonnier B, Decousus H, et al. Subcutaneous low molecular weight heparin compared with continuous intravenous unfractionated heparin in the initial treatment of proximal vein thrombosis. Arch Intern Med 1993; 153: 1541–1546

35. Lindmarker P, Holmström M, Granqvist S, Johnsson H, Lockner D. Comparison of once-daily subcutaneous Fragmin with continuous intravenous unfractionated heparin in the treatment of deep venous thrombosis. Thromb Haemost 1994; 72: 186–190

36. Luomanmäki K and the Finnish multicentre group. Low molecular weight heparin (Fragmin) once daily vs continuous infusion of standard heparin in the treatment of DVT. Haemostasis 1994; 24 (Suppl. 1): 248

37. Levine M, Gent M, Hirsh J, et al. A comparison of low-molecular-weight heparin administered primarily at home with unfractionated heparin administered in the hospital for proximal deep-vein thrombosis. N Engl J Med 1996; 334: 677–681

38. Koopman MMW, et al. Treatment of venous thrombosis with intravenous unfractionated heparin administered in the hospital as compared with subcutaneous low-molecular-weight heparin administered at home. N Engl J Med 1996; 334: 682–687

39. Fiessinger JN, Lopez-Fernandez M, Gatterer E, et al. Once-daily Subcutaneous Dalteparin, a Low Molecular Weight Heparin, for the Initial Treatment of Acute Deep Vein Thrombosis. Thromb Haemost 1996; 76: 195–199

40. Anonymous. Low-molecular-weight heparin in the treatment of patients with venous thromboembolism. The Columbus Investigators. N Engl J Med 1997; 337: 657–662

41. Simonneau G, Sors H, Charbonnier B, Page Y, Laaban J-P, Azarian R, Laurent M, Hirsch J-J, Ferrari E, Bosson J-L, Mottier D, Beau B. A comparison of low-molecular-weight heparin with unfractionated heparin for acute pulmonary embolism. N Engl J Med 1997; 337: 663–669

42. Prandoni P, Lensing AWA, Cogo A, et al. The long-term clinical course of acute deep venous thrombosis. Ann Intern Med 1996; 125: 1–7

43. Schulman S, Rhedin A-S, Lindmarker P, et al, and the Duration of Anticoagulation Trial Study Group. A comparison of six weeks with six months of oral anticoagulant therapy after a first episode of venous thromboembolism. N Engl J Med 1995; 332: 1661–1665

44. Franzeck UK, Schalch I, Jager KA, et al. Prospective 12-year follow-up study of clinical and hemodynamic sequelae after deep vein thrombosis in low risk patients. Circulation 1996; 93: 74–79

45. Hull RD, Carter CJ, Jay RM, et al. The diagnosis of acute, recurrent, deep-vein thrombosis: a diagnostic challenge. Circulation 1983; 67: 901–906

46. Schulman S, Granqvist S, Holmstrom M, et al. The duration of oral anticoagulant therapy after a second episode of venous thromboembolism. N Engl J Med 1997; 336: 393–398

47. Prandoni P, Lensing AWA, Buller HR, et al. Deep-vein thrombosis and the incidence of subsequent symptomatic cancer. N Engl J Med 1992; 327: 1128–1133

48. Simioni P, Prandoni P, Lensing AWA, et al. The risk of recurrent venous thromboembolism in patients with an Arg506_Gln mutation in the gene for factor V. N Engl J Med 1997; 336: 339–403

49. Schulman S, Svenungsson E, Granqvist S, and the Duration of Anticoagulation Study Group. Anticardiolipin antibodies predict early recurrence of thromboembolism and death among patients with venous thromboembolism following anticoagulant therapy. Am J Med 1998; 104: 332–338

50. Research Committee of the British Thoracic Society. Optimum duration of anticoagulation for deep-vein thrombosis and pulmonary embolism. Lancet 1992; 340: 873–876

51. Levine MN, Hirsh J, Gent M, et al. Optimal duration of oral anticoagulant therapy: A randomized trial comparing four weeks with three months of warfarin in patients with proximal deep vein thrombosis. Thromb Haemost 1995; 74: 606–611

52. Van den Belt AGM, Bossuyt PMM, Prins MH, Gallus AS, Büller HR. Replacing inpatient care by outpatient care in the treatment of deep venous thrombosis. An economic evaluation. Thromb Haemost 1998; 79: 259–263

VI.2 Thrombolysis for treatment of venous thromboembolism

G. Agnelli, S. Z. Goldhaber

The fibrinolytic system

The basic reaction of the fibrinolytic system is the conversion of the inactive proenzyme plasminogen to plasmin, an enzyme able to degrade fibrin into soluble fibrin degradation products. Two immunologically distinct physiological plasminogen activators (PAs) have been identified: the tissue-type PA (t-PA) and the urokinase-type PA (u-PA) [1]. The t-PA is responsible for the dissolution of fibrin in the circulation. Inhibition of the fibrinolytic system may occur either at the level of the PAs, by specific plasminogen activator inhibitors (PAIs), or at the level of plasmin, mainly by α2-antiplasmin. Physiological fibrinolysis is regulated by specific molecular interactions between its main components as well as by controlled synthesis and release of PAs, mainly t-PA, and PAIs from endothelial cells.

Structure of the main components of the fibrinolytic system

Plasminogen
Human plasminogen is a single-chain glycoprotein with Mr of 92,000; present in plasma at a concentration of 1.5 to 2 µm. It consists of 791 amino acids and contains 5 homologous triple-loop structures or "kringles" [2]. These kringles contain structures, called lysine binding sites and aminohexyl binding sites that mediate the specific binding of plasminogen to fibrin and the interaction of plasmin with by α2-antiplasmin [3]. Plasminogen is converted to plasmin by cleavage of the Arg56-Val562 peptide bond [4]. The plasmin molecule is a two-chain trypsin-like serine proteinase with an active site composed of His603, Asp646, and Ser741 [2, 4].

Tissue-type plasminogen activator (t-PA) and urokinase-type plasminogen activator (u-PA)
Human t-PA was first isolated as a single-chain serine proteinase with Mr about 70,000, consisting of 527 amino acids with Ser as the NH2-terminal amino acid. Following cleavage of the Arg278-Ile279 bond by serine proteases, particularly plasmin, single-chain t-PA is converted to a molecular form consisting of two polypeptide chains (tct-PA, two-chain tissue plasminogen activator) linked by a single disulphide bridge. The plasma concentration of t-PA antigen is about 5 ng/ml, whereas the concentration of free t-PA is probably less than 1 ng/ml, the remaining circulating bound to PAIs. The t-PA molecule contains four domains: 1) a NH2-terminal region of 47-residues (residues 4 to 50) (F-domain), homologous with the finger domain of fibronectin, which is responsible for the affinity of t-PA for fibrin; 2) residues 50 to 87 (E-domain) which are homologous with epidermal growth factor; 3) two regions comprising residues 87 to 176 and 176 to 262 (K1 and K2 domains) which share a high degree of homology with the five kringles of plasminogen; and 4) a serine proteinase domain (P, residues 276 to 527) with the active site residues His322, Asp371 and Ser478 [5]. The t-PA molecule comprises three potential N-glycosylation sites, at Asn117 (K1), Asn184 (K2) and Asn448 (P). t-PA preparations usually contain a mixture of variant I (with all three glycosylation sites) and variant II (lacking carbohydrate at Asn184) [5]. In contrast to the single-chain precursor form of most serine proteinases, single-chain t-PA is enzymatically active. The structure of t-PA is similar to that of u-PA. The only major difference is the presence in t-PA of the region similar to one of the nine regions of fibronectin, which is responsible for the affinity of t-PA for fibrin.

α2-Antiplasmin and PAIs

α2-antiplasmin is the main physiological plasmin inhibitor in human plasma, whereas plasmin formed in excess of α2-antiplasmin may be neutralised by α2-macroglobulin. α2-antiplasmin, a Mr 67,000 single-chain glycoprotein containing 464 amino acids and 13% carbohydrate, is present in plasma at a concentration of about 1 μm.

Rapid inhibition of both t-PA and u-PA in normal human plasma occurs primarily by plasminogen activator inhibitor-1 (PAI-1) [6]. In healthy individuals, highly variable plasma levels of both PAI activity and PAI-1 antigen have been observed. PAI activity ranges from 0.5 to 47 U/ml (t-PA neutralising units, 1 mg active PAI-1 corresponding to 700,000 units) with 80 percent of the values below 6 U/ml. PAI-1 antigen ranges between 6 and 85 ng/ml. PAI-1 is a single-chain glycoprotein with Mr about 52,000 consisting of 379 amino acids. Plasminogen activator inhibitor-2 (PAI-2) was first extracted from human placenta but it was later also found in leukocytes, monocytes and macrophages. PAI-2 levels in plasma are low, but are elevated during pregnancy [7]. The role of intracellular PAI-2 is unclear because its main target enzyme (u-PA) occurs extracellularly. The specific (patho)physiological role of PAI-2 remains to be determined.

Mechanisms involved in regulation of the fibrinolytic system

Fibrinolysis is mainly regulated as a result of increased or decreased synthesis and/or secretion of t-PA and of PAI-1, primarily from the vessel wall. Vascular endothelial cells synthesise and secrete t-PA in the circulating blood [8]. Stimulation of vascular endothelium by venous occlusion, infusion of a number of agents and physical exercise results in a rapid release of t-PA. This response is too rapid to represent increased synthesis and may reflect release from a cellular storage pool, although such a storage pool has not been conclusively identified. PAI-1 mRNA has been demonstrated in a large variety of tissues, suggesting that common cells in these tissues, such as endothelial or smooth muscle cells, may be the sites of production [9]. For unknown reasons PAI-1 exhibits a circadian variation; its plasma concentration is highest in the morning and lowest in the late afternoon and evening, whereas t-PA exhibits an opposite diurnal variation.

Inhibition of fibrinolysis occurs at the level of plasminogen activation or at the level of plasmin. α2-antiplasmin forms an inactive 1:1 stoichiometric complex with plasmin. The inhibition of plasmin by α2-antiplasmin can be represented by two consecutive reactions: a fast, second order reaction producing a reversible inactive complex, which is followed by a slower first-order transition resulting in an irreversible complex. The half-life of plasmin molecules on the fibrin surface, which have both their lysine binding sites and active site occupied, is estimated to be 2 to 3 orders of magnitude longer than that of free plasmin [10]. PAI-1 reacts very rapidly with single-chain and two-chain t-PA and with two-chain u-PA, with second-order inhibition rate constants of the order of 10^7 M^{-1}.s^{-1} and it does not react with scu-PA [11].

Activation of plasminogen by t-PA is enhanced in the presence of fibrin or at the endothelial cell surface. t-PA is a poor enzyme in the absence of fibrin, but the presence of fibrin strikingly enhances the activation rate of plasminogen [12]. Plasmin formed at the fibrin surface has both its lysine binding sites and active site occupied and is thus only slowly inactivated by α2-antiplasmin (half-life of about 10–100 s); in contrast, free plasmin, when formed, is rapidly inhibited by α2-antiplasmin (half-life of about 0.1 s) [10]. During fibrinolysis, fibrinogen and fibrin itself are continuously modified due to cleavage by thrombin or plasmin, yielding a number of reaction products [13]. Thrombin-catalysed formation of desA-fibrin monomer, and a certain degree of desA-fibrin polymerisation are essential for stimulation of plasminogen activation by t-PA. Kinetic data support a mechanism in which fibrin provides a surface to which t-PA and plasminogen adsorb in a sequential and ordered way yielding a cyclic ternary complex [12]. Formation of this complex results in an enhanced affinity of t-PA for plasminogen, yielding up to three orders of magnitude higher efficiencies for plasminogen activation. In agreement with this mechanism, the increase in fibrin stimulation after formation of fibrin X-polymers is associated with an enhanced binding of t-PA and plasminogen. During fibrin clot lysis, single-chain t-PA is converted to two-chain t-PA at the fibrin surface. This conversion is probably of little physiological relevance, since the activity of single-chain t-PA and two-chain t-PA is enhanced to the same extent in the presence of fibrin or fragment X-polymer [14].

Clinical pharmacology of thrombolytic agents

Table 1. Thrombolytic agents.

First generation
Streptokinase
Urokinase (double-chain u-PA)

Second generation
Tissue-type plasminogen activator (t-PA)
Pro-urokinase (single chain u-PA)
Acylated derivatives of the SK-plasminogen activator complex (APSAC)

Third generation
t-PA mutants
Chimeric plasminogen activators
Complexes of plasminogen activators + fibrin-specific monoclonal antibodies
Complexes of plasminogen activators derivatives of Desmodus Rotundus
Recombinant staphylokinase

The pharmacological agents that convert plasminogen to plasmin are known as plasminogen activators. Whatever their mechanism of action, they are able to cleave the Arg560-Val561 bond in the plasminogen molecule to give plasmin. Plasminogen activation is controlled at various levels by inhibitors that prevent massive activation of the fibrinolytic system, which could possibly lead to the degradation of clotting factors sensitive to the proteolytic action of plasmin.

The proteases involved in the activation of plasminogen are serine proteases characterised by the presence of the amino acid serine at the catalytic site. All these enzymes consist of two chains linked by one or more disulphide bridges. The amino-terminal chain, known as the A-chain, gives the enzyme affinity for a given substrate [15]. Proteases that have a rudimentary A-chain, such as trypsin, are able to break down a large number of substrates whereas the enzymes, which have a more developed A-chain, have high specificity for a given substrate. The B-chain carries the active site and is made up of about 250 amino acids without any marked differences between the various serine proteases. Although plasmin has a higher specificity for fibrin than other proteases, it can however break down other substrates of the clotting system. Degradation of some of these substances, such as fibrinogen, factor V, and factor VIII, has a negative effect on the clotting system, thus giving rise to a condition which favours bleeding.

Thrombolytic agents can be classified as first, second and third generation thrombolytic drugs (Table 1). The first generation includes streptokinase (SK) and urokinase (UK). The second generation agents include t-PA, pro-urokinase and the acylated-plasminogen-SK complex (APSAC). The third generation agents include a number of newly developed compounds; among these, reteplase, lanoteplase and TNK-tPA are the most extensively evaluated.

First generation thrombolytic agents

Streptokinase

Streptokinase (SK) was the first thrombolytic agent to be extensively evaluated in patients [16]. SK is a protein of bacterial origin prepared by purification of filtrates of cultures of certain strains of group A β-hemolytic streptococci. SK consists of a single polypeptide chain of 415 amino acids and has a molecular weight of 47,400. Unlike the other thrombolytic agents, SK is not a direct plasminogen activator but activates the fibrinolytic system by a unique mechanism: one molecule of SK combines with one molecule of plasminogen to form an SK-plasminogen complex (activator complex). It is this complex that is the true plasminogen activator. Plasmin in the SK-plasmin complex is not rapidly neutralised by α2-antiplasmin. This accounts for the hyperplasminemia observed during treatment with SK and the consequent breakdown of fibrinogen and the other clotting factors.

The elimination of SK from the circulation is biphasic with an initial half-life of 4 minutes and a terminal half-life of 30 minutes. The level of antistreptococcal antibodies influences clearance. About 350,000 IU of SK are needed to neutralise the circulating antibodies in 95 % of healthy subjects. In some cases up to 3,000,000 units may be required. A few days after treatment with SK, the level of anti-SK antibodies rises by a factor of 50 – 100 and remains raised for 4 to 6 months. The mechanisms responsible for the clearance of the SK-plasminogen complex are not fully understood.

The standard initial dose of streptokinase adopted in the treatment of deep vein thrombosis (DVT) and pulmonary embolism (PE) varies from 250,000 to 750,000 IU over 10 – 30 minutes followed by an infusion of 100,000 IU/h for one or more days. In recent years, a high dose of 1,500,000 IU infused over 60 minutes has formed the basis for the use of the thrombolytic agents in the treatment of acute myocardial infarction [17]. Several attempts have been made to reduce the duration of streptokinase infusion (30 minutes) or to increase the dose. The results obtained are not sufficiently convincing to bring out a change in the therapeutic regime currently used. As for all thrombolytic drugs, the most serious side-effect of streptokinase is bleeding. In contrast to the 'physiological' activators of fibrinolysis, such as t-PA and urokinase, streptokinase exhibits an increased incidence of allergic reactions, which are found in around 4% of patients. The incidence of anaphylactic shock is 4%. Hypotension, even marked hypotension, is common. Due to the antigenicity of SK, repeated treatment with this agent should be avoided.

Urokinase

Urokinase is a serine protease that was first identified in human urine [18] and purified for therapeutic purposes, from the urine itself or from kidney cell cultures.

The native form of single-chain urokinase (scu-PA) is converted by plasmin or kallikrein into high molecular weight double-chain urokinase (HMW-urokinase) which has a molecular weight of 54,000. In addition to HMW-urokinase, urokinase can also be obtained as a double-chain with a molecular weight of 34,000 (low molecular weight double-chain urokinase, LMW-urokinase). LMW-urokinase has a greater specific activity (200,000 IU/ mg compared with 120,000 IU/mg for HMW-urokinase). In equimolar concentrations the two forms have almost the same activity.

Urokinase has a few advantages over SK. The most important of these is that urokinase is not antigenic and, therefore, is free from the risk of allergic-type side-effects seen with SK; its lack of antigenicity allows the treatment to be repeated at short intervals. In addition, because it is a direct activator of plasminogen, the fibrino(geno)lytic effect is proportional to the dose administered.

The plasma kinetics of urokinase is bi-exponential with an identical initial phase (t 1/2 about 4 minutes) for both forms, and a terminal half-life which is shorter for the HMW form [19]. Urokinase is metabolised in the liver and excreted as an inactive form in the urine.

The conventional dosage of urokinase is 4,000 IU/Kg over 10 minutes followed by infusion of 4,000 IU/Kg/h for 12–24 hours. This is the dosage used for the treatment of PE. A more recent therapeutic regimen involves administration of 3,000,000 units over 2 h, or 1,000,000 units in the first 10 minutes followed by 2,000,000 units in 110 minutes. In myocardial infarction urokinase is most frequently given as a bolus injection

of 2,000,000 units or by infusion of 3,000,000 units over 90 minutes.

Second generation thrombolytic agents

This group of thrombolytic agents includes rt-PA, single-chain urokinase (also known as pro-urokinase or scu-PA), and the acylated derivatives of the SK-plasminogen complex or APSAC. The interest for the second generation thrombolytic agents is due to the theoretical possibility of achieving selective thrombolysis with these compounds. Initial studies with the second generation thrombolytics in man showed that the fibrin-specificity of these agents is not absolute but is closely related to the dose and the method of administration. Effective therapeutic doses cause a varying degree of fibrinogenolysis, although less extensive than that observed with SK. In addition, it should be stressed that prevention or limitation of systemic proteolysis does not necessarily result in a lower incidence of hemorrhagic complications as these are multifactorial and not exclusively due to systemic proteolysis.

Recombinant tissue plasminogen activator (rt-PA)

The structural and physico-chemical features of recombinant tissue plasminogen activator are similar to those of native t-PA and have already been described. t-PA was originally isolated from uterine tissue and melanoma cell cultures. In the early eighties the gene that controls the synthesis of t-PA was cloned and expressed in eukaryotic cells with the production of large amounts of recombinant t-PA (rt-PA) [5]. rt-PA has antigenic characteristics and biochemical and enzymatic properties similar to those of native t-PA.

Many mechanisms are involved in the removal of rt-PA from the circulation and not all are fully understood. Metabolism in the liver is the main mechanism for rt-PA clearance. Bi-exponential kinetics has been observed after infusion of rt-PA in human subjects [20]; the initial half-life is 4 minutes and the terminal half-life 46 minutes. The rapid clearance takes place almost exclusively by the hepatic route after uptake of rt-PA at the level of structures contained in the heavy chain. The biological activity of rt-PA on the thrombi appears to be longer than its half-life in the circulation. It has been shown that the administration of rt-PA to rabbits with experimental jugular thrombosis produced a thrombolytic effect lasting over 2 h, despite the fact that after 30 minutes measurable quantities of activator are no longer present in the circulation [21].

The original recommended dose of rt-PA for the treatment of acute myocardial infarction was 100 mg over 3 h: 60 mg in the first hour, of which 10 mg given as a bolus in the first 2 minutes, followed by 20 mg in the second and the third hours. More recently, a so-called 'front-loaded' treatment has been proposed, consisting of a 15 mg bolus injection, followed by 50 mg in the first 30 minutes and another 35 mg in the next 60 minutes. For the thrombolytic treatment of acute peripheral occlusion, the recommended dosage ranges from 0.05 to 0.10 mg/Kg/h given over a period of 8 hours. Recently, preliminary clinical studies have been conducted on the use of rt-PA given as a single bolus (50–70 mg) or as a 50 mg double bolus given 30 minutes apart.

Pro-urokinase

As already mentioned, the most striking structural difference between rt-PA and scu-PA concerns the A-chain which in the rt-PA molecule contains 120 additional amino. In purified system scu-PA acts like a true enzyme and is able to activate plasminogen directly. The weak activity of scu-PA in plasma has been explained by postulating the existence of a competitive inhibitor that forms an inactive but reversible complex with scu-PA. Addition of fibrin or fibrinogen degradation fragments to plasma would cause dissociation of the complex, thus unblocking the enzyme. This theory has the advantage of explaining the fibrin-specificity of scu-PA in the absence of any affinity for fibrin itself.

Acylated fibrinolytic enzymes

The agent APSAC (anistreplase) is a non-covalent equimolecular complex of human Lys-plasminogen and SK. The catalytic centre is situated in the carboxy-terminal region of the plasminogen, but the lysine binding site is situated in the amino-terminal region. Acylation of the catalytic centre is achieved by using a reversible acylated substance, p-amidinophenyl-p'-anisateHCl. SK dissociates from the plasminogen SK complex at a rate that is lower than the rate of deacylation of the complex, and therefore the activity of anistreplase is controlled by its deacylation. Anistreplase has a deacylation half-life in plasma of 105–120 minutes. In healthy volunteers anistreplase has a half-life of 70 minutes which is longer than that of the plasminogen-SK complex formed in vivo after administration of SK alone; in fact, this latter complex has a half-life of 25 minutes. The recommended dose of anistreplase for acute myocardial infarction is 30 IU (1 mg = 1 IU) given as a bolus. Thirty milligrams of anistreplase contains about 1,250,000 IU of SK.

Clinical trials with thrombolytic agents in deep vein thrombosis

Thrombolysis for DVT has been plagued by several problems unique to this patient population. First, clot dissolution with peripherally administered thrombolytics is usually accomplished successfully in only one-third to two-thirds of patients. Second, associated comorbid conditions and a lengthy thrombolytic infusion period of 24 hours or more predispose DVT patients to extensive hemorrhagic complications. Third, even when thrombolysis is effectively achieved, successful clot lysis has not been demonstrated definitively to yield a reduction in clinically important adverse events. Fourth, the population of DVT patients that is eligible for thrombolysis is quite narrow, which means that any well thought out thrombolytic strategy will only apply to a small proportion of all DVT patients. Finally, thrombolysis almost always will extend the length of hospital stay of a DVT patient. No strategy for outpatient administration of DVT thrombolysis has yet been validated. In contrast, most DVT treatment strategies for the 21st century rely upon an abbreviated hospital stay or a completely outpatient approach to DVT management. Thus, the concept of DVT thrombolysis will always confront a strong countercurrent inclined toward administration of low molecular weight heparin, given as a "bridge" to warfarin, with the intent of early hospital discharge or even obviating hospitalisation entirely. The only FDA approved dosing regimen for DVT thrombolysis is streptokinase 250,000 units as a loading dose, followed by 100,000 units per hour for 24–72 hours. No catheter-directed thrombolytic regimen has ever received FDA approval.

Efficacy and safety

In a pooled analysis of randomised trials of streptokinase plus heparin versus heparin alone, streptokinase successfully lysed clots in one-half to two-thirds of patients [22]. Thrombolytic therapy plus heparin achieved clot lysis 3.7 times more often than heparin alone. However, this benefit was offset by a 2.9 times greater rate of major hemorrhagic complications among streptokinase treated patients.

In an effort to improve efficacy and safety, trials of more fibrin specific thrombolytic agents were undertaken. The hope was that drugs such as rt-PA would improve the rate of clot dissolution and, furthermore, because of enhanced clot specificity, would decrease overall rates of hemorrhage. However, this approach, at least with peripherally administered thrombolysis, has proven disappointing so far.

Efficacy results were discouraging in a randomised controlled trial of 64 patients who were assigned to rt-PA alone, rt-PA plus heparin, or heparin alone [23]. The rt-PA infusion regimen was 0.05 mg/kg/hour for 24 hours via a peripheral vein, with a maximum dose of 150 mg. These patients were assessed with venography both at baseline and at 24–36 hours after initiation of therapy. Complete or more than 50% lysis occurred in only 28% of patients treated with rt-PA, and 29% of patients treated with rt-PA plus heparin. None of the heparin alone patients had 50% or more clot lysis. No lysis whatsoever occurred in 44% of patients treated with rt-PA plus heparin or in 83% of patients who received heparin alone. In this trial, one nonfatal intracranial hemorrhage occurred in a patient who received rt-PA alone.

The 29% rate of complete or partial clot lysis observed with rt-PA plus heparin was similar to the 21% rate of complete or partial clot lysis obtained by Turpie and colleagues in a separate DVT trial, using two 8-hour infusions of rt-PA with a "heparin recovery period" in between [24]. The authors gave heparin plus 0.5 mg/kg of rt-PA over 8 hours, continued the heparin for 24 hours, and then repeated the same heparin plus rt-PA infusion for the next 8 hours. Verhaeghe and colleagues [25] reported similar efficacy outcomes despite two clever rt-PA dosing regimens: 1) 100 mg rt-PA over 8 hours followed by heparin alone and then 50 mg over 8 hours on the second hospital day, or 2) 50 mg rt-PA over 8 hours followed by heparin alone, and then 50 mg over 24 hours on the second hospital day.

Thus, extended duration infusions of peripherally administered thrombolysis have only demonstrated modest efficacy, at a cost of substantial morbidity from hemorrhage. Subsequently, shorter durations of thrombolytic drug administration were tested, with the hope of reducing the frequency of bleeding complications while still conferring efficacy. Initially, a case series of 27 DVT patients was reported [26]. They received a novel dosing regimen of bolus urokinase: 1,000,000 units administered as a 10 minute bolus, with a total of 3 boluses given over approximately 24 hours. Patients received heparin overnight between bolus urokinase doses. Efficacy was assessed by comparing baseline and prehospital discharge vascular imaging studies. Overall, 52% of patients had clot lysis, 33% had no change, and 15% had more extensive thrombosis. There were no bleeding complications. At 24 hours after starting urokinase, mean plasma fibrinogen levels had declined 61% from baseline and mean bleeding times had increased 28% from baseline (but remained within the normal range). The mild increase in bleeding times suggested that platelet function remained unaffected. Normal platelet function, despite prolonged fibrinogenolysis, may have contributed to the absence of bleeding. The excellent safety regimen of bolus urokinase was subsequently confirmed in a randomised comparison against heparin [27]. However, the rather low efficacy rate precluded this approach from being adopted on a widespread basis.

Contemporary outcome measures

A decade ago, clinical trials in DVT thrombolysis focused upon the narrow endpoints of documenting clot dissolution while minimising the frequency of hemorrhagic complications. However, as we approach the new millennium, these immediate, short term goals are no longer considered sufficient by most clinicians in order to justify widespread use of a DVT thrombolytic strategy. As with thrombolytic trials of myocardial infarction, PE, and peripheral arterial occlusive disease, broader measures of outcome are generally demanded. For DVT, such endpoints might include reduction in the frequency of PE, reduction in the frequency of venous insufficiency, or improvement in quality of life.

Clinical practice has evolved so that patients are often active participants in decision-making for DVT thrombolysis. To use this strategy, patients are given a summary of the trade-offs for utilisation or omission of thrombolytic agents. Utilisation of thrombolytics entails a risk of major hemorrhage, including an approximate 1% risk of intracranial hemorrhage. Adverse clinical events such as intracranial hemorrhage require an adjustment of perspectives for DVT thrombolysis. DVT is not a life-threatening condition as myocardial infarction. Therefore, DVT patients selected for thrombolysis should be at lower risk for hemorrhagic complications than the overall population of myocardial infarction or PE patients who receive thrombolytic therapy. On the other hand, it is the opinion of some authors that omission of thrombolytics makes it likely that venous insufficiency will worsen over the next several years, possibly causing a major decrement in quality of life.

A contemporary approach considers the values that patients attach to clinical outcomes [28]. This method lends itself to formal decision analysis, which calculates both the probabilities of various clinical outcomes based upon published studies and patients' preferences regarding these outcomes. Using this analytic strategy, streptokinase for DVT treatment was estimated to reduce the frequency of postphlebitic syndrome by 56% overall. In this overview, severe postphlebitic syndrome was reduced from a rate of 5.6% in patients treated with heparin alone to zero in patients who received both heparin and streptokinase. However, major bleeding following DVT thrombolysis was found to be 2.9 times more common, with a 4.5 times more frequent rate of intracranial hemorrhage and a 4.0 times higher mortality rate. When patients in this study were asked to attach values to various outcomes, they were willing to accept only a small risk of death or intracranial hemorrhage to avoid the postphlebitic syndrome. However, this study was severely limited by its small size of 36 patients, only 16 of whom actually had suffered DVT. Furthermore, all patients in this study were older than 50 years of age.

Eligibility for DVT thrombolysis

A major additional hurdle is that few DVT patients are appropriate candidates for thrombolysis. Selection criteria must be especially stringent, because DVT itself is not life threatening. Most patients with DVT have important contraindications which, if ignored, might lead to major hemorrhagic complications.

In an analysis of 87 consecutive patients with venograms indicating DVT, 15 patients had DVT limited to calf veins and were therefore not candidates for thrombolysis [29]. Calf vein thrombosis rarely leads to severe postphlebitic syndrome, and the risks of thrombolysis in such patients are only rarely justified. Of the remaining 72 patients with proximal leg DVT, only one-fifth were thought to be eligible for thrombolysis. The three most common contraindications to thrombolysis were: 1) recent trauma or surgery within 14 days, 2) gastrointestinal bleeding, and 3) a history of significant bleeding diathesis or a known chronic bleeding

disorder. In a separate study of 209 DVT patients diagnosed by venous ultrasound, only 7% were assessed as being appropriate candidates for DVT thrombolysis [30]. Thus, this management strategy is quite limited in its general applicability to DVT patients and must be reserved for special subgroups.

Catheter-directed thrombolysis

Further analysis of the results of peripherally administered rt-PA to DVT patients in a prior venographic trial showed that thrombolytic therapy is much more likely to cause clot lysis in the presence of non-obstructive thrombi [31]. Of 81 obstructive venous segments in rt-PA treated patients, only 11 demonstrated 50% or greater clot lysis. It is possible that the obstructive nature of certain venous thrombi, together with the presence of collateral venous flow, may prevent systemically administered fibrinolytic agents from reaching the thrombus in sufficient amounts to cause lysis. In such patients, catheter-directed DVT thrombolysis appears to be a much more efficacious strategy.

In a case series of 174 patients from Lille, France who were treated with peripherally administered streptokinase for an average of 3 days, only 14% of patients with occlusive clots had completely successful DVT thrombolysis [32]. In contrast, completely successful clot lysis was observed in 60% of the patients with non-obstructive venous thrombi.

Actual clinical practice

In practice, DVT thrombolysis is administered for massive DVT associated with threatened arterial insufficiency or phlegmasia cerulea dolens. Furthermore, DVT thrombolysis is usually offered to young patients with iliofemoral venous thrombosis that is thought to be so extensive as to virtually guarantee subsequent venous insufficiency if managed with anticoagulation alone.

Clinical trials with thrombolytic agents with pulmonary embolism (Tables 2 and 3)

Urokinase and streptokinase

Urokinase was compared with heparin alone in 160 patients with angiographically documented PE in the Urokinase Pulmonary Embolism Trial [33]. The loading dose was 4,400 U/kg followed by 4,400 U/kg/h for 24 hours. Urokinase dissolved pulmonary arterial clot more rapidly than heparin alone and, in certain instances, reversed clinical shock. However, there was no difference in the rate of death or recurrent PE between the two groups. Furthermore, hemorrhaghic complications occurred more often among those patients randomised to urokinase.

In the Urokinase-Streptokinase Pulmonary Embolism Trial [34], 167 patients with angiographically documented PE were randomised to 1 of 3 different thrombolytic treatments: 12 hours of urokinase, 24 hours of urokinase, or 24 hours of streptokinase. There was no heparin control group. When the 3 thrombolytic regimens were compared, morbidity and mortality were similar, as was the frequency of major bleeding complications.

In a small trial, streptokinase proved lifesaving in patients with massive PE, hypotension, and heart failure who were randomised to streptokinase plus anticoagulation rather than to anticoagulation alone [35]. Due to ethical considerations resulting from a clear survival benefit in the thrombolysis group, the trial was stopped after the first 8 of 40 intended patients were enrolled. All 4 patients who received thrombolysis survived massive PE. However, of the 4 allocated to the anticoagulation alone group, all died from progressive right heart failure, and the 3 who underwent post-mortem examination had right ventricular myocardial infarction (without significant coronary arterial obstruction), undoubtedly due to massive PE.

Recombinant tissue plasminogen activator

PAIMS-2 investigators in Italy [36] randomised 36 patients with angiographically proven PE to 100 mg of rt-PA over 2 hours plus heparin or to heparin alone. Clot lysis at follow-up angiography occurred in the rt-PA group but was not observed among heparin alone patients. Mean pulmonary

Table 2. Randomised controlled trials comparing thrombolytic agents with heparin in the treatment of acute pulmonary embolism.

| | Treatment | No. | No. of deaths | No. (and %) of bleeding episodes | |
				major	minor
UPET [33]	UK	82	6 (1)	22 (27)	15 (18)
	Heparin	78	7 (3)	11 (14)	10 (13)
Tibbott [90]	SK	13	0	1 (8)	3 (32)
	Heparin	17	1 (1)	1 (6)	3 (18)
Ly [91]	SK	14	0	2 (14)	3 (21)
	Heparin	11	1 (1)	1 (9)	3 (27)
PIOPED [92]	rt-PA	9	1 (0)	1 (11)	0
	Heparin	4	0	0	0
Levine [93]	rt-PA	33	1 (1)	0	14 (45)
	Heparin	25	0	0	1 (4)
PAIMS 2 [36]	rt-PA	20	2	3 (15)	11 (55)
	Heparin	16	1	2 (12)	4 (25)
Goldhaber [44]	rt-PA	46	0	0	3 (6)
	Heparin	55	2	1 (2)	1 (2)

* = The number of deaths from PE is in parentheses.

Table 3. Randomised controlled trials comparing different thrombolytic regimes in the treatment of acute pulmonary embolism.

| | Treatment | No. | No. of deaths | No. (and %) of bleeding episodes | |
				major	minor
USPET [34]	SK	54	5 (NA)	10 (19)	NA
	UK	67	4 (NA)	10 (17)	NA
	UK	54	5 (NA)	7 (13)	NA
UKEP [94]	UK	67	4 (4)	3 (5)	13 (19)
	UK	62	3 (3)	2 (3)	16 (26)
Verstraete [55]	rt-PA (i. p.)	19	2 (2)†	5 (15)†	11 (32)†
	rt-PA (i. v.)	15			
Goldhaber [42]	rt-PA	22	1 (0)	0	1 (4)
	UK	23	2 (2)	1 (4)	7 (30)
Goldhaber [43]	rt-PA	44	2 (2)	10 (21)	NA
	UK	46	1 (1)	6 (13)	NA
Meyer [31]	rt-PA	34	3 (1)	0	14 (41)
	UK	29	1 (0)	1 (3)	17 (57)
Goldhaber [26]	rt-PA bolus	60	6	2 (3)	6 (10)
	rt-PA infusion	27	1	2 (7)	4 (15)

i. p. = intrapulmonary artery infusion

i. v. = intravenous infusion

* = The number of deaths from PE is in parentheses

NA = not available

† = These numbers were not broken down by treatment group

artery pressure decreased from 30 to 21 mm Hg in the rt-PA group, but increased in patients who received heparin alone. Two rt-PA patients died (1 from renal failure following cardiac tamponade and one from intracranial bleeding), and 1 patient who received heparin alone died from recurrent PE.

The European Cooperative Study Group Investigators compared 100 mg of rt-PA over 2 hours with a 12 hour weight adjusted infusion of urokinase (4,400 U/kg bolus, followed by 4,400 U/kg/h for 12 hours) [37]. The principal end point was reduction in total pulmonary resistance, defined as pulmonary artery mean pressure divided by cardiac index. At 2 hours, total pulmonary resistance decreased by 36% in the rt-PA group, compared with an 18% decrease in urokinase treated patients (p = 0.0009). However, by 6 hours, urokinase appeared to "catch up" to rt-PA, and hemodynamic differences between the 2 groups did not persist.

Investigators at Brigham and Women's Hospital in Boston have co-ordinated five trials of PE thrombo-

lysis, which have introduced new concepts in PE thrombolysis (Table 4).

PE Trial #1 [38, 39] was an open label study of 47 patients with angiographically documented PE. 50–90 mg of rt-PA administered over 2–6 hours caused clot lysis in 94% of cases. Hemodynamic and angiographic improvement was accompanied by recovery in pulmonary perfusion [40]. One day after rt-PA, there was a 57% increase in perfusion among those patients who had follow-up lung scans. Right ventricular function also improved [41]. Within a day of treatment, the right ventricular end-diastolic diameter was halved from an average of 3.9 to 2.0 centimetres. Rapid reversal of right heart failure – specifically, right ventricular dysfunction, right ventricular dilatation, and tricuspid regurgitation – suggested that thrombolytic agents might reduce the mortality from acute PE.

PE Trial #2 was a randomised trial comparing 100 mg of rt-PA over 2 hours vs. 4,400 U/kg of UK as a bolus followed by 4,400 U/kg/hour for 24 hours [42]. By 2 hours, 82% of rt-PA-treated

Table 4. New concepts in pulmonary embolism thrombolysis.

Variable	Old	New
Diagnosis	Mandatory pulmonary angiogram	High probability lung scan or suggestive echo-cardiogram (if hypotensive) or angiogram
Indications	Systemic arterial hypotension; hemodynamic instability	Hypotension or normotension with accompanying right ventricular hypokinesis
Time window	5 days or less	14 days or less
Agents	Streptokinase (SK) or urokinase (UK)	rt-PA or SK or UK
Dosing regimens	24h SK or 12−24h UK	100 mg/2h rt-PA
Route	Via pulmonary artery catheter	Via peripheral vein
Coagulation tests	"Coagulation tests" every 4−6h during infusion	PTT at conclusion of thrombolysis
Location	Intensive Care Unit	Intermediate Care Unit

patients showed clot lysis compared with 48 % of UK-treated patients (p = 0.0008). Thrombolysis at angiography was associated with a reduction of elevated pulmonary arterial pressures. In the dosing regimens employed, rt-PA was more rapid and safer than UK. However, at 24 hours, there was no difference in scintigraphic improvement between rt-PA and UK patients. Furthermore, at 2 and 24 hours after initiation of thrombolysis, the fibrinogen levels were similar in both treatment groups.

PE Trial #3 compressed the 24 hour dose of UK to make it more comparable to the high concentration/short infusion period that was previously used for rt-PA [43]. The novel UK dose was 3,000,000 U/2 hours, with the first 1,000,000 U given as a bolus over 10 minutes. This trial enrolled 90 patients who were randomised to UK or to rt-PA 100 mg/2 hours. Repeat pulmonary angiograms at 2 hours indicated that a 2-hour regimen of rt-PA and a new concentrated 2-hour dosing regimen of urokinase exhibited similar efficacy and safety. The one substantive difference between the two agents was that 8 of 46 urokinase patients, compared with 0 of 44 rt-PA patients, suffered rigors (p = 0.004).

PE Trial #4 tested the hypothesis that rt-PA followed by anticoagulation accelerates the improvement of right ventricular function and pulmonary perfusion more rapidly than anticoagulation alone [44]. In this multicentre randomised controlled trial, 101 "hemodynamically stable" patients were randomised: 46 to rt-PA 100 mg/2 hours followed by heparin and 55 to heparin alone. rt-PA (100 mg/2hours) followed by heparin provided striking improvement in right ventricular function and pulmonary perfusion compared with heparin anticoagulation alone. Most importantly, no clini-

cal episodes of recurrent PE occurred among rt-PA patients, but there were 5 (2 fatal and 3 nonfatal) clinically suspected recurrent PE within 14 days in patients randomised to heparin alone (p = 0.06), despite adequate anticoagulation as judged by partial thromboplastin times. All five presented initially with right ventricular hypokinesis on echocardiogram, despite normal systemic arterial pressure at baseline. Thus, echocardiography helped identify a subgroup of PE patients with impending right ventricular failure who appeared to be at high risk of adverse clinical outcomes if treated with heparin alone. The investigators concluded that such patients, in particular, may be excellent candidates for thrombolytic therapy in the absence of contraindications.

PE Trial #5 (also known as the Bolus Alteplase Pulmonary Embolism [BAPE] Trial) [45] and a consortium of French trialists [46] utilised essentially the same investigational protocol to compare the safety of reduced dose bolus rt-PA (0.6 mg/kg, with a maximum of 50 mg, administered over 15 minutes) with full dose 100 mg/2 hours rt-PA. In PE Trial #5, which enrolled 90 patients, there were 6 deaths in the first 14 days after randomisation: 5 (8 %) in the bolus group and 1 (4 %) in the 2 hours rt-PA group (p = 0.66). Efficacy, assessed by lung scanning in all patients and either by repeat angiography or repeat echocardiography (depending on the participating hospital), was similar in the two groups. There was no difference in the major bleeding rates between the two treatment arms. Patients who received reduced dose bolus rt-PA had less depression of fibrinogen levels (p = 0.007) and smaller increases in FDPs (p = 0.013) than patients who had received 100 mg/2 hours of rt-PA. Nevertheless, there was no relationship between clinical outcome or the development of bleeding complications with respect to coagulation results.

In the French trial that tested the same two dosing regimens of rt-PA, the investigators studied 53 patients with angiographically documented PE [46]. They found no significant difference between the two treatment groups when post-thrombolysis reductions in total pulmonary resistance were compared. Major bleeding occurred in 8 % of bolus rt-PA patients compared with 6 % of 2 hours rt-PA patients.

Right ventricular function, thrombolysis, and pulmonary embolism registries

Evidence now exists from three registries of PE patients that right ventricular failure is associated with a poor prognosis. The German Management and Prognosis of Pulmonary Embolism Registry (MAPPET) of 1,001 patients found that mortality increases as right ventricular dysfunction becomes more profound [47]. Furthermore, thrombolysis appeared to improve the clinical outcome of hemodynamically stable patients with major PE [48]. In MAPPET, individual physicians decided without any standardised protocol whether to administer thrombolytic therapy. The death rate at 30 days was 5 % for thrombolysis patients (versus 11 % for heparin alone patients), and the recurrent PE rate during hospitalisation was 8 % (versus 19 % for heparin alone patients). After multivariate analysis, a marked benefit persisted for the thrombolysis treated patients. The penalty for use of thrombolysis was a three-fold higher rate of major bleeding. Overall, MAPPET provides additional support for those who hypothesise that thrombolysis will benefit PE patients who present with normal systemic arterial pressure and right ventricular dysfunction.

In a Swedish Registry of 126 consecutive PE patients, right ventricular dysfunction on echocardio-graphy was associated with a 6-fold increase in in-hospital death and a 3-fold increase in mortality at 1 year [49]. During the hospitalisation for PE, no patient with normal right ventricular function died.

The largest PE Registry, the International Cooperative Pulmonary Embolism Registry (ICOPER), enrolled 2,454 patients [50]. In this Registry, 47 % of patients underwent echocardiography. Of these patients, 40 % had right ventricular hypokinesis. Overall, the mortality rate in ICOPER was 17 % at 3 months: 21 % in those with right ventricular hypokinesis and 15 % in those with normal right ventricular function. Multivariate analysis demonstrated that right ventricular hypokinesis was associated with a 2-fold increase in risk of death at 3 months.

Bleeding complications

The most feared complication is intracranial hemorrhage. Among the 312 patients receiving thrombolysis for PE in 5 clinical trials, there was a 1.9 % risk (95 % CI, 0.7 to 4.1 %) of intracranial bleeding [51]. Two of the six patients had pre-existing known intracranial disease and received thrombolysis in violation of the protocol. Two of the six intracranial hemorrhages probably were due to administration of heparin and not thrombolysis because they occurred late, 62 and 157 hours after thrombolysis. Diastolic blood pressure on admission was significantly elevated in patients who developed intracranial hemorrhage compared with those who did not (90.3 vs. 77.6 mm Hg; $p = 0.04$). Of the 312 patients, no one under age 55 suffered intracranial bleeding. However, these data indicate that meticulous patient screening is imperative before administering thrombolysis. Other risk factors associated with bleeding after thrombolysis include increasing age and increasing body mass index [52].

Local versus systemic thrombolysis

For DVT thrombolysis, systemically administered drug is probably only worthwhile when thrombus is documented as non-obstructive. Otherwise, it is unlikely that this approach will succeed. Among appropriately selected patients with obstructive ilio-femoral venous thrombosis, local, catheter-directed thrombolysis is usually effective and safe [53]. This strategy can be combined with venous thrombec-tomy [54]. For PE thrombolysis, rt-PA administered locally within the pulmonary artery appears to confer no advantage over peripheral administration of the drug [55]. This might be due to the presence of the bronchial collateral circulation that ensures some blood flow to pulmonary thromboemboli and also because thromboemboli from PE rarely cause complete obstruction of the pulmonary artery.

Third generation thrombolytic agents

This group consists of agents developed in an attempt to improve the characteristics of the first and second generation thrombolytic agents. The third generation thrombolytic agents are obtained by genetic engineering. The majority of these agents are not destined for clinical development but, instead, will remain tools to study and understand the correlations between structure and function of plasminogen activators. Only a few of the third generation thrombolytic agents have started undergoing clinical studies in man after extensive in vitro or animal studies. The third generation thrombolytic agents include: t-PA mutants with modified functional properties, chimeric plasminogen activators, complexes of plasminogen activators with fibrin-specific monoclonal antibodies, and recombinant staphylokinase.

Mutant variants of t-PA with modified functional properties

t-PA mutants with modified functional properties include t-PA mutants with increased affinity for fibrin, t-PA mutants resistant to plasmin, t-PA mutants with increased catalytic efficiency in the presence of fibrin, t-PA mutants resistant to the inhibitory action of PAI-I and t-PA mutants with a long plasma half-life.

t-PA mutants with increased affinity for fibrin
Structure-function correlation studies have indicated that the finger and epidermal growth factor domains in the t-PA molecule must remain intact for the activator to display a high level of binding to fibrin [56]. Attempts to clone t-PA mutants with greater affinity for fibrin than the wild-type t-PA have proved disappointing and it appears very difficult to 'improve' t-PA as far as this particular property is concerned [57]. Non-glycosylated mutant variants of t-PA have been produced and results are encouraging. These agents are based on evidence that certain oligosaccharide chains, especially those containing sialic acid, reduce the affinity of t-PA for fibrin [58]. Another approach is to substitute kringle 1 with one or more kringle 2's in order to increase the number of lysine-binding sites within the molecule [59].

Plasmin resistant t-PA mutants
The objective of forming mutants of this type is to avoid conversion of single-chain t-PA into double-chain t-PA in order to increase specificity for fibrin. Some of these variants have a lower capacity to activate plasminogen in the absence of fibrin. This capacity is rapidly recovered in the presence of fibrin [60, 61]. An agent of particular interest appears to be a plasminogen activator isolated from the saliva of the so-called vampire bat Desmodus rotundus [62]. This activator, known as Bat-PA, has many similarities with human t-PA but does not have the kringle 2 and the plasmin cleavage site for conversion to a double chain. In animal experiments Bat-PA exhibits greater affinity for fibrin than t-PA.

t-PA mutants with increased catalytic efficiency in the presence of fibrin
The activation of t-PA by fibrin relies on structural sites located in kringle 2 and, less importantly, in the finger domain. Attempts to improve t-PA by functionally exposing the kringle 2 structure have only given modest results.

Mutant variants of t-PA resistant to PAI-I
The plasminogen activators are inhibited in plasma by specific inhibitors (PAI). In particular, PAI-I inhibits single-chain and double-chain t-PA and urokinase. Mutant variants of t-PA have been developed resistant to the inhibition of PAI-I [63 – 66]. As a result of the resistance of the inhibitory action of PAI-I, these compounds have a longer plasma half-life compared with that of t-PA. One of these mutants has been shown to have a prolonged plasma half-life and high thrombolytic activity [66]. Since, during thrombolytic treatment, there is an excess of circulating t-PA over PAI-I, it is not certain whether mutants resistant to PAI-I have significant advantages compared with t-PA. Nevertheless, the relative concentrations of plasminogen activator and PAI-I could be of critical importance several hours after administration of the thrombolytic agent by bringing about the phenomenon of reocclusion. t-PA mutants resistant to PAI-I might, therefore, be more effective than t-PA for the short-term prevention of reocclusion.

t-PA with a long plasma half-life
t-PA has a short half-life in vivo. The structures responsible for the rapid clearance of t-PA are located on the A (or heavy) chain and structure-function correlation studies have indicated that these are the finger and epidermal growth factor domains. Structure-function correlation studies show that, in the finger domain, in the epidermal growth factor domain and in kringle 1, are located the structures responsible for the rapid clearance of

t-PA, and related to this is the component in carbohydrates located at the level of the epidermal growth factor domain and in kringle 1. Mutants without one or more of the three domains mentioned above have a half-life 5 or 10 times longer than native t-PA [64, 67 – 77]. Removal of carbohydrates may occur by means of point mutagenesis of enzymatic deglycosylation.

The longer half-life of these compounds enables them to be administered as a single or repeated bolus. The advantages of the mutants with long half-lives compared with t-PA still have to be proved. Encouraging results have been obtained with reteplase, a non-glycosylated t-PA mutant composed of kringle 2 and the light chain [73 – 77]. The plasma half-life of reteplase is around 5 times longer than that of t-PA [74].

Chimeric plasminogen activators

By forming chimeric variants of the plasminogen activators it is hoped to combine, in a single molecule, the positive characteristics of a number of different activators. Consequently, most of the chimeric activators produced consist of the A-chain of t-PA and the chain of scu-PA [78 – 82]. The t-PA structures responsible for its affinity for fibrin reside in the A-chain whereas the ability of scu-PA to be activated by fibrin is independent of this chain. These hybrid plasminogen activators have a longer half-life than t-PA and weaker affinity for fibrin, while retaining the ability to be activated by fibrin. The good results obtained in animal studies need to be confirmed in man. In particular, in animal experiments, K_2tu-PA, a hybrid composed of the kringle 2 of t-PA and the β-chain of scu-PA, administered as a bolus, inhibits the deposition of newly formed fibrin on the thrombus more effectively than rt-PA, raising the possibility that it may have greater efficacy in preventing rethrombosis [82].

Chimeric plasminogen activators, which combine in the same molecule several advantageous characteristics of individual agents such as a high affinity or fibrin, a long-life and resistance to inhibition by PAI-I, have been recently developed [66, 83 – 84].

Complexes of plasminogen activators and fibrin-specific monoclonal antibodies

In order to target thrombolytic agents to the thrombus, plasminogen activators have been conjugated with murine monoclonal antibodies directed against components of the thrombus [85 – 86]. Use of antibodies with specificity for the components of the thrombus combined with plasminogen activators allows these thrombolytic substances to be concentrated on the surface of the thrombus. As far as conjugation with anti-fibrin antibodies is concerned, the principal problem lies in the need to use antibodies that do not cross-react with fibrinogen. When using anti-platelet antibodies a different approach is needed because the monoclonal antibodies must be directed against epitopes present on the surface of activate platelets, but not against those present on resisting platelets. This discriminatory capacity is essential if the thrombolytic agent is to be directed at the surface of the thrombus without interacting with the circulating platelets. The use of plasminogen activators conjugated with antiplatelet antibodies or anti-fibrin antibodies appear to be a very promising idea, but their clinical use is still a long way off [85 – 87].

Staphylokinase

Staphylokinase is a 136 amino acid protein derived by certain strains of staphylococci that is now produced by routine recombinant DNA technology [88]. Staphylokinase has a unique structure, mechanism of action and fibrin specificity. The clinical experience to date is encouraging although limited. Further studies are required in order to determine the optimal dose and mode of administration, the optimal conjunctive therapy and the merits in terms of efficacy and safety relative to established and new thrombolytic agents.

Emerging strategies in thrombolytic therapy

It is evident that patients with massive PE, cardiogenic shock, or overt hemodynamic instability should receive thrombolytic therapy or, if contraindications exist, embolectomy. Suggested but not proven is that patients with normal systemic arterial pressure and moderate or marked right ventricular dysfunction (usually documented by echocardiogram) should also be treated with thrombolysis.

It appears that among such patients, rapid improvement of right ventricular function and pulmonary perfusion, accomplished with thrombolytic therapy followed by heparin, may lead to a lower rate of death and recurrent PE. Three possible mechanisms may be operative. 1) Thrombolysis may function as a "medical embolectomy", with lysis of massive pulmonary arterial thrombus, thereby preventing the downhill spiral of right heart failure. 2) Among patients with anatomically smaller PE, thrombolysis may prevent the continued release of serotonin and other neurohumoral factors, which might otherwise lead to worsening pulmonary hypertension. 3) Thrombolysis may dissolve much of the source of the thrombus in the pelvic or deep leg veins, thereby decreasing the likelihood of recurrent PE (Table 5).

Of the three FDA-approved thrombolytic regimens for PE (Table 6), rt-PA appears to be the most effective and safe, based upon clinical trial reports. Importantly, the time window for PE thrombolysis is quite wide [89]. In addition, practical steps can be taken to streamline PE thrombolysis, thus making this process more efficient, more economical, and safer. For example, costs can be controlled by omitting testing of fibrinogen, fibrin(ogen) split products, and thrombin time, all of which are generally unnecessary for clinical management.

Finally, the role of DVT thrombolysis will require further clarification. For now, its use should be concentrated among patients with threatened limbs, extensive iliofemoral venous thrombosis, or moderate thrombosis that does not appear to be improving with standard anticoagulation.

Table 5. Advantages of thrombolysis.

Proven

Accelerate clot lysis
Accelerate pulmonary tissue reperfusion
Accelerate reversal of right heart failure
Improve pulmonary capillary blood volume

Possible

Reduce mortality
Reduce recurrent PE
Minimise adverse neurohumoral effects
Reduce chronic pulmonary hypertension
Improve the quality of life

Table 6. FDA-approved thrombolytic regimens for PE.

STREPTOKINASE: 250,000 IU as a loading dose over 30 minutes, followed by 100,000 U/hr for 24 hours – approved in 1977.

UROKINASE: 4,400 IU/kg as a loading dose over 10 minutes, followed by 4,400 IU/kg/hr for 12 – 24 hours – approved in 1978.

rt-PA: 100 mg as a continuous peripheral intravenous infusion administered over 2 hours – approved in 1990.

References

1. Collen D. On the regulation and control of fibrinolysis. Thromb Haemost 1980; 43: 77–89

2. Forsgren M, Raden B, Israelsson M, et al. Molecular cloning and characterization of a full-length cDNA clone for human plasminogen. FEBS Lett 1987; 213: 254–260

3. Collen D, Lijnen HR. Basic and clinical aspects of fibrinolysis and thrombolysis. Blood 1991; 78: 3114–3124

4. Robbins KC, Summaria L, Hsieh B, Shah RJ. The peptide chains of human plasmin. Mechanism of activation of human plasminogen to plasmin. J Biol Chem 1967; 242: 2333–2342

5. Pennica D, Holmes WE, Kohr WJ, et al. Cloning and expression of human tissue-type plasminogen activator cDNA in E. coli. Nature 1983; 301: 214–221

6. Kruithof EKO. Plasminogen activator inhibitors – a review. Enzyme 1988; 40: 113–121

7. Kruithof EKO, Gudinchet A, Bachmann F. Plasminogen activator inhibitor 1 and plasminogen activator inhibitor 2 in various disease states. Thromb Haemostas 1988; 59: 7–12

8. Van Hinsbergh VWM, Kooistra T, Emeis JJ, Koolwijk P. Regulation of plasminogen activator production by endothelial cells: role in fibrinolysis and local proteolysis. J Biol Chem 1989; 60: 261–272

9. Loskutoff DJ. Regulation of PAI-1 gene expression. Fibrinolysis 1991; 5: 197–206

10. Wiman B, Collen D. On the kinetics of the reaction between human antiplasmin and plasmin. Eur J Biochem 1978; 84: 573–578

11. Thorsen S, Philips M, Selmer J, et al. Kinetics of inhibition of tissue-type and urokinase-type plasminogen activator by plasminogen-activator inhibitor type 1 and type 2. Eur J Biochem 1988; 175: 33–39

12. Hoylaerts M, Rijken DC, Lijnen HR, Collen D. Kinetics of the activation of plasminogen by human tissue plasminogen activator. Role of fibrin. J Biol Chem 1982; 257: 2912–2919

13. Thorsen S. The mechanism of plasminogen activation and the variability of the fibrin effector during tissue-type plasminogen activator-mediated fibrinolysis. Ann NY Acad Sci 1992; 667: 52–63

14. Andreasen PA, Petersen LC, Danø K. Diversity in catalytic properties of single-chain and two-chain tissue-type plasminogen activator. Fibrinolysis 1991; 5: 207–215

15. Muelleretz S. Fibrinolysis. General aspects, characteristic features and perspectives. Fibrinolysis 1987; 1: 3–12

16. Tillet WS, Garner RL. The fibrinolytic activity of hemolytic streptococci. J Exp Med 1933; 68: 485–502

17. White HD, Norris RM, Brown MA, et al. Effect of intravenous streptokinase on left ventricular function and early survival after acute myocardial infarction. New Engl J Med 1987; 317: 850–855

18. MacFarlane RG, Pilling J. Fibrinolytic activity in normal urine. Nature 1947; 159: 779

19. Schneider P, Bachmann F, Sauser D. Urokinase: a short review of its properties and of its metabolism. In: D'Angelo A, Mannucci PM (eds). Urokinase: basic and clinical aspects. Londra: Academic Press, 1982; 1–15

20. Verstraete M, Bounameaux H, De Cock F e coll. Pharmacokinetics and systemic fibrinogenolytic effects of recombinant human tissue-type plasminogen activator (rt-PA) in humans. J Pharmacol Exp Ther 1985; 235: 506–12

21. Agnelli G, Buchanan MR, Fernandez F, et al. Sustained thrombolysis with DNA-recombinant tissue-type plasminogen activator in rabbits. Blood 1985; 66: 399–401

22. Goldhaber SZ, Buring JE, Lipnick RJ, Hennekens CH. Pooled analyses of randomised trials of streptokinase and heparin in phlebographically documented acute deep venous thrombosis. Am J Med 1984; 76: 393–397

23. Goldhaber SZ, Meyerovitz MF, Green D, Vogelzang RL, Citirin P, Heit JA, Sobel M, Wheeler HB, Plante D, Kim H, Hopkins A, Tufte M, Stump D, Braunwald E. Randomised controlled trial of tissue plasminogen activator in proximal deep venous thrombosis. Am J Med 1990; 88: 235–240

24. Turpie AGG, Levine MN, Hirsh J, et al. Tissue plasminogen activator (rt-PA) versus heparin in deep vein thrombosis: Results of a randomised trial. Chest 1990; 97: 172S–175S

25. Verhaeghe R, Besse P, Bounameaux H, Marbet GA: Multicenter pilot study of the efficacy and safety of systemic rt-PA administration in the treatment of deep vein thrombosis of the lower extremities and/or pelvis. Thromb Res 1989; 55: 5–11

26. Goldhaber SZ, Polak JF, Feldstein ML, Meyerovitz MF, Creager MA. Efficacy and safety of repeated boluses of urokinase in the treatment of deep venous thrombosis. Am J Cardiol 1994; 73: 75–79

27. Goldhaber SZ, Hirsch DR, MacDougall RC, Polak JF, Creager MA. Bolus recombinant urokinase versus heparin in deep venous thrombosis: A randomised controlled trial. Am Heart J 1996; 132: 314–318

28. O'Meara JJ III, McNutt RA, Evans AT, Moore SW, Downs SM. A decision analysis of streptokinase plus heparin as compared with heparin alone for deep-vein thrombosis. N Engl J Med 1994; 330: 1864–1869

29. Brown WD, Goldhaber SZ. How to select patients with deep vein thrombosis for tPA therapy. Chest 1989; 95: 276S–278S

30. Markel A, Manzo RA, Strandness DE JR. The potential role of thrombolytic therapy in venous thrombosis. Arch Intern Med 1992; 152: 165–1267

31. Meyerovitz MF, Polak JF, Goldhaber SZ. Short-term response to thrombolytic therapy in deep venous thrombosis: Predictive value of venographic appearance. Radiology 1992; 184: 345–348

32. Théry C, Bauchart JJ, Lesenne M, Asseman P, Flajollet J-G, Legghe R, Marache P. Predictive factors of effectiveness of streptokinase in deep venous thrombosis. Am J Cardiol 1992; 69: 117–122

33. The Urokinase Pulmonary Embolism Trial. A national cooperative study. Circulation 1973; 47: II-1–108

34. The Urokinase-Streptokinase Embolism Trial. Phase 2 results. A cooperative study. JAMA 1974; 229: 1606–1613

35. Jerjes-Sanchez C, Ramirez-Rivera A, Garcia M de L, Arriaga-Nava R, Valencia S, Rosado-Buzzo A, Pierzo JA, Rosas E. Streptokinase and heparin versus heparin alone in massive pulmonary embolism: A randomised controlled trial. J Thrombosis and Thrombolysis 1995; 2: 227–229

36. Dalla-Volta S, Palla A, Santolicandro A, et al. PAIMS 2: Alteplase combined with heparin versus heparin in the treatment of acute pulmonary embolism. Plasminogen Activator Italian Multicenter Study 2. J Am Coll Cardiol 1992; 20: 520–526

37. Meyer G, Sors H, Charbonnier B, Kasper W, Bassand J-P, Kerr IH, Lesaffre E, Vanhove P, Verstraete M on behalf of the European Cooperative Study Group for Pulmonary Embolism. Effects of intravenous urokinase versus alteplase on total pulmonary resistance in acute massive pulmonary embolism: A European multicenter double-blind trial. J Am Coll Cardiol 1992; 19: 239–245

38. Goldhaber SZ, Vaughan DE, Markis JE, Selwyn AP, Meyerovitz MF, Loscalzo J, Kim DS, Kessler CM, Dawley DL, Sharma GVRK, Sasahara A, Grossbard EB, Braunwald E. Acute pulmonary embolism treated with tissue plasminogen activator. Lancet 1986; 2: 886–889

39. Goldhaber SZ, Meyerovitz MF, Markis JE, Kim D, Kessler CM, Sharma GVRK, Vaughan DE, Selwyn AP, Dawley DL, Loscalzo J, Sasahara A, Grossbard EB, Braunwald E, on behalf of the Participating Investigators. Thrombolytic therapy of acute pulmonary embolism: Current status and future potential. JACC 1987; 10: 96B–104B

40. Parker JA, Markis JE, Palla A, Goldhaber SZ, Royal HD, Tumeh S, Kim D, Rustgi AK, Holman BL, Kolodny GM, Braunwald E, on behalf of the Participating Investigators. Early improvement in pulmonary perfusion after rt-PA therapy for acute embolism: Segmental perfusion scan analysis. Radiology 1988; 166: 441–445

41. Come PC, Kim D, Parker JA, Goldhaber SZ, Braunwald E, Markis JE and Participating Investigators. Early reversal of right ventricular dysfunction in patients with acute pulmonary embolism after treatment with intravenous tissue plasminogen activator. J Am Coll Cardiol 1987; 10: 971–978

42. Goldhaber SZ, Kessler CM, Heit J, Markis J, Sharma GVRK, Dawley D, Nagel JS, Meyerovitz M, Kim D, Vaughan DE, Parker JA, Tumeh SS, Drum D, Loscalzo J, Reagan K, Selwyn AP, Anderson J, Braunwald E. A randomised controlled trial of recombinant tissue plasminogen activator versus urokinase in the treatment of acute pulmonary embolism. Lancet 1988; 2: 293–298

43. Goldhaber SZ, Kessler CM, Heit JA, Elliott CG, Friedenberg WR, Heiselman DE, Wilson DB, Parker JA, Bennett D, Feldstein ML, Selwyn AP, Kim D, Sharma GVRK, Nagel JS, Meyerovitz MF. Recombinant tissue-type plasminogen activator versus a novel dosing regimen of urokinase in acute pulmonary embolism: A randomised controlled multicenter trial. J Am Coll Cardiol 1992; 20: 24–30

44. Goldhaber SZ, Haire WD, Feldstein ML, Miller M, Toltzis R, Smith JL, Taveira da Silva AM, Come PC, Lee RT, Parker JA, Mogtader A, McDonough TJ, Braunwald E. Alteplase versus heparin in acute pulmonary embolism: randomised trial assessing right ventricular function and pulmonary perfusion. Lancet 1993; 341: 507–511

45. Goldhaber SZ, Agnelli G, Levine MN, on behalf of the Bolus Alteplase Pulmonary Embolism Group. Reduced dose bolus alteplase vs conventional alteplase infusion for pulmonary embolism thrombolysis. An international multicenter randomised trial. Chest 1994; 106: 718–724

46. Sors H, Pacouret G, Azarian R, Meyer G, Charbonnier B, Simonneau G. Hemodynamic effects of bolus vs 2-h infusion of alteplase in acute massive pulmonary embolism. A randomised controlled multicenter trial. Chest 1994; 106: 712–717

47. Konstantinides S, Geibel A, Kasper W, Olschewski M, Kienast J, Iversen S, Grosser KD. Predictors of in-hospital mortality in patients with acute massive pulmonary embolism: Results of the Management and Prognosis of Pulmonary Embolism Registry. Circulation 1996; 94 (suppl I): I–572 (Abstract)

48. Konstantinides S, Geibel A, Olschewski M, Heinrich F, Grosser K, Rauber K, Iversen S, Redecker M, Kienast J, Just H, Kasper W. Association between thrombolytic treatment and the prognosis of hemodynamically stable patients with major pulmonary embolism. Results of a Multicenter Registry. Circulation 1997; 96: 882–888

49. Ribeiro A, Lindmarker P, Juhlin-Dannfelt A, Johnsson H, Jorfeldt L. Echocardiography-Doppler in pulmonary embolism: Right ventricular dysfunction as a predictor of mortality. Am Heart J 1997 (in press)

50. Goldhaber SZ, De Rosa M, Visani L. International Cooperative Pulmonary Embolism Registry. Circulation 1997 (in press, abstract)

51. Kanter DS, Mikkola KM, Patel SR, Parker JA, Goldhaber SZ. Thrombolytic therapy for pulmonary embolism. Frequency of intracranial haemorrhage and associated risk factors. Chest 1997; 111: 1241–1245

52. Mikkola KM, Patel SR, Parker JA, Grodstein F, Goldhaber SZ. Increasing age is a major risk factor for haemorrhagic complications following pulmonary embolism thrombolysis. Am Heart J 1997 (in press)

53. Bjarnason H, Kruse JR, Asinger DA, Nazarian GW, Dietz CA Jr, Caldwell MD, Key NS, Hirsch AT, Hunter DW. Iliofemoral deep venous thrombosis: Safety and efficacy outcome during 5 years of catheter-directed thrombolytic therapy. J Vasc Interv Radiol 1997; 8: 405–418

54. Comerota AJ, Aldridge SC, Cohen G, Ball DS, Pliskin M, White JV. A strategy of aggressive regional therapy for acute iliofemoral venous thrombosis with contemporary venous thrombectomy or catheter-directed thrombolysis. J Vasc Surg 1994; 20: 244–254

55. Verstraete M, Miller GAH, Bounameaux H, Charbonnier B, Colle JP, Lecorf G, Marbet GA, Mombaerts, P, Olsson CG. Intravenous and intrapulmonary recombinant tissue-type plasminogen activator in the treatment of acute massive pulmonary embolism. Circulation 1988; 77: 353–360

56. Johannessen M, Diness V, Pingel K, et al. Fibrin affinity and clearance of t-PA deletion and substitution analogues. Thromb Haemostasis 1990; 63: 54–59

57. Collen D, Lijnen HR, Vanlinthout I, et al. Thrombolytic and pharmacokinetic properties of human tissue-type plasminogen activator variants, obtained by deletion and/or duplication of structural/functional domains, in a hamster pulmonary embolism model. Thromb Haemostasis 1991; 65: 174–80

58. Wilhelm J, Kalyan NK, Lee SG, et al. Deglycosylation increases the fibrinolytic activity of a deletion mutant of tissue-type plasminogen activator. Thromb Haemostasis 1990; 63: 464–471

59. Kalyan NK, Wilhelm J, Lee SG, et al. Construction, expression and biochemical characterisation of a novel triskringle plasminogen activator gene. Fibrinolysis 1990; 4: 79–86

60. Urano S, Metzger AR, Castellino FJ. Plasmin-mediated fibrinolysis by variant recombinant tissue-type plasminogen activators. Proc Natl Acad Sci USA 1989; 68: 2568–2571

61. Petersen LC, Johannessen M, Foster D, et al. The effect of polymerised fibrin on the catalytic activities of one-chain tissue-type plasminogen activator as revealed by an analogue resistant to plasmin cleavage. Biochim Biophys Acta 1988; 952: 245–254

62. Gardell SJ, Duong LT, Diehl RE, York JD, Hare TR, Register RB, Jacobs JW, Dixon RA, Friedman PA. Isolation, characterization, and cDNA cloning of a vampire bat salivary plasminogen activator. J Biol Chem 1989; 264: 7947–7952

63. Haigwood NL, Mullenbach GT, Moore GK, et al. Variants of human tissue-type plasminogen activator substituted at the protease cleavage site and glycosylation sites, and truncated at the N- and C-termini. Protein Eng 1989; 2: 611–620

64. Johannesson M, Diness V, Pingel K, Petersen LC, Rao D, Lioubin P, O'Hara P, Mulvihill E. Fibrin affinity and clearance of t-PA delation and substitution analogues. Thrombosis Haemostas 1990; 63: 54–59

65. Shohet RV, Spitzer S, Madison EL, Bassel-Duby R, Gething M-J, Sambrook JF. Inhibitor-resistant tissue-type plasminogen activator: an improved thrombolytic agent in vitro. Thrombosis Haemostas 1994; 71: 124–128

66. Collen D, Stassen JM, Yasuda T, et al. Comparative thrombolytic properties of tissue-type plasminogen activator (rt-PA) and a plasminogen activator inhibitor-resistant glycosylation variants in a combined arterial and venous thrombosis model in the dog. Thromb Haemost 1994; 72: 98–104

67. Cambier P, Van de Werf F, Larsen GR, Collen D. Pharmacokinetics and thrombolytic properties of a non-glycosylated mutant of human tissue-type plasminogen activator, lacking the finger and growth factor domains, in dogs with copper coil-induced coronary artery thrombosis. J Cardiovasc Pharmacol 1988; 11: 468–472

68. Collen D, Stassen J-M, Larsen G. Pharmacokinetics and thrombolytic properties of delation mutants of human tissue-type plasminogen activator in rabbits. Blood 1988; 71: 216–219

69. Larsen GR, Metzger M, Hensen K, Blue Y, Horgan P. Pharmacokinetics and distribution analysis of variant forms of tissue-type plasminogen activator with prolonged clearance in rat. Blood 1989; 73: 1842–1850

70. Jackson CV, Crowe VG, Craft TJ, Sundboom JL, Grinnell BW, Bobbitt JL, Burck PJ, Quay JF, Smith GF. Thrombolytic activity of a novel plasminogen activator, LY210 825, compared with recombinant tissue-type plasminogen activator in a canine model of coronary artery thrombosis. Circulation 1990; 82: 930–940

71. Collen D, Lijnen HR, Vanlinthout I, Kieckens L, Nelles L, Stassen JM. Thrombolytic and pharmacokinetic properties of human tissue-type plasminogen activators variants, obtained by delation and/or duplication of structural/functional domains, in a hamster pulmonary embolism model. Thrombosis Haemostas 1991; 65: 174–180

72. Nicolini FA, Nichols WW, Metha JL, Saldeen TGP, Schofield R, Ross M, Player DW, Pohl GB, Mattsson C. Sustained reflow in dogs with coronary thrombosis with K2P, a novel mutant of tissue-plasminogen activator. JACC 1992; 20: 228–235

73. Martin U, Sponer G, Strein K. Evaluation of thrombolytic and systematic effects of the novel recombinant plasminogen activator BM 06.022 compared with alteplase, anistreplase, streptokinase and urokinase in a canine model of coronary artery thrombosis. JACC 1992; 19: 433–440

74. Martin U, Köhler J, Sponer G, Strein K. Pharmacokinetics of the novel recombinant plasminogen activator BM 06.022 in rats, dogs, and non-human primates. Fibrinolysis 1992; 6: 39–43

75. Tebbe U, von Essen R, Smolarz A, Limbourg P, Rox J, Rustige J, Vogt A, Wagner J, Meyer-Sabellek W, Neuhaus K-L. Open, non-controlled dose-finding study with a novel recombinant plasminogen activator (BM 06.022) given as a double bolus in patients with acute myocardial infarction. Am J Card 1993; 72: 518–523

76. Neuhaus K-L, von Essen R, Vogt A, Tebbe U, Rustige J, Wagner H-J, Appel K-F, Stienen U, König R, Meyer-Sabellek W. Dose finding with a novel recombinant plasminogen activator (BM 06.022) in patients with acute myocardial infarction: Results of the German Recombinant Plasminogen Activator (GRECO) Study. J Am Coll Cardiol (in press)

77. Smalling RW, Bode C, Kalbfleisch J, Sen S, Feldman R, Mann D, Limbourg P, Odenheimer DJ, Meyer-Sabellek W and the RAPID Investigators. Effects of reteplase and alteplase on speed and completeness of coronary artery patency. Eur Heart J 1994; 15: 527

78. Wilson S, Cronk DW, Dodd I, Esmail AF, Kalindjian SB, McMurdo L, Browne MJ, Smith RAG, Robinson JH. The use of active centre acylation to control the pharmacokinetic profile of a recombinant chimaeric plasminogen activator. Thrombosis Haemostas 1993; 70: 984–988

79. Pièrard L, Jacobs P, Gheysen D, et al. Mutant and chimeric recombinant plasminogen activators: production in eukaryotic cells and preliminary characterization. J Biol Chem 1987; 262: 11 771–11 778

80. Gheysen D, Lijnen HR, Pièrard L e coll. Characterization of a recombinant fusion protein of the finger domain of tissue-type plasminogen activator with a truncated single chain urokinase-type plasminogen activator. J Biol Chem 1987; 262: 11 779–11 784

81. Agnelli G, Pascucci C, Colucci M, et al. Thrombolytic activity of two chimeric recombinant plasminogen activators (FK$_2$tu-PA and K$_2$tu-PA) in rabbits. Thromb Haemostasis 1992; 68: 331–335

82. Agnelli G, Pascucci C, Nenci GG, Mele A, Bürgi R, Heim J. Thrombolytic and haemorrhagic effects of bolus doses of tissue-type plasminogen activator and a hybrid plasminogen activator with prolonged plasma half-life (K$_2$tu-PA: CGP 42 935). Thrombosis and Haemostasis 1993; 70: 294–300

83. Paoni NF, Keyt BA, Refino CJ, Chow AM, Nguyen HV, Berleau LT, Badillo J, Peña LC, Brady K, Wurm FM, Ogez J, Bennet WF. A slow clearing, fibrin-specific, PAI-1 resistant variant of t-PA (T103N, KHRR 296–299 AAAA). Thrombosis Haemostas 1993; 70: 307–312

84. Refino CJ, Paoni NF, Keyt BA, Pater CS, Badillo JM, Ogez J, Bennet WF. A variant of t-PA (T103N, KHRR 296–299 AAAA) that, by bolus, has increased potency and decreased systemic activation of plasminogen. Thrombosis Haemostasis 1993; 70: 313–319

85. Bode C, Matsueda G, Hui KY, Haber E. Antibody-directed urokinase: a specific fibrinolytic agent. Science 1985; 229: 765–767

86. Runge MS, Bode C, Matsueda GR, Haber E. Conjugation to an antifibrin monoclonal antibody enhances the fibrinolytic potency of tissue plaminogen activator in vitro. Biochemistry 1988; 27: 1153–1157

87. Bode C, Meinhardt G, Runge MS, et al. Conjugation of urokinase to an antiplatelet antibody results in a more potent fibrinolytic agent. Thromb Haemostasis 1989; 62: 483

88. Vanderschueren S, Van de Werfe F, Collen D. Recombinant staphylokinase for thrombolytic therapy. Fibrinol Proteol 1997, Suppl 2: 39–44

89. Daniels LB, Parker JA, Patel SR, Grodstein F, Goldhaber SZ. Relation of duration of symptoms with response to thrombolytic therapy in pulmonary embolism. Am J Cardiol 1997; 80: 184–188

90. Tibbutt DA, Davies JA, Anderson JA, et al. Comparison by controlled clinical trial of streptokinase and heparin in treatment of life-threatening pulmonary embolism. Br Med J 1974; i: 343–347

91. Ly B, Arnesen H, Eie H, Hol R. A controlled clinical trial of streptokinase and heparin in the treatment of major pulmonary embolism. Acta Med Scand 1978; 203: 465–470

92. Anonymous. Tissue plasminogen activator for the treatment of acute pulmonary embolism. A collaborative study by the PIOPED investigators. Chest 1990; 97: 528–533

93. Levine M, Hirsh J, Weitz J, et al. A randomized trial of a single bolus dosage regimen of recombinant tissue plasminogen activator in patients with acute pulmonary embolism. Chest 1990; 98: 1473–1479

94. Anonymous. The UKEP study: multicentre clinical trial on two local regimens of urokinase in massive pulmonary embolism. The UKEP Study Research Group. Eur Heart J 1987; 8: 2–10

VI.3 Surgical intervention in the treatment of pulmonary embolism and chronic thromboembolic pulmonary hypertension

D. P. Kapelanski, J. A. Macoviak, S. W. Jamieson

Operative management of acute pulmonary embolism

The annual prevalence of deep venous thrombosis in the United States has been estimated at approximately 2 million cases [1]. Within this cohort, pulmonary embolism (PE) occurs in nearly one-third, accounting for an annual occurrence of somewhat more than 600,000 cases [2]. Of these 600,000 individuals with acute PE, the embolism is the immediate cause of death in 8 to 12 % of patients, or about 60,000 individuals yearly [3]. By way of comparison, motor vehicle related deaths claimed 43,536 individuals and firearm-related deaths claimed 38,317 individuals in the United States during 1991 [4].

When acute PE is fatal, in approximately 35 % of cases this is within the initial hour, and it is not unreasonable to conclude that the majority in this cohort will almost always be beyond the hope of intervention [2, 5]. Of those who survive longer than one hour, a correct diagnosis is made and the appropriate treatment initiated in only 29 %, and even in hospitalised patients, the recognition rate is not significantly higher [2, 6–10]. Conversely, even a worst case estimate suggests that in about 12,000 instances annually, a patient with an acute PE survives longer than one hour, is correctly diagnosed, is provided with appropriate treatment, yet nevertheless succumbs [11].

Although fatal PE is often the terminal event in hospitalised patients with advanced malignancy or end stage heart and lung disorders, in as many as 40 % intermediate term survival is jeopardised solely by the PE [10–13]. If one adopts the more conservative estimate, that only 20 % would have been long term survivors in the absence of the embolism, this cursory analysis implies that in the United States annually no fewer than 2,400 otherwise healthy individuals might benefit from more aggressive management of their acute embolic disease than is presently practised [13]. Although this is a substantial number, this same analysis suggests that an alternative to current treatment algo-

rithms would be required in somewhat fewer than 2 % of the patients who are both diagnosed with acute PE, and who have survived the initial hour. The remaining patients would either survive anyway or be disqualified from more aggressive intervention by virtue of concurrent disease.

At the present time, three treatment modalities that may be beneficial in this subgroup are available: thrombolysis (see Chapter VI.2); catheter embolectomy or dispersion (see Chapter VI.4); and operative embolectomy. The first two interventions are discussed in depth elsewhere in this volume; the initial portion of this chapter will focus on the third.

In 1908, Trendelenberg reported his initial experience with operative management of acute PE [14]. Although none of his three patients survived, the important concept of immediate restitution of pulmonary blood flow gained rapid acceptance. However, even though the technical aspects of embolectomy were readily mastered, clinical diagnosis was infrequent prior to circulatory collapse, and in the absence of suitable resuscitation techniques, hypoxic brain injury was almost certain. Long term survival with complete functional recovery was therefore not reported until 1924 [15]. In 1960, Allison successfully used total body hypothermia and circulatory arrest for this operation [16], though the advantages of this technique were rapidly superseded by those afforded by cardiopulmonary bypass [17]. Even within the past decade, however, embolectomy with inflow occlusion has been advocated as a life-saving alternative when extracorporeal support is not readily available [18].

Despite the feasibility of embolectomy, its role in the management of acute PE has long been contested, and we are unaware of persuasive new data that might permit resolution of this debate. Suffice it to say, so long as patients die of acute PE, the method will justifiably have adherents.

Furthermore, two techniques may well compel increasing consideration of embolectomy. First, as described in Chapter IV.2, echocardiography with Doppler interrogation offers a rapid, non-invasive method to screen for pulmonary hypertension, and can demonstrate centrally located pulmonary arterial thrombi, as well as thrombi in transit through the right heart [19–21]. Of perhaps greater importance, the echocardiographic demonstration of indices of imminent right ventricular failure may allow efficient stratification of patients and allow identification of a higher risk group that would benefit from urgent right ventricular decompression. In this group, there will always be a proportion for which thrombolytic agents pose an excessive hazard [22–27]. Second, the advent of percutaneous circulatory support systems may improve the success of resuscitation in hospitalised patients with circulatory collapse, offering an opportunity for diagnosis in a group already proven to be at increased risk [27, 28].

Operative technique

In those patients not already sustained by extracorporeal support, circulatory stability is precarious. Under such circumstances, the hazards implicit in any delay in operation must be balanced by the advantages that might accrue with the provision of additional invasive monitoring prior to induction. At the minimum, the surface electrocardiogram, cutaneous oximetry, and arterial pressure should be monitored.

Our colleagues currently prefer etomidate (0.2 mg/kg, i.v.) to other agents for anesthetic induction; if clinically warranted, supplemental fentanyl citrate (10–40 µg/kg, i.v.) can be cautiously administered. Neuromuscular blockade can be achieved by administration of pipecuronium bromide (10 mg, i.v.).

Median sternotomy provides rapid access for central cannulation and is the incision of choice. Even in those patients stabilised by extracorporeal assistance preoperatively, it is advantageous to convert to a conventional circuit during the embolectomy. While peripheral arterial cannulation would be acceptable, the complete diversion of venous blood provided by separate caval cannulation facilitates visibility within the pulmonary arterial tree, and permits removal of thrombus in transit within the right heart or central veins [29]. The addition of a heat exchanger to the extracorporeal circuit will allow the induction of modest systemic hypothermia, increasing the tolerance for limited intervals of reduced flow or circulatory arrest. De-

compression of the left ventricle is desirable, since bronchial flow may inhibit inspection of the distal pulmonary arteries.

An anterior incision in the main pulmonary artery, extending from 1 cm distal to the valve to the bifurcation, provides adequate visibility. Unless operation has been delayed for several days, the embolic material is not adherent and can be easily extracted. Because some fragmentation may have occurred, either preoperatively or during the evacuation, it is essential to inspect the distal vessels to ensure patency. Extracorporeal flow can be transiently reduced or interrupted to facilitate this examination. Any thrombotic material encountered can generally be removed with forceps or suction; gentle, manual inflation of the lungs may dislodge more distal fragments, and by propelling them centrally allow easy retrieval. The distal right pulmonary artery is not readily inspected through an incision in the main pulmonary artery, and accordingly, an additional arteriotomy on the anterior surface of the right main pulmonary artery, between the ascending aorta and the superior vena cava, will prove helpful. Alternatively, fiberoptic angioscopy can be used to examine the distal vessels, though the instrumentation is not routinely available [30]. Once distal patency is confirmed, both arteriotomies are repaired with continuous monofilament suture. If intraoperative transesophageal echocardiography demonstrates thrombus in transit, a limited right atriotomy allows removal, and is similarly repaired. Extracorporeal support is thereafter weaned in standard fashion.

Results

Not unexpectedly, perioperative mortality following embolectomy for acute PE is related to the severity of preoperative disability, and to a lesser extent on the operative technique. Relatively few patients (26%) withstand normothermic arrest with inflow occlusion when operation follows a preoperative arrest, though in experienced hands this same technique affords excellent survival (97%) when undertaken in patients with lesser degrees of impairment [18]. In patients undergoing embolectomy with the assistance of cardiopulmonary bypass, the influence of preoperative arrest on anoxic neurologic injury is comparable, and in its absence survival in excess of 80% can be achieved [31–39]. With either method, operation is easier and the outcome better when the emboli are encountered centrally [37, 39–41].

Late evaluation of survivors indicates the initial hemodynamic improvements are generally sustained and functional impairment is rare in the absence of recurrent embolisation. Concurrent disease, primarily malignancy, is the most important determinant of late survival [31, 39, 41].

Chronic thromboembolic pulmonary hypertension

Epidemiology and the natural history of the disease

In the overwhelming majority of treated patients who survive the acute episode, pulmonary emboli resolve without apparent clinical or physiologic sequelae, and it has been estimated that chronic thromboembolic disease will develop in only 0.5% of patients with a clinically recognised acute PE [42, 43]. Based on the prevalence of PE, these data suggest that approximately 2,500 individuals may progress to chronic thromboembolic pulmonary hypertension in the United States each year [44]. However, because many patients diagnosed with chronic thromboembolic disease have no antecedent history of acute embolism, the true incidence of this disorder may well be somewhat greater. In one large, unselected autopsy series, the prevalence of chronic major vessel thrombi was as high as 1%, suggesting that chronic thromboembolic disease might afflict as many as 100,000 individuals in the United States [45].

Although various theories have been advanced, in the preponderance of patients the etiology of unresolved or chronic thromboembolic disease is unknown [46, 47]. In those patients with persistent defects on serial perfusion scans, only a minority have a recognised disorder of the coagulation or thrombolytic cascades; among the more commonly identified are the presence of a lupus anticoagulant or deficiencies of protein C or antithrombin [48].

In the absence of operation, the prognosis of patients with chronic thromboembolic disease and pulmonary hypertension is poor. Survival is inversely related to the severity of pulmonary hypertension at diagnosis; fewer than 10% survive five years when the pulmonary artery pressure exceeds 50 mm Hg [49]. Chronic anticoagulation represents the mainstay of the medical regimen. Though anticoagulation is primarily employed to forestall future embolic episodes, it also serves to limit the development of thrombus in regions of low flow within the pulmonary vasculature. Inferior vena caval filters are routinely employed to prevent recurrent embolisation. If caval filtration and anticoagulation fail to prevent recurrent emboli, immediate thrombolysis may prove useful, but it must be noted that lytic agents are incapable of altering the chronic component of the disease.

The symptomatic manifestations of right ventricular failure are conventionally treated with diuretics and vasodilators, and while improvement may ensue, the effect is generally transient unless the fundamental pathophysiologic process is addressed [50, 51].

Clinical evaluation

In the initial phase, chronic thromboembolic pulmonary vascular disease may pose a difficult diagnostic problem. The cardinal symptom is progressive exercise intolerance, typically characterised as exertional breathlessness, although chest discomfort may also be described, and syncope is an infrequent index occurrence [42, 45]. In young individuals, the development of dyspnea generally prompts an aggressive evaluation. In the middle-aged and elderly, however, and in particular when a prior embolism has not been documented, the development of mild dyspnea or vague exertional chest discomfort is often initially ascribed to maladies more frequent in that population, including among others emphysema, coronary atherosclerosis, and simple physical deconditioning.

A careful examination in the early stages of the disease may reveal prolongation of the second heart sound with an invariant, accentuated P2. Murmurs caused by turbulent flow in partially obstructed lobar and segmental pulmonary arteries may occasionally be appreciated posteriorly over the lung fields. With increasing right ventricular compromise, jugular venous distension with prominence of the A and V waves may be evident, and generally precedes the identification of a murmur of tricuspid regurgitation and the development of a right ventricular lift. Peripheral oedema is a variable finding, and the association with right-sided failure may be especially difficult to discern in the patient with chronic lower extremity venous stasis. As right-sided failure progresses, cyanosis, hepatomegaly, and ascites are signs forewarning limited survival.

The electrocardiogram is generally featureless; however, right ventricular hypertrophy or strain are the characteristic patterns if pathologic variations are found. Usually, spirometry is also unexceptional; when noted, the typical anomaly is of mild to moderate restriction as a result of prior infarction and parenchymal scarring [52]. Rarely, mild obstruction is noted, and when present has been attributed to the development of an exuberant bronchial collateral circulation with hyperemia of the distal airways. Maximum minute ventilation is frequently elevated to compensate for the increase in dead space; not unexpectedly, the latter abnormality is exacerbated with exercise. While the majority of patients exhibit a reduction in carbon monoxide diffusion capacity, this feature is neither invariant nor specific. Concordant with the above, hypoxemia at rest is distinctly less frequent than during exercise, and hypercapnia altogether uncommon.

Although the chest roentgenogram is not typically diagnostic, right ventricular prominence is a frequent finding, as are enlargement or asymmetry of the main pulmonary arteries (Fig. 1). Similarly, a pattern of asymmetric perfusion associated with pruning of the pulmonary vascular markings is commonplace. Peripheral scarring and regional pleural thickening attributable to prior pulmonary infarction are occasionally identified.

Given the relatively indistinct characteristics of early and limited disease, it is not surprising that chronic thromboembolic pulmonary hypertension

is rarely the initial diagnosis considered, and it is frequent for patients to solicit the opinion of several consultants before the process is accurately identified. As indicated above, this is particularly problematic when a prior history of acute embolism is lacking. Whenever the diagnosis of chronic thromboembolic pulmonary hypertension is carefully thought about, the most useful screening studies are two-dimensional surface echocardiography with Doppler imaging and radionuclide ventilation-perfusion scanning [51, 53–56].

The echocardiogram typically demonstrates right-sided chamber enlargement and right ventricular hypertrophy. The interventricular septum may appear flattened and often exhibits paradoxical motion. Tricuspid regurgitation is a common finding. The main pulmonary artery is generally enlarged, and Doppler imaging demonstrates an increase in pulmonary artery pressure. Exercise characteristically increases the pulmonary hypertension, and should routinely be employed whenever the disease is suspected but the resting echocardiogram demonstrates only subtle abnormalities. The typical radionuclide ventilation perfusion scan demonstrates one or more unmatched lobar or segmental perfusion defects. While not frequently available, prior studies provide an important basis for comparison, particularly when the studies suggest limited, rather than absent segmental perfusion. Because radionuclide perfusion scans characteristi-

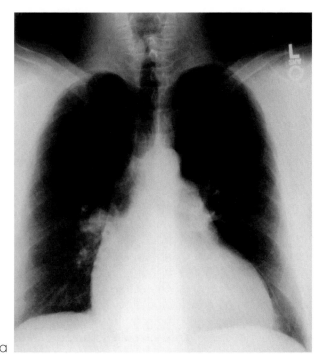
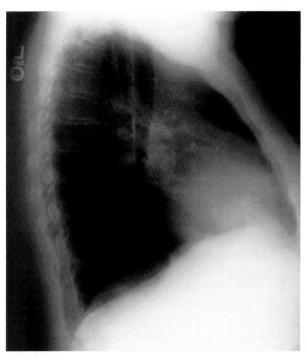

a   b

Fig. 1a, b. PA (a) and lateral (b) radiographs reveal severe cardiomegaly with right ventricular enlargement. There is enlargement of the main, right and left pulmonary arteries.

385

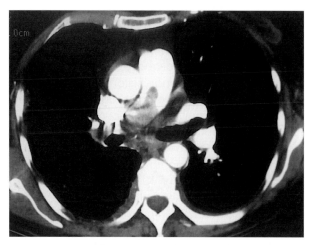

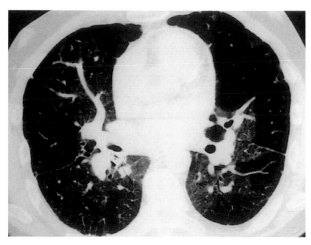

Fig. 2a. CT scan demonstrating enlargement of the main pulmonary artery and thrombus in the main pulmonary artery extending into the proximal right pulmonary artery.

Fig. 2b. CT scan demonstrating mosaic oligemia characteristic of chronic thromboembolic pulmonary disease.

cally underestimate the extent of disease demonstrated by angiography and defined at operation, an equivocal scan in a patient with other features suggestive of chronic thromboembolic disease should not preclude additional evaluation [57].

Recently, computed tomography (CT) and magnetic resonance imaging (MRI) have been advocated as screening techniques for the diagnosis of chronic thromboembolic pulmonary hypertension [58–62]. Thrombus within the central pulmonary arteries is better demonstrated by helical CT than either conventional CT or MRI, though the absence of thrombus proximal to the segmental pulmonary arteries is not a valid exclusionary criterion, nor does its presence exclude other pulmonary hypertensive disorders (Fig. 2). Helical CT may also demonstrate enlarged bronchial arteries or a pattern of mosaic oligemia; the latter appears to be a relatively specific marker for chronic thromboembolic disease [62]. The adjunct visualisation of other thoracic structures with either method may suggest other causes of pulmonary hypertension, including mediastinal fibrosis and neoplasia. At present, however, neither MRI or CT has sufficient accuracy to establish an unequivocal diagnosis of chronic thromboembolic pulmonary hypertension, nor does either method provide sufficient information to define operative candidacy accurately. Accordingly, we do not routinely utilise either as screening methods in our own practice.

The combination of right heart catheterisation and selective pulmonary arteriography is the accepted standard with which to establish the diagnosis of chronic thromboembolic pulmonary hypertension. The angiographic features include the presence of scalloped intimal irregularities; pouch-like defects; abrupt reductions in vessel calibre, up to and in-

cluding complete obstruction of segmental and more proximal arteries, or the presence of bands traversing the vessel lumen (Fig. 3) [63]. Although digital subtraction angiography can be employed as a screening examination, the resolution is only rarely adequate to determine operative candidacy, and we do not employ this method in our own practice. If pulmonary pressures and resistance are only modestly elevated at right heart catheterisation, but other studies, including arteriography, are concordant with the diagnosis of chronic thromboembolic disease, hemodynamics should be reassessed during exercise or pharmacological stress to ascertain if flow limitation ensues. Coronary cineangiography is also routinely attained at this time in individuals with the appropriate risk profile. Because patency of the distal pulmonary vasculature is rarely a consideration in the absence of prior infarction, selective bronchial artery angiography is not indicated [64].

Percutaneous fiberoptic pulmonary angioscopy is reserved for those instances in which pulmonary arteriography reveals equivocal features [65]. Angioscopy is most frequently employed when typical angiographic features are identified solely in segmental and more peripheral pulmonary artery branches. Other, less common indications include an apparent unilateral process or disease in which the clinical features appear disproportionately more severe than the apparent extent of angiographic involvement. The characteristic angioscopic findings in chronic thromboembolic pulmonary disease are precisely those encountered at operation, specifically intimal thickening and irregularity, and the presence of pouches, bands and webs.

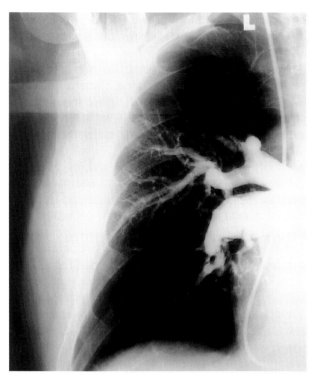

Fig. 3a. Right pulmonary angiogram depicting markedly diminished flow to lower lobe, with preservation of some perfusion to the upper and middle lobes. Multiple pouches and webs are evident. Same patient as in Fig. 1.

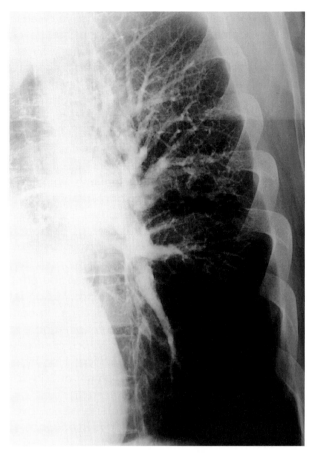

Fig. 3b. Left pulmonary angiogram demonstrates reduced flow to lower lobe, with irregularity of the descending pulmonary artery and band formation. There is relative preservation of flow to apico-posterior and anterior segments of the upper lobe. Same patient as in Fig. 1.

Operative management of chronic thromboembolic pulmonary hypertension

Hollister first proposed thromboendarterectomy for chronic thromboembolic pulmonary hypertension in 1956 [66]. Over the following two decades, the procedure was attempted only sporadically. In a 1984 review, the aggregate world experience was 85 patients, with a perioperative mortality rate of 22% [16, 67–71]. The team at the University of California, San Diego Medical Center, has benefited from an institutional experience of nearly 900 operative cases over the past 27 years [72–75]. Our current approach, described below, has been continuously refined while accumulating a personal experience presently in excess of 700 procedures [76].

Pulmonary thromboendarterectomy is indicated for symptomatic individuals with proven or strongly suspected chronic thromboembolic disease amenable to operative correction. The majority of patients are within New York Heart Association class III or class IV at the time of operation. However, we do not exclude patients with lesser disability, since the natural history of this disease suggests that inexorable deterioration is the rule and our present experience allows operation to be tendered at an acceptably low risk. In general, the pulmonary vascular resistance in minimally symptomatic individuals exceeds 300 dynes/sec/cm^5 at rest or during stress. There is no upper limit of pulmonary vascular resistance that would exclude patients from operation.

The criteria defining operative accessibility encompass both anatomy and operative experience. We are confident in our ability to recognise the various endovascular manifestations of this disease, and can readily initiate a plane of dissection within the individual segmental pulmonary arteries if necessary. Thus it is our feeling that pulmonary hypertension as a result of emboli is always operable. However, it can be quite arduous to discriminate between chronic thrombo-obliterative disease and the chronic, atheromatous changes that develop secondary to long-standing pulmonary hypertension, particularly when the pathologic changes are encountered at relatively distal levels. It is worth emphasising that at whatever level the obstruction begins, success can be assured only if the most distal tendrils of the propagated thrombus are removed. Operation is almost inevitably lethal whenever a significant improvement in pulmonary flow is not achieved in those patients with high preoperative pulmonary vascular resistance.

Our screening evaluation comprises the assessment previously elaborated, as well as any additional studies necessary to fully assess risk in an individual destined to undergo a major operation. Advanced chronological age is not considered a barrier, and we have successfully operated on individuals well within their eighth decade. In contrast, co-morbid disorders that are not amenable to correction prior to operation, and which are likely to increment operative risk significantly or independently limit functional improvement or survival are generally a basis for exclusion.

If not previously implanted, an inferior vena caval filter is routinely placed several days in advance of operation.

Operative technique

Routine monitoring for anesthetic induction consists of the surface electrocardiogram, cutaneous oximetry, and radial and pulmonary artery pressures. Apprehensive patients may be pre-medicated with midazolam hydrochloride (1–4 mg, i. v.) or fentanyl citrate (50–100 µg, i. v.). In the majority of patients, anesthesia is induced with fentanyl (20–40 µg/kg, i. v.). If cardiac function is satisfactory, midazolam (2–10 mg, i. v.) is added. Neuromuscular blockade is achieved by administration of pipecuronium bromide (10 mg, i. v.).

Following induction and intubation and prior to incision, monitoring is supplemented by the addition of capnography, transesophageal echocardiography and electro-encephalography. Because gradients frequently develop between central and peripheral arterial pressure during the rewarming period, femoral arterial pressure monitoring is our customary practice. Body temperature is assessed using thermistors incorporated in the pulmonary artery and bladder catheters. Left atrial pressure is not regularly determined.

If the patient maintains permissive hemodynamics following the induction of anesthesia, up to 500 ml

of autologous whole blood is withdrawn for later use, and the volume deficit replaced with crystalloid.

Because chronic thromboembolic pulmonary hypertension is almost uniformly a bilateral process, the ideal exposure is obtained with a median sternotomy incision. Venous inflow to the heart-lung machine is achieved by trans-atrial insertion of separate superior and inferior vena caval cannulae, while arterialised blood is returned through a conventional cannula in the ascending aorta. Immediate decompression of the heart is attained by insertion of a vent catheter in the main pulmonary artery. Once ventricular fibrillation ensues during systemic hypothermia, additional decompression is achieved with a vent catheter placed in the right superior pulmonary vein and directed across the mitral valve into the left ventricle. Caval snares are placed and tightened to completely divert systemic venous return.

The conduct of cardiopulmonary bypass has been previously described [77]. Beef lung heparin sodium (400 units/kg, i. v.) is administered to prolong the activated clotting time beyond 400 seconds, and supplemental heparin is administered as required to maintain this level of anticoagulation. An asanguinous prime (Plasma-Lyte, 1600 ml) is supplemented with albumin (25 g), mannitol (12.5 g), methylprednisolone sodium succinate (30 mg/kg) and additional heparin (100 units/kg). Moderate hemodilution (hematocrit 18–25%) is standard. Phenytoin sodium (15 mg/kg, i. v., maximum 1,000 mg) is administered at the onset of cardiopulmonary bypass to reduce the risk of perioperative seizure. Aprotinin is strictly avoided to obviate the potential for early thrombotic occlusion in the endarterectomised vessels. In patients with documented heparin-induced platelet aggregation, an infusion of epoprostenol sodium (100 ng/kg/min, i. v.) is started prior to intraoperative heparin administration, and this infusion is maintained for the initial 24 hours following operation. The intense vasodilatation ordinarily induced by this agent is effectively countered by titrated administration of phenylephrine hydrochloride.

Core cooling to a target temperature of 20°C, assessed at multiple sites, is initiated at the inception of cardiopulmonary bypass. The gradient between core and blood temperature is maintained at less than 10°C. Additional conductive cooling is provided with a thermostatically controlled blanket on the operating table, and radiant heat loss is encouraged by maintenance of the operating room temperature below 20°C. Ice packs are dispersed over the cranium.

While the patient is being cooled on bypass the superior vena cava is mobilised by dissection of the investing pericardium with cautery, avoiding entry into the right pleural space and either traction or thermal injury to the right phrenic nerve. The cephalad limit of this dissection is the azygos vein postero-laterally and the junction of the superior vena cava with the innominate vein antero-medially. If during this mobilisation the postero-medial dissection strays from the superior vena cava, the nodal tissue at the tracheo-bronchial angle may inadvertently be traversed, engendering immediate hemorrhage from enlarged bronchial collaterals, or promoting prolonged lymphatic drainage after operation. A modified cerebellar retractor is used to displace the superior vena cava laterally and the ascending aorta medially, thus facilitating separation of the right main pulmonary artery from the left atrium, and permitting antero-lateral exposure of the origin of the ascending lobar artery and the medial segmental artery.

Once the targeted core temperature is attained, the anterior surface of the right main pulmonary artery is incised. The medial extent of this incision is approximately 1 cm lateral to the adventitial fusion of the ascending aorta and right main pulmonary artery, and readily allows reconstruction. The incision is continued laterally along the anterior aspect of the descending pulmonary artery, terminating immediately proximal to the origin of the medial segmental artery.

Despite complete diversion of systemic venous return and both right and left sided venting, the extensive bronchial collateral flow only occasionally allows intravascular dissection at this juncture. Whenever blood obscures the pulmonary artery lumen, the aorta is clamped, and cold blood cardioplegia (10 ml/kg, maximum 1,000 ml) is instilled proximal to the aortic clamp. Following administration of cardioplegia, blood is evacuated from the left heart by gentle aspiration applied to the cardioplegia delivery catheter. Additional cardioplegia is never administered. A recirculating cooling jacket prevents myocardial rewarming. Cerebral electrical quiescence is induced at this time by titrated administration of thiopental sodium (500 – 1,000 mg, i. v.).

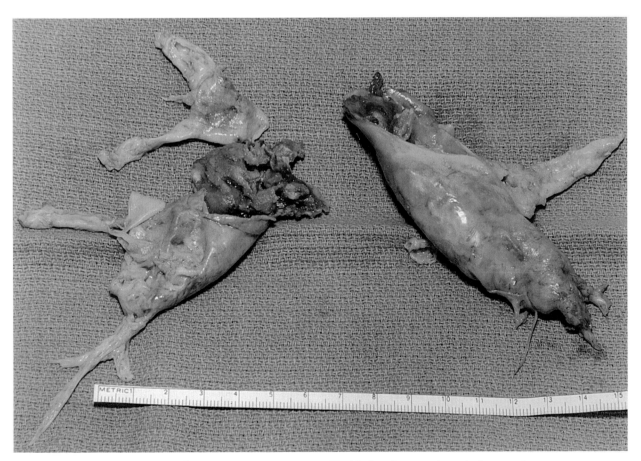

Fig. 4. Operative specimen arrayed in anatomic position. Laminated friable thrombus is evident in both main pulmonary arteries. Abrupt termination of both descending pulmonary arteries can be seen. The thickened, fibrous layer is characteristic of remodelled thrombus. Same patient as in Fig. 1.

Circulatory arrest is then initiated, and the patient exsanguinated. Gentle repeated manual inflation of the lungs simplifies the evacuation of blood from within the pulmonary vessels and permits further dissection under conditions of ideal visibility. Any loose, thrombotic debris encountered is first removed. Then, a microtome knife is used to develop the endarterectomy plane posteriorly, since any inadvertent egress at this site could be readily repaired. The plane is developed laterally and anteriorly with a specially designed aspirating dissector, preserving the full thickness of the artery immediately adjacent to the arteriotomy, which facilitates a hemostatic closure. The medial endpoint of the dissection is carefully trimmed; retrograde dissection within the right pulmonary artery is only sporadically required to restore an effective lumen. Dissection within the descending pulmonary artery is rendered easier if the endarterectomy plane is developed circumferentially directly beyond the distal extent of the arteriotomy. It is generally simplest to complete the dissection of the ascending artery before initiating the dissection of the descending artery. Visibility within both major branches is ordinarily superb with this approach, and only rarely is the arteriotomy extended superiorly to enhance exposure within the ascending artery. With care and experience, the eversion dissection ordinarily allows removal of chronic, thromboembolic material at least two branching generations distal to the origin of the segmental arteries (Fig. 4). At the completion of the dissection, the lumen is carefully inspected and any residual debris evacuated. In spite of the relatively tenuous nature of the distal pulmonary artery branches, disruption or perforation has not been problematic.

Ordinarily, the thromboendarterectomy can be completed on either side during a single circulatory arrest period less than 20 minutes in duration. If, after that interval, it appears certain that the dissection could be concluded within an additional five minutes, the arrest period is extended by just that amount. Conversely, if the dissection is unlikely to be completed within 25 minutes or less of circulatory arrest, a reperfusion interval of not less than 10 minutes is provided, and circulation is not again interrupted until the saturation of mixed venous blood exceeds 90%. We believe that strict adherence to this regimen has minimised the occurrence of anoxic neurological complications, although in our experience multiple arrest periods are only infrequently required.

Once the right thromboendarterectomy is completed, the arteriotomy is repaired with a continuous monofilament suture. A meticulously constructed, tension-free, hemostatic closure is essential, since hemorrhage from either pulmonary arteriotomy is unlikely to be reparable without resumption of cardiopulmonary bypass.

Endovascular exposure of the left pulmonary artery is then begun. Inferior and right lateral displacement of the heart enhances visibility of the intrapericardial extent of the left pulmonary artery. The pulmonary vent catheter is withdrawn, and the arteriotomy extended laterally to the pericardial reflection, avoiding entry into the left pleural space. Additional lateral dissection does not enhance intraluminal visibility, and may endanger the left phrenic nerve. Since the preceding dissection has generally re-established normal arterial patency on the right side, with resulting back flow from the bronchial circulation, dissection within the left pulmonary artery is usually impossible without the induction of circulatory arrest and exsanguination, as described above.

The left-sided dissection is virtually analogous in all respects to that accomplished on the right. As on the right, the thromboendarterectomy plane is initiated posteriorly, and distal dissection is facilitated by circumferential development of the plane distal to the arteriotomy. In distinction to the right-sided dissection, that on the left can ordinarily be initiated beyond the arteriotomy; if this proves impossible, preservation of a full thickness margin immediately adjacent to the arteriotomy will aid the subsequent repair. Although the left main bronchus frequently hinders visibility of the basilar segmental arteries, this is easily remedied by the careful application of lateral pressure with the aspirating dissector, displacing the bronchus medially. Any attempt to improve exposure by lateral pressure of the basilar vessels is likely to endanger them. The duration of circulatory arrest intervals during performance of the left-sided dissection is subject to the identical restrictions previously described.

With completion of thromboendarterectomy on the left, cardiopulmonary bypass is re-instituted. Simultaneously, supplemental methylprednisolone (500 mg, i. v.) and mannitol (12.5 g, i. v.) are administered. The pulmonary vent catheter is replaced, and the distal arteriotomy is repaired, using the technique formerly used on the right. Rewarming is initiated with the resumption of extracorporeal circulation. As during cooling, the thermal gradient between blood and core temperature is maintained at less than 10°C. The cranial ice-packs are discarded, and additional heat transfer is afforded by the thermostatically controlled blanket. Sodium nitroprusside is routinely administered to promote vasodilatation and ensure homogeneous rewarming.

If indicated, myocardial re-vascularisation or intra-cardiac procedures are routinely accomplished during the re-warming interval. With the restoration of normal pulmonary artery pressures, tricuspid valve regurgitation is invariably and rapidly rectified, and accordingly, tricuspid valve reconstruction is not attempted [55]. The foramen ovale, if open, is routinely closed. We preferentially employ a one centimetre lateral incision, immediately cephalad to the inferior vena cava, in order to minimise the risk of postoperative atrial dysrhythmias. Myocardial cooling is discontinued once all cardiac procedures have been concluded. The caval snares are released, and air assiduously displaced from within the heart, lungs and aorta prior to the restoration of coronary perfusion.

Lidocaine hydrochloride (200 mg, i. v.) is administered at the onset of myocardial reperfusion, and calcium chloride (1 g, i. v.) is given approximately 20 minutes later. The left-sided vent is removed prior to defibrillation, while the right-sided vent is maintained until the cessation of assisted circulation. A vent in the ascending aorta is maintained throughout the rewarming interval to allow the unhampered egress of air.

The extensive intra-pericardial dissection, in concert with the rapid resumption of systemic anticoagulation, has in the past been associated with an appreciable incidence of delayed tamponade. To minimise this, a posterior pericardial window can readily be created on the left side prior to termination of extracorporeal support. Alternatively, a malleable, closed drainage system is placed intraoperatively and retained until the risk of delayed tamponade is diminished.

Discontinuation of extracorporeal support is accomplished using conventional criteria. Dopamine hydrochloride is routinely administered at renal doses, while other inotropic agents and vasodilators are titrated as necessary to sustain acceptable hemodynamics. Temporary atrial and ventricular epicardial pacing wires are customarily placed. Despite the duration of extracorporeal circulation, hemostasis is readily achieved, and homologous platelets or coagulation factors are infrequently utilised. We do not customarily administer e-aminocaproic acid or desmopressin acetate. The techniques employed for mediastinal drainage and wound closure do not vary from those employed in other patients we attend.

Post operative care

In most respects, the postoperative management of patients undergoing thromboendarterectomy does not differ from that of other patients undergoing major cardiac operations in our institution. Intermittent pneumatic calf compression is requisite until discharge. Once the risk of perioperative hemorrhage has abated, heparin prophylaxis is initiated. Warfarin is restarted once central venous and arterial catheters have been removed, with a target International Normalised Ratio (INR) of 2.5 to 3 times the control value. In addition to particular concern for the risk of recurrent venous thromboembolism in these patients, three phenomena are distinct to this procedure and merit specific mention: residual pulmonary hypertension, pulmonary steal, and pulmonary reperfusion injury.

Persistent pulmonary hypertension is the most vexing of these problems, since at first glance a flaw in the preoperative evaluation and in the operative conduct seems implicit, but foremost because survival is unlikely. We do operate on some very ill patients in whom we think that the underlying lesion may be primary pulmonary hypertension. The justification is that occasionally we cannot be certain and we do not believe that they will survive until a donor could be found – transplantation otherwise being the only therapy. In our most recent 330 patients, 36.4% of perioperative deaths were directly attributable to the problem of inadequate relief of pulmonary artery hypertension. Attempts at pharmacological manipulation of high residual pulmonary vascular resistance with sodium nitroprusside, epoprostenol sodium, or inhaled nitric oxide have not been efficacious, nor have we salvaged any with the creation of a controlled aperture atrial septal defect to allow right ventricular decompression. Because our experience has demonstrated the residual hypertensive defect is fixed, we do not advocate the use of mechanical circulatory support.

Pulmonary steal is largely an epiphenomenon. It was initially recognised when postoperative perfusion scans depicted regions of reduced perfusion suggestive of recurrent embolism or thrombosis [78]. Subsequent pulmonary arteriograms failed to demonstrate new defects, but instead indicated a redistribution of pulmonary flow to those segments rendered patent at operation. It is not yet certain if this pattern of preferential flow results from an unmasking of impaired arteriolar regulatory capability when chronic proximal flow limitation is alleviated, or if the steal identifies a component of arteriopathy in those segments with persistent preoperative flow and chronic exposure to elevated pulmonary pressures. Because the steal largely dissipates over time, the net consequences are insignificant [79]. However, in the perioperative period, the pattern of abnormal flow distribution has important consequences for the evolution and management of pulmonary reperfusion injury. Pulmonary reperfusion injury occurs in virtually all operated patients, although the clinical manifestations are highly variable, ranging from a mild, perioperative hypoxemia readily managed with supplemental oxygen to a fulminant variant in which hemorrhagic oedema fluid rapidly compromises effective gas exchange [80]. The features are those of a non-cardiogenic oedema initially confined to those segments in which normal antegrade pulmonary blood flow has been reconstituted at operation. Because of the steal phenomenon, the consequent ventilation : perfusion unbalance cannot be compensated for by normal physiologic auto-regulatory mechanisms, compounding the severity of the gas exchange abnormality. As with many other forms of acute lung injury, leukocytes appear to play a permissive role in the development and expression of this disorder [81, 82].

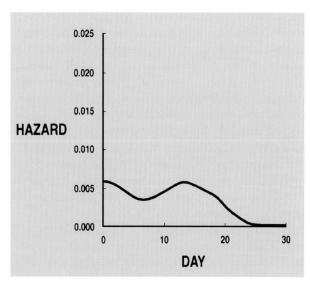

Fig. 5. The instantaneous hazard function for death in hospital within the initial 30 days following pulmonary thromboendarterectomy was estimated using the SPSS procedure SURVIVAL. Surviving patients were censored at hospital discharge. The hazard function was smoothed over the 30 day interval using distance weighted least squares (SYSTAT procedure PLOT). An initial peak hazard associated primarily with residual pulmonary hypertension occurred on postoperative day two (0.0154 ± 0.007) (mean ± SE). A second relative maximum extended from postoperative days 14 (0.0172 ± 0.012) through day 18 (0.0190 ± 0.019). and reflected the influence of other causes of mortality, predominately reperfusion injury.

The management principles in severe reperfusion injury are not substantially different from those supportive measures employed in other forms of acute lung injury, including a careful titration of positive end-expiratory pressure, the progressive transition from volume-limited to pressure-limited, inverse ratio ventilation, and the judicious acceptance of moderate hypercapnia. Assiduous fluid management is essential, transfusing homologous blood as necessary to maintain effective systemic oxygen delivery. Albeit limited, our recent experience suggests inhaled nitric oxide may prove useful. When hypoxemia has been refractory to these measures, and provided cardiac output is not limited by residual pulmonary hypertension, we have successfully employed veno-venous extracorporeal carbon dioxide removal (ECCO2R).

Results

Over the most recent three calendar years (1/1/1994 – 31/12/1996), our team has performed 330 pulmonary thromboendarterectomies. The mean patient age was 52 ± 15 years (mean ± standard deviation). The youngest in this series was 16, and the oldest 85. There was a slight male predominance, with 178 men and 152 women.

In nearly one-third of these cases, at least one additional cardiac procedure was performed during the same anesthetic; most commonly, the adjunct procedure was closure of a persistent foramen ovale (86 patients, 26.1 %) or coronary artery bypass grafting (27 patients, 8.2 %). There was one instance each of aortic, mitral, and tricuspid valve replacement for calcific stenosis, myxomatous degeneration, and endocarditis with vegetation, respectively. One patient suffered an intra-operative aortic dissection and received a prosthetic graft. An open lung biopsy and a breast biopsy were each performed once, in separate patients. The average operative procedure was completed in 6.7 ± 1.1 hours, and required 245 ± 46 minutes of cardiopulmonary bypass and 97 ± 25 minutes of myocardial ischemia. The average, cumulative circulatory arrest time required to perform bilateral thromboendarterectomy was 35 ± 13 minutes.

Operative mortality

Twenty-two patients (6.7 %) did not survive operation. The instantaneous hazard function for hospital mortality is represented in Figure 5. Among those who died, residual pulmonary hypertension was the proximate cause in eight (2.5%). The median survival for patients dying as a consequence of persistent pulmonary hypertension was two days (5 ± 7), including one intra-operative death. In each instance, severe right ventricular failure was rapidly followed by progressive renal and hepatic dysfunction.

Eight deaths (2.5%) were attributable to severe reperfusion injury. Perioperative myocardial infarction, global neurological injury and septicemia each occurred in separate patients within this group, and were important factors contributing to postoperative death. One patient with severe reperfusion injury and modest residual pulmonary hypertension was initially stabilised and was improving while on ECCO2R, but suffered a cardiac arrest during an oxygenator exchange, at which time the family elected to terminate support. In contrast to the fairly rapid demise of patients dying from residual pulmonary hypertension, the median postoperative survival in this group was nine days (18 ± 22).

In the remaining six patients, the causes of death were diverse. The patient who had received the prosthetic aortic graft developed tamponade after the withdrawal of temporary epicardial pacing leads on postoperative day four; cardiac function did not recover despite open resuscitation. One patient developed delayed tamponade and died on postoperative day seven when right ventricular perforation occurred during an attempted therapeutic pericardiocentesis. One patient with pre-operative renal and hepatic impairment who underwent urgent operation to alleviate right ventricular failure died on postoperative day 13; despite an improvement in hemodynamics, multiorgan failure was not reversed. The patient who had undergone tricuspid valve replacement died with multisystem organ failure on postoperative day 13. One patient died on postoperative day 41 of severe pancreatitis complicated by multi-system failure. One patient with moderate emphysema and chronic steroid medication died of intractable respiratory failure after 97 days; this patient had also developed a sternal wound dehiscence.

Operative morbidity

Severe reperfusion injury was the single most frequent complication, occurring in 34 instances (10.3%). As indicated above, eight patients with severe reperfusion injury did not survive; each of the remaining 26 patients required prolonged mechanical ventilatory support, and one was salvaged only by the utilisation of ECCO2R. Septic

episodes complicated the post-operative course in two patients who survived despite their reperfusion injury. Extended ventilator support necessitated tracheostomy in 10 patients in this group. The median postoperative hospitalisation in patients who survived after developing severe reperfusion injury was 35 days (39 ± 24).

Relatively few respiratory complications developed in the absence of reperfusion injury. Pneumonia developed in two patients, and there was one instance each of pneumothorax, symptomatic pleural effusion requiring thoracentesis, and lobar atelectasis requiring bronchoscopy. One patient developed sub-glottic oedema that did not improve with corticosteroids, and was managed by elective tracheostomy.

Non-fatal neurological complications occurred in five patients, for a cumulative neurological morbidity of 1.8%. Two patients with focal infarcts had completely recovered at the time of hospital discharge, while one patient with multiple embolic infarcts had residual disability at discharge, but full recovery was anticipated. One patient with transient hemiparesis on the second postoperative day was found to have a chronic subdural hematoma; the radiographic and clinical features were indeterminate for acute extension. This patient experienced complete recovery with conservative management and deferral of postoperative anticoagulation for a three week period. One patient who had undergone repair of an atrial septal aneurysm suffered a transient ischemic episode on the second postoperative day. A comprehensive evaluation was consistent with an embolism originating from the atrial suture line. No additional symptoms occurred following anticoagulation.

Early postoperative hemorrhage required re-exploration in eight patients (2.5%). Hospitalisation was prolonged in only one, and in that instance was attributable to the concomitant development of severe reperfusion injury. Six patients (1.8%) developed sternal wound complications, including sterile dehiscence in five and mediastinitis in one. The patient with mediastinitis survived, as did four of the patients with sterile dehiscence. Delayed tamponade developed in three patients (0.9%), and proved fatal in two, as described above. The third patient recovered following sub-xiphoid drainage.

Isolated cardiac complications were few. Supraventricular tachycardia requiring cardioversion occurred in four patients (1.2%). A permanent pacemaker was implanted in one patient who developed complete heart block after operation.

In the majority of patients (n = 246, 74.5%), the postoperative course was uneventful, and the median hospitalisation was a comparatively brief 10 days (11 ± 4). In contrast, the median hospital stay in survivors was prolonged to 20 days (28 ± 21) once any complication had developed.

Hemodynamic results

In this as well as prior groups, a reduction in pulmonary pressures and resistance to normal levels and the corresponding improvement in pulmonary blood flow have been both immediate and sustained [76, 83]. In addition to the hemodynamic benefits, echocardiographic studies have demonstrated that with the elimination of chronic pressure overload, right ventricular geometry rapidly reverts toward normal, and the concomitant elimination of pathological septal motion quickly restores normal left ventricular diastolic function [55, 84]. Intermediate term analyses (less than two years) within this institutional series indicate more than 90% of operative survivors will attain NYHA function class I or II status [83, 85]. While anecdotal reports describing sustained hemodynamic and functional improvement after thromboendarterectomy have been presented, a comprehensive examination of the late functional and hemodynamic status has not hitherto been feasible, since relatively few operative survivors were at risk [86]. Figure 6 demonstrates that only within the past

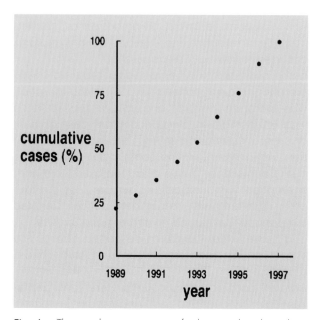

Fig. 6. The cumulative proportion of pulmonary thromboendarterectomies performed at UCSD Medical Center over the past 25 years. Fewer than 20% of the total number of procedures were performed in the 17 years prior to 1989, while more than half have been undertaken within the past five years.

few years has sufficient experience been accumulated to allow a late analysis of a suitably large sample in which perioperative mortality is not a confounding factor. This analysis is currently in progress.

Future challenges

In the majority of patients, the development of chronic thromboembolic pulmonary hypertension signifies a medical failure, initially in the prophylaxis and management of venous thrombosis, and secondarily in the recognition, treatment, and follow-up surveillance of those patients developing an acute PE. The appropriate remedies are elaborated elsewhere in this book. Those observations notwithstanding, acute embolism is clinically occult in a significant proportion of patients diagnosed with chronic thromboembolic disease, and in an even greater proportion of individuals, the disorder altogether eludes diagnosis during life. It can be assumed that within the latter population, chronic thromboembolic disease caused significant disability and contributed to premature death, even though an effective surgical therapy was available. Increased awareness of the prevalence of this disease and its many manifestations should reduce the likelihood that this disorder escapes ante-mortem detection, even in an era in which economic constraints increasingly influence clinical practice. However, even when the full array of methods presently available is employed by an experienced group, some residual diagnostic uncertainty persists in between 10 and 20% of patients, and in most such instances "operative accessibility" of the disease is the usual basis for concern. It is our opinion that all thromboembolic disease is reachable at operation – however, there may be other factors (such as irreversible small vessel pulmonary hypertensive changes) which are inoperable. At this time, the sole therapeutic alternative to pulmonary thromboendartectomy is pulmonary transplantation. Because many of the patients in whom the wisdom of operation is deemed equivocal are by virtue of age or other restrictions ineligible for transplantation, it is inevitable that we will continue to offer operation at an assumed higher risk to some patients for whom this judgement is in retrospect erroneous. The less palatable alternative is to exclude all such patients from consideration, even while recognising that many might benefit from the operation. Based on our present experience, we anticipate that in the future this hazard will continue to account for an operative mortality of between 2 and 4%.

The successive improvements in technique developed over the four decades since the initial operative attempts allow pulmonary thromboendarterectomy to be offered now to patients with an acceptable mortality and excellent anticipation of clinical improvement. Over this same period substantial improvements in anesthetic management, perioperative monitoring, and in the methods of extracorporeal circulatory assistance have effected a significant overall reduction in the risk of open cardiac procedures. Former patients have benefited from these developments, and we will continue to incorporate important new refinements.

The principal remaining challenge in this patient population lies in the management and ultimately in the prevention of reperfusion injury. In contrast to many other forms of acute lung injury, and notwithstanding the systemic inflammatory response inaugurated by extracorporeal circulation, the anatomic basis of this process is focal, the inciting stimulus is temporally discrete, and sepsis is not an imminent consideration. Furthermore, cardiopulmonary physiology is exceptionally well documented in these patients prior to operation. Accordingly, this population offers a unique opportunity to enhance our understanding of the pathophysiology of acute lung injury. More importantly, these patients comprise an increasingly large and relatively homogeneous group within which the efficacy of promising new interventions can be assessed. Even though acute lung injury currently represents an innate and often formidable hazard of pulmonary thromboendarterectomy, these patients are likely to be among the first that pharmacological intervention will ultimately help.

References

1. Hirsh J, Hoak J. Management of deep vein thrombosis and pulmonary embolism. A statement for healthcare professionals. Council on Thrombosis (in consultation with the Council on Cardiovascular Radiology), American Heart Association. Circulation 1996; 93 (12): 2212–2245

2. Dalen JE, Alpert JS. Natural history of pulmonary embolism. Prog Cardiovasc Dis 1975; 17: 257–270

3. Soskolne CL, Wong AW, Lilienfeld DE. Trends in pulmonary embolism death rates for Canada and the United States, 1962–1987. Can Med Assoc J 1990; 142: 321–324

4. MMWR Morb Mortal Wkly Rep 1994; 43: 37–42

5. Marzegalli M, Rietti P, Chirico MA, et al. Heart arrest in acute pulmonary embolism. An anatomo-clinical study. G Ital Cardiol 1994; 24: 21–26

6. Rubinstein I, Murray D, Hoffstein V. Fatal pulmonary emboli in hospitalized patients. An autopsy study. Arch Intern Med 1988; 148: 1425–1426

7. Goldhaber SZ, Hennekens CH, Evans DA, Newton EC, Godleski JJ. Factors associated with correct antemortem diagnosis of major pulmonary embolism. Am J Med 1982; 73: 822–826

8. Walden R, Bass A, Modan R, Adar R. Pulmonary embolism in post-mortem material with clinical correlations in 425 cases. Int Angiol 1985; 4: 469–473

9. Morpurgo M, Schmid C. The spectrum of pulmonary embolism. Clinicopathologic correlations. Chest 1995; 107: 18S–20S

10. Mandelli V, Schmid C, Zogno C, Morpurgo M. "False negatives" and "false positives" in acute pulmonary embolism: a clinical-postmortem comparison. Cardiologia 1997; 42: 205–210

11. Carson JL, Kelley MA, Duff A, et al. The clinical course of pulmonary embolism. N Engl J Med 1992; 326: 1240–1245

12. Alpert JS, Smith R, Carlson J, et al. Mortality in patients treated for pulmonary embolism. JAMA 1976; 236: 1477–1480

13. Morpurgo M, Schmid C. Clinico-pathological correlations in pulmonary embolism: a-posteriori evaluation. Prog Respir Dis 1980; 13; 8–15

14. Trendelenburg F. Ueber die operative behandlung der Embolie der Lungenarterie. Arch Klin Chir 1908; 86: 686–700

15. Kirschner M. Ein durch die Trendelenburgsche Operation genheilter Fall von Embolie der Arterien pulmonalis. Arch Klin Chir 1924; 133: 312

16. Allison PR, Dunnill MS, Marshall R. Pulmonary embolism. Thorax 1960; 15: 273–283

17. Sharp EH. Pulmonary embolectomy: Successful removal of a massive pulmonary embolus with the support of cardiopulmonary bypass: A case report. Ann Surg 1962; 156: 1

18. Clarke DB, Abrams LD. Pulmonary embolectomy: a 25 year experience. J Thorac Cardiovasc Surg 1986; 92: 442–445

19. Barton CW, Eisenberg MJ, Schiller N. Transesophageal echocardiographic diagnosis of massive pulmonary embolism during cardiopulmonary resuscitation. Am Heart J 1994; 127: 1639–1642

20. Casazza F, Centonze F, Chirico M, et al. The early echocardiographic diagnosis of a massive pulmonary embolism. G Ital Cardiol 1994; 24: 483–490

21. Ohteki H, Norita H, Sakai M and Narita Y. Emergency pulmonary embolectomy with percutaneous cardiopulmonary bypass. Ann Thorac Surg 1997; 63: 1584–1586

22. Fang BR, Chiang CW, Lee YS. Echocardiographic detection of reversible right ventricular strain in patients with acute pulmonary embolism: report of 2 cases. Cardiology 1996; 87: 279–282

23. Lualdi JC, Goldhaber SZ. Right ventricular dysfunction after acute pulmonary embolism: pathophysiologic factors, detection, and therapeutic implications. Am Heart J 1995; 130: 1276–1282

24. Meneveau N, Bassand JP, Schiele F, et al. Safety of thrombolytic therapy in elderly patients with massive pulmonary embolism: a comparison with nonelderly patients. J Am Coll Cardiol 1993; 22: 1075–1079

25. Severi P, Lo Pinto G, Poggio R and Andrioli G. Urokinase thrombolytic therapy of pulmonary embolism in neurosurgically treated patients. Surg Neurol 1994; 42: 469–470

26. Mikkola KM, Patel SR, Parker JA, Grodstein F and Goldhaber SZ. Increasing age is a major risk factor for hemorrhagic complications after pulmonary embolism thrombolysis. Am Heart J 1997; 134: 69–72

27. Kanter DS, Mikkola KM, Patel SR, Parker JA, Goldhaber SZ. Thrombolytic therapy for pulmonary embolism. Frequency of intracranial hemorrhage and associated risk factors. Chest 1997; 111: 1241–1245

28. Davies MJ, Arsiwala SS, Moore HM, et al. Extracorporeal membrane oxygenation for the treatment of massive pulmonary embolism. Ann Thorac Surg 1995; 60: 1801–1803

29. Jakob H, Vahl C, Lange R, et al. Modified surgical concept for fulminant pulmonary embolism. Eur J Cardiothorac Surg 1995; 9: 557–560

30. Morshuis WJ, Jansen EW, Vincent JG, Heystraten FJ, Lacquet LK. Intraoperative fiberoptic angioscopy to evaluate the completeness of pulmonary embolectomy. J Cardiovasc Surg (Torino) 1989; 30: 630–634

31. Glassford DM, Alford WC, Burrus GR, Stoney WS, Thomas CS. Pulmonary embolectomy. Ann Thorac Surg 1981; 32: 28–32

32. Mattox KL, Feldtman RW, Beall AC, DeBakey ME. Pulmonary embolectomy for acute massive pulmonary embolism. Ann Surg 1982; 195: 726–731

33. Robison RJ, Fehrenbacher J, Brown JW, Madura JA, King H. Emergent pulmonary embolectomy: the treatment for massive pulmonary embolus. Ann Thorac Surg 1986; 42: 52–55

34. Lund O, Nielsen TT, Schifter S, Roenne K. Treatment of pulmonary embolism with full-dose heparin, streptokinase or embolectomy – results and indications. Thorac Cardiovasc Surg 1986; 34: 240–246

35. Gray HH, Morgan JM, Paneth M, Miller GA. Pulmonary embolectomy for acute massive pulmonary embolism: an analysis of 71 cases. Br Heart J 1988; 60: 196–200

36. Gulba DC, Schmid C, Borst HG, et al. Medical compared with surgical treatment for massive pulmonary embolism. Lancet 1994; 343: 576–577

37. Stulz P, Schlapfer R, Feer R, Habicht J, Gradel E. Decision making in the surgical treatment of massive pulmonary embolism. Eur J Cardiothorac Surg 1994; 8: 188–193

38. Jakob H, Vahl C, Lange R, et al. Modified surgical concept for fulminant pulmonary embolism. Eur J Cardiothorac Surg 1995; 9: 557–560

39. Doerge HC, Schoendube FA, Loeser H, Walter M, Messmer BJ. Pulmonary embolectomy: review of a 15-year experience and role in the age of thrombolytic therapy. Eur J Cardiothorac Surg 1996; 10: 952–957

40. Soyer R, Brunet AP, Redonnet M, et al. Follow-up of surgically treated patients with massive pulmonary embolism – with reference to 12 operated patients. Thorac Cardiovasc Surg 1982; 30: 103–108

41. Lund O, Nielsen TT, Ronne K, Schifter S. Pulmonary embolism: long-term follow-up after treatment with full-dose heparin, streptokinase or embolectomy. Acta Med Scand 1987; 221: 61–71

42. Benotti JR, Ockene IS, Alpert JS, Dalen JE. The clinical profile of unresolved pulmonary embolism. Chest 1983; 84: 669–678

43. Dalen JE, Banas JS, Brooks HL, et al. Resolution rate of acute pulmonary embolism in man. N Engl J Med 1969; 280: 1194–1199

44. Fedullo PF, Auger WR, Channick RN, Moser KM, Jamieson SW. Chronic thromboembolic pulmonary hypertension. Clin Chest Med 1995; 16: 353–374

45. Presti B, Berthrong M, Sherwin RM. Chronic thrombosis of major pulmonary arteries. Hum Pathol 1990; 21: 601–606

46. Moser KM, Auger WR, Fedullo PF. Chronic major-vessel thromboembolic pulmonary hypertension. Circulation 1990; 81: 1735–1743

47. Shure D, Bloor CM. Heparin prevents pulmonary artery remodelling in postobstructive pulmonary arteriopathy in dogs. Chest 1988; 93: 154S–155S

48. Auger WR, Permpikul P, Moser KM. Lupus anticoagulant, heparin use and thrombocytopenia in patients with chronic thromboembolic pulmonary hypertension: a preliminary report. Am J Med 1995; 99: 3920–3926

49. Riedel M, Stanek V, Widimsky J and Prerovsky I. Longterm follow-up of patients with pulmonary thromboembolism. Late prognosis and evolution of hemodynamic and respiratory data. Chest 1982; 81: 151–158

50. Dantzker DR, Bower JS. Partial reversibility of chronic pulmonary hypertension caused by pulmonary thromboembolic disease. Am Rev Respir Dis 1981; 124: 129–131

51. Rich S, Levitsky S and Brundage BH. Pulmonary hypertension from chronic pulmonary thromboembolism. Ann Intern Med 1988; 108: 425–434

52. Morris TA, Auger WR, Ysrael MZ, et al. Parenchymal scarring is associated with restrictive spirometric defects in patients with chronic thromboembolic pulmonary hypertension. Chest 1996; 110: 399–403

53. D'Alonzo GE, Bower JS, Dantzker DR. Differentiation of patients with primary and thromboembolic pulmonary hypertension. Chest 1984; 85: 457–461

54. Chow LC, Dittrich HC, Hoit BD, Moser KM, Nicod PH. Doppler assessment of changes in right-sided cardiac hemodynamics after pulmonary thromboendarterectomy. Am J Cardiol 1988; 61: 1092–1097

55. Dittrich HC, Nicod PH, Chow LC, et al. Early changes of right heart geometry after pulmonary thromboendarterectomy. J Am Coll Cardiol 1988; 11: 937–943

56. Moser KM, Page GT, Ashburn WL, Fedullo PF. Perfusion lung scans provide a guide to which patients with apparent primary pulmonary hypertension merit angiography. West J Med 1988; 148: 167–170

57. Ryan KL, Fedullo PF, Davis GB, et al. Perfusion scans understate the severity of angiographic and hemodynamic compromise in chronic thromboembolic pulmonary hypertension. Chest 1988; 93: 1180–1185

58. Gefter WB, Hatabu H, Holland GA, et al. Pulmonary thromboembolism: recent developments in diagnosis with CT and MR imaging. Radiology 1995; 197: 561–574

59. Bergin CJ, Rios G, King MA, et al. Accuracy of high-resolution CT in identifying chronic pulmonary thromboembolic disease. Am J Roentgenol 1996; 166: 1371–1377

60. Bergin CJ, Hauschildt J, Rios G, et al. Accuracy of MR angiography compared with radionuclide scanning in identifying the cause of pulmonary arterial hypertension. Am J Roentgenol 1997; 168: 1549–1555

61. Bergin CJ, Sirlin CB, Hauschildt JP, et al. Chronic thromboembolism: diagnosis with helical CT and MR imaging with angiographic and surgical correlation. Radiology 1997; 204: 695–702

62. King MA, Bergin CJ, Yeung DW, et al. Chronic pulmonary thromboembolism: detection of regional hypoperfusion with CT. Radiology 1994; 191: 359–363

63. Auger WR, Fedullo PF, Moser KM, Buchbinder M, Peterson KL. Chronic major-vessel thromboembolic pulmonary artery obstruction: appearance at angiography. Radiology 1992; 182: 393–398

64. Mills, Jackson DC, Sullivan DC, et al. Angiographic evaluation of chronic pulmonary embolism. Radiology 1980; 136: 301–308

65. Shure D, Gregoratos G, Moser KM. Fiberoptic angioscopy: role in the diagnosis of chronic pulmonary artery obstruction. Ann Intern Med 1985; 103: 844–850

66. Hollister LE, Cull VL. The syndrome of chronic thromboembolism of the major pulmonary arteries. Am J Med 1956; 21: 312–320

67. Hurwitt ES, Schein CJ, Rifkin H, Lebendiger A. A surgical approach to the problem of chronic pulmonary artery obstruction due to chrombosis or stenosis. Ann Surg 1958; 147: 157–165

68. Houk VN, Hufnagel CA, McClenathan JE, Moser KM. Chronic thrombosis obstruction of major pulmonary arteries. Report of a case successfully treated by thromboendarterectomy and review of the literature. Am J Med 1963; 35: 269–282

69. Castleman B, McNeely BU, Scannell G. Case records of the Massachusetts General Hospital. Case 32–1964. N Engl J Med 1964; 271: 40–50

70. Cabrol C, Cabrol A, Acar J, et al. Surgical correction of chronic postembolic obstructions of the pulmonary arteries. J Thorac Cardiovasc Surg 1978; 76: 620–628

71. Chitwood WR, Sabiston DC, Wechsler AS. Surgical treatment of chronic unresolved pulmonary embolism. Clin Chest Med 1984; 5: 507–536

72. Moser KM, Braunwald NS. Successful surgical intervention in severe chronic thromboembolic pulmonary hypertension. Chest 1973; 64: 29–35

73. Utley JR, Spragg RG, Long WB, Moser KM. Pulmonary endarterectomy for chronic thromboembolic obstruction: recent surgical experience. Surgery 1982; 92: 1096–1102

74. Daily PO, Dembitzsky WP, Iversen S, Moser KM, Auger W. Current early results of pulmonary thromboendarterectomy for chronic pulmonary embolism. Eur J Cardiothorac Surg 1990; 4: 117–121

75. Daily PO, Dembitsky WP, Iversen S, Moser KM, Auger W. Risk factors for pulmonary thromboendarterectomy. J Thorac Cardiovasc Surg 1990; 99: 670–678

76. Jamieson SW, Auger WR, Fedullo PF, et al. Experience and results with 150 pulmonary thromboendarterectomy operations over a 29-month period. J Thorac Cardiovasc Surg 1993; 106: 116–126

77. Winkler MH, Rohrer CH, Ratty SC, et al. Perfusion techniques of profound hypothermia and circulatory arrest for pulmonary thromboendarterectomy. J Extracorporeal Tech 1990; 22: 57–60

78. Olman MA, Auger WR, Fedullo PF, Moser KM. Pulmonary vascular steal in chronic thromboembolic pulmonary hypertension. Chest 1990; 98: 1430–1434

79. Moser KM, Metersky ML, Auger WR, Fedullo PF. Resolution of vascular steal after pulmonary thromboendarterectomy. Chest 1993; 104: 1441–1444

80. Levinson RM, Shure D, Moser KM. Reperfusion pulmonary edema after pulmonary artery thromboendarterectomy. Am Rev Respir Dis 1986; 134: 1241–1245

81. Auger WR, Moser KM, Comito RM, et al. Efficacy of intravenous ICI 200, 880 in the prevention of adult respiratory distress syndrome in patients undergoing pulmonary thromboendarterectomy. Am Rev Respir Crit Care Med 1994; 149: A1032

82. Kerr KM, Auger WR, Marsh JJ, et al. Selectin blockade with CY-1503 may prevent reperfusion lung injury following pulmonary thromboendarterectomy. Am Rev Respir Crit Care Med 1997; 155: A898

83. Fedullo PF, Auger WR, Channick RN, Moser KM, Jamieson SW. Surgical management of pulmonary embolism. In: Morpurgo M (ed). Pulmonary Embolism. New York: Marcel Dekker Inc, 1994: 223–240

84. Dittrich HC, Chow LC, Nicod PH. Early improvement in left ventricular diastolic function after relief of chronic right ventricular pressure overload. Circulation 1989; 80: 823–830

85. Moser KM, Daily PO, Peterson K, et al. Thromboendarterectomy for chronic, major-vessel thromboembolic pulmonary hypertension. Immediate and long-term results in 42 patients. Ann Intern Med 1987; 107: 560–565

86. Sabiston DC, Wolfe WG, Oldham HN, et al. Surgical management of chronic pulmonary embolism. Ann Surg 1977; 185: 699–712

VI.4 Interventional techniques for venous thrombosis

J. A. Reekers, M. W. Mewissen, H. J. Baarslag

Introduction

Acute treatment of venous thrombosis is in most instances less mandatory compared to arterial thrombosis. It is only in special circumstances that an acute intervention is performed.

Interventional techniques for venous thrombosis are performed by either local administration of thrombolytic agents, mechanical thrombectomy or surgery. The aims of treatment of venous thrombosis are different for specific locations. In massive pulmonary embolism (PE) a rapid restoration of flow is important to prevent death or late sequelae like pulmonary hypertension. On the other hand, an indwelling line-related thrombosis is treated to preserve this line or to maintain the venous entry-site for future therapy; late sequelae are less prominent. The aim of treating DVT with local lytic drugs is to prevent late complications like venous insufficiency or to treat a possible underlying lesion, like the May-Turner syndrome.

Percutaneous interventions in pulmonary embolism

Immediate mortality due to PE is about 10%. Especially when PE is severe or happens in a patient with underlying cardiopulmonary disease, the hemodynamics will be compromised due to increased ventricular afterload. In these patients rapid restoration of pulmonary blood flow and reduction of the thrombus bulk is mandatory.

ase: 2,000 IU/lb loading dose over 10 min followed by 2,000 IU/lb/h for 12–24 hours: or 100 mg rt-PA as a continuous infusion over 2 hours. The contraindications to systemic thrombolysis are stroke, recent major surgery, intracranial neoplasm, abdominal or gastrointestinal bleeding.

Intravenous thrombolysis

Systemic thrombolysis by injection of the lytic drug into a peripheral vein is still often used. Within fourteen days after the onset of complaints, fibrinolysis can still be applied [1]. It has been shown that with peripheral lytic therapy there is an improvement in perfusion of lung scans compared with heparin alone [2, 3]. This therapy can be life-saving in patients with massive PE, cardiogenic shock or hemodynamic instability [4]. The disadvantage of this technique is the time delay between the beginning of the therapy and the actual clot lysis. There is also an increase in bleeding complications with systemic lysis. The most used intravenous thrombolytic regimens are [5]: Urokin-

Catheter-directed thrombolysis

With this technique the thrombolytic drug is infused directly into the pulmonary artery. This technique can be performed immediately after a diagnostic angiography. There is some discussion whether the tip of the catheter should be in the main pulmonary artery or imbedded into the thrombus. The most used drugs are Urokinase or Rt-PA. After puncture of a femoral vein the catheter tip is positioned into the clot, followed by a bolus of 250,000 IU Urokinase. This is followed by an infusion of 100,000 IU/h for 12–24 hours. The patient is also heparinised to maintain a PTT at 1.5 to 2.5 times the normal limits. For rt-PA a bolus of 10 mg is followed by 20 mg/h over 2 hours.

Although hemorrhagic bleeding complications might be fewer with low dose catheter-directed thrombolysis due to decreasing the activity of systemic fibrinolysis, with the catheter in the PE, there are no data demonstrating decrease of complications. A study by Verstraete et al., using rtPA, did not show any significant benefit of local intrapulmonary infusion over the intravenous route [6].

In the UPET study the rate of major bleeding complications was 6% for rt-Pa and 12%–27% for Urokinase [7]. But clot lysis is time-consuming and when pulmonary blood flow is not restored quickly the outcome may still be fatal.

Additional mechanical clot fragmentation with a catheter, a balloon catheter or other devices may increase the velocity of thrombolysis. Increase of the clot surface, and in this way enhanced exposure of the lytic drug due to the larger surface area, is probably the mechanism of improved lysis. The effectiveness of combined clot fragmentation and local thrombolysis has been demonstrated in several studies [8 – 11].

Although it is reasonable to assume that early clot lysis and reperfusion will give a better early and long-term outcome concerning survival, there are no randomised studies to prove this.

Thromboembolectomy

In recent years a variety of devices have been developed for local embolectomy or thrombectomy. Some of these devices will retrieve clots while others use mechanical fragmentation, sometimes in combination with aspiration. Although there is almost never a total removal of thrombus, debulking in combination with fragmentation can be very beneficial. The rationale for this is that the volume of the peripheral pulmonary circulation is two times that of the central pulmonary arteries. Fragmentation and redistribution of central clot into the peripheral pulmonary arteries may improve pulmonary blood flow and, in this way, prevent right heart failure.

Whether mechanical thrombectomy can work as a stand-alone technique in massive PE, or if a combination with local lysis is superior, has to be proven. A theoretical advantage of not using lytic drugs is the reduction of hemorrhagic complications.

Thromboembolectomy devices

There are devices which are specially dedicated to treatment of PE. All the other currently available devices are designed for thromboembolectomy in general.

Dedicated thromboembolectomy devices

The Greenfield embolectomy device
This device, which is specially designed for treatment of PE, works with suction alone for soft and non-wall adherent thrombus. The device needs a venotomy or a 24 Fr sheath for the introduction [12]. Besides the good results of the inventor, there are no other data available [13].

Impeller basket device
This device was designed for the treatment of PE. The device is formed by a flexible wire shaft inside a 7 Fr catheter with a small impeller mounted on the wire and in the centre of a metallic self-expandable basket. The impeller is connected through the wire to an external electric motor, which can rotate at 100,000 rpm. The impeller creates a vortex inside the vessel lumen and pulls the thrombus into the basket, causing fragmentation of the clots. The basket protects the vessel wall from the rotational impeller [14]. The device has limited steerability and is stiff. There is also a modified impeller device [15]. There is besides experimental animal data some human experience [16]. It is very doubtful if this device will ever play a role in the treatment of PE.

Rotatable pigtail catheter
The rotatable pigtail catheter is modelled on a custom-made high torque pigtail catheter with a diameter of 5 Fr, a length of 110 cm, 10 side ports and a radiopaque tip. With a straightened stiff wire, through the oval side hole in the pigtail curve, the catheter is connected to an electric motor (max 500 rpm). During rotation the pigtail can be advanced or withdrawn over the wire as a guide rail [17]. In dogs this device seems to work. No human data available.

Reekers PE-hydrolyser catheter

(custom-made Cordis, Rhoden, The Netherlands)
A 90 cm long, 7 Fr hydrolyser catheter (description of functioning see under general thrombectomy devices) with a fixed pigtail tip. The wire cannot enter this pigtail tip. The catheter is introduced through a 9 Fr guiding catheter in the main pulmonary artery (Fig. 1).

General thromboembolectomy devices

There are two different, more or less evaluated, types of mechanical thrombectomy devices available: devices which have a mechanical, external motor-driven, rotating action for fragmentation of the clot, and devices whose functioning is based on a modified water-pump whereby the principal action is thrombosuction.

Rotating devices

The two commercially available and FDA-approved rotating devices are the Amplatz Clot Buster and the Trerotola device. The main action of both of these devices is fragmentation of thrombus, which can in some instances be followed by aspiration. The Trerotola device has never been reported for pulmonary use and will, therefore, not be discussed here.

The Amplatz thrombectomy device

(Microvena, Minneapolis, USA)
This device was first reported in 1989 [18]. It is an 8 Fr rapidly spinning helical screw propeller which is housed in an 8 Fr short metal protective capsule. The metal capsule has several side ports allowing for recirculation and remaceration of thrombotic material. The capsule is attached to a 100 cm long catheter. Torque to the helix is transmitted by a cable driven by an air motor at ap-

proximately 100,000 rpm. Liquification of clot produces particles ranging in size from 13 to 1,000 um [19]. The device was studied for a possible hemolytic effect, which showed to be definite but transient and related to the activation time [20]. The FDA only approved this device for thrombosed dialysis fistulae. There is one publication on pulmonary application of this device for massive PE in critically ill patients but the series that is published is too small to draw any definite conclusions on clinical efficacy [21]. The main disadvantages of this device are the French-size (8 Fr) and that it cannot be guided over a wire. A 6 Fr device is currently under evaluation. To date there is no information regarding possible vessel wall damage.

Hydrodynamic devices

The two commercially available hydrodynamic devices are the Hydrolyser and the Possis-device (Angiojet), which are currently both in the process of acquiring FDA approval. The main action of these devices is the mobilising of fresh clot and its subsequent removal by suction.

The Hydrolyser

(Cordis, Rhoden, The Netherlands)
The Hydrolyser is a 6 or 7 Fr double lumen catheter with a small injection lumen and a larger exhaust lumen. The exhaust lumen is connected to a collection bag. The device is activated with a standard contrast injection pump filled with saline. For the 7 Fr device a flow of 4 ml/ sec at 750 psi through the injection lumen is required [22]. The device, which is available in different lengths, can be guided over a 0.025" wire through the exhaust lumen. The latest version of the 6 Fr device is a flexible triple lumen catheter with a separate 0.020" guide wire lumen and can be applied safely in vessels between 3 – 8 mm.

Fig. 1a – d. 42-year-old female with progressive dyspnea over a period of 5 days. No haemodynamic problems. The VQ scan showed no perfusion over the left lung.
(a) Pulmonary angiography with catheter tip in pulmonary trunk. Occlusion of the left main pulmonary artery. **(b)** Reekers-PE Hydrolyser catheter introduced through a long 9 Fr sheath at the origin of the left pulmonary artery. **(c)** After 3 runs with the device there was no further angiographic improvement. Major debulking of thrombus in the left pulmonary artery. There was an instant improvement both clinically and regarding the O2 demand. Treatment was continued with systemic low-molecular heparin for 1 week followed by coumarin. **(d)** Control angiography at 6 months shows further improvement, but part of the lingula branch is still missing. The patient is clinically symptom-free.

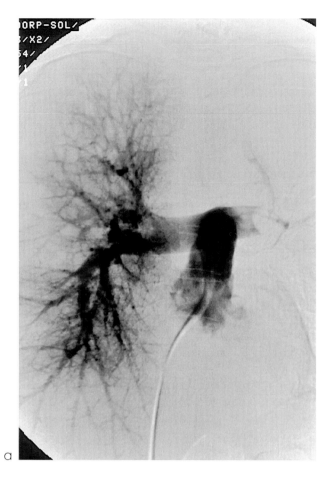

a

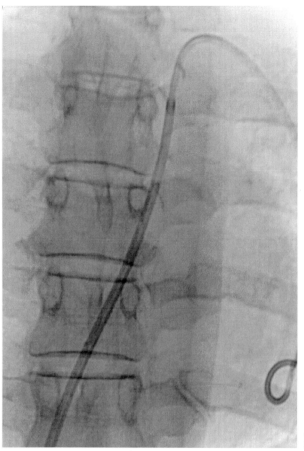

b

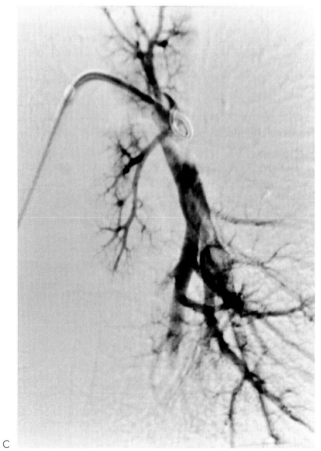

c

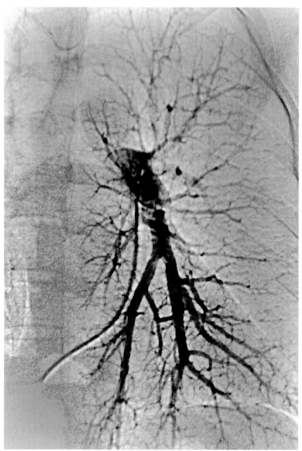

d

It has been shown in vivo that the Hydrolyser gives no vessel wall reaction [23]. The main disadvantage of this catheter, as is the case for all hydrodynamic systems, is that it only works effectively in fresh clot, which means an arterial clot no older than about 10 days. The great advantage of the Hydrolyser system is that no investments are required for an extra pump or other hardware, it is simply a catheter. There is some clinical experience with this device in PE, which reports good results [24, 25]. A special PE-hydrolyser design is described above.

The Possis rheolytic catheter
(Possis Medical, Minneapolis, USA)

The device consists of a 4–6 Fr dual lumen tubing. There is an injection lumen and a larger exhaust lumen. At the catheter tip there are three holes through which water jets exit perpendicularly, with a pressure of about 1–2 psi. Additionally, three water jets with a pressure of 1,000 psi are directed into the catheter lumen to remove fragmented thrombus with the aid of the venturi effect. To work this device a special pump is necessary which can provide a pressure of 10,000–15,000 psi to the catheter. The catheter can be guided over a wire. Some clinical data are available concerning this device and PE [26].

Stents for massive pulmonary embolism

There have been a few reports about treatment of otherwise therapy-resistant, wall-adherent, massive PE, in critically ill patients, with stents [27, 28]. In both reports this treatment was used as a final emergency option after all other available techniques were used. The stents were placed in the main pulmonary artery, and a rapid reperfusion with immediate relief of complaints was seen. One of the patients was free of symptoms at 8 months [27]. Although there is a lot of experience with stents at other arterial and venous locations, with the current available data this technique can only be advised in a bail-out situation.

Percutaneous interventions for subclavian vein thrombosis

Subclavian vein thrombosis

It is generally believed that subclavian thrombosis does not produce a long-term disability due to good collateral circulation. Nevertheless, a post thrombotic arm syndrome can be recognised in up to 70% of patients with a subclavian vein effort thrombosis [29]. Data are not available that prove the need for more invasive therapy for all subclavian thrombosis, like local thrombolysis or percutaneous thrombectomy. However, there seem to be some indications for treatment of subclavian vein thrombosis that have literature support. Early clot removal for active healthy patients with a need to use the limbs in sport and work is favoured by a panel of experts of American vascular surgeons. They promote catheter-directed thrombolysis as initial therapy [30].

Subclavian vein effort thrombosis

Thrombosis of the subclavian vein is often seen in combination with a costoclavicular compression syndrome. Compression of the vein at the thoracic outlet is the etiology for this problem. In the acute phase, history of thrombosis shorter than 2 weeks, local catheter-directed thrombolytic therapy followed by operation is the first choice [31, 32]. The aim of lytic therapy is to prevent chronic fibrous obliteration of the subclavian vein. The outcome for patients with spontaneous subclavian vein thrombosis, treated with heparin and oral anticoagulants alone, is inferior to lytic therapy, both for recanalisation and symptom resolution [33].

Subclavian vein thrombosis with indwelling lines

Indwelling subclavian lines for dialysis, chemotherapy and nutrition have a high risk for thrombosis. The primary treatment target is not prevention of post-thrombotic problems but preservation of the line and/or venous excess for future use. Catheter-directed thrombolysis can be used, but also percutaneous thrombectomy devices might play a future role here. Especially the short treatment time and the absence of lytic drugs is theoretically promising (Fig. 2).

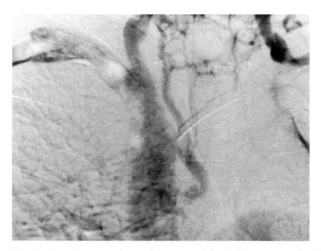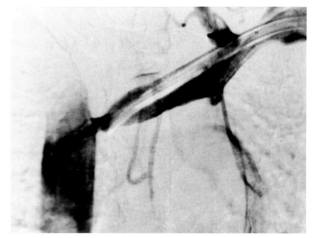

Fig. 2a, b. Patient with a catheter in the left subclavian artery for dialysis. Acute swelling of the left arm and dysfunction of the subclavian line.
(a) Thrombosis of the left subclavian and brachiocephalic vein. **(b)** After mechanical thrombectomy with a 7 Fr hydrolyser, through the left basilic vein. Total removal of thrombus and re-functioning of the line. Stenosis at the junction of the left brachiocephalic vein and the VCS. This stenosis was treated by PTA from the right femoral vein.
Conclusion: Venous entrée in the left subclavian vein saved for future treatment. No line change was necessary. Treatment of clinical symptoms.

Catheter-directed thrombolysis for lower extremity deep vein thrombosis

Introduction

The therapeutic goals for treating the patient with acute DVT include preventing PE, restoration of unobstructed blood flow through the thrombosed segment, prevention of recurrent thrombosis and preservation of venous valve function. Success in achieving these clinical goals will minimise the morbidity and mortality of PE and will also diminish the sequelae of the postthrombotic syndrome (PTS). As shown by Johnson, it is the combination of reflux and obstruction that correlates with the severity of PTS, as opposed to either alone [34]. Up to two-thirds of the patients with iliofemoral DVT will develop edema and pain, with 5 % developing ulcers in spite of adequate anticoagulation [35].

The standard of care at the moment includes systemic anticoagulation with heparin followed by coumadin therapy [36]. Such a regimen, however, does not promote lysis to reduce the thrombus load nor does it contribute to restoration of venous valvular function. Anticoagulation alone, therefore, does not protect the limb from PTS, which can occur months to years following the acute thrombotic event [35].

Thrombolysis is a potentially attractive form of therapy since it provides the opportunity for promptly restoring venous patency and preserving venous valve function. This therapy provides the potential for preventing the long-term sequelae of DVT. There is published evidence that thrombolytic agents, even administered systemically, are superior to standard anticoagulation therapy in achieving early lysis of thrombus. In a pooled analysis of thirteen randomised studies, Comerota and Aldridge found that only 4 % of patients treated with heparin had significant or complete lysis compared to 45 % of patients randomised to systemic streptokinase therapy [37]. Similarly, in reviewing pooled data from six trials judged to have proper randomisation, systemic thrombolysis was 3.7 times more effective in producing some degree of lysis than was heparin [38]. In spite of these results, progress was hindered, probably because of the use of systemic administration where the drug does not reach the thrombus in sufficient concentration to provide optimal results.

The report by Semba and Dake in 1994 provided the first insight on the potential role of catheter-directed thrombolytic (CDT) techniques [39]. They reported complete lysis in 72 % of the patients with concomitant resolution of symptoms. Only one patient suffered a bleeding complication of hemi-positive stools. After the drug was discontinued, there were no significant adverse sequelae. Delivering the thrombolytic agent directly into the thrombus offers significant advantages over systemic therapy, which may fail to reach and penetrate an occluded venous segment. Because throm-

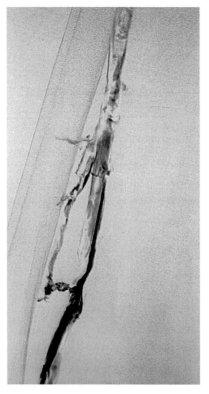

a

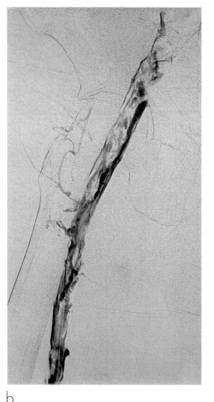

b

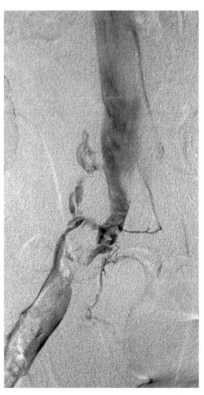

c

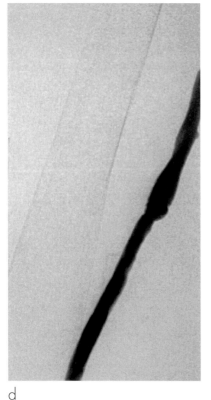

d

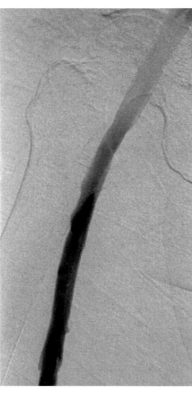

e

Fig. 3a – g. Thirty-five-year-old man who presented with a one week history of worsening pain and swelling of the right lower extremity, following repair of an inguinal hernia. Duplex study revealed DVT extending from the popliteal vein to the common iliac vein. Following catheterisation of the right popliteal vein under ultrasound guidance, the non-invasive studies are confirmed at venography. There is thrombosis of the superficial femoral, common femoral, external and common iliac veins **(a, b, c)**. Following administration of 4.3 million units of Urokinase over 36 hours directly into the thrombus with a 5 Fr coaxial infusing system, there is complete lysis demonstrated in all previously thrombosed veins **(d, e, f)**. Note uncovered stenosis in proximal common iliac vein **(f**, black arrows), successfully treated with a Wallstent **(g**, black arrows). At one-year follow-up, the deep veins remain patent and the patient is asymptomatic.

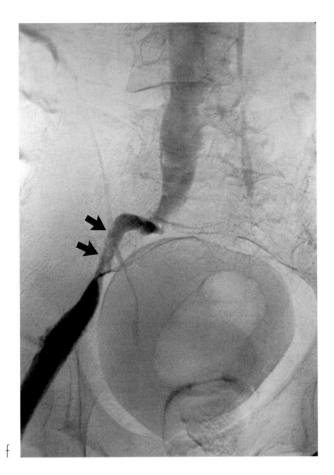

f

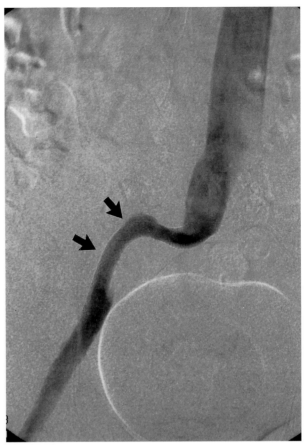

g

bolytic agents activate plasminogen within the thrombus, delivery of the drug to that site enhances its effectiveness. By focusing the delivery of higher concentrations of drug, lysis rates can be improved, the duration of treatment can be reduced, and complications associated with the exposure of the patient to systemic thrombolytic therapy may be reduced. The progress of CDT can be monitored by direct imaging techniques, and lesions potentially contributing to the thrombosis can be identified. These defects, such as stenosis of the common iliac vein, can be treated by balloon angioplasty with or without the placement of endovascular stents (Fig. 3).

Technique of catheter-directed lysis

With the patient prone on the angiographic table, we prefer the ipsilateral popliteal venous approach, because it is often difficult to penetrate an occluded superficial femoral vein from the internal jugular vein or the contralateral common femoral vein, because of venous valves that may prevent safe catheter and guide wire manipulations. The popliteal vein should be accessed under ultrasound guidance with a small gauge echogenic needle to avoid inadvertent puncture of the popliteal artery. A 5 Fr short sheath is then introduced, via which all subsequent catheters can be exchanged. Following baseline venography obtained via the popliteal sheath, the occluded vein is crossed with a straight-tip 5 Fr catheter and a 0.035 inch curved-tip guide wire. Venography is then repeated to confirm intraluminal passage of the catheter, which is then exchanged for a 5 Fr infusing coaxial system, consisting of a proximal multi-sidehole catheter and a distal infusing wire. It is critical to position the system directly into the thrombus, to maximise plasminogen activation at the site of obstruction. Urokinase therapy is initiated at 150,000–200,000 units per hour, evenly split between the infusing ports. As a general practice, we rarely employ a total Urokinase dose of greater than 200,000 units per hour regardless of the thrombus burden. Intravenous heparin is concomitantly administered via the popliteal sheath at a rate of 500–1,000 units per hour following a 5,000-unit bolus of heparin. Patients are monitored in the ICU or a step-down unit, similar to those receiving thombolytic treatment for acute PE or an arterial occlusion. Because the duration of therapy may excess 48 hours, it is not necessary to frequently assess the progress of lysis. The frequency of follow-up venograms should be every 12 hours, primarily to reposition the infusion devices into the remaining thrombus. Gentle thrombus maceration with a 6 mm balloon angioplasty catheter may be helpful, particularly in the superficial femoral vein, where focal narrowings are at times encountered, probably representing sites of organised thrombus. Typically, unless a complication would dictate otherwise, lytic therapy should be continued until complete lysis is achieved, unless no discernible progress is venographically demonstrated from the previous venogram obtained 12 hours prior. Since the grade of thrombolysis has been shown in the Registry to be a strong predictor of continued patency, it is critical that a complete lysis on the venogram is achieved. Lesions uncovered in the iliac venous segments should probably be treated with stents, although the long-term benefits of such devices are not known. However, if left untreated, there appears to be a significant risk of early rethrombosis.

The venous registry: overview and early results

Clearly, the initial report by Semba and Dake suggested that CDT can be effective in achieving significant lysis of thrombus and may be associated with low complication rates [39]. This experience stimulated the development of a multicentre registry, which was recently closed after enrolment of almost 500 patients within over 50 Northern American centres. The results have not yet been published but have been presented at several meetings, the last in San Diego on September 13, 1997 [40]. Complete data with follow-up of at least 6 months were available on nearly 300 patients, 70% of which had ilio-femoral DVT (IFVT). Treatment duration averaged more than 48 hours with close to 7 million units of Urokinase administered in those with direct intrathrombus delivery. One third of the patients received adjunctive stenting for residual narrowing, but this was close to 40% in the IFVT group and close to half of those with left-sided involvement. Lysis was graded as I < 50%, II > 50% and III = 100%. Grade II and III lysis were achieved in over 80% of cases. Complete lysis was achieved in close to one third. The degree of lysis was found to be a significant predictor of early and continued patency. Seventy-five percent of limbs with complete lysis remained

patent at one year, compared to only 32% for limbs with insignificant lysis (< 50%). In general, acute DVT (< 10 days) predicted a better lysis grade when compared to chronic DVT (> 10 days), although significant lysis could be achieved in patients with chronic IFDVT. When isolated FPDVT was present for more than 10 days, none achieved complete lysis. Reflux at 6 months follow-up was less than 30% in those with complete lysis, around 45% in those with > 50% lysis, but over 60% in those with < 50% initial lysis, again showing the greater protective effect of complete clot removal. Longer follow-up, including those who still had incomplete data at six months, should provide more definitive recommendations based on careful subgroup analysis and functional evaluation. There were only 2 deaths in the entire study (0.4%), one from intracranial hemorrhage and one of the six patients who suffered a PE (1.2%).

Because the Registry was not designed to be a controlled trial, no restrictions were imposed on patient enrolment such as duration of symptoms, location of thrombus, prior history of DVT or technique of thrombolysis. Therefore, patients with a variety of these features were prospectively enrolled. This may help explain a relatively low overall yield of complete lysis (31%). However, when analysed by subgroups, several important observations can be made. For example, for a patient with acute IFDVT and no prior history of previous DVT, when CDT was performed via the popliteal vein (without a pedal infusion), complete lysis occurred 65% of the time and the 1-year patency was 96%. At the other extreme, complete lysis never occurred in any patients with chronic FPDVT. Analysis of groups with particular combinations of features, while not always numerous for statistical comparison, provides a useful perspective of what can be expected from CDT in different settings and can serve as a guide to patient selection for this potentially effective form of treatment.

In conclusion, CDT can safely and effectively dissolve thrombus from the deep veins of identifiable groups of patients with symptomatic lower limb DVT. The best results can be anticipated in patients with acute symptoms without a prior history of DVT, who are treated with CDT without systemic infusion. The long-term benefits of this form of therapy are not yet known and cannot be conclusively derived from this study. The Registry data should help design the protocol of a controlled trial comparing CDT and anticoagulation which will be necessary to validate the long-term benefits of CDT and its application for the prevention of the post-thrombotic syndrome.

References

1. Daniels LB, Parker JA, Patel SR, Grodstein F, Goldhaber SZ. Relation of duration of symptoms with response to thrombolytic therapy in pulmonary embolism. Am J Cardiol 1997; 80: 184–188

2. Tow DE, Wagner HN. Urokinase pulmonary embolism trial: Phase I results. JAMA 1970; 214: 2163–2172

3. Urokinase-Streptokinase pulmonary embolism trial: Phase 2 results. JAMA 1974; 229: 1606–1613

4. Jerjes-Sanchez C, Ramirez-Rivera A, Garcia MI, et al. Streptokinase and heparin versus heparin alone in massive pulmonary embolism: a randomized controlled trial. J Thromb Thrombolysis 1995; 2: 227–229

5. Goldhaber Sz. Thrombolytic therapy for pulmonary embolism. Semin Vasc Surg 1992; 5: 69–75

6. Verstraete M, Miller GAH, Bounameux H, et al. Intravenous and intrapulmonary recombinant tissue-type plasminogen activator in the treatment of acute massive pulmonary embolism. Circulation 1988; 77: 353–360

7. The Urokinase pulmonary embolism trial: a national cooperative study. Circulation 1973; 47: 1–108

8. Brady AJ, Crake T, Oakley CM. Percutaneous catheter fragmentation and distal dispersion of proximal pulmonary embolus. Lancet 1991; 338: 1186–1189

9. Essop MR, Middlemost S, Skoularigis J, Sareli P. Simultaneous mechanical clot fragmentation and pharmacologic thrombolysis in acute massive pulmonary embolism. Am J Cardiol 1992; 70: 427–430

10. Fava M, Loyola S, Flores P, Huete I. Mechanical fragmentation and pharmacologic thrombolysis in massive pulmonary embolism. J Vasc Intervent Radiol 1997; 8: 261–266

11. Stock KW, Jacob AL, Schnabel KJ, Bongartz G, Steinbrich W. Massive pulmonary embolism: Treatment with thrombus fragmentation and local fibrinolysis with recombinant human-tissue plasminogen activator. Cardiovasc Intervent Radiol 1997; 20: 364–368

12. Greenfield LJ, Kimmel D, McCurdy WC. Transvenous removal of pulmonary emboli by vacuum-cup transcatheter technique. J Surg Res 1969; 9: 347–352

13. Greenfield LJ, Proctor MC, Williams DM, Wakefield TW. Long-term experience with transvenous catheter pulmonary embolectomy. J Vasc Surg 1993; 18: 450–456

14. Schmitz-Rode T, Vorwerk D, Guenther RW, et at. Percutaneous fragmentation of pulmonary emboli in dogs with the impeller basket catheter. Cardiovasc Intervent Radiol 1993; 16: 234–242

15. Schmitz-Rode T, Adam G, Kilbingr M, et al. Fragmentation of pulmonary emboli: in vivo experimental evaluation of 2 high-speed rotating catheters. Cardiovasc Intervent Radiol 1996; 19: 165–169

16. Schmitz-Rode T, Guenther RW. New device for percutaneous fragmentation of pulmonary emboli. Radiology 1991; 180: 135–137

17. Schmitz-Rode T, Guenther RW, Pfeffer JG, et al. Acute massive pulmonary embolism: use of a rotatable pigtail catheter for diagnosis and fragmentation therapy. Radiology 1995; 197: 157–162

18. Bildsoe MC, Moradian GP, Hunter DW, et al. Mechanical clot dissolution: New concept. Radiology 1989; 171: 231–233

19. Yasui K, Qian Z, Nazarian GK, et al. Recirculation-type Amplatz clot macerator: Determination of particle size and distribution. J Vasc Intervent Radiol 1993; 4: 275–278

20. Nazarian GK, Qian Z, Coleman CC, et al. Hemolytic effect of the Amplatz thrombectomy device. J Vasc Intervent Radiol 1994; 5: 155–160

21. Uflacker R, Strange C, Vujic I. Massive pulmonary embolism: preliminary results of treatment with the Amplatz thrombectomy device. J Vasc Intervent Radiol 1996; 7: 19–28

22. Reekers JA, Kromhout JG, van der Waal K. Catheter for percutaneous thrombectomy: first clinical experience. Radiology 1993; 188: 871–874

23. Van Ommen V, van der Veen FH, Daemen MJ, et al. In vivo evaluation of the Hydrolyser hydrodynamic thrombectomy catheter. J Vasc Intervent Radiol 1994; 5: 823–826

24. Henry M, Amor M, Henry I, Tricoche O, Allaoui M. The hydrolyser thrombectomy catheter: a single center experience. J Endovasc Surg 1998; 5: 24–31

25. Michalis LK, Tsetis DK, Rees MR. Percutaneous removal of pulmonary artery thrombus in a patient with massive pulmonary embolism using the hydrolyser catheter: the first human experience. Clinical Radiology 1997; 52: 158–161

26. Koning R, Cribier A, Gerber L, et al. A new treatment for severe pulmonary embolism: percutaneous rheolytic thrombectomy. Circulation 1997; 96: 2498–2500

27. Haskal ZJ, Soulen MC, Huettl EA, Palevsky HI, Cope C. Life-threatening pulmonary emboli and cor pulmonale: Treatment with percutaneous pulmonary artery stent placement. Radiology 1994; 191: 473–475

28. Koizumi J, Kusano S, Akima T, et al. Emergent Z stent placement for treatment of cor pulmonale due to pulmonary emboli after failed lytic treatment: Technical considerations. Cardiovasc Intervent Radiol 1998; 21: 254–257

29. Rochester JR, Beard JD. Acute management of subclavian vein thrombosis. Br J Surg 1995; 82: 433–434

30. Rutherford RB, Hurlbert SN. Primary subclavian-axillary vein thrombosis: Consensus and commentary. Cardiovasc Surg 1996; 4: 420–423

31. Molina JE. Need for emergency treatment in subclavian vein effort thrombosis. J Am Col Surg 1995; 181: 414–420

32. Sheeran SR, Hallisey MJ, Murphy TP, et al. Local thrombolytic therapy as part of a multidisciplinary approach to acute axillosubclavian vein thrombosis (Paget-Schroeter syndrome). J Vasc Intervent Radiol 1997; 8: 253–260

33. AbuRahma AF, Short YS, White JF III, Boland JP. Treatment alternatives for axillary subclavian vein thrombosis: long-term follow up. Cardiovasc Surg 1996; 4: 783–787

34. Johnson BF, Manzo RA, Bergelin RO, Srandness DE Jr. Relationship between changes in the deep venous system and the development of the post-thrombotic syndrome after an acute episode of lower limb deep venous thrombosis: A one-to-six year follow-up. J Vasc Surg 1995; 21: 307

35. Strandness DE, Langlois Y, Cramer M, Randkett A, et al. Long-term sequelae of acute venous thrombosis. JAMA 1983; 250: 1289–1292

36. Hull RD, Raskob GE, Rosenbloom D, Panju AA, Brill-Edwards P, Ginsberg JF, Hirsch J, Martin GJ, Green D. Heparin for 5b days as compared with 10 days in the initial treatment of proximal venous thrombosis. N Engl J Med 1990; 322 (18): 1260–1264

37. Comerota A, Aldridge SC. Thrombolytic therapy for deep venous thrombosis: a clinical review. Can J Surg 1993; 36: 359–364

38. Goldhaber SZ, Buring JE, Lipchick RJ, et al. Pooled analysis of randomized trials of streptokinase and heparin in phlebographically documented acute deep venous thrombosis. Am J Med 1984; 76: 393–397

39. Semba CP, Dake MD. Catheter directed thrombolysis for iliofemoral venous thrombosis. Radiology 1994; 191: 487–494

40. Mewissen MW: Venous Registry Investigators meeting held in San Diego, CA. October 1997

Chapter VII
Management Strategies

VII.1 Management strategies in patients with suspected pulmonary embolism

M. Oudkerk, E. J. R. van Beek, W. L. J. van Putten, F. F. H. Rutten

Introduction

Clinicians frequently encounter patients in whom symptoms and signs suggest a diagnosis of venous thromboembolism. In the western world, approximately 2 to 3 per 1,000 inhabitants are yearly investigated for this disease. These estimates stem from population-based hospital studies [1–3] and questionnaires among physicians [4]. The epidemiology of venous thromboembolism is discussed in more detail in Chapter I.

The aim of any diagnostic management strategy is to adequately rule out pulmonary embolism (PE) in order to safely withhold anticoagulants. At the same time, patients with emboli need to be identified in order to initiate anticoagulant therapy, since missing this disease has severe repercussions in terms of recurrent thromboembolism which may be fatal or could lead to the development of pulmonary hypertension or respiratory disability. The importance of this division is related to two major factors. First, of all patients who are suspected of venous thromboembolism, the disease is proven in only approximately 30%, whereas the remaining patients suffer from illnesses which do not require anticoagulation [5–11]. Second, the use of anticoagulants, whether this is fibrinolytic therapy or heparinoids and oral anticoagulation,

is associated with considerable mortality and morbidity (as discussed in Chapters VI.1 and VI.2) [12–17].

The diagnostic evaluation of patients with suspected pulmonary thromboembolism starts with taking a clinical history, performing a physical examination, and laboratory investigations, electrocardiography and chest radiography (see Chapters II and IV.2). Although these investigations are all useful for the assessment of the patient's general condition and for the detection of other conditions that may mimic PE (the differential diagnosis is very extensive indeed!), these investigations are very limited in their ability to identify patients who require anticoagulant therapy from those in whom this treatment should be withheld. Hence, objective diagnostic tests are required to reach a definitive diagnosis in patients with suspected PE. The variety of available diagnostic tests has been discussed in the preceding chapters, and one can easily imagine that a great number of diagnostic strategies are in use, under investigation or could be thought up. The primary goal of this chapter is to compare various diagnostic strategies that may be used in the diagnostic management of patients with suspected PE.

Assumptions for natural history, evaluated diagnostic tests and therapy

Several assumptions have to be made when building a model for cost-effectiveness analysis purposes. These relate to the prevalence of disease in the population which is suspected of having the illness under investigation, the influence of therapeutic interventions on the natural course of the illness, the adverse events due to therapeutic interventions, the performance of diagnostic tests and the overall costs of diagnostic and therapeutic

management. For the model that was constructed, we performed a Medline search to obtain baseline data on these parameters. Furthermore, a cost-assessment was performed both in academic and non-academic institutions in The Netherlands and several hospitals in Europe, Canada and the USA. This approach allowed the following assumptions to be made.

Prevalence

In our analysis we assumed that among the patients suspected of PE 9% have emboli limited to the subsegmental vessels and 21% in segmental or greater vessels, while 70% have no PE. Of the patients with PE 70% were assumed to also have deep vein thrombosis (DVT). The proportion of patients suspected of PE that only have DVT was assumed to be very low and set at 0.1%.

The prevalence of angiographically proven PE, in patients with clinical suspicion thereof, is approximately 30% [5–11]. More recently, some studies have revealed that the emboli are limited to subsegmental vessels and segmental or greater vessels in 9% and 21%, respectively [18, 19]. Venous thromboembolism is regarded as one clinical entity. This is based on several studies, which evaluated the presence of PE in patients with proven DVT. These studies demonstrated that PE may be shown in 50% of patients with proven DVT [20–23]. Furthermore, several studies which evaluated the presence of DVT in patients with proven PE demonstrated an incidence of 35% to 90%, depending on whether ultrasonography [24–30] or contrast venography [31, 32] was performed.

Natural history and anticoagulant therapy

The natural course of venous thromboembolism has been evaluated rather sparsely. The only randomised trial dates back to 1960, which showed a mortality of 30% [33]. Later studies showed that the use of anticoagulant therapy reduced this mortality to approximately 5% [34–38].

Anticoagulant therapy is routinely started by instituting intravenous heparin therapy while the patient undergoes objective diagnostic tests [39, 40]. If a diagnosis of venous thromboembolism is proven, heparin therapy is continued for approximately 7 days [41, 42]. Oral anticoagulants are titrated to obtain an INR of 2–3 and continued for a period of 3 months [14]. More recently, intravenous heparin is being replaced by subcutaneous low-molecular weight heparins [15, 16]. However, the impact of low-molecular weight heparins in patients with PE has been much less than in patients with DVT [15, 16, 43]. Anticoagulant therapy is correlated with fatal bleeding complications, which occur in approximately 0.75% of patients receiving adequate anticoagulant therapy. Furthermore, non-fatal major bleeding complications occur in 5% of anticoagulated patients [12]. Some of the costs of diagnosis and therapy and some mortality despite adequate treatment are un-

Table 1. Average costs of diagnostics and therapy in patients suspected of PE*.

Category costs	Costs per unit (Euro)
Diagnostics	
Ultrasound	47
Clinical decision rule	18
Perfusion scan	120
Ventilation scan	186
VQ scan (1.2 x P, 1 x V)**	373
Spiral CT	216
Angiography	598
D-dimer	7
Therapy 120	
Hospitalisation day	168
Heparin (UFH)	10
Heparin (LMWH)	12
Clinical recurrent thrombosis	2,142
Bleeding costs	3,524
Monthly costs Coumarin including thrombosis unit	20

* = Costs are taken from the Dutch ANTELOPE study [76].

** = If more than two days have passed between the first perfusion scan and the planned ventilation scan, the perfusion scan should be repeated.

avoidable with any diagnostic strategy (Table 1). Unavoidable costs are the costs for one day hospital admission (Euro 168, Dfl 369) ($ 1 = Euro 0.86; Euro 1 = $ 1.32) for diagnostic tests and one day of intravenous heparin (Euro 10, Dfl 23) for all patients with suspected PE. In addition to these unavoidable costs for testing come the costs for the anticoagulant therapy that should be given to the patients with PE or DVT: 6 days hospitalisation (Euro 168, Dfl 369 per day) and intravenous heparin (Euro 10, Dfl 23 per day) and 3 months of oral anticoagulant therapy with regular monitoring (Euro 20, Dfl 44 per month). In 5% of the patients with anticoagulant therapy a major bleeding complication is expected, the costs of which were calculated from a large multicentre study (Euro 3,515, Dfl 7,732) [44].

Unavoidable mortality consists of the mortality due to deep vein thrombosis or PE despite adequate treatment, which is assumed to be 5% of the patients treated correctly, and mortality due to fatal bleeding complications by the anticoagulant treatment, which is assumed to occur in 0.75% of the patients receiving anticoagulant treatment [37–40].

With a prevalence of 30% PE or DVT the unavoidable costs are Euro 571 (Dfl 1,257) and the unavoidable mortality amounts to 1.7 % per patient with suspected PE.

Diagnostic strategies are compared not with respect to the unavoidable costs and mortality, but with respect to the excess or avoidable costs and mortality. Excess costs are the costs due to prolonged hospital stay and anticoagulant treatment due to longer testing or due to an inadequate treatment. In all treatment strategies studied it was assumed that the testing could be completed in one day unless a ventilation scintigraphy or more than 3 different tests were required, in which case it was assumed that the testing could be completed in two days. The costs of the separate tests are specified in the sections below. The excess costs due to treatment of a patient without DVT or PE consist of the costs of 6 days heparin treatment and 3 months of oral anticoagulant treatment and the costs of major bleedings occurring in 5 % of these patients. These costs amount to Euro 1,305 (Dfl 2,872) per patient with unnecessary anticoagulant treatment. The excess costs due to non-treatment of a patient in whom the diagnosis of DVT or PE was missed are assumed to be Euro 45 (Dfl 100) for a patient with DVT without PE, Euro 91 (Dfl 200) for a patient with subsegmental PE and Euro 182 (Dfl 400) for a patient with segmental or greater PE. Any savings due to not spending money on required anticoagulant therapy are ignored, since many of these patients may receive treatment later on in case of recurrent signs or symptoms of non-fatal PE.

Excess mortality is the mortality due to testing or inadequate treatment. Of all tests considered only the pulmonary angiography is assumed to be associated with a low risk of procedural mortality (0.1 %). The mortality due to anticoagulant treatment of a patient without PE or DVT is assumed to be 0.75 %. Excess mortality due to fatal recurrence in patients with PE or DVT in which the diagnosis was missed and anticoagulant treatment was not given is assumed to be 5 % for patients with DVT only, 10 % for patients with subsegmental PE and 20 % for patients with segmental or greater PE.

Diagnostic tests

The strategies we evaluated were constructed using six diagnostic tests, which have been evaluated to a reasonable extent in the literature and are commonplace in clinical practice. These tests are perfusion and ventilation scintigraphy, ultrasound of the legs, pulmonary angiography, spiral CT and D-dimer.

Although other diagnostic modalities, such as echocardiography, contrast venography, EBT and MRI are available for the diagnosis of PE, these are not employed in large cohorts. Furthermore, their evaluation in large studies is lacking. A main problem, which has been getting attention only in recent years, is related to the distribution of PE. It is obvious that diagnostic tests will be more sensitive as emboli are larger. However, the literature does not give detailed information on the exact distribution of emboli. Nevertheless, we have estimated sensitivity and specificity of diagnostic tests separately for emboli that are confined to subsegmental vessels and for those that are segmental or larger.

Pulmonary angiography

Pulmonary angiography is generally regarded as the reference method for the diagnosis of PE. This creates the problem of setting appropriate sensitivity and specificity estimates. The clinical validity of a normal pulmonary angiogram has been demonstrated in several large clinical studies, which performed follow-up of 3 months or more [9, 31, 45–47]. From these data, it was estimated that the sensitivity of pulmonary angiography was very high. However, some inter- and intraobserver variability exists, hence a sensitivity of 100 % is not a realistic estimate [5, 19, 48]. Since the observer variability increases with a decrease in embolus size, we have separated these estimates into two categories: for subsegmental emboli we assumed a sensitivity of 95 %, while this was estimated to be 98 % for segmental or greater emboli. A specificity of 96 % was assumed.

Pulmonary angiography is an invasive technique, which is correlated with some morbidity and mortality. However, of these, only mortality was regarded as a significant parameter in this setting. Several large studies have addressed the complication rate of pulmonary angiography in recent years. From these, we estimated a procedure-related mortality of 0.1 % [47, 49–52].

The costs for pulmonary angiography were estimated at Euro 598 (Dfl 1,316).

Lung scintigraphy

Lung scintigraphy consists of two separable parts: perfusion and ventilation scintigraphy. Ventilation scintigraphy is only useful in case of segmental defects on the perfusion scan. Based on the PIOPED study, the chances of obtaining various perfusion-ventilation lung scan results are described in Table 2 [5]. A normal perfusion lung scan is considered to exclude the presence of PE, and anticoagulants may be withheld [53 – 55]. At the other end of the spectrum, a high probability lung scan result is considered as sufficient proof to warrant institution of long-term anticoagulant therapy [5, 6, 9, 10, 56 – 62]. Mortality as a complication of lung scintigraphy is considered to be negligible.

The costs for perfusion and ventilation scintigraphy were estimated to be Euro 120 (Dfl 263) and Euro 186 (Dfl 409), respectively.

Table 2. Chances of lung scan results in absence of pulmonary embolism or presence of subsegmental or segmental emboli.

| | Pulmonary thromboembolism | | |
	absent	subseg-mental	segmen-tal or larger
	(percentages)		
Perfusion lung scan			
• normal	20	0.55	0.05
• subsegmental defects	62	74.45	29.24
• segmental defects	18	25.00	70.71
Ventilation lung scan*			
• match	89	85	19.36
• mismatch	11	15	80.64
Combination PV scan			
• normal	20.00	0.55	0.05
• non-diagnostic	78.02	95.60	42.93
• high probability	1.98	3.75	57.02

* = Only performed if segmental defects are detected on perfusion lung scan.

Spiral computed tomography (spiral CT)

Spiral CT is a relatively new diagnostic modality for PE. It has been shown to be accurate in the diagnosis of segmental or larger emboli, but has shown suboptimal sensitivity for thrombi at the subsegmental level [63 – 72]. The interobserver variability is dependent on observer experience and also increases with smaller emboli, thus reducing the sensitivity and, to a lesser extent, the specificity [71, 73, 74]. Furthermore, the clinical validity has been evaluated in only one medium-sized study in selected patients [75]. Nevertheless, its availability, non-invasive nature and the early indications of high accuracy parameters require spiral CT to be included into this cost-effectiveness analysis.

The sensitivity of spiral CT for segmental or larger emboli and thrombi at subsegmental level was assumed at 90 % and 40 %, respectively. The specificity was assumed to be 86 % [76].

Mortality due to spiral CT is considered negligible for this analysis. The costs of spiral CT were estimated to be Euro 216 (Dfl 475).

Ultrasonography of the leg veins

Ultrasonography of the leg veins for the diagnosis of PE is related to the notion that DVT coexists in up to 90 % of patients with proven pulmonary emboli [31, 32]. This led to the investigation of ultrasonography in patients who presented with chest symptoms, which revealed that the sensitivity and specificity were in the order of 35 % and 99 %, respectively [24 – 30].

Mortality due to ultrasonography is considered negligible. The costs for ultrasonography of the leg veins were estimated to be Euro 47 (Dfl 104).

M. Oudkerk, E. J. R. van Beek, W. L. J. van Putten, F. F. H. Rutten

Plasma D-dimer measurements

Table 3. Variables in the baseline analysis and the range used in the sensititivy analysis.

	base-line	sensitivity analysis
Prevalence of PE	30%	20%–40%
– subsegmental PE	9%	6%–12%
– segmental PE	21%	14%–28%
Pulmonary angiography		
– mortality	0.1%	0%–0.2%
– specificity	96%	not varied
– sensitivity subsegmental PE	95%	90%–97%
– sensitivity segmental PE	98%	96%–99%
Lung scintigraphy		
– specificity	see Table 2	not varied
– sensitivity	see Table 2	not varied
Spiral CT		
– specificity	86%	80%–95%
– sensitivity subsegmental PE	40%	not varied
– sensitivity segmental PE	90%	not varied
Ultrasonography		
– specificity[1]	99%	not varied
– sensitivity[2]	35%	not varied
D-dimer		
– specificity[3]	50%	40%–60%
– sensitivity[4]	95%	90%–99%
Mortality due to missed diagnosis		
– deep vein thrombosis	5%	2.5%–10%
– subsegmental PE	10%	5%–20%
– segmental PE	20%	10%–40%
Mortality due to bleeding complications[5]	0.75%	0.5%–1%

[1] for patients without DVT, irrespective of PE

[2] for patients with DVT, irrespective of PE

[3] for patients without DVT and without PE

[4] for patients with PE or DVT

[5] excess mortality in patients without PE or DVT, but treated with anticoagulants

D-dimer is a break-down product of cross-linked fibrin [77]. Increased levels of plasma D-dimer may be encountered with the break-down of thrombi, although many other causes of intravascular thrombosis (such as sepsis, pregnancy, or post-operative state) yield similar results [78, 79]. Plasma D-dimer levels may be measured by a variety of methods. Latex agglutination methods have proved to be insufficiently sensitive for clinical application [80–82]. Enzyme-linked immunosorbent assays have shown sufficient detection capabilities; however, these tests are time-consuming and have limited applicability in individual patients [78, 80–88]. More recently, a number of fast, individual techniques based on monoclonal antibody reactions have been investigated and shown promising results [89–92]. Several studies have shown the sensitivity of these new tests to be over 90%, while the specificity ranges between 30% and 50% [89–92]. Some clinical management studies have been conducted in patients with suspected venous thromboembolism [93–95], but only one of these was exclusively in patients with suspected PE [93]. It has become clear that the sensitivity will have to be very high, if D-dimer measurement is going to be of value, i. e. safe, in the management of venous thromboembolism [96]. In the present analysis, we assumed a sensitivity of 95% and a specificity of 50%.

The mortality due to D-dimer testing is considered negligible. The costs for a fast D-dimer test were estimated to be Euro 7 (Dfl 16).

Sensitivity analysis

The baseline analysis has made use of the assumptions stated above. To test the influence of changing parameters on the final outcome of the analysis, we performed sensitivity analyses by changing one parameter or set of parameter values at a time. The parameters are summarised in Table 3, which shows the range over which the sensitivity analyses were carried out.

Evaluated diagnostic strategies

A total of 41 diagnostic strategies were evaluated using a mathematical model. These strategies were:

1. *Clairvoyant:* this strategy assumes that the clinician would always be correct in diagnosing patients with venous thromboembolism and institute or withhold anticoagulant therapy correctly in all patients.
2. *Treat all:* this strategy is based on complete absence of diagnostic tests and all patients with suspected venous thromboembolism receiving anticoagulant therapy. This is a reference strategy: no pulmonary emboli remain untreated.
3. *Treat none:* this strategy may be regarded as a baseline (natural course of the disease), and is included as a matter of reference.
4. *Perfusion scintigraphy (P):* this strategy is based on withholding anticoagulant therapy in patients with a normal perfusion lung scan, and treating all others.
5. *Perfusion ventilation scintigraphy, ultrasonography and angiography (PVUA):* in this strategy patients are initially managed on the basis of the lung scan (anticoagulants are withheld or instituted in case of a normal perfusion scan or high probability scan, respectively). In patients with non-diagnostic lung scan results, ultrasonography of the leg veins is performed for potential presence of DVT (and these patients receive anticoagulant therapy). In patients in whom ultrasonography is normal, pulmonary angiography is performed as the final diagnostic test.
6. *Ultrasonography and angiography (UA):* patients with suspected PE undergo ultrasonography of the leg veins for detection of DVT (and are treated if abnormal). In the remainder, pulmonary angiography is carried out.
7. *Perfusion ventilation scintigraphy and angiography (PVA):* this strategy is similar to strategy 5, but all patients with non-diagnostic lung scan results undergo pulmonary angiography.
8. *Perfusion scintigraphy and angiography (PA):* anticoagulants are withheld in patients with a normal perfusion lung scan, the remainder undergo pulmonary angiography.
9. *Angiography (A):* all patients undergo pulmonary angiography.
10. *Perfusion ventilation scintigraphy and ultrasonography (PVU):* this strategy is similar to strategy 5, but here all patients with normal ultrasonography findings remain untreated.
11. *Perfusion ventilation scintigraphy (PV):* in this strategy, management relies solely on the lung scan findings: patients with a high probability lung scan are treated with anticoagulants, while patients with other lung scan findings remain untreated.
12. *D-dimer (D):* venous thromboembolism is excluded if a normal plasma D-dimer concentration is measured, the remainder receive anticoagulant therapy.
13. *D-dimer and perfusion scintigraphy (DP):* venous thromboembolism is excluded if a normal plasma D-dimer level exists. In the remainder, perfusion lung scan is used to further exclude PE. In patients with abnormal D-dimer levels and non-normal perfusion scintigram, anticoagulant therapy is given.
14. *D-dimer, perfusion-ventilation scintigraphy, ultrasonography and angiography (DPVUA):* venous thromboembolism is considered excluded by either a normal D-dimer test or a normal perfusion lung scan, whereas anticoagulant therapy is instituted in patients with either a high probability lung scan or abnormal compression ultrasonogram. In the remaining patients, angiography serves as the final test.
15. *D-dimer, perfusion-ventilation scintigraphy and angiography (DPVA):* similar to strategy 14, but no ultrasonography performed.
16. *D-dimer, perfusion scintigraphy and angiography (DPA):* similar to strategy 14, but neither ventilation scintigraphy nor ultrasonography performed.
17. *D-dimer and angiography (DA):* PE excluded by normal D-dimer levels, the remainder undergo pulmonary angiography.
18. *Ultrasonography, D-dimer and perfusion scintigraphy (UDP):* venous thromboembolism proven by ultrasonography, the remainder undergo D-dimer testing. Thromboembolism excluded by normal D-dimer test or normal perfusion lung scan. The remaining patients are treated with anticoagulants.
19. *D-dimer, perfusion-ventilation scintigraphy (DPV):* venous thromboembolism excluded by normal D-dimer, and proven by high probability lung scan. Patients with abnormal D-dimer values and normal or non-diagnostic lung scan findings remain untreated.

20. *Perfusion-ventilation scintigraphy, spiral CT and angiography (PVSA):* venous thromboembolism excluded by normal perfusion scan and proven by high probability lung scan. In patients with other lung scan findings, spiral CT is performed. If pulmonary emboli are shown, patients are treated with anticoagulants. Patients with normal spiral CT scans undergo pulmonary angiography.

21. *Perfusion-ventilation scintigraphy, ultrasonography, spiral CT and angiography (PVUSA):* similar to strategy 20, but ultrasonography performed prior to spiral CT for detection of DVT.

22. *Perfusion scintigraphy, ultrasonography, spiral CT and angiography (PUSA):* patients with normal perfusion lung scan remain untreated. The remaining patients undergo ultrasonography. If ultrasonography shows DVT, patients receive anticoagulant therapy. Patients with normal ultrasound results undergo spiral CT and pulmonary angiography if spiral CT is normal (similar to strategy 20).

23. *Perfusion scintigraphy, spiral CT and angiography (PSA):* venous thromboembolism excluded by normal perfusion scan. The remaining patients undergo spiral CT. In patients with normal spiral CT findings, pulmonary angiography is performed.

24. *Spiral CT and angiography (SA):* venous thromboembolism proven by spiral CT. If spiral CT does not show thrombi, pulmonary angiography is performed.

25. *Ultrasonography, spiral CT and angiography (USA):* venous thromboembolism proven by either abnormal ultrasound findings or spiral CT demonstrated thrombi. In the remaining patients, angiography performed as final test.

26. *Perfusion scintigraphy and spiral CT (PS):* venous thromboembolism excluded by normal perfusion lung scan. The remaining patients undergo spiral CT. Patients with normal spiral CT findings remain untreated.

27. *Ultrasonography, perfusion scintigraphy and spiral CT (UPS):* similar to strategy 26, but ultrasonography used as initial screening test for detection of DVT.

28. *Perfusion-ventilation scintigraphy and spiral CT (PVS):* initial management is based on the lung scan (normal perfusion excludes venous thromboembolism, high probability scan result proves disease). In patients with non-diagnostic lung scan findings, spiral CT is used to prove venous thromboembolism. Patients with normal spiral CT remain untreated.

29. *Spiral CT (S):* all management is based solely on spiral CT.

30. *D-dimer, perfusion-ventilation scintigraphy, spiral CT and angiography (DPVSA):* similar to strategy 20, but D-dimer used as initial screening test. In patients with normal D-dimer results, no further diagnostic tests are performed and these remain untreated.

31. *D-dimer, perfusion-ventilation scintigraphy, ultrasonography, spiral CT and angiography (DPVUSA):* similar to strategy 21, but D-dimer used as initial screening test for exclusion of venous thromboembolism.

32. *D-dimer, perfusion scintigraphy, ultrasonography, spiral CT and angiography (DPUSA):* similar to strategy 22, but D-dimer as initial test for exclusion of venous thromboembolism.

33. *D-dimer, perfusion scintigraphy, spiral CT and angiography (DPSA):* similar to strategy 23, but D-dimer used as initial screening test.

34. *D-dimer, spiral CT and angiography (DSA):* similar to strategy 24, but D-dimer used as initial screening test.

35. *D-dimer, ultrasonography, spiral CT and angiography (DUSA):* similar to strategy 25, but D-dimer used as initial screening test.

36. *D-dimer, perfusion scintigraphy and spiral CT (DPS):* similar to strategy 26, but D-dimer used as initial screening test.

37. *Ultrasonography, D-dimer, perfusion scintigraphy and spiral CT (UDPS):* similar to strategy 26, but ultrasonography and D-dimer used as initial screening tests for proof or exclusion of venous thromboembolism, respectively.

38. *D-dimer, perfusion-ventilation scintigraphy and spiral CT (DPVS):* similar to strategy 28, but D-dimer used as initial screening test.

39. *Perfusion-ventilation scintigraphy, D-dimer and spiral CT (PVDS):* similar to strategy 28, but D-dimer used to exclude venous thromboembolism in patients with non-diagnostic lung scan results. Patients with non-diagnostic lung scan results and abnormal D-dimer levels undergo spiral CT.

40. *D-dimer and spiral CT (DS):* venous thromboembolism excluded by normal D-dimer test. In the remaining patients, spiral CT is used as final test (similar to strategy 29).

41. *Perfusion scintigraphy, ultrasonography and angiography (PUA):* similar to strategy 5, but no ventilation scintigraphy performed. Hence, all patients with non-normal perfusion lung scan undergo ultrasonography. Angiography is performed as final test in those with normal ultrasonography results.

Outcome measures

It was assumed that the outcomes of all tests are independent conditional on the true state of the patient. The primary outcome measures for each strategy were the average mortality and costs per patient, defined as the excess mortality and costs compared to the optimal (clairvoyant) strategy and treatment. Secondary parameters of interest were the proportions of patients with inadequate treatment decision. A cost-effectiveness analysis was performed in which for each strategy the costs per life saved were calculated compared to the natural course of pulmonary embolism (no treatment strategy).

Results

Outcome of the various strategies

Table 4 gives an overview of the results of the various strategies. The clairvoyant strategy made use of no diagnostic tests, for the remaining strategies the percentages of patients requiring to undergo the various diagnostic tests is listed in Table 4a.

The excess mortality, excess costs (as compared to the clairvoyant strategy) and inadequate treatment decisions are listed in the Table 4b. The strategies are listed in order of increasing mortality (Table 4c). Some interesting results will be highlighted.

Excess mortality is lowest in strategies that use pulmonary angiography as a final diagnostic test. Strategy 5 has the lowest mortality of all angiography strategies. This is mainly the result of adequate use of other non-invasive tests, which reduce the number of patients requiring angiography.

With the exception of strategy 5, the performance of spiral CT prior to pulmonary angiography generally leads to a reduction in mortality (i.e. strategies 23 vs. 8, 20 vs. 7, 25 vs. 6 and 22 vs. 41). However, this slightly better performance in terms of mortality is correlated with performance of spiral CT in more than two-thirds of patients for a reduction in pulmonary angiography of only approximately 25%. Furthermore, the number of inadequate treatment decisions increases three-fold, largely as a result of overtreatment. These changes in strategies result in increased costs with the incorporation of spiral CT prior to pulmonary angiography.

Strategies which incorporate plasma D-dimer measurement for the exclusion of venous thromboembolism result in a two-fold or more increase in mortality when compared to other strategies using pulmonary angiography. There is a major cost reduction, but this is largely due to the inadequate withholding of anticoagulant therapy in patients with venous thromboembolism.

Strategies which solely rely on non-invasive techniques all lead to a three to four-fold increase in mortality when compared to strategies 5 or 23. It is clear that this is mainly related to increasing numbers of patients who do not receive anticoagulant therapy despite the presence of venous thromboembolism. The costs of these strategies are all much lower than strategies containing angiography, but the mortality is deemed unacceptably high.

Figure 1 shows a plot of the various strategies in terms of mortality versus costs. It becomes obvious that some strategies, although relatively cheap, result in mortality rates which are almost 6 times higher if one compares, for instance, the cost-effectiveness ratio of strategy 40 with strategy 5. Figure 1a shows a plot of those strategies that result in excess mortality of less than 0.3%. Clearly strategy 5 dominates with the lowest mortality, while it is also one of the cheapest. For comparison, the strategy that performs angiography in all patients (9) is cheaper, but it also results in a higher procedure-related mortality. This illustrates the notion that it is worthwhile to reduce the number of patients that require pulmonary angiography as long as these non-invasive diagnostic tests carry sufficient sensitivity, such that not too many patients with pulmonary thromboembolism remain untreated. From this figure it is easy to select the most cost-effective strategies, which are those that are nearest to the axes of the plot. Other strategies are dominated, e.g. they have both higher mortality and higher costs. For instance, strategy 5 dominates strategies 20–25.

Table 4a. Outcome of the various strategies in terms of tests required.

Strategy*	Test performed (% of patients)**					
	P-scan	V-scan	US	Angio	D-dimer	SVCT
1. clairvoyant	–	–	–	–	–	–
2. treat all	–	–	–	–	–	–
3. treat none	–	–	–	–	–	–
4. perfusion	100	–	–	–	–	–
5. PVUA	100	30	72	67	–	–
6. UA	–	–	100	92	–	–
7. PVA	100	30	–	72	–	–
8. PA	100	–	–	86	–	–
9. Angio	–	–	–	100	–	–
10. PVU	100	30	72	–	–	–
11. PV	100	30	–	–	–	–
12. D-dimer	–	–	–	–	100	–
13. DP	64	–	–	–	100	–
14. DPVUA	64	23	44	40	100	–
15. DPVA	64	23	–	44	100	–
16. DPA	64	–	–	56	100	–
17. DA	–	–	–	46	100	–
18. UDP	56	–	100	–	92	–
19. DPV	64	23	–	–	100	–
20. PVSA	100	30	–	53	–	72
21. PVUSA	100	30	72	51	–	67
22. PUSA	100	–	86	53	–	78
23. PSA	100	–	–	56	–	86
24. SA	–	–	–	68	–	100
25. USA	–	–	100	65	–	92
26. PS	100	–	–	–	–	86
27. UPS	92	–	100	–	–	78
28. PVS	100	30	–	–	–	72
29. Spiral CT	–	–	–	–	–	100
30. DPVSA	64	23	–	29	100	44
31. DPVUSA	64	23	44	28	100	40
32. DPUSA	64	–	56	29	100	49
33. DPSA	64	–	–	31	100	56
34. DSA	–	–	–	37	100	64
35. DUSA	–	–	64	35	100	56
36. DPS	64	–	–	–	100	56
37. UDPS	56	–	100	–	92	49
38. DPVS	64	23	–	–	100	44
39. VDS	100	30	–	–	72	44
40. DS	–	–	–	–	100	64
41. PUA	100	–	86	78	–	–

* = For description of strategy see Materials and Methods section.

** = Perfusion scan, ventilation scan, ultrasonography of leg veins, pulmonary angiography, D-dimer test, spiral volumetric computed tomography.

Table 4b. Outcome of the various strategies in terms of mortality, average costs per patient and inadequately treated patients (in order of increasing mortality).

Strategy*	Mortality (%)	Extra costs** (Euro)	Inadequate treatment decisions (%)	
			treatment withheld	treated***
1. clairvoyant	0.000	0	0.00	0.00
5. PVUA	0.174	683	0.59	4.09
23. PSA	0.175	766	0.46	9.75
20. PVSA	0.181	806	0.42	10.90
25. USA	0.190	803	0.29	12.77
22. PUSA	0.192	857	0.36	10.21
21. PVUSA	0.193	882	0.33	11.35
7. PVA	0.196	672	0.77	3.57
24. SA	0.199	780	0.39	12.19
41. PUA	0.206	664	0.78	2.77
6. UA	0.218	643	0.72	3.47
8. PA	0.243	664	1.02	2.24
9. Angio	0.255	636	0.97	2.80
31. DPVUSA	0.368	510	1.82	5.67
32. DPUSA	0.370	498	1.84	5.11
34. DSA	0.376	450	1.88	6.10
30. DPVSA	0.377	507	1.90	5.45
33. DPSA	0.380	497	1.94	4.88
35. DUSA	0.382	502	1.78	6.38
14. DPVUA	0.391	456	2.06	2.04
15. DPVA	0.402	424	2.23	1.78
18. UDP	0.410	493	1.19	28.38
4. perfusion	0.427	850	0.08	55.92
16. DPA	0.454	439	2.48	1.12
17. DA	0.456	409	2.42	1.40
13. DP	0.473	451	1.58	27.96
12. D-dimer	0.517	466	1.50	34.95
2. treat all	0.524	913	0.00	69.90
28. PVS	0.781	471	6.22	9.02
27. UPS	0.791	442	5.72	8.45
39. PVDS	0.852	368	6.79	5.20
37. UDPS	0.931	334	6.56	4.57
38. DPVS	0.965	296	7.41	4.51
26. PS	1.027	416	7.62	7.83
29. Spiral CT	1.038	352	7.59	9.79
36. DPS	1.205	267	8.74	3.91
40. DS	1.208	219	8.71	4.89
10. PVU	2.035	271	13.39	1.93
11. PV	2.693	236	17.79	1.38
19. DPV	2.806	169	18.40	0.69
3. treat none	5.105	46	30.10	0.00

* = For description of strategy see Materials and Methods section.

** = Clairvoyant strategy reflects the absolute threshold for necessary diagnostic and treatment costs (Euro 580, Dfl 1,275).

*** = In patients who receive anticoagulants, 5% will have major bleeding complications.

Table 5. Mortality and cost-effectiveness in terms of life saved as compared to natural course of pulmonary embolism.

Strategy*	mort	cost	ls	ec	cpls
5. PVUA	1.74	683	49.31	637	12,791
23. PSA	1.75	766	49.30	719	14,589
20. PVSA	1.81	806	49.24	760	15,425
25. USA	1.90	803	49.15	756	15,385
22. PUSA	1.92	857	49.13	810	16,494
21. PVUSA	1.93	882	49.12	836	17,013
7. PVA	1.96	672	49.09	626	12,747
24. SA	1.99	780	49.06	734	14,960
41. PUA	2.06	664	48.99	617	12,597
6. UA	2.18	643	48.87	596	12,202
8. PA	2.43	664	48.62	618	12,705
9. angio	2.55	636	48.50	589	12,154
31. DPVUSA	3.68	510	47.37	464	9,795
32. DPUSA	3.70	498	47.35	451	9,535
34. DSA	3.76	450	47.29	403	8,526
30. DPVSA	3.77	507	47.28	460	9,735
33. DPSA	3.80	497	47.25	450	9,529
35. DUSA	3.82	502	47.23	456	9,651
14. DPVUA	3.91	456	47.14	409	8,685
15. DPVA	4.02	424	47.03	378	8,033
18. UDP	4.10	493	46.95	447	9,519
4. perfusion	4.27	850	46.78	803	17,172
16. DPA	4.54	439	46.51	393	8,445
17. DA	4.56	409	46.49	363	7,802
13. DP	4.73	451	46.32	404	8,726
12. D-dimer	5.17	466	45.88	419	9,143
2. treat all	5.24	913	45.81	866	18,907
28. PVS	7.81	471	43.24	425	9,819
27. UPS	7.91	442	43.14	396	9,175
39. PVDS	8.52	368	42.53	321	7,555
37. UDPS	9.31	334	41.74	288	6,899
38. DPVS	9.65	296	41.40	249	6,021
26. PS	10.27	416	40.78	370	9,066
29. spiral CT	10.38	352	40.67	306	7,524
36. DPS	12.05	267	39.00	221	5,655
40. DS	12.08	219	38.97	173	4,429
10. PVU	20.35	271	30.70	224	7.310
11. PV	26.93	236	24.12	189	7,851
19. DPV	28.06	169	22.99	123	5,330
3. treat none	51.05	46	–	–	–

*	=	For description of strategy see Materials and Methods section.
mort	=	mortality per 1,000
cost	=	costs (Euro) per patient)
ls	=	lives saved per 1,000 compared to no treatment strategy
ec	=	extra costs (Euro) compared to no treatment strategy
cpls	=	costs per life saved compared to no treatment

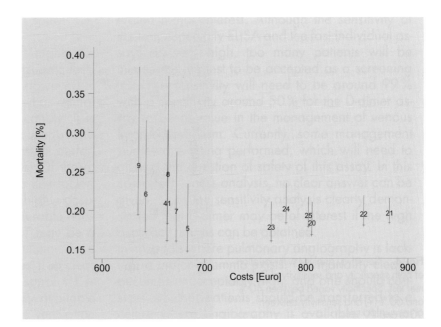

Fig. 2. Sensitivity analysis for selected strategies. Variation of sensitivity of pulmonary angiography between 90 % and 97 % (+) for subsegmental and 96 % and 99 % (+) for segmental emboli.

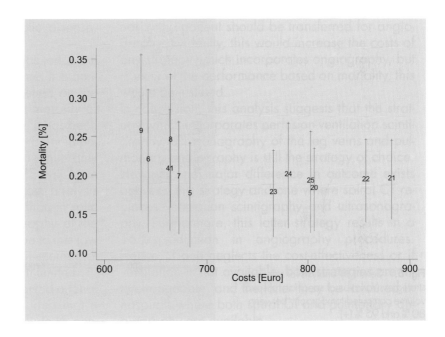

Fig. 3. Sensitivity analysis for selected strategies. Variation of mortality of pulmonary angiography between 0 % and 0.2 % (+).

strategies which require most patients to undergo pulmonary angiography (Figure 3). Strategy 23 and strategy 5 remain the best strategies over the range tested.

D-dimer had a baseline sensitivity of 95 % and specificity of 50 %, but this seemed insufficient. In Figure 4, it becomes evident that D-dimer measurement may be highly cost-effective if the sensitivity is increased to 99 % and the specificity to 60 %. Under those circumstances, strategies using D-dimer as an initial screening test would have to be favoured.

The effects of increasing specificity of spiral CT are shown in Figure 5. Clearly, with increasing specificity fewer patients would require unnecessary anticoagulant therapy. Hence, both mortality and costs would decrease, and the mortality of strategies 20 – 25 would become less than that of strategy 5.

The remaining factors which were addressed in the sensitivity analysis did not lead to a change in order of the best strategies. Changes in prevalence had a minimal effect, while an increase in bleeding complications resulted in worse performance of strategies with a high number of patients

References

1. Kierkegaard A. Incidence of acute deep venous thrombosis in two districts. A phlebographic study. Acta Chir Scand 1980; 146: 267–269

2. Anderson FA, Wheeler HB, Goldberg RJ. A population-based perspective of the hospital incidence and case-fatality rates of deep vein thrombosis and PE. The Worcester DVT study. Arch Intern Med 1991; 151: 933–938

3. Silverstein MD, Heit JA, Mohr DN, Petterson TM, O'Fallon WM, Melton LJ III. Trends in the incidence of deep vein thrombosis and pulmonary embolism: a 25-year population-based study. Arch Intern Med 1998; 158: 585–593

4. Van Beek EJR, Büller HR, Van Everdingen JJE, Zwijnenburg A, ten Cate JW. Diagnostic management of suspected pulmonary embolism in the Netherlands: results from a questionnaire. Thromb Haemostas 1991; 65: 1171

5. The PIOPED investigators. Value of the ventilation/perfusion scan in acute pulmonary embolism: results of the prospective investigation of pulmonary embolism diagnosis (PIOPED). JAMA 1990; 263: 2753–2759

6. Biello DR, Mattar AG, McKnight RC, Siegel BA. Ventilation-perfusion studies in suspected pulmonary embolism. Am J Radiol 1979; 133: 1033–1037

7. McNeil BJ. Ventilation-perfusion studies and the diagnosis of pulmonary embolism: concise communication. J Nucl Med 1980; 21: 319–323

8. Hull RD, Raskob GE, Coates G, Panju AA, Gill GJ. A new noninvasive management strategy for patients with suspected pulmonary embolism. Arch Intern Med 1989; 149: 2549–2555

9. Cheely R, McCartney WH, Perry JR, et al. The role of noninvasive tests versus pulmonary angiography in the diagnosis of pulmonary embolism. Am J Med 1981; 70: 17–22

10. McBride K, LaMorte WW, Menzoian JO. Can ventilation-perfusion scans accurately diagnose acute pulmonary embolism? Arch Surg 1986; 121: 754–757

11. Van Beek EJR, Kuijer PMM, Büller HR, Brandjes DPM, PMM Bossuyt, ten Cate JW. The clinical course of patients with suspected pulmonary embolism. Arch Intern Med 1997; 157: 2593–2598

12. Levine MN, Raskob G, Landefeld SC, Hirsh J. Hemorrhagic complications of anticoagulant treatment. Chest 1995; 108 (Suppl. 4): 276–289

13. Hirsh J. Heparin. N Engl J Med 1991; 324: 1565–1574

14. Hirsh J. Oral anticoagulant drugs. N Engl J Med 1991; 324: 1865–1875

15. The Columbus investigators. Low molecular weight heparin in the treatment of patients with venous thromboembolism. N Engl J Med 1997; 337: 657–662

16. Simonneau G, Sors H, Charbonnier B, et al. A comparison of low-molecular-weight heparin with unfractionated heparin for acute pulmonary embolism. N Engl J Med 1997; 337: 663–669

17. Dalen JE, Alpert JS, Hirsch J. Thrombolytic therapy for pulmonary embolism: is it effective? Is it safe? When is it indicated? Arch Intern Med 1997; 157: 2550–2556

18. Oser RF, Zuckerman DA, Gutierrez FR, Brink JA. Anatomic distribution of pulmonary emboli at pulmonary angiography: implications for cross-sectional imaging. Radiology 1996; 199: 31–35

19. Van Beek EJR, Bakker AJ, Reekers JA. Interobserver variability of pulmonary angiography in patients with non-diagnostic lung scan results: conventional versus digital subtraction arteriography. Radiology 1996; 198: 721–724

20. Huisman MB, Büller HR, ten Cate JW, et al. Unexpected high prevalence of silent pulmonary embolism in patients with deep venous thrombosis. Chest 1989; 95: 498–502

21. Dorfman GS, Cronan JJ, Tupper TB, Messersmith RN, Denny DP, Lee CH. Occult pulmonary embolism: a common occurrence in patients with deep venous thrombosis. Am J Roentgenol 1987; 148: 263–266

22. Doyle DJ, Turpie AGG, Hirsh J, et al. Adjusted subcutaneous heparin or continuous intravenous heparin in patients with acute deep vein thrombosis. Ann Intern Med 1987; 107: 441–445

23. Parcouret G, Alison D, Pootier JM, Bertrand P, Charbonnier B. Free-floating thrombus and embolic risk in patients with angiographically confirmed proximal deep venous thrombosis. Arch Intern Med 1997; 157: 305–308

24. Hull RD, Raskob GE, Ginsberg JS, et al. A non-invasive strategy for the treatment of patients with suspected pulmonary embolism. Arch Intern Med 1994; 154: 289–297

25. Schiff MJ, Feinberg AW, Naidich JB. Noninvasive venous examinations as a screening test for pulmonary embolism. Arch Intern Med 1987; 147: 505–507

26. Killewich LA, Nunnelee JD, Auer AI. Value of lower extremity venous duplex examination in the diagnosis of pulmonary embolism. J Vasc Surg 1993; 17: 934–939

27. Quinn RJ, Nour R, Butler SP, et al. Pulmonary embolism in patients with indeterminate probability lung scans: diagnosis with Doppler venous US and D-dimer measurements. Radiology 1994; 190: 509–511

28. Smith LL, Iber C, Sirr S. Pulmonary embolism: confirmation with venous duplex US as adjunct to lung scanning. Radiology 1994; 191: 143–147

29. Christiansen F, Kellerth B, Anderson T, Ragnarson A, Hjortevang F. Ultrasound at scintigraphic "intermediate probability of pulmonary embolism". Acta Radiol 1996; 37: 14–17

30. Turkstra F, Kuijer PMM, van Beek EJR, Brandjes DPM, Büller HR, Ten Cate JW. Value of compression ultrasonography for the detection of deep venous thrombosis in patients suspected of having pulmonary embolism. Ann Intern Med 1997; 126: 775–781

31. Hull RD, Hirsh J, Carter CJ, et al. Pulmonary angiography, ventilation lung scanning and venography for clinically suspected pulmonary embolism with abnormal perfusion lung scan. Ann Intern Med 1983; 98: 891–899

32. Kruit WHJ, de Boer AC, Sing AK, van Roon F. The significance of venography in the management of patients with clinically suspected pulmonary embolism. J Intern Med 1991; 230: 333–339

33. Barritt DW, Jordan SC. Anticoagulant drugs in the treatment of pulmonary embolism. A controlled study. Lancet 1960; i: 1309–1312

34. Carson JL, Kelley MA, Duff A, et al. The clinical course of pulmonary embolism. N Engl J Med 1992; 326: 1240–1245

35. Douketis JD, Kearon C, Bates S, Duku EK, Ginsberg JS. Risk of fatal pulmonary embolism. JAMA 1998; 279: 458–462

36. Monreal M, Ruiz J, Salvador R, Morera J, Arias A. Recurrent pulmonary embolism. A prospective study. Chest 1989; 95: 976–979

37. Prandoni P, Lensing AWA, Cogo A, et al. The long-term clinical course of acute deep venous thrombosis. Ann Intern Med 1996; 125: 1–7

38. Beyth RJ, Cohen AM, Landefeld CS. Long term outcomes of deep vein thrombosis. Arch Intern Med 1995; 155: 1031–1037

39. Gallus A, Tillett J, Jackson J, Mills W, Wycherley A. Safety and efficacy of warfarin started early after submassive venous thrombosis or pulmonary embolism. Lancet 1986; ii: 1293–1296

40. Hull R, Delmore T, Genton E, et al. Warfarin-sodium versus low-dose heparin in the long-term treatment of venous thrombosis. N Engl J Med 1979; 301: 855–858

41. Hull RD, Raskob GE, Rosenbloom D, et al. Heparin for 5 days as compared with 10 days in the initial treatment of proximal vein thrombosis. N Engl J Med 1990; 322: 1260–1264

42. Brandjes DPM, Heyboer H, Büller HR, De Rijk M, Jagt H, Ten Cate JW. Aceno-coumarol and heparin compared with acenocoumarol alone in the initial treatment of proximal vein thrombosis. N Engl J Med 1992; 327: 1485–1489

43. Kuijer PMM, Prins MH, Büller HR. Low-molecular weight heparins: treatment of venous thromboembolism. In: Sasahara AA, Loscalzo J (eds.). New therapeutic agents in thrombosis and thrombolysis. Marcel Dekker Inc, New York, 1997: 127–142

44. Michel BC, Seerden RJ, Van Beek EJR, Büller HR, Rutten FFH. A modelling approach towards the evaluation of the cost-effectiveness of diagnostic strategies in pulmonary embolism. Health Economics 1996; 5: 307–318

45. Novelline RA, Baltarowich OH, Athanasoulis CA, et al. The clinical course of patients with suspected pulmonary embolism and a negative pulmonary arteriogram. Radiology 1978; 126: 561–567

46. Henry JW, Relyea B, Stein PD. Continuing risk of thromboemboli among patients with normal pulmonary angiograms. Chest 1995; 107: 1375–1378

47. Van Beek EJR, Reekers JA, Batchelor D, Brandjes DPM, Peeters FLM, Büller HR. Feasibility, safety and clinical utility of angiography in patients with suspected pulmonary embolism and non-diagnostic lung scan findings. Eur Radiol 1996; 6: 415–419

48. Quinn MF, Lundell CJ, Klotz TA, et al. Reliability of selective pulmonary arteriography in the diagnosis of pulmonary embolism. Am J Radiol 1987; 149: 469–471

49. Stein PD, Athanasoulis C, Alavi A, et al. Complications and validity of pulmonary angiography in acute pulmonary embolism. Circulation 1992; 85: 462–468

50. Van Rooij WJJ, Den Heeten GJ, Sluzewski M. Pulmonary embolism: diagnosis in 211 patients with use of selective pulmonary digital subtraction angiography with a flow-directed catheter. Radiology 1995; 195: 793–797

51. Hudson ER, Smith TP, McDermott VG, et al. Pulmonary angiography performed with iopamidol: complications in 1434 patients. Radiology 1996; 198: 61–65

52. Nilsson T, Carlsson A, Mare K. Pulmonary angiography: a safe procedure with modern contrast media and technique. Eur Radiol 1998; 8: 86–89

53. Kipper MS, Moser KM, Kortman KE, Ashburn WL. Longterm follow-up of patients with suspected pulmonary embolism and a normal lung scan. Chest 1982; 82: 411–415

54. Hull RD, Raskob GE, Coates G, Panju AA. Clinical validity of a normal perfusion lung scan in patients with suspected pulmonary embolism. Chest 1990; 97: 23–26

55. Van Beek EJR, Kuyer PMM, Schenk BE, Brandjes DPM, Ten Cate JW, Büller HR. A normal perfusion lung scan in patients with clinically suspected pulmonary embolism: frequency and clinical validity. Chest 1995; 108: 170–173

56. Hull RD, Hirsh J, Carter CJ, et al. Diagnostic value of ventilation-perfusion lung scanning in patients with suspected pulmonary embolism. Chest 1985; 88: 819–828

57. Hull RD, Raskob GE, Carter CJ, et al. Pulmonary embolism in outpatients with pleuritic chest pain. Arch Intern Med 1988; 148: 838–844

58. Alderson PO, Biello DR, Sachariah KG, Siegel BA. Scintigraphic detection of pulmonary embolism in patients with obstructive pulmonary disease. Radiology 1981; 138: 661–666

59. Spies WG, Burstein SP, Dillehay GL, Vogelzang RL, Spies SM. Ventilation-perfusion scintigraphy in suspected pulmonary embolism: correlation with pulmonary angiography and refinement of criteria for interpretation. Radiology 1986; 159: 383–390

60. Gray HW, McKillop JH, Bessent RG, Fogelman I, Smith ML, Moran F. Lung scanning for pulmonary embolism: clinical and pulmonary angiographic correlations. Q J Med 1990; 77: 1135–1150

61. McNeil BJ. A diagnostic strategy using ventilation-perfusion studies in patients suspected for pulmonary embolism. J Nucl Med 1976; 17: 613–616

62. Fischer KC, McNeil BJ. The indeterminate lung scan: its characteristics and its association with pulmonary embolism. Eur J Nucl Med 1979; 4: 49–53

63. Remy-Jardin M, Remy J, Wattinne L, Giraud F. Central pulmonary thromboembolism: diagnosis with spiral volumetric CT with the single breath-hold technique – comparison with pulmonary angiography. Radiology 1992; 185: 381–387

64. Dresel S, Stäbler A, Scheidler J, Hozknecht N, Tatsch K, Hahn K. Diagnostic approach in acute pulmonary embolism: perfusion scintigraphy versus spiral computed tomography. Nucl Med Comm 1995; 16: 1009–1015

65. Blum AG, Delfau F, Grignon B, et al. Spiral-computed tomography versus pulmonary angiography in the diagnosis of acute massive pulmonary embolism. Am J Cardiol 1994; 74: 96–98

66. Steiner VP, Wesner PD, Lund GK, et al. Primärdiagnostik und Verlaufskontrolle der akuten Lungenembolie: Vergleich zwischen digitaler Subtraktionsangiographie und Spiral-CT. Fortschr Röntgenstr 1994; 161: 285–291

67. Goodman LR, Curtin JJ, Mewissen MW, et al. Detection of pulmonary embolism in patients with unresolved clinical and scintigraphic diagnosis: helical CT versus angiography. Am J Roentgenol 1995; 164: 1369–1374

68. Drucker EA, Rivitz SM, Shepard JO, Boiselle PM, Trotman-Dickenson B, McLoud TC. Assessment of helical CT in the diagnosis of acute pulmonary embolism. Radiology 1996; 201(P): 303

69. Remy-Jardin M, Remy J, Deschildre F, et al. Diagnosis of pulmonary embolism with spiral CT: comparison with pulmonary angiography and scintigraphy. Radiology 1996; 200: 699–706

70. Van Rossum AB, Treurniet FEE, Kieft GJ, Smith SJ, Schepers-Bok R. Role of spiral volumetric computed tomographic scanning in the assessment of patients with clinical suspicion of pulmonary embolism and an abnormal ventilation/perfusion lung scan. Thorax 1996; 51: 23–28

71. Van Rossum AB, Pattynama PMT, Tjin A Ton ER, et al. Pulmonary embolism: validation of spiral CT angiography in 149 patients. Radiology 1996; 201: 467–470

72. Mayo JR, Remy-Jardin M, Müller N, et al. Pulmonary embolism: prospective comparison of spiral CT with ventilation-perfusion scintigraphy. Radiology 1997; 205: 447–452

73. Remy-Jardin M, Remy J, Artaud D, Deschildre F, Duhamel A. Peripheral pulmonary arteries: optimization of the spiral CT acquisition protocol. Radiology 1997; 204: 157–163

74. Van Rossum AB, van Erkel AR, van Persijn van Meerten EL, Tjin A Ton ER, Rebergen SA, Pattynama PMT. Accuracy of helical CT for acute pulmonary embolism: ROC-analysis of observer performance related to clinical experience. Eur Radiol 1998; 8: 1160–1164

75. Ferretti GR, Bosson JL, Buffaz PD, et al. Acute pulmonary embolism: role of helical CT in 164 patients with intermediate probability at ventilation-perfusion scintigraphy and normal results at duplex US of the legs. Radiology 1997; 205: 453–458

76. Dutch ANTELOPE study (to be published).

77. Gaffney PJ. Distinction between fibrinogen and fibrin degradation products in plasma. Clin Chim Acta 1975; 65: 109–115

78. Demers C, Ginsberg JS, Johnston M, Brill-Edwards P, Panju A. D-dimer and thrombin-antithrombin III complexes in patients with clinically suspected pulmonary embolism. Thromb Haemostas 1992; 67: 408–412

79. Raimondi P, Bongard O, de Moerloose P, Reber G, Waldvogel F, Bounameaux H. D-dimer plasma concentration in various clinical conditions: implications for the use of this test in the diagnostic approach of venous thromboembolism. Thromb Res 1993; 69: 125–130

80. Leitha T, Speiser W, Dudczak R. Pulmonary embolism: efficacy of D-dimer an thrombin-antithrombin III complex determinations as screening tests before lung scanning. Chest 1991; 100: 1536–1541

81. Ginsberg JS, Brill-Edwards PA, Demers C, Donovan D, Panju A. D-dimer in patients with clinically suspected pulmonary embolism. Chest 1993; 104: 1679–1684

82. Van Beek EJR, Van den Ende B, Berckmans RJ, et al. A comparative analysis of D-dimer assays in patients with clinically suspected pulmonary embolism. Thromb Haemostas 1993; 70: 408–413

83. Bounameaux H, De Moerloose P, Perrier A, Reber G. Plasma measurement of D-dimer as diagnostic aid in suspected venous thromboembolism: an overview. Thromb Haemostas 1994; 71: 1–6

84. Elias A, Appel I, Huc B, et al. D-dimer test and diagnosis of deep vein thrombosis: a comparative study of 7 assays. Thromb Haemostas 1996; 76: 518–522

85. Goldhaber SZ, Vaughan DE, Tumeh SS, Loscalzo J. Utility of cross-linked fibrin degradation products in the diagnosis of pulmonary embolism. Am Heart J 1989; 116: 505–508

86. Bounameaux H, Schneider PA, Slosman D, De Moerloose P, Reber G. Plasma D-dimer in suspected pulmonary embolism: a comparison with pulmonary angiography and ventilation-perfusion scintigraphy. Blood Coag Fibrinol 1990; 1: 577–579

87. Rowbotham BJ, Egerton-Vernon J, Whitaker AN, Elms MJ, Bunce IH. Plasma cross-linked fibrin degradation products in pulmonary embolism. Thorax 1990; 45: 684–687

88. Goldhaber SZ, Simons GR, Elliott CG, et al. Quantitative plasma D-dimer levels among patients undergoing pulmonary angiography for suspected pulmonary embolism. JAMA 1993; 270: 2819–2822

89. Ginsberg JS, Wells PS, Brill-Edwards P, et al. Application of a novel and rapid whole blood assay for D-dimer in patients with clinically suspected pulmonary embolism. Thromb Haemostas 1995; 73: 35–38

90. Turkstra F, Van Beek EJR, Ten Cate JW, Büller HR. Reliable rapid blood test for the exclusion of venous thromboembolism in symptomatic outpatients. Thromb Haemostas 1996; 76: 9–11

91. De Moerloose P, Desmarais S, Bounameaux H, et al. Contribution of a new, rapid individual and quantitative automated D-dimer ELISA to exclude pulmonary embolism. Thromb Haemostas 1996; 75: 11–13

92. Rowe CA, Bolitho JS, Jane A, et al. Rapid detection of D-dimer using a fiber optic biosensor. Thromb Haemostas 1998; 79: 94–98

93. Perrier A. Bounameaux H, Morabia A, et al. Diagnosis of pulmonary embolism by a decision analysis-based strategy including clinical probability, D-dimer levels, and ultrasonography: a management study. Arch Intern Med 1996; 156: 531–536

94. Bernardi E, Prandoni P. Compression ultrasound and D-dimer in the management of patients with clinically suspected deep-vein thrombosis. Thromb Haemostas 1997 (Suppl): 767

95. Kraayenhagen RA, Koopman MMW, Bernardi E, et al. Simplification of the diagnostic management of outpatients with symptomatic deep vein thrombosis with D-dimer measurements. Thromb Haemostas 1997 (Suppl): 159

96. Van Beek EJR, Schenk BE, Michel BC, Van den Ende A, Van der Heide YT, Brandjes DPM, Bossuyt PMM, Büller HR. The role of plasma D-dimer concentration in the exclusion of pulmonary embolism. Br J Haematol 1996; 92: 725–732

97. Oudkerk M, Van Beek EJR, Van Putten WLJ, Büller HR. Cost-effectiveness analysis of various strategies in the diagnostic management of pulmonary embolism. Arch Intern Med 1993; 153: 947–954

98. Perrier A, Bounameaux H, Morabia A, et al. Contribution of D-dimer plasma measurement and lower-limb venous ultrasound to the diagnosis of pulmonary embolism: a decision analysis model. Am Heart J 1994; 127: 624–635

99. Van Erkel AR, Van Rossum AB, Bloem JL, Kievit J, Pattynama PMT. Spiral CT angiography for suspected pulmonary embolism: a cost-effectiveness analysis. Radiology 1996: 201: 29–36

100. Hull RD, Feldstein W, Stein PD, Pineo GF. Cost-effectiveness of pulmonary embolism diagnosis. Arch Intern Med 1996; 156: 68–72

101. Van Rossum AB, van Houwelingen HC, Kieft GJ, Pattynama PMT. Prevalence of deep vein thrombosis in suspected and proven pulmonary embolism. A meta-analysis. Br J Radiol 1998

VII.2 Management of venous thromboembolism in pregnancy

W. S. Chan, J. Ginsberg

Introduction

Venous thromboembolism (VTE) is an uncommon but important cause of maternal mortality [1 – 5]. When VTE is suspected during pregnancy, objective testing must be done for definitive diagnosis. Radiological procedures expose the developing foetus to small amounts of radiation, which is a concern to patients and their physicians.

In this chapter, we will review the pathophysiology of VTE during pregnancy, propose guidelines for diagnosis, which minimise radiation exposure to the foetus, and discuss the immediate and long-term management of this disease. Our discussion of therapeutic options will include the use of low molecular weight heparins (LMWHs), a group of agents which are being used with increasing frequency.

Epidemiology

Early studies reporting the incidence of deep venous thrombosis (DVT) in pregnancy were based on clinical diagnosis alone and, therefore, are probably inaccurate [6 – 8]. When objective testing with venography was used, Bergqvist et al. [8] and Kierkegaard et al. [9] reported that the frequency of antepartum DVT was 0.7/1,000 and 0.13/1,000, respectively. Pregnancy-related DVT occurs 3 to 5.5 times more commonly in the postpartum than the antepartum period [9 – 12]. With Caesarean section, the risk of DVT increases to 1.8 % [13], or as high as 20 times the risk associated vaginal delivery [12]. The risk associated with Caesarean section has been decreasing, possibly due to early mobilisation and the increased use of prophylactic anticoagulation [12].

Pulmonary embolism (PE) remains the most important preventable cause of maternal death [1 – 5]. The incidence of PE is estimated at 0.3 to 1.3 % of all pregnancies [14]; in non-pregnant patients, approximately 50 % of patients with DVT have silent PE [15], and so the true rate of PE in pregnancy is probably higher.

Pathophysiology of VTE in pregnancy

Pregnancy increases the risk of venous thrombosis. The physiological changes that occur in pregnancy to promote thrombosis include at least two of Virchows triad, stasis and hypercoagulability, and possibly the third, endothelial damage.

Venous stasis of the lower limbs occurs during pregnancy. Measurements of femoral venous flow by Doppler ultrasound [16] and the transit time of radiolabelled sodium [17], both demonstrated reduced venous flow, particularly in the third trimester. The probable reason for this stasis is the enlargement of the uterus and the engagement of the foetal head within the pelvic brim. A decrease in venous tone as a result of hormonal influences might be a contributing factor [18]. Whether the degree of reduction of venous flow is similar in both legs – to explain the predominance of DVT in the left leg [19] – is unclear. A possible explanation for this clinical observation is the compression of the left iliac vein by the right iliac artery [20].

If venous stasis alone was an important factor, then a preponderance of DVT should be seen during the third trimester. This was not the observation made in 60 pregnancies [19] in which the distribution of DVT in the first, second, and third trimester was 24%, 47%, and 29%, respectively. Hypercoagulability in pregnancy has a role in promoting venous thrombosis. Coagulation factors II, VII, VIII: C, VIII: Ag, X and fibrinogen increase by the third trimester [21–23], resulting in a shortened activated partial thromboplastin time (aPTT) and prothrombin time (PT) [24]. Coagulation inhibitors such as antithrombin have been reported to be normal [25–27] or decreased [28–30]. Protein C levels are normal [28, 30], whereas free and total protein S decrease [28, 31, 32]. A decrease in plasma fibrinolytic activity, measured by the euglobulin lysis time, is seen in pregnancy [11, 25, 33]. Plasminogen levels increase in pregnancy [29, 33, 34], but the relative level of tissue plasminogen activator activity is disputed [33–35]. Overall, these changes in the hemostatic and fibrinolytic systems promote thrombosis during pregnancy. They revert to the non-pregnant state two weeks after delivery [32].

The third factor in Virchows triad that may contribute to thrombosis during pregnancy is endothelial injury following delivery as a result of placental separation or if a Caesarean section is performed [36].

Diagnosis

As in non-pregnant patients, diagnosis of DVT and PE in the pregnant population requires accurate objective testing. The main barrier to objective testing is the fear, by physicians and patients, of radiation exposure to the developing foetus. Ginsberg et al. [37] calculated radiation doses to the foetus associated with various diagnostic tests for VTE. A careful review of the literature demonstrated that at most, a doubling in the incidence of childhood cancers may occur with foetal exposure of less than 5 rads; there should be no increase in congenital malformations. In clinical practice, a radiation exposure dose limited to < 0.5 rads is usually possible in diagnosing VTE (Table 1).

Diagnostic tests for DVT

Contrast Venography

Contrast venography is the reference standard test for the diagnosis of VTE [38–40]. The test is diagnostic for DVT when an intraluminal filling defect is seen in multiple projections, whereas DVT is excluded if the deep veins of the calf and proximal veins are normal. The radiation exposure required for visualisation of the venous system can be minimised by lead-shielding and performing limited venography [37].

IPG

Occlusive cuff impedance plethysmography, IPG, is an accurate test for the detection of proximal DVT (popliteal or more proximal veins) in non-pregnant patients [41–44]. This technique measures the capacity of the venous system to fill and empty in response to temporary venous outflow obstruction. The sensitivity of IPG for calf vein

Table 1. Estimates of amount of radiation absorbed by the foetus for different procedures.

Procedure	Estimated Foetal Radiation (rads)
Bilateral venography without abdominal shield	0.628
Unilateral venography without abdominal shield	0.314
Limited venography, abdominal shielded	< 0.050
Pulmonary angiography via femoral route	0.405
Pulmonary angiography via brachial route	< 0.050
Perfusion lung scan using ^{99m}TcMAA	
3mCi	0.018
1–2 mCi	0.006–0.012
Ventilation lung scan	0.004–0.019
Using ^{133}Xe	
Using ^{99m}TC DTPA	0.007–0.035
Using ^{99m}TC SC	0.001–0.005
Radioisotope venography	0.205
Radioactive fibrinogen uptake scanning	2.000
Chest radiography	< 0.001

From: Ginsberg JS, Hirsh J, Rainbow AJ, et al. Risks to the foetus of radiologic procedures used in the diagnosis of maternal venous thromboembolic disease. Thromb Haemost 1989; 61: 189–196; with permission.

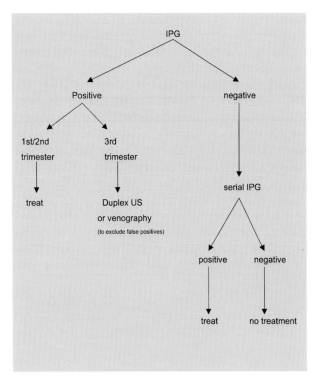

Fig. 1. Diagnosis of clinically suspected DVT in pregnancy with IPG.

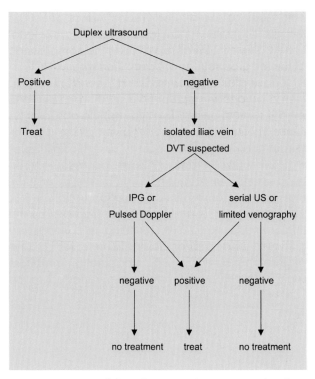

Fig. 2. Diagnosis of clinically suspected DVT using Duplex ultrasound.

thrombosis is poor [43]. During pregnancy, the gravid uterus can obstruct venous outflow in the iliac veins and cause false positive results. Therefore, to eliminate false positives, modification of the technique should be done by positioning the patient in the lateral decubitus position for 20 to 30 minutes prior to performing the test [7, 45]. Hull et al. [7] evaluated IPG in pregnancy and showed that anticoagulation can be safely withheld if serial testing by IPG (Days 1, 3, 5, 7, 10 and 14) was normal.

Duplex ultrasound
Real time duplex ultrasound is widely available in many centres for diagnosis of DVT. The test is highly sensitive and specific for proximal vein thrombosis [46], but relatively insensitive for calf DVT. Lensing et al. demonstrated that the single criterion of vein compressibility is sufficient for accurate detection of proximal DVT. In the pregnant population, this test is limited in its inability to detect isolated iliac vein thrombosis [47]. Some investigators [48–50] have reported that direct visualisation of iliac vein thrombosis is possible, but unfortunately, this technique of detection is very much operator dependent.

Diagnostic approach to DVT

Reasonable diagnostic approaches to patients with suspected DVT during pregnancy are summarised in Figures 1 and 2. IPG can be used for initial testing and if the results are positive, treatment should be initiated, except in the third trimester when false positives can occur. If the results are negative, serial testing with IPG should be done. Alternatively, duplex ultrasound can be used.

Diagnostic tests for pulmonary embolism

Clinical diagnosis of PE during pregnancy is inaccurate. Therefore, when suspected, objective testing should be performed to avoid unnecessary anticoagulation of patients without PE and to ensure appropriate treatment of patients with PE. Pulmonary angiography is the reference standard for the diagnosis of PE [51, 52], but is invasive and expensive. Radiation exposure to the developing foetus can be minimised by performing angiography via the brachial route [37]. The initial approach in diagnosis of PE during pregnancy remains ventilation-perfusion lung scanning. A high probability lung scan provides sufficient grounds to diagnose PE, whereas a normal perfusion scan rules out PE [53]. When the lung scan is non-diagnostic, further testing is required [51, 54, 55], and IPG or duplex ultrasound should be performed because the detection of DVT in a patient with suspected PE provides grounds for anticoagulation. However, if IPG or Duplex are normal, PE cannot be excluded and pulmonary angiography should be considered if clinical suspicion remains high.

Our approach to the diagnosis of PE in pregnancy is summarised in Figure 3.

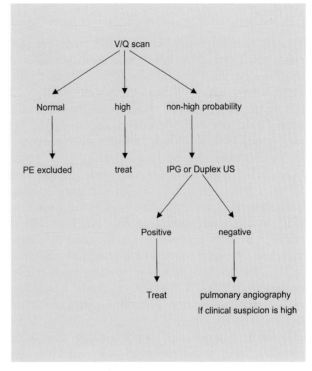

Fig. 3. Diagnosis of clinically suspected PE during pregnancy.

Treatment

Once venous thromboembolism is diagnosed, treatment should be instituted. The selection of an anticoagulant for treatment in pregnancy is made by considering foetal exposure risks and potential maternal side-effects. Heparin (unfractionated or low molecular weight heparin) is the treatment of choice in the antepartum period because it is safe for the foetus, although it can cause maternal complications. Warfarin should be avoided during pregnancy as it crosses the placenta and is associated with embryopathy and foetal wastage.

Heparin

The treatment of choice for pregnant patients with VTE is heparin [56–59]. Unfractionated heparin (UH) is a glycosaminoglycan that potentiates the activity of antithrombin to inactivate thrombin, factor Xa and factor IXa. UH does not cross the placenta and is safe for the foetus.

Maternal side-effects associated with UH use include bleeding [60], heparin-induced thrombocytopenia (HIT) [61–63] and osteoporosis [64–66]. HIT is IgG-mediated and can be associated with thrombotic complications. When this complication occurs, heparin therapy should be stopped and alternative therapy with danaparoid sodium should be considered [67]. Osteoporosis resulting from heparin use is particularly relevant to women who are treated with prolonged heparin therapy during pregnancy. In a retrospective analysis of 184 women, Dahlman and colleagues [64] reported that symptomatic osteoporotic vertebral fractures occurred at a frequency of 2.2%. These fractures occurred in women treated with UH doses as low as 15,000 U/day, for as short a duration as 7 weeks. Of additional concern is the subclinical reduction in bone density that can occur in about one quarter of pregnant heparin-treated women [65, 66]. The mechanism of heparin-induced bone loss is unknown [68]. Heparin-treated patients should be advised to consume recommended doses of calcium and vitamin D during pregnancy.

Warfarin

Vitamin K antagonists like warfarin cross the placenta and are associated with embryopathy if used during the first trimester [69–72], and central nervous system (CNS) abnormalities if used during any trimester [70, 73]. Pregnancy loss also seems to occur with increased frequency during pregnancy [73, 74]. Typical warfarin embryopathy is characterised by stippled epiphyses, nasal hypoplasia, eye abnormalities, and developmental retardation, and occurs with exposure to warfarin between six and nine weeks of gestation [73]. In one study, embryopathy was reported to occur in 30% of pregnancies associated with warfarin use between six and nine weeks of gestation [75]. Other studies, however have reported a lower incidence [76]. CNS abnormalities, consisting of hydrocephalus, dorsal midline dysplasia characterised by agenesis of the corpus callosum, Dandy-Walker malformation, and mid-line cerebellar atrophy, have been reported with warfarin use during any trimester [73], but the incidence is likely to be low.

In view of the relatively high incidence of problems with warfarin, the use of warfarin for the treatment of VTE during pregnancy is difficult to justify. Warfarin is however, the treatment of choice in the postpartum period, even with breastfeeding, since drug activity is detected at insignificantly low quantities in breast milk [77, 78].

LMWH

Low molecular weight heparins (LMWHs) are effective in preventing and treating VTE in non-pregnant patients [79–83]. These agents have the potential to become an important treatment option in the pregnant population.

LMWHs are obtained by the enzymatic cleavage or chemical depolymerisation of unfractionated heparin, producing molecules with an average molecular weight of 4,000 to 6,000 daltons. Due to their molecular weight, the relative anti-factor Xa to anti-factor IIa ratio is higher (2–4 : 1) compared to UH (1 : 1). In addition, they show decreased binding to endothelial surfaces and platelets, and predictable pharmacokinetic action [63]. The risks of bleeding and thrombocytopenia associated with UH are reduced with LMWH use [79–83]. Importantly, the risk for osteoporosis may be reduced with LMWH compared to UH [84].

LMWHs do not cross the placenta [85–90]. The literature available to date on the effectiveness of LMWH for thromboprophylaxis and treatment of VTE in pregnancy is limited. Four studies [88, 91–93] have reported the use of LMWHs for thromboprophylaxis in 79 pregnant patients. There were no clinical recurrences of VTE. The doses of LMWH used were variable; the dose of dalterparin ranged from 2,500 U once daily to 22,500 U once daily. When anti-factor Xa levels were measured, trough levels of 0.15–0.25 u/ml prior to injection [88, 93] and peak levels of 0.2–0.5 u/ml 2–6 hours after administration [91] were targeted. The pharmacokinetics of LMWHs change as gestation progresses; Sturridge et al. [92] showed that anti-factor Xa levels decreased with the same dose of enoxaparin after 20 weeks, suggesting that upward dose adjustments may be needed if target anti-Xa levels are to be achieved. It is unknown whether these dose adjustments influence clinical outcomes.

LMWHs have advantages over UH. The risks of bleeding, thrombocytopenia, and possibly, osteoporosis are lower compared to UH. The need for aPTT assays for dose adjustment is also eliminated. However, more studies are required to determine if doses used in non-pregnant patients apply to pregnant patients, and to determine if LMWHs are just as effective as UH in prophylaxis and treatment of VTE in pregnancy.

Thrombolytic therapy and caval filters

Thrombolytic agents, like tissue plasminogen activator, urokinase, and streptokinase, activate plasminogen, which converts fibrin into soluble peptides [94]. Thrombolytic agents are used in selected non-pregnant patients with acute massive PE with hemodynamic compromise [94] and with extensive DVT, to reduce the subsequent incidence of post-phlebitic syndrome. Pregnancy is a relative contra-indication to thrombolytic therapy, and experience with their use during pregnancy is limited to case reports [95–99]. Until their safety is demonstrated, these agents should only be considered in pregnant women with hemodynamic instability from massive PE.

The mainstay of therapy for VTE is anticoagulation; inferior vena cava filters have been used for the prevention of PE in pregnancy [100–104]. Experience during pregnancy is mostly with the Greenfield filter [105], although a newer removable filter, FCP 2002 has also been used. The use of these devices during pregnancy should follow similar indications in non-pregnant patients. These include: 1) acute VTE and one or more absolute contraindications to anticoagulation and 2) failure of anticoagulation [67].

Management of long-term anticoagulation started prior to pregnancy

When patients are on oral anticoagulation prior to pregnancy, either for prosthetic heart valves or for treatment of VTE, two approaches can be undertaken. The first option is to convert oral anticoagulation therapy to adjusted-dose subcutaneous injections of heparin prior to conception; the second option is to wait until conception occurs, as indicated by positive blood pregnancy test before switching. The first option avoids exposure of the foetus to any warfarin at all and hence prevents the possibility of embryopathy, the second option minimises maternal osteoporosis as a consequence of prolonged heparin therapy. Since warfarin embryopathy is not likely to result from warfarin exposure before 6 weeks, we usually adopt the latter approach.

Management of anticoagulation during pregnancy

Antepartum

Once VTE is diagnosed during pregnancy, the patient should receive intravenous UH therapy initiated by a bolus of 5,000 U followed by an infusion of 30,000 U to 35,000 U/24h for 5–10 days [106, 107], with the aPTT adjusted to 1.5 to 2.5 times control, or more precisely, aPTT values corresponding to plasma heparin levels of 0.2–0.4 U/ml by protamine assay [108].

Subsequently, the patient is discharged on twice daily subcutaneous injections of UH, the dose of which is adjusted by keeping the mid-interval aPTT 1.5 to 2.5 times control [59]. The aPTT should be checked at regular intervals as pregnancy progresses. If LMWH is used in pregnancy, the dose should be either 200 IU/kg once a day or 100 IU/kg twice a day. As pregnancy progresses, it is not known whether adjustment of LMWH, based on anti-Xa activity, is needed [92].

Peripartum

Ideally at term, the last dose of subcutaneous unfractionated heparin should be given no later than 24 hours prior to active labour. To achieve this, induction of labour is planned at term. This approach is based on the observation that some patients have a prolonged aPTT more than 20 hours after the last dose of subcutaneous UH [109]. If pre-term labour occurs or if C-section is required urgently, rapid reversal of heparin activity can be achieved with protamine. For patients who developed VTE within the last 3 months, the risk of recurrence may be sufficiently high to warrant using intravenous heparin during the peripartum period. The infusion can then be discontinued 4–6 hours prior to the expected time of delivery or when active labour begins.

The half-life of LMWH is 3–4 hours [63]. Unlike unfractionated heparin, protamine reverses anti-Xa activity by 50%. A reasonable approach to avoid delay of epidural procedures and potential bleeding is to induce labour at term, with the last administered dose 12 to 24 hours prior to elective induction of labour.

Postpartum

After hemostasis is achieved, intravenous or subcutaneous administration of UH or LMWH is resumed. Oral anticoagulation with warfarin can also be started at this time. Once a therapeutic International normalised ratio (INR) of 2.0–3.0 is achieved, heparin is discontinued and the patient kept on warfarin for 4–6 weeks thereafter. Breastfeeding is safe while on warfarin and should be encouraged [77, 78].

Implications of VTE diagnosed in pregnancy

After a patient is diagnosed with VTE in pregnancy, and given appropriate treatment, counselling regarding future pregnancy risks should be given. Unfortunately, reliable rates of the risk of recurrence in future pregnancies are unavailable. The estimated rates are 0 to 15% [110, 111]. With the lack of definitive trials, approaches to future pregnancies vary from no anticoagulation and close surveillance, to low dose heparin in early trimesters, escalating to full doses near term [59]; the correct approach is unknown. Studies are currently underway to address rates of recurrences in these patients.

Thrombophilias

The thrombophilias include deficiencies of protein C, S or antithrombin [116–118], activated protein C-resistance [119–121], hyperhomocysteinemia [122, 123], plasminogen deficiency [124] and phospholipid antibodies [125]. One of these abnormalities occurs in about one quarter of patients under age 45 with DVT [112, 113] and in 50% of those with recurrent thrombosis [114, 115].

The risk of developing VTE in previously asymptomatic individuals during pregnancy is not known [126, 127]. Therefore, the decision to use prophylaxis in asymptomatic carriers requires a careful discussion with the patient, weighing the risks of anticoagulation and maternal morbidity and mortality from thrombosis.

Antithrombin, Protein C, and Protein S deficiencies

Deficiency of antithrombin (AT) is inherited in an autosomal dominant fashion, with a prevalence of 1:5,000 [114]. Fifty percent of affected individuals experience one episode of thrombosis by age 21 [133]. AT deficiency has been repeated to be present in 18–40% of women with VTE during pregnancy, and in 11–13% who developed these events in the postpartum period [127, 133]. A recent study, however, identified that only 3% of previously asymptomatic patients with AT develop VTE during pregnancy [126]. While prophylaxis of individuals with AT deficiency with previous VTE is advised, need for prophylaxis of asymptomatic individuals is unknown.

Homozygous protein C deficiency presents in the new-born period as neonatal purpura fulminans [134]. The heterozygous state occurs at a frequency of 1 in 200–500 [135, 136]. The risk of thrombosis in this group is higher when compared to their non-deficient relatives (hazard ratio 8.8) [137]. Protein C deficiency has been repeated to be present in 15–24% of individuals with VTE during pregnancy [127, 133]. However, only 1.7% of protein C deficient patients develop VTE during pregnancy [126].

Deficiency of protein S is associated with increased risk of VTE [138–140]. Hereditary protein S deficiency is an autosomal dominant trait, with variable penetrance, with an estimated frequency in the normal population of 1 in 16,000 [118]. The frequency of protein S deficiency in individuals with thrombosis in pregnancy has been repeated to be 16–27% [127, 133]. This may only represent 6.6% of previously asymptomatic protein S patients who become pregnant [126].

Activated Protein C (APC)-resistance

APC-resistance as an important and common inheritable cause of thrombophilia [128]. The prevalence of APC-resistance in the population is about 5–7% [119, 132]. In patients with diagnosed VTE, 16–36% have APC-resistance [119–121]. The risk of VTE conferred by this thrombophilia is seven to eight-fold greater than the normal population [119, 129]. The prevalence of APC-resistance in woman who develop DVT in pregnancy is high; between 17% and 60% [130, 131].

There are no studies defining risks of VTE in previously asymptomatic pregnant individuals. The approach of careful clinical surveillance during pregnancy is reasonable if patients are also educated regarding the symptoms of VTE. Alternatively, heparin can be used.

Antiphospholipid antibodies

Antiphospholipid antibodies (APLA) are a heterogeneous group of antibodies directed against phospholipids. They can be detected as lupus anticoagulants (LA) in clotting assays and as anticardiolipin antibodies (ACLA) in immunoassays. These antibodies can occur in patients with systemic lupus erythematosus (SLE), with the use of certain drugs, and in other systemic diseases [141]. In patients with SLE, these antibodies are associated with thrombosis and foetal loss [141]. In non-SLE patients, LA itself is strongly associated with thrombosis, but ACLA might not be [125].

In patients with LA and no history of VTE, close surveillance is a reasonable approach, whereas those with previous VTE should probably receive heparin. For patients with recurrent foetal losses, current evidence suggests that aspirin plus heparin is useful in preventing pregnancy loss.

Puerperal ovarian vein thrombophlebitis

Puerperal ovarian vein thrombophlebitis (POVT) is a distinct presentation of pelvic vein thrombophlebitis [142]. The incidence of POVT is 0.05% – 0.18% [143 – 145]. The mechanism of POVT is probably injury to the vascular endothelium, resulting in bacterial invasion [142, 143]. The incidence of diagnosed endometritis in cases of POVT has been reported to be 45% [143, 146]. Unlike DVT, there is a right-sided preponderance of POVT; 90% of cases occur in the right side. This likely results from retrograde flow in the left ovarian vein, towards the uterus [143].

POVT is most commonly associated with forceps delivery and Caesarean section [143]. It occurs 2 – 4 days after delivery and affected patients can present with right lower quadrant pain, fever, nausea, and vomiting. Examination can reveal a rope-like mass in the right lower quadrant, and paralytic ileus [142, 143, 146]. Evidence for systemic

septic embolism has been reported in up to 32 – 38% of patients [145, 147].

Diagnosis of POVT is definitively done at laparotomy [146]. Non-surgical diagnosis of POVT has been done with venogram [148], excretory urogram [144, 149], CT, MRI [150 – 153], and US [146, 155, 156]. A reasonable initial approach to diagnosis would be the use of US to rule out other diagnoses such as abscesses and appendicitis, followed by CT or MRI if necessary.

Medical treatment is the mainstay of POVT therapy. Patients should be given broad spectrum antibiotics to cover anaerobic and aerobic streptococcus, Proteus, staphylococcus, yeast, and bacteroides, and IV anticoagulation for 7 – 10 days [142, 145]. Long-term anticoagulation in the absence of IVC thrombus or pulmonary emboli, is probably not required.

Conclusions

VTE is an important disease to recognise, diagnose and treat during pregnancy. The importance in using objective testing before initiating therapy

cannot be overemphasised because of the significant side-effects associated with anticoagulation therapy.

References

1. Sachs BP, Brown DA, Driscoll ST, et al. Maternal mortality in Massachusetts. Trends and Prevention. N Engl J Med 1987; 316: 607 – 672
2. Report on Confidential Inquiries into Maternal Deaths for England and Wales 1979 – 1981. London HMSO, 1986
3. Kaunitz AM, Hughes JM, Grimes DA, et al. Causes of Maternal mortality in the US. Obstet Gynecol 1985; 65: 605 – 612
4. Rochat RW, Koorin LM, Atrash HK, et al. Maternal mortality in the United States: Report from the Maternal Mortality Collaborative. Obstet Gynecol 1988; 72: 91 – 97
5. Mclean R, Mattison ET, Cochrane NE. Maternal mortality study annual report 1970 – 1976. NY State J 1979; 79: 39 – 46
6. Villasanta U. Thromboembolic disease in pregnancy. Am J Obstet Gynecol 1965; 93: 142 – 160
7. Hull RD, Raskob GE, Carter CJ. Serial impedance plethysmography in pregnant patients with clinically suspected deep vein thrombosis. Ann Intern Med 1990; 112: 663 – 667
8. Bergqvist D, Hedner U. Deep vein thrombosis during pregnancy. Acta Obstet Gynecol Scand 1983; 62: 239 – 243
9. Kierkegaard A. Incidence and diagnosis of deep vein thrombosis associated with pregnancy. Acta Obstet Gynecol Scand 1983; 62: 239 – 243
10. Aaro KA, Jeurgens JL. Thrombophlebitis associated with pregnancy. Am J Obstet Gynecol 1971; 109: 1128 – 1136
11. Douketis JD, Ginsberg JS. Diagnostic Problems with venous thromboembolic disease in pregnancy. Haemost 1995; 25: 58 – 71
12. Treffers PE, Huidekoper BL, Weenink GH, et al. Epidemiological observations of thromboembolic disease during pregnancy and in the puerperium in 56,022 women. Int J Gynaecol Obstet 1983, 21: 3237 – 331
13. Bergqvist A, Bergqvist D, Hallbook T. Acute deep vein thrombosis after caesarian section. Acta Obstet Gynecol Scand 1979; 58: 473 – 476
14. Rutherford SF, Phelan JP. Thromboembolic disease in pregnancy. Clin Perinatol 1980; 13: 719 – 739

15. Huisman MV, Buller HR, ten Cate JW et al. Unexpected high prevalence of silent pulmonary embolism in patients with deep vein thrombosis. Chest 1989; 95: 498–502

16. Ikard RW, Ueland K, Folse K. Lower limb venous dynamics in pregnant women. Surg Gyneol Obstet 1971; 132: 483–488

17. Wright HP, Osborn SB. Changes in the rate of flow of venous blood in the leg during pregnancy, measured with radioactive sodium. Surg Gynecol Obstet 1950; 90: 481–485

18. Goodrich SM, Wood JE. Peripheral venous distensibility and velocity of venous blood flow during pregnancy or during oral contraceptive therapy. Am J Obstet Gynecol 1964; 90: 740–744

19. Ginsberg JS, Brill-Edwards P, Burrows RF, et al. Venous thrombosis during pregnancy: leg and trimester of presentation. Thromb Haemost 1992; 67: 519–520

20. Cockett FB, Thomas ML. The iliac compression syndrome. Br J Surg 1965; 52: 816–821

21. Bonnar J. Blood coagulation fibrinolysis in obstetrics. Clin Hemotol 1973; 12: 58–63

22. Bonnar J. The blood coagulation and fibrinolytic systems in the newborn and mother at birth. Br J Obstet Gynaecol 1971; 78: 355–360

23. Daniel DG. Estrogens and puerperal thromboembolism. Am Heart J 1969; 78: 720–722

24. Reid DE, Frigoletto FD, Tullis JL. Hypercoagulable states in pregnancy. Am J Obstet Gynecol 1971; 111: 493–504

25. Stirling Y, Woolf L, North WRS, et al. Hemostasis in normal pregnancy. Thromb Haemost 1984; 52: 176–182

26. Weenink GH, Treffers PE, Kahle LH, et al. Antithrombin III in normal pregnancy. Thromb Res 1982; 26: 281–287

27. Weiner CP, Brandt J. Plasma antithrombin III activity in normal pregnancy. Obstet Gynecol 1984; 64: 46–48

28. De Boer K, ten Cote JW, Stark A, et al. Enhanced thrombin generation in normal and hypertensive pregnancy. Am J Obstet Gynecol 1989; 160: 95–100

29. Gjonnaess FI, Fagerhol MK. Studies in coagulation and fibrinolysis in pregnancy. Acta Obstet Gynecol Scand 1975; 54: 363–367

30. Gonzalez R, Alberca I, Vicente V. Protein C levels in late pregnancy, postpartum and in women on oral contraceptives. Thromb Res 1985; 39: 637–640

31. Comp PC, Thurnau GR, Welsh J, et al. Functional and immunologic protein S levels are decreased during pregnancy. Blood 1986; 68: 881–885

32. Demers C, Ginsberg JS. Deep venous thrombosis and pulmonary embolism in pregnancy. Clin Chest Med 1992; 23: 645–656

33. Wright JG, Cooper P, Astedt B, et al. Fibrinolysis during human pregnancy: complex interrelationships between plasma levels of tissue plasminogen activator and inhibitors and the euglobulin clot lysis time. Br J Haematol 1988; 69: 253–258

34. Kruithof EKO, Tran-Thang C, Gudinchet A, et al. Fibrinolysis in pregnancy: a study of plasminogen activator inhibitors. Blood 1987; 69: 460–466

35. Ballegeer V, Mombaerts P, Declerk PJ. Fibrinolytic response to venous occlusion and fibrin fragment D-dimer levels in normal and complicated pregnancy. Thromb Heremost 1987; 58: 1030–1032

36. Barbour L, Pickard J. Conroversies in thromboembolic disease during pregnancy: a critical review. Obstet Gynecol 1995; 86: 621–636

37. Ginsberg JS, Hirsh J, Rainbow AJ, Coates G. Risks to the foetus of radiologic procedures used in the diagnosis of maternal venous thromboembolic disease. Thromb Haemost 1989; 61: 189–196

38. Hull R, Hirsh J, Sackett DL, et al. Clinical validity of a negative venogram in patients with clinically suspected venous thrombosis. Circulation 1981; 64: 622–625

39. Rabinov K, Paulin S. Roentgen diagnosis of venous thrombosis in the leg. Arch Surg 1972; 104: 134–144

40. Thomas ML. Phlebography. Arch Surg 1972; 104: 145

41. Hull RD, Von Aker WG, Hirsh H, et al. Impedance plethysmography using the occlusive cuff technique in the diagnosis of venous thrombosis. Circulation 1976; 53: 696–700

42. Hull RD, Taylor DW, Hirsh J, et al. Impedance plethysmography: the relationship between venous filling and sensitivity and specificity for proximal vein thrombosis. Circulation 1978; 58: 898–902

43. Hull RD, Hirsh J, Carter CJ, et al. Diagnostic efficacy of impedance plethysmography for clinically suspected deep-vein thrombosis. A randomized trial. Ann Intern Med 1985; 102: 21–28

44. Huisman MV, Buller HR, ten Cate JW, et al. Serial impedance plethsmography for suspected deep venous thrombosis in outpatients. The Amsterdam general practitioner study. N Engl J Med 1986; 314: 823–828

45. Ginsberg J, Turner C. Brill-Edwards P, et al. Pseudothrombosis in pregnancy. CMAJ 1988; 139: 409–410

46. Lensing AWA, Prandoni P, Brandjes D, et al. Detection of deep vein thrombosis by real time B-mode ultrasonography. N Engl J Med 1989; 320: 342–345

47. Duddy MJ, McHugo JM. Duplex ultrasound of the common femoral vein in pregnancy and the puerperium. Br J Radiol 1991; 64: 785–791

48. Frede TE, Ruthberg BN. Sonographic demonstration of iliac vein thrombosis in the maternity patient. J Ultrasound Med 1988; 7: 33–37

49. Polak JF, O'Leary DH. Deep vein thrombosis in pregnancy: non-invasive diagnosis. Radiology 1988; 166: 377–379

50. Greer IA, Barry J, Mackon N, et al. Diagnosis of deep venous thrombosis in pregnancy: a new role for diagnostic ultrasound. Br J Obstet Gynaecol 1990; 97: 53–57

51. Hull RD, Hirsh J, Carter CJ, et al. Pulmonary angiography, ventilation scanning and venography for clinically suspected pulmonary embolism with abnormal perfusion lung scan. Ann Intern Med 1983; 98: 891–899

52. Goodman PC. Pulmonary angiography. Clin Chest Med 1984; 5: 465–477

53. Rosenow EC. Venous and pulmonary thromboembolism: and algorithmic approach to diagnosis and management. Mayo Clin Proc 1995; 70: 45–49

54. Hull RD, Raskob GE, Ginsberg JS. A non-invasive strategy for the treatment of patients with suspected pulmonary embolism. Arch Intern Med 1994; 154: 289–297

55. The PIOPED investigators. Value of the ventilation/perfusion scan in acute pulmonary embolism: results of the Prospective Investigation of Pulmonary Embolism Diagnosis (PIOPED). JAMA 1990; 263: 2753–2759

56. Maternal and neonatal haemostasis working party of the haemostasis and thrombosis task guidelines on the prevention, investigations and management of thrombosis associated with pregnancy. J Clin Pathol 1993; 46: 489–496

57. Toglia MR, Weg JG. Venous thromboembolism during pregnancy. N Engl J Med 1996; 335: 108–114

58. Rutherford SE, Phelan JP. Thromboembolic disease in pregnancy. Clin Perinatal 1986; 13: 719–739

59. Ginsberg JS, Hirsh JS. Use of antithrombotic agents during pregnancy. Chest 1995; 108: 3055–3115

60. Ginsberg JS, Kowalchuk G, Hirsh J, et al. Heparin therapy during pregnancy: risk to the foetus and mother. Arch Intern Med 1989; 149: 2233–2236

61. King DJ, Kelton JG. Heparin-associated thrombocytopenia. Ann Intern Med 1984; 100: 535–540

62. Warkentin TE, Kelton JG. Heparin-induced thrombocytopenia. Ann Rev Med. Palo Alto, California: Annual Reviews Inc, 1989: 31–44

63. Hirsh J, Raschke R, Warkentin TE, et al. Heparin: mechanism of action pharmacokinetics, dosing considerations, monitoring, efficacy, and safety. Chest 1995; 108: 258s–275s

64. Dahlman TC. Osteoporotic fractures and the recurrence embolism during pregnancy and the puerperium in 184 women undergoing thromboprophylaxis with heparin. Am J Obst Gynecol 1993; 168: 1265–1270

65. Barbour L, Kick S, Steiner J, et al. A prospective study of heparin induced osteoporosis in pregnancy using bone densitometry. Am J Obstet Gynecol 1994; 770: 862–869

66. Ginsberg JS, Kowalchuk G, Hirsh J, et al. Heparin effect on bone density. Thromb Haemost 1990; 64: 286–289

67. Ginsberg JS. Management of venous thromboembolism. N Eng J Med 1996; 335: 1816–1828

68. Dahlman T, Sjoberg HE, Hellgren M, et al. Calcium homeostasis in pregnancy during long-term heparin treatment. Br J Obstet Gynecol 1992; 99: 412–416

69. Shaul WJ, Emery H, Hall JG. Chondrodysplasia Punctata and maternal warfarin use during pregnancy. Am J Dis Child 1975; 360–362

70. Shaul W, Hall JG. Multiple congenital anomalies associated with oral anticoagulants. Am J Obstet Gynecol 1976; 127: 191–198

71. Raivio KO, Ikonen E, Saarikoski S. Fetal risks due to warfarin therapy during pregnancy. Acta Paediatr Scand 1977; 66: 735–739

72. Becker MH, Genieser NB, Finegold M, et al. Chondrodysplasia Punctata. Am J Dis Child 1975; 129: 356–359

73. Hall JG, Pauli RM, Wilson KM. Maternal and fetal sequelae of anticoagulation during pregnancy. Am J Med 1980; 68: 122–140

74. Ginsberg JS. Hirsh J, Turner DC, et al. Risks to the foetus of anticoagulant therapy during pregnancy. Thromb Haemost 1989; 61: 197–203

75. Iturbe-Alessio I, Fonesca MC, Mutchinik O, et al. Risks of anticoagulant therapy in pregnant women with artificial heart valves. N Eng J Med 1986; 315: 1390–1393

76. Cortufo M, de Luca TSL, Calabro R, et al. Coumarin anticoagulation during pregnancy in patients with mechanical valve prostheses. Cardiothorac Surg 1991; 5: 300–305

77. Mckenna R, Cole ER, Vasan U. Is warfarin sodium contraindicated in the lactating mother? J Ped 1983; 103: 325–327

78. Orme ML'e, Lewis PJ, De Swiet M, et al. May mothers given warfarin breastfeed their infants? Br Med J 1977; 1: 1564–1565

79. Siragusa S, Cosmi B, Piovella F, et al. Low molecular weight heparin and unfractionated heparin in the treatment of patients with acute venous thromboembolism: results of a meta-analysis. Am J Med 1996; 100: 269–277

80. Koopman MMW, Prandoni P, Piovella F. Treatment of venous thrombosis with intravenous unfractionated heparin administered in the hospital as compared with subcutaneous low-molecular weight heparin administered at home. N Engl J Med 1996; 334: 682–687

81. Leizovovicz A, Simmonneau G, Deousus H, et al. Comparison of efficacy and safety of low molecular weight heparin and unfractionated heparinn in initial treatment of deep venous thrombosis: a meta-analysis. B Med J 1994; 309: 299–304

82. Lensing AWA, Prins MH, Davidson BL, et al. Treatment of deep venous thrombosis with low-molecular-weight heparins: a meta-analysis. Arch Intern Med 1995; 155: 601–607

83. Levine MN, Hirsh J. An overview of clinical trials of low molecular weight heparin fractions. Acta Chir Scand Suppl 1988; 543: 73–80

84. Monreal M, Lafoz E, Olive A, et al. Comparison of subcutaneous unfractionated heparin with a low molecular weight heparin (Fragmin) in patients with venous thromboembolism and contraindications for coumadin. Thromb Haemost 1994; 71: 7–11

85. Forestier F, Daffos F, Capella-Padovsky M. LMW heparin does not cross the placenta during the second trimester of pregnancy. Thromb Res 1984; 34: 557–560

86. Forestier F, Sole Y, Aiach M, et al. Absence of transplacental passage of fragmin (Kabi) during the second and third trimesters of pregnancy. Thromb Haemost 1992; 607: 180–181

87. Matzsch T, Bergqvist D, Bergqvist A. No transplacental passage of heparin of an enzymatically depolymerised LMW heparin. Blood Coagul Fibrinol 1991; 2: 273

88. Melissari E, Parker CJ, Wilson NV, et al. Use of LMW heparin in pregnancy. Thromb Haemost 1992; 68: 652–656

89. Harenberg J, Schneider D, Heilman L, et al. Lack of anti-Xa activity in umbilical cord vein sample after subcutaneous administration of heparin or low molecular mass heparin in pregnant women. Haemost 1993; 23: 314–320

90. Omri A, Delaloye JF, Anderson H, et al. Low molecular weight heparin novo (LHN-1) does not cross the placenta during the second trimester of pregnancy. Thromb Haemost 1987; 57: 234

91. Rasmussen C, Wadt J, Jacobsen B. Thromboembolic prophylaxis with low molecular weight heparin during pregnancy. Int J Obstet Gynecol 1994; 47: 121–125

92. Sturridge F, De Swiet M, Letsky E. The use of low molecular weight heparin for thromboprophlaxis in pregnancy. Br J Obstet Gynecol 1994; 101: 69–71

93. Hunt BJ, Doughty HA, Majumdar G, et al. Thromboprophylaxis with low molecular weight heparin (Fragmin) in high risk pregnancies. Thromb Haemost 1997; 77: 39–43

94. Hyers TM, Hull RD, Weg JG. Antithrombotic therapy for venous thromboembolic disease. Chest 1995; 108: 335S–351S

95. Kramer WB, Belfort M, Saade GR, et al. Successful urokinase treatment of massive pulmonary embolism in pregnancy. Obstet Gynecol 1995; 86: 660–662

96. McTaggert DR, Ingram TG. Massive pulmonary embolism during pregnancy treated with streptokinase. Med J Aust 1977; 1: 18–20

97. Delclos GL, Davila F. Thrombolytic therapy for pulmonary embolism in pregnancy; a case report. Am J Obstet Gynecol 1986; 155: 375–376

98. Mazeika PK, Oakley CM. Massive pulmonary embolism in pregnancy treated with streptokinase and percutaneous catheter fragmentation. Eur Heart J 1994; 15: 1281–1283

99. Flossdorf T, Breulmann M, Hopf HB. Successful treatment of massive pulmonary embolism with recombinant tissue type plasminogen activator (rt-PA) in a pregnant woman with intact gravidity and preterm labor. Int Care Med 1990; 16: 454–456

100. Scurr J, Stannard P, Wright J. Extensive thromboembolic disease in pregnancy treated with a Kimray Greenfield vena cava filter. Br J Obstet Gynecol 1981; 88: 778–780

101. Hux CH, Wapner RJ, Chayer B, et al. Use of the Greenfield filter for thromboembolic disease in pregnancy. Am J Obstet Gynecol 1986; 155: 734–737

102. Banfield PJ, Pittam M, Marwood R. Recurrent pulmonary embolism in pregnancy managed with the Greenfield vena cava filter. Int J Gynecol Obstet 1990; 33: 275–278

103. Arbogast JD, Blessed WB, Lacoste H, et al. Use of the Greenfield cava filter to prevent recurrent pulmonary embolism in a heparin allergic gravida. Obstet Gynecol 1994; 4: 653–654

104. Aburahma AF, Bastug DF, Tiley EH 3rd, et al. Management of deep vein thrombosis of the lower extremity in pregnancy. W U Med J 1993; 89: 445–447

105. Greenfield LJ, Michna BA. Twelve year clinical experience with the Greenfield vena caval filter. Sur 1988; 104: 706–712

106. Hull RD, Raskob GE, Hirsh J, et al. Continuous intravenous heparin compared with intermittent subcutaneous heparin in the initial treatment of proximal-vein thrombosis. N Eng J Med 1986; 315: 1109–1114

107. Hull RD, Raskob GE, Rosenbloom D, et al. Heparin for 5 days as compared with 10 days in the initial treatment of proximal venous thrombosis. N Engl J Med 1990; 322: 1260–1264

108. Brill-Edwards P, Ginsberg JG, Johnston M. Establishing a therapeutic range for heparin. Ann Intern Med 1993; 119: 104–109

109. Anderson DR, Ginsberg JS, Burrows R, et al. Subcutaneous heparin during pregnancy: a need for concern at the time of delivery. Thromb Haemost 1991; 65: 248–250

110. De Sweit M, Floyd E, Letsky E. Low risk of recurrent thromboembolism in pregnancy (letter). Br J Hosp Med 1987; 38: 264

111. Tengborn L. Recurrent thromboembolism in pregnancy and puerperium: is there a need for thromboprophylaxis? Am J Obstet Gynecol 1989; 160: 90–94

112. Tabernero MD, Tomas JF, Alberca I, et al. Incidence and clinical characteristics of hereditary disorders associated with venous thrombosis. Am J Hematol 1991; 36: 249–254

113. Heijboer H, Brandjes DMP, Buller HR, et al. Deficiencies of coagulation inhibiting and fibrinolytic proteins in outpatients with deep-vein thrombosis. N Engl J Med 1990; 323: 1512–1516

114. Vittore CP, Demos TC. Hereditary deficiency of protein C, protein S, and antithrombin III. Can Assoc Rad J 1996; 47: 251–256

115. Hajjar KA. Factor V Leiden – an unselfish gene? New Engl J Med 1994; 331: 1585–1587

116. Hirsh J, Piovella F, Pini M. Congenital antithrombin III deficiency. Am J Med 1989; 87 (suppl 3B): 345–385

117. Svensson PJ, Dahlback B. Resistance to activated protein C as a basis for venous thrombosis. N Engl J Med 1994; 330: 517–521

118. Gladson CL, Scharrer I, Hach V, et al. The frequency of type I heterozygous protein S and protein C deficiency in 141 unrelated young patients with venous thrombosis. Thromb Haemost 1988; 59: 18–22

119. Koster T, Rosendaal FR, Ronde H, et al. Venous thrombosis due to poor anticoagulant response to activated protein C: Leiden thrombophilia study. Lancet 1993; 342: 1503–1506

120. Gillespie DL, Carrington LR, Griffin JH, et al. Resistance to activated protein C: a common inherited cause of venous thrombosis. Ann Vas Surg 1996; 10: 174–177

121. Simioni P, Prandoni P, Lensing AWA, et al. The risk of recurrent venous thromboembolism in patients with an Arg 506 Glu mutation in the gene for factor V (Factor V Leiden). N Engl J Med 1997; 336: 399–403

122. Fermo I, Vigaro D'Angelo S, Paroni R, et al. Prevalence of moderate hyperhomocysteinemia in patients with early-onset venous and arterial occlusive disease. Ann Int Med 1995; 123: 747–753

123. Den Heijer M, Blom HJ, Gerrits WJ, et al. Is hyperhomocystaeinemia a risk factor for recurrent thrombosis? Lancet 1995; 345: 882–885

124. Scharrer I, Hach-Wurderle V, Aygoren E, et al. Frequency and clinical manifestations of congenital plasminogen and fibrinogen deficiency compared to AT III – PC – and PS – deficiency inn patients suffering from thromboses. Fibrinolysis 1988; 2 (suppl 2): 16–17

125. Ginsberg JS, Wells PS, Brill-Edwards P, et al. Antiphospholipid antibodies and venous thromboembolism. Blood 1995; 86: 3685–3691

126. Friederich PW, Sanson BJ, Simioni P, et al. Frequency of pregnancy related venous thromboembolism in anticoagulant factor deficient women: implications for prophylaxis. Ann Int Med 1996; 125: 955–960

127. Conard J, Horellou MH, Van Dreden P, et al. Thrombosis and pregnancy in congenital deficiencies in AT III, protein C, and Protein S: a study of 78 women. Thromb Haemost 1990; 63: 319–320

128. Zoller B, Dahlback B. Linkage between inherited resistance to activated protein C and factor V gene mutation in venous thrombosis. Lancet 1994; 343: 1536–1538

129. Vandenbroucke JP, Koster T, Briet E, et al. Increased risk of venous thrombosis in oral contraceptive users who are carriers of factor V Leiden mutation. Lancet 1994; 344: 1453–1457

130. Hirsch DR, Mikkola KM, Merles PW, et al. Pulmonary embolism and deep venous thrombosis during pregnancy or oral contraceptive use: prevalence of factor V Leiden. Am Heart J 1996; 131: 1145–1148

131. Hellgren M, Tengborn L, Abildgaard U. Pregnancy in women with congential antithrombin III deficiency: experience of treatment with heparin and antithrombin. Gynecol Obstet Invest 1982; 14: 127–141

132. Ben Tal O, Zivelin A, Seligsohn U. The relative frequency of hereditary thrombotic disorders among 107 patients with thrombophilia in Israel. Thromb Haemost 1989; 61: 50–54

133. Pabinger I, Kyrle PA, Heistinger M, et al. The risk of thromboembolism in asymptomatic patients with protein C and protein S deficiency; a prospective cohort study. Thromb Haemost 1994; 71: 441–445

134. Seligsohn U, Berger A, Abend M, et al. Homozygous protein C deficiency manifested by massive venous thrombosis in the newborn. N Engl J Med 1984; 310: 559–562

135. Tait RC, Walker ID, Reitsma PH, et al. Prevalence of protein C deficiency in the healthy population. Thromb Haemost 1995; 73: 87–93

136. Miletich J, Sherman L, Broze G Jr. Absence of thrombosis in subjects with heterozygous protein C deficiency. N Engl J Med 1987; 317: 991–996

137. Allaart CF, Poort SR, Roserdaal FR, Reitsman PH, et al. Increased risk of venous thrombosis in carriers of hereditary protein C deficiency defect. Lancet 1993; 341: 134–138

138. Comp PCC, Nixon RR, Cooper MR, Esman CT. Familial protein S deficiency is associated with recurrent thrombosis. J Clin Invest 1984; 74: 2082–2088

139. Wilkerson DK, Burrell L, Cisar LA, et al. Hereditary protein S deficiency in a large New Jersey kindred. J Vas Surg 1993; 18: 932–938

140. Engesser L, Broekmans AW, Briet E, et al. Hereditary protein S deficiency: clinical manifestations. Ann Intern Med 1987; 106: 677–682

141. Love PE, Santoro SA. Antiphospholipid antibodies: anticardiolipin and the lupus anticoagulant in systemic lupus erythematosis (SLE) and in non-SLE disorders. Ann Intern Med 1990; 112: 682–698

142. Duff P, Gibbs RS. Pelvic vein thrombophlebitis: diagnostic dilemma and therapeutic challenge. Obstet Gynecol Surv 1983; 38: 365–373

143. Brown TK, Mursick RA. Puerperal ovarian vein thrombophlebitis: a syndrome. Am J Obstet Gynecol 1971; 109: 263–273

144. Derrick FC, Turner WR, House EE, et al. Evidence of right ovarian syndrome in pregnant females. Obstet Gynecol 1970; 35: 37–38

145. Josey WE, Staggers SR Jr. Heparin therapy in septic pelvic thrombophlebitis: a study of 46 cases. Am J Obstet Gynecol 1974; 120: 228–233

146. Munsick RA, Gillanders LA. A review of the syndrome of puerperal ovarian vein thrombophlebitis. Obstet Gynecol Surv 1981; 36: 57–66

147. Maull KI, Van Nagell JR, Greenfield LJ. Surgical implications of ovarian vein thrombosis. Am Surg 1978; 44: 727–733

148. Salzer RB, Abas S. Ovarian vein phlebography in postpartum patients. Obstet Gynecol 1970; 35: 270–277

149. Dykhuizen RF, Roberts JA. The ovarian vein syndrome. Surg Gynecol Obstet 1970; 130: 443–452

150. Savador SJ, Otero RR, Savador BL. Puerperal ovarian vein thrombosis: evaluation with CT, US and MR imaging. Radiology 1988; 167: 637–639

151. Angel JL, Knuppel RA. Computed tomography in diagnosis of puerperal ovarian vein thrombosis. Obstet Gynecol 1984; 63: 61–64

152. Ross MG, Mintz, Tuomala R, et al. The diagnosis of puerperal ovarian vein thrombophlebitis by computed axial tomography scan. Obstet Gynecol 1983; 62: 131–133

153. Brown CEL, Love TW, Cunningham FG, et al. Puerperal pelvic thrombophlebitis: impact on diagnosis and treatment using xray computed tomography and magnetic resonance imaging. Obstet Gynecol 1986; 68: 789–794

154. Mintz MC, Levy DW, Axel L, et al. Puerperal ovarian vein thrombosis: MR diagnosis. Am J Roentgenol 1987; 149: 1273–1274

155. Baka JJ. Ovarian vein thrombosis with atypical presentation: role of sonography and duplex Doppler. Obstet Gynecol 1989; 73: 887–889

156. Rudoff JM, Astrausleas KJ, Rudoff JC, et al. Ultrasonographic diagnosis of septic pelvic thrombophlebitis. J Ultrasound Med 1988; 7: 287–291

VII.3 Management of pulmonary embolism in childhood

C. H. van Ommen, P. Monagle, M. Peters, M. Andrew

Introduction

Pulmonary embolism (PE) is a well-recognised cause of morbidity and mortality in adults, especially amongst hospitalised patients [1, 2]. There have been numerous large multicentre trials aimed at improving the diagnosis and management of adults with PE [3–7]. The earliest described case of PE in childhood dates back to 1861 when Löschner reported a PE in a 9-year old child [8], which had developed in association with a fractured tibia. Despite this, over 130 years later, the number of cases of PE in children reported in the literature number only in the few hundreds, restricted mostly to case reports and series. The incidence, risk factors and clinical presentation remain poorly described. Recently, pharmacokinetic and dosefinding studies were performed with standard heparin [9, 10], low molecular weight heparin [11] and oral anticoagulants [12, 13], which allowed a few specific guidelines for antithrombotic therapy in newborns and children to be published [14].

Tremendous improvements in tertiary pediatric care over the last decade have led to a dramatic increase in survival for children with previously fatal primary disorders [15]. The aggressive surgical and pharmacological approaches which have led to this increased survival have only been possible with the improved ability to provide adequate supportive care to critically ill children. For example, the use of central venous lines (CVLs) permits the administration of fluids, nutrition and life-saving drugs to children in whom adequate venous access would not be possible. Similarly, the increased use of extracorporeal circulation techniques permits children to be sustained through acute reversible cardiorespiratory insults which were previously not survivable. Paradoxically, the improved survival of children with serious primary problems is associated with the development of secondary complications, some of which were rarely seen in children previously [16]. Thromboembolic disease, which includes PE, is one of the most frequent and serious secondary complications, occurring disproportionately in children successfully treated for congenital heart disease and cancer [17]. The increasing incidence of PE in children warrants a systematic review of the available information on diagnosis and treatment as well as the development of strategies to prevent and improve care of this thrombotic complication.

The following chapter focuses on PE in children and summarises available information. Medline searches of the literature were conducted from 1966 to 1998 using combinations of key words and supplemented by additional references located through the bibliographies of listed articles. All articles were evaluated for the strength of the study design using standardised criteria [18]. Results from studies with stronger study designs were priorised over results from studies with weaker study designs. Information on the incidence, clinical presentation, diagnostic strategies, risk factors and management strategies, and outcome in children with PE are described. Future studies required to improve the diagnosis and management of PE in children are discussed.

Incidence

The current incidence of PE in children is unknown and likely changing, reflecting rapid changes in tertiary care pediatrics and the evolution of secondary complications. Overall, the incidence of PE in children is decreased compared to adults, due to the decreased risk of thrombotic complications in general in children. There are a variety of physiological mechanisms that likely provide protection to children from thrombotic complications.

A number of retrospective autopsy studies have estimated the overall incidence of PE in children to be 0.05% – 4.2% [19 – 22]. The variation in results of autopsy studies probably reflects patient selection and the various techniques used to detect PE. Large macroscopic emboli were unlikely to be missed at post mortem examination, but the rate of PE rose considerably if microscopic techniques were used. The largest retrospective chart review, of adolescents who were admitted to an inner city referral and teaching hospital in the Bronx, New York, reported an incidence of PE of 78 per 100,000 hospitalised adolescents [23].

The first multicentre prospective registry of PE in children aged between 1 month and 18 years reported an incidence of PE of 8.6 per 100,000 pediatric admissions [24]. The decreased index of clinical suspicion for PE in children and absence of standardised diagnostic techniques suggests that clinical studies provide a minimal estimate of the incidence of PE in pediatric patients. Table 1 summarises the studies that reported on the incidence of PE.

Clinical presentation

The clinical diagnosis of PE lacks both sensitivity and specificity. In a prospective study of 173 consecutive adult patients arriving at the emergency room with pleuritic chest pain, signs and symptoms, when used alone to diagnose PE, at best had a sensitivity of 85%, but a specificity of only 37% [25]. Clinical signs, however, are usually the first reason why patients are suspected of having the disorder and may serve as a basis for selecting patients who require further diagnostic studies.

There are only a few studies available on clinical presentation of PE in children. PE is frequently clinically silent or with minimal symptoms which can be explained by other co-morbid conditions [26]. In a retrospective series by Buck et al., only 50% of children with clinically significant PE had clinical symptoms which were attributable to PE. The clinical diagnosis of PE was considered in only 15% of these children [19]. Other authors reported on the subtlety of symptoms in PE in children [27, 28]. In teenagers the most classic complaint was (pleuritic) chest pain, noted in 84%. Other frequently occurring complaints included dyspnea, cough and hemoptysis. Common findings were hypoxemia, tachypnea and fever [23]. In children receiving artificial ventilation, the most obvious indication of PE is a marked increase in oxygen requirements [26]. Other signs which have been reported to occur in children with acute PE are acute right heart failure, cyanosis, hypotension, arrhythmia, pallor, syncope, tachycardia and sweating [19, 21, 27, 29 – 33]. Recurrent acute PE may remain undetected until a child presents with chronic pulmonary hypertension or cardiac failure [34 – 36].

Although many of the clinical features of PE in children are similar to those in adults, the diagnosis is often unnecessarily delayed. The clinical symptoms of PE are often confused with the clinical symptoms of the underlying disorder, or thought to represent cardiorespiratory deterioration due to other causes, such as sepsis of cardiac failure in critically ill children [26]. The same population of children is likely at increased risk for PE due to the presence of multiple risk factors for thrombotic complications. PE should be considered in the differential diagnosis of cardiorespiratory deterioration in all critically ill children.

Special attention should be given to the group of children and adolescents with indwelling central venous catheters, as 25 – 46% of all deep venous thrombosis (DVT) and/or PE are secondary to these catheters [24, 37 – 39]. Especially children with central venous catheters receiving long-term parenteral nutrition who develop unexplained dyspnea, fever or exhaustion should be screened for PE both clinically and with objective diagnostic tools [40, 41].

Table 1. Incidence of PE in childhood.

Author	Year	Study type	Total n	Age	Diagnostic method	Incidence PE
A. Autopsy						
Emery [20]	1962	retrospective	2,000	0–7	autopsy	1.25%
Jones [21]	1966	retrospective	10,000	0–16	autopsy	0.73%
Sanerkin [186]	1966	retrospective	330	newborn	autopsy	14%
Buck [19]	1981	retrospective	–	0–19	autopsy	4.2%
Byard [22]	1990	retrospective	17,500	0–13	autopsy	0.05%
B. Clinical diagnosis						
Jones [179]	1975	retrospective case reports	36	0–15	clinical	–
Bernstein [23]	1986	retrospective chart review	24,250	12–21	angiography, V/Q, autopsy	0.078%
Andrew [24]	1994	prospective	–	1m–18	V/Q	0.0086%
C. In selected diseases						
Raman [184]	1971	prospective	30 adults and children	Guillain-Barré syndrome	clinical/autopsy	33%
Egli [180]	1974	retrospective review	3377	nephrotic syndrome	clinical	1.8%
Hoyer [181]	1986	retrospective review	26	asymptomatic nephrotic syndrome	routine V/Q	28%
Desai [29]	1989	retrospective review	178	fatal burns	autopsy	1.7%
Piatt [185]	1989	retrospective review	32	VA shunts	clinical	3%
Hsu [182]	1991	cross sectional	62	pre-cardiac transplant	V/Q/ angiography	31%
Marraro [183]	1991	prospective	205	acute leukemia	digital angiography/ perfusion scans	3.4%
Uderzo [187]	1993	retrospective review	67	BMT for leukemia	angiography/ V/Q	4.5%
McBride [132]	1994	retrospective review	28,692	trauma	clinical	0.0069%
Dollery [53]	1994	cross sectional	34	long-term TPN	V/Q, CXR	32%
Nuss [38]	1995	retrospective review	61	thrombosis	V/Q	20%
Derish [26]	1995	retrospective review	21	ICU deaths	autopsy	24%
Adams [39]	1997	prospective registry	243	CVL-related thrombosis	clinically indicated V/Q	10.7%

PE = pulmonary embolism
n   = number
TPN = total parenteral nutrition
CXR = chest X-ray
V/Q = ventilation/perfusion scan
CVL = central venous line
ICU = intensive care unit
BMT = bone marrow transplant

Diagnosis

In reports published before 1975, PE was usually either a surgical or a pathological diagnosis. Since 1975, 66% of reported pediatric cases have been diagnosed with lung scan and/or angiography. However, the details of lung scan patterns were not always obtained [37].

Individual radiographic tests that are used to diagnose PE in children are the same as those used for adults and consist of pulmonary angiogram, ventilation perfusion scan, magnetic resonance imaging (MRI), helical computerised tomography (Spiral CT), echocardiogram and others. The clinical utility of these radiographic tests has been studied extensively in adults resulting in useful diagnostic approaches to adult patients with suspected PE while reducing costs and risks to patients [3–6]. There are few studies in children addressing either the specificity and sensitivity of specific investigations or diagnostic strategies. The following section discusses the radiographic tests currently used to diagnose PE in children and provides a diagnostic approach to PE in pediatric patients. Extrapolations from the adult literature are made where relevant.

The current reference standard for the ante-mortem diagnosis of PE in adults is *pulmonary angiography*. This technique has several disadvantages, such as invasiveness, high costs and limited availability. Pulmonary angiography requires selective catheterisation of the pulmonary arteries and injection of radio-opaque contrast media [5]. Catheter placement may be technically difficult in small children or those with complex cardiac lesions. In addition, critically sick children may be at increased risk for complications from the procedure. Small pulmonary emboli which cause subsegmental perfusion lung scan defects may also go undetected. Furthermore, the relatively high radiation dose necessary for pulmonary angiography prevents its use as a screening test. Other risks of pulmonary angiography include a) consequences due to sedation or anaesthesia, b) embolism, if unstable right arterial thrombi are dislodged, and c) pulmonary hypertensive crises, in the case of chronic obstruction. In adult patients, morbidity and mortality is 3% and 0.2% respectively [42]. The mortality and morbidity in pediatric patients is unknown. In order to minimise these risks, pulmonary angiography should be restricted to specialist centres, where experience in catheterisation of small children and interpretation of pulmonary angiograms is available.

Ventilation/perfusion scan (V/Q Scan) is the most accurate non-invasive test for predicting pulmonary emboli, with a positive predictive value of 88% in the adult population [3]. Segmental or greater defect in perfusion with normal ventilation is considered as a "high probability lung scan" [3–7]. Ventilation scanning is performed by inhalation of a radioactive gas mixed with air, usually Xenon 133, Technetium 99 (^{99}Tc) or Krypton-81. Older children are able to co-operate by holding their breath. In young infants and neonates reliable images can be obtained through continuous tidal breathing with little or no co-operation [43] (Fig. 1). Age and weight specific isotope doses have been calculated. The radiation exposure to critical organs as a result of the procedure is minimal [43, 44]. Perfusion scanning is performed by injecting particles labelled with radioactive isotope, most commonly ^{99}Tc. Macro-aggregated Albumin (MAA) is the most widely used particulate material [45]. Perfusion scanning is very safe in patients of all ages, however the technique of temporary obstruction of capillaries used for perfusion scanning has important implications for children [43]. Adult lungs contain over 290×10^9 capillaries and the number of particles injected ranges from 2×10^5 to 10^6. Neonates have greatly reduced numbers of pulmonary capillaries. The number of alveoli and small pulmonary arteries increases rapidly during early infancy. Adult levels are probably reached around the end of the first decade. The injection of 2×10^5 to 10^6 particles of MAA into a neonate would cause increased occlusion of capillaries and potentially cause severe hypoxia. The risk of perfusion scan induced hypoxia is accentuated in children with severe diffuse pulmonary disease and advanced pulmonary hypertension [43]. Severe pulmonary hypertension results in arterial thickening and reduction in vessel lumen size, such that higher order arterioles may be occluded by the MAA particles. Although such adverse reactions are exceptionally rare, a fatal reaction has been reported in a 7-year-old child [46]. A similar theoretical concern exists in children with right to left cardiac shunts [43]. MAA particles may pass across the shunt and be lodged in the cerebral circulation.

The classification of V/Q results in children is similar to and extrapolated from diagnostic studies in adults. There are some unique underlying diseases that may influence the interpretation of V/Q scans in children. For example, V/Q scans may be difficult in children with congenital heart disease char-

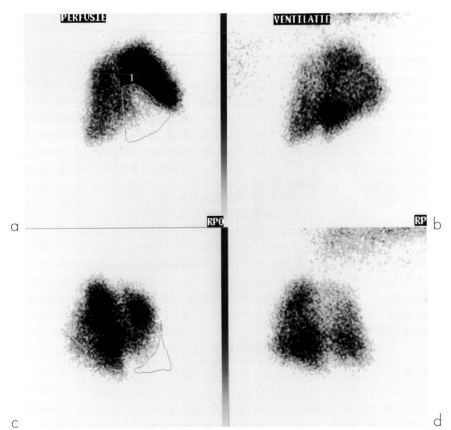

Fig. 1a–d. Right and left posterior oblique ventilation **(b, d)** and perfusion lung scans **(a, c)** of a two-week-old infant, showing well-matched defects in the right lower lobe.

acterised by imbalanced pulmonary blood flow between the left and right lungs, or even within each lung [47]. Children with left to right shunts will have variable distribution of the isotope due to the mixture of arterial blood in the pulmonary arteries [47]. In addition, coexistent peripheral pulmonary artery stenosis may be confused with multiple pulmonary emboli [45]. Finally, there have been reports of normal V/Q scans in children with large central pulmonary emboli [48].

Two-dimensional and Doppler echocardiography may be helpful in diagnosing PE as well [49]. Echocardiographic diagnosis of PE depends on direct imaging of pulmonary arterial thrombi. As this technique is only capable of evaluating the central pulmonary arteries, indirect indices of increased right ventricular volume or pressure have been used to establish the diagnosis and have been shown very sensitive in adults [50, 51]. In children the presence of structural cardiac defects makes these findings less specific. Furthermore echocardiography is of value in detecting intracardiac thrombi which may be a source of PE, and so provide indirect supportive evidence for the diagnosis of PE. One study used echocardiography to establish the prevalence of PE in 21 children with age

ranging from 5 to 132 months with central venous lines inserted longer than 3 months. Seven out of eight children with abnormal electrocardiograms (ECGs) had increased right ventricular end diastolic diameter (> 2SD above the mean value for age) by echocardiography which was suspicious for PE. Unfortunately the diagnosis was not confirmed with V/Q scan [52]. In 34 children receiving parenteral nutrition the occurrence of thrombosis and PE was evaluated by echocardiography and V/Q scan. PE was found in 9 children by V/Q scan, of which four children had normal echocardiograms [53].

Another technique is the *pulmonary arterial flow study*, an extension of nuclear angiocardiography, using ^{99}mTc-diethylenetriamine penta-acetic acid (DTPA), in which perfusion delays can be seen indicating incomplete obstruction of the central pulmonary arteries [48]. This method is not widely used.

Magnetic resonance imaging (MRI) and helical computerised tomography (Spiral CT) are generally useful in evaluating abnormalities of the pulmonary vasculature. These diagnostic modalities are currently being evaluated in adults and no studies in children have been published [54–56].

The disadvantages of MRI are that the patients' heart rate must be less than 100 beats/minute and it requires a 30-minute stay in the scanner room with limited access to the patient for monitoring [57].

Electrocardiograms (ECG) are useful in excluding other entities that present with a clinical picture of PE, such as pericarditis and acute myocardial infarction. In most cases of PE, the ECG shows nonspecific changes demonstrating sinus tachycardia or evidence of heart strain (Table 2). Although the presence of multiple abnormalities on ECG has been suggested to increase the diagnostic specificity of ECG, this approach has not gained widespread acceptance [52].

Several studies in adults have demonstrated that *D-dimer assays*, which measure fibrin degradation products, have potential clinical utility in excluding PE [58–60]. There have been no studies demonstrating the validity of D-dimers to exclude thromboembolic disease in children. The majority of children with thromboembolic disease have serious systemic illnesses such as cancer or cardiac disease. The usefulness of D-dimers in the diagnosis of thromboembolic disease in children is therefore likely considerably less than for adult patients.

Additional investigations such as blood gas analysis and chest radiography cannot be used to prove or to exclude the diagnosis of PE, but do give some additional information about the cardiorespiratory system.

Diagnostic strategy for PE in children: The accurate diagnosis of PE in children is important, because untreated PE has a significant mortality and the use of anticoagulants, in the absence of PE, exposes children to the unnecessary risk of bleeding associated with their use.

The pre-test probability has a major influence on the diagnostic process. Although some of the adult guidelines for pre-test clinical probability of PE will likely also apply to children, there are many age-dependent differences in risk for PE which necessitate separate guidelines for children. For example, a child with a CVL-related thrombosis is probably a high clinical risk patient, regardless of the presence or absence of clinical symptoms. Increasing appreciation of the subtle signs associated with PE in children and current ongoing studies will hopefully improve the clinical accuracy in predicting PE in children.

Even in the absence of prospective studies a practical approach to the diagnosis of PE in children is possible using the same principles as for adults. Figure 2 provides a suggested algorithm for diagnosing PE in children. In children with suspected PE, a V/Q scan should be performed whenever

Table 2. Electrocardiogram abnormalities possibly associated with PE in children [52].

S > 1.5 mm in I and aVL or R/S < 1

Q in III and aVF, but not II

Negative T in III, aVF, V1–V5

Right bundle branch block

ST elevation in V1

Upright T waves in V1

QRS < 5 mm in all limb leads

Transition in V5 or V6

Frontal QRS > 90°

Indeterminate axis

Right atrial hypertrophy

Atrial arrhythmia

feasible. If the V/Q scan is high probability for PE, this can be generally accepted as diagnostic for PE and anticoagulant therapy should be instituted. If the V/Q scan is normal, this can be generally accepted as diagnostic for the absence of PE. If the V/Q scan is indeterminate, further tests are required. If a CVL is in place in the upper venous system, a venogram (Fig. 3) or compression ultrasound of the jugular veins should be performed. If a thrombus is detected, anticoagulation therapy should be instituted. If there is no CVL in the upper venous system, ultrasound can be used to screen the lower proximal venous system for DVT. If the ultrasounds are normal, either follow-up ultrasounds or bilateral venograms should be considered depending on the strength of the clinical concern for PE. Serial testing is usually not required for venogram negative patients. In addition, an echocardiogram should be considered, particularly if there is underlying congenital or acquired heart disease.

Other tests are used to detect DVT but are relatively insensitive. For example, ultrasound, although useful for examining neck veins and lower proximal venous system, is relatively insensitive for DVT in the upper central venous system. Linograms (contrast injected through a CVL) (Fig. 4) are also insensitive in diagnosing CVL-related thrombosis [9]. ECG and D-dimers may add further useful information, but are unlikely to positively confirm the diagnosis of PE.

If the V/Q scan is uninterpretable due to abnormal pulmonary blood flow secondary to cardiac disease, either structural of functional, then the de-

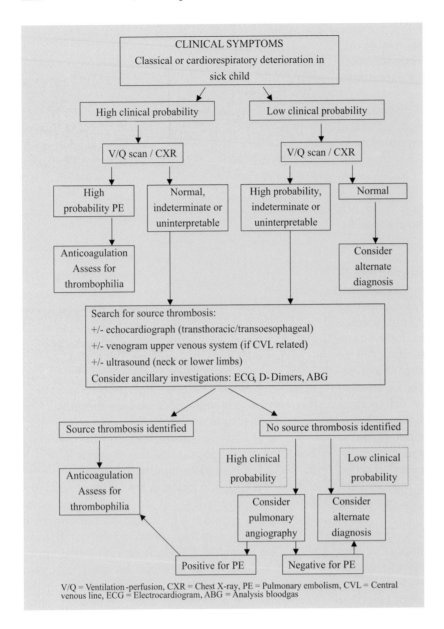

CLINICAL SYMPTOMS
Classical or cardiorespiratory deterioration in sick child

High clinical probability

Low clinical probability

V/Q scan / CXR

V/Q scan / CXR

High probability PE

Normal, indeterminate or uninterpretable

High probability, indeterminate or uninterpretable

Normal

Anticoagulation Assess for thrombophilia

Consider alternate diagnosis

Search for source thrombosis:
+/- echocardiograph (transthoracic/transoesophageal)
+/- venogram upper venous system (if CVL related)
+/- ultrasound (neck or lower limbs)
Consider ancillary investigations: ECG, D-Dimers, ABG

Source thrombosis identified

No source thrombosis identified

High clinical probability

Low clinical probability

Anticoagulation Assess for thrombophilia

Consider pulmonary angiography

Consider alternate diagnosis

Positive for PE

Negative for PE

V/Q = Ventilation -perfusion, CXR = Chest X-ray, PE = Pulmonary embolism, CVL = Central venous line, ECG = Electrocardiogram, ABG = Analysis bloodgas

Fig. 2. Suggested algorithm for diagnosis of PE in children.

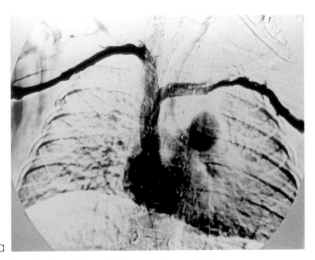
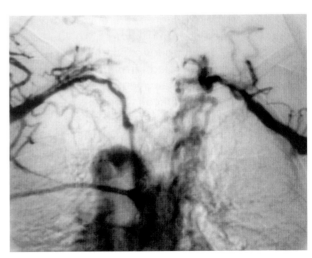

a

b

Fig. 3a, b. Normal (a) versus abnormal (b) venogram.

monstration of a source thrombosis associated with clinical symptoms of PE is usually enough to warrant a positive diagnosis and subsequent therapy. In some instances pulmonary angiography is necessary to establish the diagnosis.

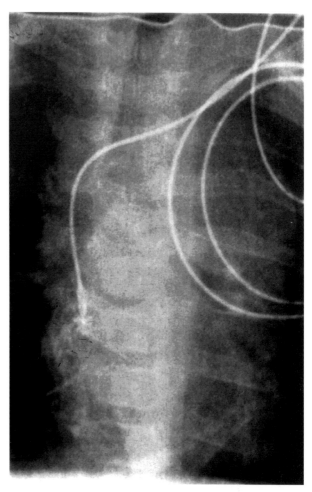

Fig. 4. An abnormal linogram.

Risk factors

In almost all children with PE, DVT or both, one or more acquired or congenital risk factors can be found. The results of studies concerning risk factors vary enormously, depending on the design (retro- or prospective), the age and the size of the study population. Other factors influencing the results include the source of the data, whether they were obtained by registry, survey or autopsy. Table 3 summarises the risk factors in pediatric patients. In the first prospective Canadian registry study 96% of the children with DVT, PE or both had one or more risk factors [24]. Only one risk factor was found in 12%; two and three risk factors were present in 39% and 35%, respectively. In about 10% of the children even four risk factors could be found.

The pediatrician must be aware that some acute or chronic diseases in childhood may disturb the normal hemostatic balance, causing a "hypercoagul-

able" or "prethrombotic state", increasing the risk of thrombotic complications. For instance, a varicella-infection may be accompanied by a severe acquired protein S deficiency, sometimes causing a thromboembolic complication [61–65].

In addition to DVT, PE in neonates and children may also consist of other pathological or iatrogenic materials [66]. PE in children and neonates can consist of air [67–69], tumour [70, 71] (especially Wilms tumour), brain tissue [72], necrotic liver tissue [73], teflon [74], intralipid [75–76], right ventricular myxoma [77, 78], fat, and bone marrow [79]. The clinical scenario should alert clinicians to the possibility of PE secondary to these materials. Unlike PE comprised of fibrin, anticoagulation is not likely necessary in PE comprised of other materials.

In the next section the most frequent acquired and inherited risk factors are described.

Table 3. Risk factors in children with thromboembolic complications.

Acquired risk factors	Hereditary risk factors
Central venous line [19, 23, 24, 26, 37–40, 83, 94, 123, 124, 179, 202]	Protein S deficiency [24, 37, 38, 108, 124]
Infection [19, 22–24, 37, 38, 45, 61–65, 123, 124, 172, 179]	Protein C deficiency [24, 37, 38, 105–107, 115, 124]
Renal disease [23, 24, 27, 37, 38, 120, 123, 124, 188, 189]	Antithrombin deficiency [24, 37, 38, 109, 110, 124, 125]
Malignancy [19, 22–24, 31, 34, 37, 38, 183, 188]	Factor V mutation [111, 112, 117–122, 124–126, 130]
Cardiac disease [19, 21, 23, 24, 37, 38, 95–99, 174, 179, 182, 190–193]	Factor II mutation [127]
Antiphospholipid antibodies [38, 99–104, 124]	Homocystinuria [37, 129–131, 201]
Dehydration [23]	Lipoprotein (a) [128]
Inflammatory bowel disease [37, 188]	Plasminogen deficiency [37, 124]
Systemic lupus erythematosus [23, 24, 37, 38]	Dysfibrinogenemia [37, 103, 124]
Obesity [23, 24, 37]	Heparin cofactor II deficiency [37, 124]
Surgery [22–24, 30, 37, 179, 194, 195]	
Immobilisation [19, 23, 37, 38, 179]	
Trauma [19, 23, 37, 38, 132, 179, 188]	
Sickle cell anemia [24, 37, 38, 196, 206]	
Medication:	
• Oral anticonceptives [23, 24, 37, 38, 188]	
• High dose estrogen to reduce height [197, 198, 205]	
• L-Asparaginase [203, 204]	
Ventriculo atrial shunts [19, 23, 37, 185, 199]	
Major burns [29]	
Liver transplantation [37, 200]	

Acquired risk factors

a) Central venous line

CVLs have become an important component in the treatment of preterm neonates and children with primary diseases such as cancer, malabsorption and cardiac diseases. Complications of indwelling central lines include infection, bleeding and catheter-related thrombosis. CVLs are thrombogenic because of disturbance of bloodflow, damage of the vessel wall and the thrombogenic material. Substances infused through the CVL, especially total parenteral nutrition (TPN) can also contribute to the damage of the vessel wall. In two registry studies, 25 to 46% of all children with thromboembolic complications had a CVL, and 10–20% of these children developed PE [38, 39, 80]. PE may occur while the CVL is in situ, during removal of the CVL, or from residual thrombus following CVL removal

[81]. About 90% of all thromboembolic complications in newborns are catheter-related, commonly accompanied by infections [82].

The reported incidences of thrombosis associated with CVL vary from about 1% to 67% [40, 52, 53, 83–94]. These differences are probably due to diverse patient populations studied and the frequency and indication of radiological investigation. For instance, in one study radiological tests were performed in patients with clinical suspicion of thrombosis and in others the tests were done if no blood samples could be drawn from CVLs or if signs of sepsis were present. The choice of radiographic test (linogram, echocardiography, ultrasonography or venography) to detect a thromboembolic complication will also influence the observed frequency.

The incidence of thrombosis diagnosed by ultrasonography ranged from 3.5% to 36% in 5 different prospective studies, including children with femoral catheters [87–89, 92, 93]. No investigation was performed to detect PE.

Children on long-term TPN form a special high risk group. A total of 34 children and adolescents with gut failure, who all received long-term TPN (duration 2 months to 9 years), were studied by means of clinical events, ventilation perfusion scans and echocardiography [53]. Sixteen thrombotic events (10 PE, 5 right atrial thrombi, and 1 caval vein obstruction) were identified in 12 patients, of whom 4 died. A relation between TPN use and thrombosis was also found in other studies [40, 52, 94]. Using venography, even 67% of 12 children on TPN, in whom a total of 49 central venous lines were placed, showed major venous obstruction [40]. The high prevalence of thrombosis in patients with CVL and TPN suggests a need for a multicentre randomised, controlled trial to determine the benefit of low-dose oral anticoagulant therapy in this group of patients.

b) Cardiac disease

Thrombotic events are well-known complications of congenital or acquired heart diseases, attributed mainly to low flow states, contact activation or a disturbed flow pattern as observed in prosthetic valve replacements [95]. The frequency of thromboembolic complications after Fontan or modified Fontan procedures is likely at least 20%. Fontan or modified Fontan procedures are the treatment of choice for many congenital heart defects including tricuspid atresia, double-inlet ventricle and hypoplastic left heart syndrome [96–98]. Thromboembolic disease following Fontan procedures has recently been reviewed [99].

c) Antiphospholipid antibodies

Antiphospholipid antibodies are auto-antibodies directed against certain phospholipid-binding plasma proteins such as β2-glycoprotein I (β2GPI), prothrombin, protein C and protein S. Some patients have antibodies against all four of the proteins, whereas other patients have antibodies against one, two or three of these proteins in different combinations [100, 101]. The association of antiphospholipid antibodies with arterial thrombosis, venous thrombosis, recurrent foetal loss or thrombocytopenia is termed Antiphospholipid antibody syndrome (APS). Secondary APS occurs in patients with systemic lupus erythematosus or other auto-immune disease. When antiphospholipid antibodies are found in the absence of an associated autoimmune disease, it is called primary APS. Possible mechanisms whereby these antibodies predispose to thrombosis are inhibition of

protein C/protein S-mediated inactivation of factors Va and VIIIa, enhanced platelet activation and enhanced factor Xa generation by platelets [102]. One specific group of antiphospholipid autoantibodies are lupus anticoagulants. These antibodies inhibit certain in vitro phospholipid-dependent coagulation reactions, such as the conversion of prothrombin to thrombin. The anticoagulant activity of these antibodies is accentuated by lowering the phospholipid concentration in the dilute Russell's viper venom time assay. Mixing patient plasma with normal plasma does not correct the prolongation of the coagulation reaction. Lupus anticoagulants are heterogeneous, including autoantibodies to at least 2 phospholipid bound plasma proteins (prothrombin or β2GPI) [100].

In 1991 a retrospective French collaborative study was performed including 120 children with SLE [103]. Eleven of these children had 16 thrombotic episodes. In 4 cases PE was diagnosed. Lupus anticoagulant was present in eight of 11 patients (72%) with thrombosis and in only 13% of the patients without history of thrombosis. These antibodies are an important acquired risk factor as in one study in children with PE, an incidence of 45% was noted [104].

Congenital risk factors

In general, congenital heterozygous deficiency of protein C [105–107], protein S [108], antithrombin [109, 110] or the presence of factor V Leiden [111, 112] are associated with venous thrombosis in early adulthood [113, 114]. A homozygous form of protein C deficiency or protein S deficiency usually causes neonatal purpura fulminans, although later onset childhood thrombosis is a well-described clinical presentation [115].

In three surveys on thromboembolic complications in children and new-borns protein C deficiency was found in 13 to 20% and protein S deficiency in 6 to 13%, which are higher percentages than those reported in adults [24, 38, 113, 116]. Antithrombin deficiency was infrequently seen. Factor V Leiden is reported in 20–25% of the children with thrombosis. These prevalences are similar to those found in adults [111, 117–121].

In most cases these genetic defects become clinically apparent in childhood when additional congenital or acquired risk factors are present [24, 117, 122]. This implies that in children it is worthwhile to investigate defects in hemostasis, even if acquired risk factors such as CVLs seem to explain the thrombotic event [123, 124] (Table 4). Furthermore, a combination of gene defects or "double

Table 4. Recommended laboratory evaluation of pediatric patients with pulmonary embolism (PE).

First step	Second step
Antithrombin	Plasminogen
Protein C and S	Factor II mutation
Factor V mutation	Homocystinuria
Thrombin time	Lipoprotein (a)
Anti-phospholipid antibodies	Heparin cofactor II

hit" results in a much higher risk for thrombosis and at a younger age than a single defect [122]. In families in which both antithrombin deficiency and factor V Leiden were found, thrombosis occurred in 50% of the carriers of antithrombin deficiency, in 20% of the carriers of factor V Leiden and in 92% of the carriers of both defects [125]. Recently, new risk factors such as factor II mutation and lipoprotein (a) (Lp(a)) have been described. Factor II mutation is a G to A transition at nucleotide position 20210 in the 3' untranslated region of the prothrombin gene, associated with increased levels of prothrombin activity and risk of thrombosis [126, 127]. Elevated Lp(a) of more than 50 mg/dl was found in 25% of 36 children with arterial thrombosis and in about 14% of 36 children with venous thrombosis [128]. However, the role of factor II mutation and Lp(a) as contributing factor to thrombosis in children is not completely elucidated.

Hereditary homocystinuria is caused by deficient activity of one of the enzymes in methionine metabolism. Clinical signs in patients, homozygous for this disease, are mental retardation, ectopia lentis, skeletal abnormalities and life-threatening thromboembolic events. These events occur in about one third of the homozygous patients [129]. Coexistence with factor V Leiden results in an increased risk of thrombosis [130]. Acquired hyperhomocysteinemia can exist due to deficiency of vitamin B6, folate or vitamin B12 and is an important risk factor for thrombosis in adults [131]. In children it is seldom found.

Treatment

Treatment of PE can be subdivided into a) primary prophylaxis, and b) treatment of the acute event.

a) Primary prophylaxis

The overall incidence of PE in almost 29,000 pediatric trauma patients was 0.007%, and 1.85% for children with paralysis from spinal cord injury [132]. From these data the prophylaxis for PE recommended for adult trauma patients appears unwarranted in injured children. In adolescents with paraplegia, however, prophylaxis should be considered if confounding associated risk factors are present.

In general, heparin prophylaxis must be considered in children if more than two risk factors are present, especially when one of the risk factors is an indwelling venous catheter (Table 3). In individual cases, the risk of thrombosis should be weighed against the risk of antithrombotic prophylaxis.

It is obvious that more research is needed before firm guidelines concerning the indications, efficiency and safety of primary prophylaxis in this population can be made.

b) Treatment of acute event

The treatment of acute PE has two components, supportive care and specific therapy for the PE.

Supportive care

Acute massive PE causing cardiovascular collapse should initially be treated with resuscitation, endotrachial intubation and mechanical ventilation to ensure adequate tissue oxygenation and CO_2 removal. The difficulty in providing proper oxygenation and ventilation in PE is that there can be a significant increase in airway resistance and decrease in lung compliance, leading to the use of high positive and expiratory pressure (PEEP). This can in turn impair venous return to the heart in an already hemodynamically comprised patient [133]. As the mortality rate of PE is high within the first 2–3 hours of symptoms, intravenous treatment of antithrombotic therapy should be started without delay.

Antithrombotic therapy

Anticoagulation remains the mainstay of therapy for PE in children [134]. From the Canadian registry of venous thromboembolism it was clear that children with DVT, PE or both were receiving a variety of therapeutic intervention [24]. Anticoagulation therapy with heparin was the most common form of initial treatment and was used in 85% of the 137 children. Initial thrombolytic therapy (streptokinase, urokinase or tissue plasminogen activator) was administered in 15 children (10%) for extension of their original thrombus or to clear blocked central venous lines, following a variety of protocols, and with variable success. Maintenance therapy with heparin was administered to 74% of the children. The length of heparin administration varied considerably from 1 to 62 days (median 14 days). Maintenance therapy with oral anticoagulants was administered in 103 children (75%), usually overlapping the heparin therapy for a few days. Nineteen children received less than 3 months of therapy. The 60 children treated for more than 3 months had persistent underlying risk factors. The guidelines for treatment of thromboembolic complications in children were initially directly extrapolated from recommendations for adults due to lack of large prospective studies in children.

Heparin

Heparin is currently the preferred anticoagulant for the initial treatment of thromboembolic complication in pediatric patients. So far, only one prospective cohort study has been performed in which the effect of heparin in children has been evaluated [9]. After an initial injection of 50 U/kg, only 39% of the children achieved a minimal level of activated partial thromboplastin time (APTT). In most children the rate at which therapeutic heparin values were achieved was much slower than that reported for adults. This reflected the likely need for a higher initial and maintenance dose of heparin for younger children. Several studies in adults with DVT have shown that achieving a therapeutic APTT within 48 hours of initiating treatment significantly reduces the rate of recurrence [135]. Therefore, pending additional studies, the following guidelines for treatment of thrombotic complication in children are recommended [14, 134, 136].

Heparin therapy is initiated with a loading dose of 75 U/kg (maximum 5,000 U) intravenously over 10 minutes, followed by an infusion, beginning at a heparin dose of 28 U/kg/hr for infants younger than 1 year and 20 U/kg/hr for infants older than 1 year. Heparin activity is measured 4 to 6 hours after the initial dose, by determination

Table 5. Heparin nomogram for children [14, 134].

APTT (s)	Bolus (units/kg)	Hold (min)	Rate change (units/kg/hr)	Repeat APTT
< 50	50	0	↑10%	4 hrs
50–59	0	0	↑10%	4 hrs
60–85	0	0	0	24 hrs
86–95	0	0	↓10%	4 hrs
96–120	0	30	↓10%	4 hrs
> 120	0	60	↓15%	4 hrs

APTT = activated partial thromboplastin time
Reproduced with permission.

of APTT or by heparin level. Adjustments are made rapidly to achieve the therapeutic range as quickly as possible. The APTT therapeutic range is 1,5 to 2 times the initial value, which corresponds to a heparin level of 0.2–0.4 U/ml. APTT must be checked at least on a daily basis and 4–6 hours after any adjustment of the heparin concentration. Depending on the result of APTT, heparin must be adjusted accordingly (Table 5). The duration of heparin treatment for (massive) PE is 7 to 14 days.

In a prospective study on heparin therapy in pediatric patients, bleeding complications were seen in 0–2% of the patients [9, 24]. Regular monitoring of platelets during heparin therapy is required because some case reports mention heparin-induced thrombocytopenia [137, 138]. The platelet count fall begins between five and eight days after starting heparin therapy (occasionally later) [139].

Oral anticoagulant therapy

Treatment with an oral anticoagulant can be initiated 2 to 5 days after the start of heparin therapy. The loading dose is 0.2 mg/kg orally, with a maximum of 10 mg, as a single daily dose [12–14, 37, 140, 141]. Subsequent loading doses are based on the results of International Normalised Ratio (INR) response (Table 6) [14]. The therapeutic range for pediatric patients with DVT and/or PE or both is an INR of 2 to 3. The loading period is approximately 3–5 days for most patients before a stable maintenance phase is achieved. The amount of oral anticoagulant required to achieve INRs of 2 to 3 decreases with increasing age [12]. Heparin therapy should be continued until the maintenance phase is reached. Precaution is

Table 6. Oral anticoagulant nomogram for children.

I. Oral anticoagulant loading doses on day 2–4, based on INR response [14, 134]

INR	Oral anticoagulant adjustment
1.1–1.4	repeat initial loading dose
1.5–1.9	50% of initial loading dose
2.0–3.0	50% of initial loading dose
3.1–3.5	25% of initial loading dose
> 3.5	hold until INR < 3.5, then restart at 50% less than the previous dose

II. Long-term oral anticoagulant dose guidelines [14, 134]

INR	Oral anticoagulant adjustment
1.1–1.4	increase by 20% of dose
1.5–1.9	increase by 10% of dose
2.0–3.0	no change
3.1–3.5	decrease by 20% of dose
> 3.5	hold dose, check INR daily until INR < 3.5, then restart at 20% less than the previous dose

INR = International Normalized Ratio
Reproduced with permission.

needed in the following specific patient groups [14, 96, 141 – 143]:

- The loading doses must be lowered to 0.1 mg/kg in patients with liver dysfunction or patients who have had a Fontan procedure.
- If the patient is receiving total parenteral nutrition, vitamin K must be removed from the amino acid solution.
- If the patient is receiving medication which interferes with oral anticoagulants, such as antibiotics or anticonvulsion therapy, the loading dose may require adjustment.
- Breast milk contains very low levels of vitamin K, therefore new-borns fed with breast milk require a very low dose of oral anticoagulant. In contrast, most formulae contain high concentrations of vitamin K (30 – 150 ug/L). Thus new-borns on formulae need a higher dose of oral anticoagulant.
- Oral anticoagulation for patients with gut failure may be problematic due to poor absorption and repeated INR tests are necessary.
- During the first month of life levels of vitamin K-dependent coagulant factors are approximately 50% of adult values. Oral anticoagulant therapy is avoided as much as possible in this period because of bleeding risk.

Oral anticoagulant treatment may be discontinued after 3 months, unless an underlying cause of the thromboembolic complication is still present or the process is recurrent.
The hemorrhagic risk of oral anticoagulant therapy in children appears to be comparable to that in adults [12, 13].

Low molecular weight heparin
Clinical trials in adults have established that low molecular weight heparin (LMWH) offers several advantages over standard heparin that may benefit children [144 – 147]. First, the pharmacokinetics of LMWH are more predictable than standard heparin, minimising the frequency of monitoring [144]. Second, LMWHs are at least as effective as standard heparin. Third, the frequency of bleeding complications with LMWH is likely less than that with standard heparin. The use of LMWH is particularly helpful in patients who require antithrombotic protection but who are particularly vulnerable to bleeding complications [148]. Treatment of many children requiring anticoagulant therapy can be problematic because of the seriousness of their underlying disorders. These same patients may have acquired bleeding disorders (such as thrombocytopenia, disseminated intravascular coagulation, and liver disease), and poor venous access that limits monitoring [9]. Fourth, LMWH can be administered subcutaneously every 12 hours, eliminating the need for continuous venous access devoted to standard heparin administration. A subcutaneous catheter (Insuflon; Viggo-Spectramed, PO Box 631, S-251 06 Helsingborg, Sweden) can further reduce the number of needle sticks for administration of LMWH from 14 per week to one per week [11]. EMLA cream can be used as local anaesthesia.
So far, only one dose finding study of LMWH (Enoxaparin) in children has been performed [11]. Fourteen of 25 children included in this study had DVT or PE. These children were selected because they had a potential bleeding risk or they bled while receiving standard heparin therapy. A dose of 1.0 mg/kg every 12 hours subcutaneously was sufficient to achieve a 4-hour therapeutical anti-Xa level between 0.5 and 1.0 U/ml. New-borns younger than 2 months required a higher dosage; an average of 1.6 mg/kg twice a day was required to achieve the above described anti-Xa levels (Table 7). In the near future the results of a multicentre randomised controlled trial comparing LMWH with standard heparin and oral anticoagulant therapy in pediatric patients with venous thromboembolism will provide us with more information on the efficiency and side-effects of LMWH in pediatric patients.

Thrombolytic therapy

In most adults with PE thrombolytic therapy is not indicated because their clinical outcome with anticoagulant therapy alone is good and thrombolytic therapy is associated with increased cost and risk of bleeding. Thrombolysis is usually only considered in adults with massive PE, where syncope, hypotension, severe hypoxemia or heart failure are present [149]. Similarly patients with submassive embolism but with severe underlying cardiac or respiratory disease may derive lifesaving benefit from thrombolytic therapy [2]. The guidelines for the use of thrombolytic therapy in adults with PE are based on randomised controlled trials assessing the efficacy and safety of thrombolytic therapy [149–152]. Corresponding studies in infants and children have not been conducted due to the relative paucity of clinical events, resulting in the extrapolation of adult guidelines. This approach may not be optimal because of age-dependent differences in the fibrinolytic system, which influences the response to thrombolytic agents [153–159]. As well, risk factors for haemorrhagic complications of thrombolytic agents are age dependent. The risk/benefit ratio of thrombolytic therapy for PE in pediatric patients remains unknown. Several case reports and small case series have reported successful thrombolysis in children using streptokinase, urokinase or tissue plasminogen activator [160–169]. The thrombolytic agents were administered either by local pulmonary artery directed catheters or systemic intravenous infusions and were generally used in combination with heparin therapy. The optimal dose and duration of thrombolytic therapy is unknown and there is a wide range of published dose schedules, usually supported by only individual case reports. The bleeding risk from thrombolytic therapy in children depends on the underlying clinical disease and likely the duration of thrombolytic therapy. A review of the literature and a large single centre study on the use of thrombolytic therapy in general in pediatric patients reported that major bleeding occurs in approximately 30 % of pediatric patients [170, 171]. The most frequent problem was bleeding at sites of invasive procedures which required treatment with blood products. Although the incidence of bleeding into the central nervous system could not be accurately determined from the literature, it was reported in less than 3 % of patients [170, 171]. There have been no trials to compare thrombolytic therapy to anticoagulation alone in children. At the present time, thrombolytic therapy cannot be generally recommended as first line therapy for PE in all children. The decision to use thrombolytic therapy should be individualised and

considered in children with large, new PE, particularly if the PE is hemodynamically compromising the patient. Concurrent anticoagulation therapy with either standard heparin or LMWH should be considered. Table 8 provides guidelines for the use of thrombolytic therapy in children.

Embolectomy

Embolectomy is reported as successful therapy in premature neonates and children as young as 6 days old [172, 173]. Embolectomy is often used following major cardiac surgery [174]. For exam-

Table 7. Low molecular weight heparin (enoxaparin) nomogram for children [14].

Anti-Xa level (U/ml)	Hold next dose	Dose change	Repeat anti-Xa level
< 0.35 U/ml	no	↑ 25 %	4 hrs post next dose
0.35–0.49 U/ml	no	↑ 10 %	4 hrs post next dose
0.50–1.0 U/ml	no	no	Once per week at 4hrs post
1.1–1.5 U/ml	no	↓ 20 %	4 hrs post next dose
1.6–2.0 U/ml	no	↓ 30 %	4 hrs post next dose
> 2.0 U/ml	until anti-Xa < 0.5 U/ml	↓ 40 %	Before next dose; repeat q 12 hrs until < 0.5 U/ml

Reproduced with permission.

Table 8. Thrombolytic therapy dose guidelines for children [14, 134].

	Loading dose	Maintenance dose
Streptokinase	2000–4000 U/kg IV over 10 min (max. 250,000 U)	2000 U/kg/hr IV for 6–12 hrs
Urokinase	4000 U/kg IV over 10 min	4000 U/kg/hr IV for 6–12 hrs 0.1 mg/kg/hr
rTPA	none	0.1–0.6 mg/kg/hr IV for 6 hrs starting at 0.1 mg/kg/hr

Note: Start heparin therapy either during or *immediately* upon completion of thrombolytic therapy. A loading dose of heparin may be omitted.

Reproduced with permission.

ple, embolectomy may be performed following Fontan surgery, when the cause of obstructed pulmonary blood flow is not clear and exploratory surgery is required. In other circumstances, embolectomy should be considered in massive PE when pulmonary circulation is severely compromised. Embolectomy should always be followed by an appropriate period of anticoagulation.

Caval filters

Anticoagulation therapy, the standard treatment of PE, may be contra-indicated in patients with recent trauma or operation, intracranial tumours or those with other diseases, complicated by potential haemorrhage. In adults, the Greenfield-filter placed in the inferior vena cava is an alternative to anticoagulation for prevention of primary or recurrent PE [175]. Caval filters can be used in children, although obviously decreasing age and size increase the technical challenge. However, the usefulness of caval filters in children is limited by the fact that the majority of DVT associated with PE are not in the lower limbs. Temporary filters are used in children and removed when the source of PE is gone [176].

The standard adult filter has also been used in 10 adolescent patients aged 13 to 18 years. After a follow-up period from 1 to 11 years, an objective documented caval patency without clinical sequelae was present in all 10 adolescents [177]. However, in a recent study in adults, filters appear to prevent PE primarily when they were used in combination with anticoagulant medication. After cessation of anticoagulation, they do not seem to prevent PE and may actually predispose patients to symptomatic deep vein thrombosis [178].

Outcome

Some authors have suggested that the mortality from PE may be less in children compared to adults due to a superior physiological tolerance to PE [1, 19]. However, in the Canadian registry, 10% of the 22 children diagnosed with PE died as a result of the PE. Very few children in the registry were investigated for PE, so the results are likely biased towards the more severe PE [24]. Chronic pulmonary hypertension and resultant cardiac failure are well described clinical presentations of multiple undiagnosed PE in children [34, 35]. The recurrence rate for PE in children is uncertain, but likely depends upon the underlying risk factors, the effectiveness of primary antithrombotic treatment, and the duration of therapy. There is no data on the long-term effects of PE on pulmonary function in children.

Conclusions

1. The frequency of PE is likely underestimated in children.
2. Children with PE often have multiple thrombotic risk factors, which may consist of clinical diseases, therapies and/or underlying hypercoagulable conditions. The most important clinical risk factor identified is the presence of CVL-related thrombosis.
3. The clinical features of PE in children are often subtle, or masked by their primary illness. Increased diagnostic suspicion is required to prevent mortality and morbidity from undiagnosed PE.

4. Diagnostic strategies for PE in children are extrapolated from studies in adults. The positive and negative predictive values of a number of investigations may be reduced in children, due to physiological and pathophysiological differences between child and adult.
5. Anticoagulation is the mainstay of therapy for children with PE, based mostly on extrapolation from data in adults; however, therapy needs to be individualised.
6. The outcome for children with PE is uncertain; however, the mortality is probably similar to that reported in adults with PE.

Future directions

Our knowledge about all aspects of PE in children has increased dramatically over recent years, however many questions remain unanswered. The incidence of PE in many clinical situations, and hence the role of primary prophylaxis, is uncertain. Studies to determine guidelines for clinically predicting the probability of PE in children are required. Diagnostic and management strategies need to be validated in children. Currently a number of multicentre studies designed to answer some of these issues are ongoing. However, further international collaborative efforts will be required to substantially improve the care of children with PE in the future.

Acknowledgements:
This work is supported by a grant-in-aid from the Heart and Stroke Foundation of Ontario.
Dr Andrew is a Career Investigator of the Heart and Stroke Foundation of Canada.

References

1. Carson JF, Kelley MA, Duff A, Weg JG, Fulkerson WJ, Palevsky HI, Schwartz JS, Thompson BT, Popovich J, Hobbins TE, Spera MA, Alavi A, Terrin ML. The clinical course of pulmonary embolism. N Engl J Med 1992; 326:1240–1245

2. Hirsh J, Hoak J. Management of deep vein thrombosis and pulmonary embolism: A statement for healthcare professionals. From the Council on Thrombosis (in consultation with the Council on Cardiovascular Radiology), American Heart Association. Circulation 1996; 93: 2212–2245

3. The PIOPED Investigators. Value of the ventilation/perfusion scan in acute pulmonary embolism. Results of the prospective investigation of pulmonary embolism diagnosis. JAMA 1990; 263: 2573–2759

4. The PISA-PED Investigators. Invasive and noninvasive diagnosis of pulmonary embolism. Preliminary results of the prospective investigative study of acute pulmonary embolism diagnosis (PISA-PED). Chest 1995; 107: 33–38

5. Hull RD, Hirsh J, Carter CJ, Jay RM, Dodd PE, Ockelford PA, Coates G, Gill GJ, Turpie AG, Doyle DJ, Buller HR, Raskob GE. Pulmonary angiography, ventilation lung scanning and venography for clinically suspected pulmonary embolism with abnormal perfusion lung scan. Ann Intern Med 1983; 98: 891–899

6. Hull RD, Raskob GE, Coates G, Panju AA, Gill GJ. A new noninvasive management strategy for patients with suspected pulmonary embolism. Arch Intern Med 1989; 149: 2549–2555

7. Hull RD, Raskob GE, Ginsberg JS, Panju AA. A noninvasive strategy for the treatment of patients with suspected pulmonary embolism. Arch Intern Med 1994; 154: 289–297

8. Stevenson GF, Stevenson FL. Pulmonary embolism in childhood. J Pediatr 1949; 34: 62–69

9. Andrew M, Marzinotto V, Massicotte P, Blanchette V, Ginsberg JS, Brill-Edwards P, Burrows P, Benson L, Williams W, David M, Poon A, Sparling K. Heparin therapy in pediatric patients: A prospective cohort study. Pediatr Res 1994; 35: 78–83

10. Schmidt B, Ofosu FA, Mitchell L, Brooker LA, Andrew M. Anticoagulant effects of heparin in neonatal plasma. Pediatr Res 1989; 25: 405–408

11. Massicotte P, Adams M, Marzinotto V, Brooker LA, Andrew M. Low-molecular-weight heparin in pediatric patients with thrombotic disease: A dose finding study. J Pediatr 1996; 128: 313–318

12. Andrew A, Marzinotto V, Brooker LA, Adams M, Ginsberg J, Freedom R, Williams W. Oral anticoagulation therapy in pediatric patients: a prospective study. Thromb Haemost 1994; 71: 265–269

13. Tait RC, Ladusans EJ, El-Metaal M, Patel RG, Will AM. Oral anticoagulation in paediatric patients: dose requirements and complications. Arch Dis Child 1996; 74: 228–231

14. Andrew M, deVeber G, eds. Pediatric thromboembolism and stroke protocols. Hamilton, BC Decker Inc, 1997. ISBN 1-550009-055-0

15. Andrew M, Montgomery RR. Acquired disorders of hemostasis. In: Nathan DG, Orkin SH, eds. Nathan and Oski's Hematology of infancy and childhood. Philadelphia: WB Saunders Company 1998:1677–1717

16. Massicotte MP, Brooker LA, Andrew M. Hemorrhagic and thrombotic complications in children with cancer. In: Children's Cancer Group, eds. The supportive care manual in pediatric malignancy. In press

17. Andrew M, Schmidt B. Hemorrhagic and Thrombotic Complications in Children. In: Andrew M, Schmidt B, Colman RW, Hirsh J, Marder V, Salzman EW, eds. Hemostasis and Thrombosis: Basic Principles and Clinical Practice, 3rd ed. Philadelphia: J.B. Lippincott Company, 1994; 989–1000

18. Cook DJ, Guyatt GH, Laupacis A, Sackett DL, Goldberg RJ. Clinical recommendations using levels of evidence for antithrombotic agents. Chest 1995; 108: 227–230

19. Buck JR, Connor RH, Cook WW, Weintraub WH, Wesley JR, Coran AG. Pulmonary embolism in children. J Pediatr Surg 1981; 16: 385–391

20. Emery JL. Pulmonary embolism in children. Arch Dis Child 1962; 37: 591–595

21. Jones RH, Sabiston DC. Pulmonary embolism in childhood. Monogr Surg Sci 1966; 3: 35–51

22. Byard RW, Cutz E. Sudden and unexpected death in infancy and childhood due to pulmonary thromboembolism. Arch Pathol Lab Med 1990; 114: 142–144

23. Bernstein D, Coupey S, Schonberg K. Pulmonary embolism in adolescents. Am J Dis Child 1986; 140: 667–671

24. Andrew M, David M, Adams M, Ali K, Anderson R, Barnard D, Bernstein M, Brisson L, Cairney B, DeSai D, Grant R, Israels S, Jardine L, Luke B, Massicotte P, Silva M. Venous thromboembolic complications (VTE) in children: First analyses of the Canadian registry of VTE. Blood 1994; 83: 1251–1257

25. Hull RD, Raskob GE, Carter CJ, Coates G, Gill GJ, Sackett DL, Hirsh J, Thompson M. Pulmonary embolism in outpatients with pleuritic chest pain. Arch Intern Med 1988; 148: 838–844

26. Derish MT, Smith DW, Frankel LR. Venous catheter thrombus formation and pulmonary embolism in children. Pediatr Pulmonol 1995; 20: 349–354

27. Jones GL, Hebert D. Pulmonary thrombo-embolism in the nephrotic syndrome. Pediatr Nephrol 1991; 5: 56–58

28. Dye CL. Pulmonary embolism in a child. JAMA 1968; 204: 1144–1145

29. Desai MH, Linares HA, Herndon DN. Pulmonary embolism in burned children. Burns 1989; 15: 376–380

30. Goodman NW, Falkner MJ. Massive intraoperative pulmonary embolism in a child. Br J Anaesth 1987; 59: 1059–1062

31. Bulas DI, Thompson R, Reaman G. Pulmonary emboli as a primary manifestation of Wilms tumor. Am J Roentgenol 1991; 56: 155–156

32. Nichols MM, Tyson KRT. Saddle embolus occluding pulmonary arteries. Am J Dis Child 1978; 132: 926

33. Matthew DJ, Levin M. Pulmonary thromboembolism in children. Intensive Care Med 1986; 12: 404–406

34. Soares EA, Landell GA, de Oliveira JA. Subacute cor pulmonale in children: Report of two cases. Pediatr Pulmonol 1992; 12: 52–57

35. McMahon DP, Aterman K. Pulmonary hypertension due to multiple emboli. J Pediatr 1978; 92: 841–845

36. Woodruff WW, Merten DF, Wagner ML, Kirks DR. Chronic pulmonary embolism in children. Radiol 1986; 159: 511–514

37. David M, Andrew M. Venous thromboembolic complications in children. J Pediatr 1993; 123: 337–346

38. Nuss R, Hays T, Manco-Johnson M. Childhood Thrombosis. Pediatrics 1995; 96: 291–294

39. Adams M, Massicotte MP, Andrew M. Central venous catheter related thrombosis (CVLT) in children: Analysis of the Canadian registry of venous thromboembolic complications. Thromb Haemost 1997; 78: 397

40. Andrew M, Marzinotto V, Pencharz P, Zlotkin S, Burrows P, Ingram J, Adams M, Filler R. A cross-sectional study of catheter-related thrombosis in children receiving total parenteral nutrition at home. J Pediatr 1995; 126: 358–363

41. Dollery CM. Pulmonary embolism in parenteral nutrition. Arch Dis Child 1996; 74: 95–98

42. Mills SR, Jackson DC, Older RA, Heaston DK, Moore AV. The incidence, etiologies and avoidance of complications of pulmonary angiography in a large series. Radiol 1980; 136: 295–299

43. Papanicolaou N, Treves S. Pulmonary scintigraphy in pediatrics. Semin Nucl Med 1980; 10: 259–285

44. Gordon I, Helms P, Frazio F. Clinical applications of radionuclide lung scanning in infants and children. Br J Radiol 1981; 54: 576–585

45. Hurley RJ, Wesselhoeft H, James AE. Use of nuclear imaging in the evaluation of pediatric cardiac disease. Semin Nucl Med 1972; 2: 353–372

46. Vincent WR, Goldberg SJ, Desilets D. Fatality immediately following rapid infusion of macroaggregates of ^{99m}Tc albumin (MAA) for lung scan. Radiology 1968; 91: 1180–1184

47. Mishkin F, Knote J. Radioisotope scanning of the lungs in patients with systemic pulmonary anastomoses. Am J Roentgen Rad Ther Nucl Med 1968; 102: 267–273

48. Hackbarth R, Kuhns L, Sarnaik A. Central pulmonary embolism with normal ventilation perfusion scan-Diagnosis by nuclear pulmonary artery flow studies. Ann Emerg Med 1991; 20: 95–97

49. Gleason MM, White MG, Myers JL. Echocardiographic diagnosis of pulmonary embolism in childhood. J Am Soc Echocardiogr 1995; 8: 100–102

50. Cheriex EC, Sreeram N, Eussen YFJM, Pieters FAA, Wellens HJJ. Cross sectional Doppler echocardiography as the initial technique for the diagnosis of acute pulmonary embolism. Br Heart J 1994; 72: 52–57

51. Sreeram N, Cheriex E, Eussen Y, Pieters FA, Wellens HJJ. Two-dimensional Doppler echocardiography as the initial diagnostic tool for acute pulmonary embolism. J Am Coll Cardiol 1994; 23: 95A

52. Pollard AJ, Sreeram N, Wright JG, Beath SV, Booth IW, Kelly DA. ECG and echocardiographic diagnosis of pulmonary thromboembolism associated with central venous lines. Arch Dis Child 1995; 73: 147–150

53. Dollery CM, Sullivan ID, Bauraind O, Bull C, Milla PJ. Thrombosis and embolism in long-term central venous access for parenteral nutrition. Lancet 1994; 344: 1043–1045

54. Meaney JFM, Weg JG, Chenvert TL, Stafford-Johnson D, Hamilton BH, Prince MR. Diagnosis of pulmonary embolism with magnetic resonance angiography. N Engl J Med 1997; 336: 1422–1427

55. Rossum van AB, Treurniet FEE, Kieft GJ, Smith SJ, Schepers-Bok R. Role of spiral volumetric computed tomography scanning on the assessment of patients with clinical suspicion of pulmonary embolism and an abnormal ventilation/perfusion lung scan. Thorax 1996; 51: 23–28

56. Gefter WB, Hatabu H, Holland GA, Gupta KB, Henschke CI, Palevsky HI. Pulmonary thromboembolism: recent development in diagnosis with CT and MR Imaging. Radiol 1995; 197: 561–574

57. Evans DA, Wilmott RW. Pulmonary embolism in children. Pediatr Clin N Amer 1994; 41: 569–584

58. Ginsberg JS, Brill-Edwards PA, Demers C, Donavan D, Panju A. D-dimer in patients with clinically suspected pulmonary embolism. Chest 1993; 104: 1679–1684

59. De Moerloose P, Desmarais S, Bounameaux H, Reber G, Perrier A, Dupuy G, Pittet JL. Contribution of a new, rapid, individual and quantitative automated D-dimer Elisa to exclude pulmonary embolism. Thromb Haemost 1996; 75: 11–13

60. Demers C, Ginsberg JS, Johnston M, Brill-Edwards PA, Panju A. D-Dimer and Thrombin-Antithrombin III complexes in patients with clinically suspected pulmonary embolism. Thromb Haemost 1992; 67: 408–412

61. Manco-Johnson MJ, Nuss R, Key N, Moertel C, Jacobson L, Meech S, Weinberg A, Lefkowitz. Lupus anticoagulant and protein S deficiency in children with postvaricella purpura fulminans or thrombosis. J Pediatr 1996; 128: 319–323

62. D'Angelo A, Della Valle P, Crippa L, Pattarini E, Grimaldi L, D'Angelo SV. Brief report: Autoimmune protein S deficiency in a boy with severe thromboembolic disease. N Engl J Med 1993; 328: 1753–1757

63. Buffaz PD, Brut A. Clinically silent pulmonary embolism due to transient protein S deficiency. Clin Nucl Med 1995; 20: 1016–1017

64. Nguyên P, Reynaud J, Pouzol P, Munzer M, Richard O, François P. Varicella and thrombotic complications associated with transient protein C and S deficiencies in children. Eur J Pediatr 1994; 153: 646–649

65. Levin M, Eley B, Louis J, Cohen H, Young L, Heyderman R. Postinfectious purpura fulminans caused by an autoantibody directed against protein S. J Pediatr 1995; 127: 355–363

66. Williams RA. High incidence of pulmonary foreign body embolism. Pediatr Pathol 1992; 12: 479–480

67. Fenton TR, Bennet S, McIntosh N. Air embolism in ventilated very low birthweight infants. Arch Dis Child 1988; 63: 541–543

68. Lee SK, Tanswell AK. Pulmonary vascular air embolism in the newborn. Arch Dis Child 1989; 64: 507–510

69. Leicht CH, Waldman J. Pulmonary air embolism in the pediatric patient undergoing central catheter placement: A report of two cases. Anesthesiology 1986; 64: 519–521

70. Zakowski MF, Edwards RH, McDonough ET. Wilms' tumor presenting as sudden death due to tumor embolism. Arch Pathol Lab Med 1990; 114: 605–608

71. Booth AJ, Tweed CS. Case report: Fatal pulmonary embolism due to osteogenic sarcoma in a child. Clin Radiol 1989; 40: 533–535

72. Pillay SV. Pulmonary embolism of cerebral tissue in a neonate. A case report. S Afr Med J 1980; 58: 498

73. Brooks SEH, Taylor E, Golden MHN, Golden BE. Electron microscopy of herpes simplex hepatitis with hepatocyte pulmonary embolization in kwashiorkor. Arch Pathol Lab Med 1991; 115: 1247–1249

74. Weingarten J, Kauffman SL. Teflon embolization to pulmonary arteries. Ann Thorac Surg 1977; 23: 371–373

75. Hulman G, Levene M. Intralipid microemboli. Arch Dis Child 1986; 61: 702–703

76. Mughal MZ, Robinson MJ, Duckworth W. Neonatal fat embolism and agglutination of Intralipid. Arch Dis Child 1984; 59: 1098–1099

77. Gonzalez A, Altieri PI, Marquez E, Cox RA, Castillo M. Massive pulmonary embolism associated with a right ventricular myxoma. Am J Med 1980; 69: 795–798

78. Parker KM, Embry JH. Sudden death due to tricuspid valve myxoma with massive pulmonary embolism in a 15-month old male. J Forens Sci 1997; 42: 524–526

79. Allen BT, Day DL, Dehner LP. CT demonstration of asymptomatic pulmonary emboli after bone marrow transplantation: case report. Pediatr Radiol 1987; 17: 65–67

80. Adams M, Monagle P, Ali K, Barnard D, Bernstein M, Brisson L, Coppes M, David M, DeSai D, Grant R, Halton J, Israels S, Jardine L, Massicotte P, McCusker P, Silva M, Wu J. Long term outcome of paediatric thromboembolic disease: A report from the Canadian Childhood Thrombophilia Registry. Thromb Haemost 1997; 78: 398

81. Rockoff MA, Gang DL, Vacanti JP. Fatal pulmonary embolism following removal of a central venous catheter. J Pediatr Surg 1984; 19: 307–309

82. Schmidt B, Andrew M. Neonatal thrombosis: Report of a prospective Canadian and international registry. Pediatr 1995; 96: 939–943

83. Selldén H, Lannering B, Marky I, Nilsson K. Long-term use of central venous catheters in paediatric oncology treatment. Acta Anaesthesiol Scand 1991; 35: 315–319

84. Darbyshire PJ, Weightman NC, Speller DCE. Problems associated with indwelling central venous catheters. Arch Dis Child 1985; 60: 129–134

85. Stockwell M, Adams M, Andrew M, Cameron G, Pai K. Central venous catheters for out-patient management of malignant disorders. Arch Dis Child 1983; 58: 633–635

86. Korones DN, Buzzard CJ, Asselin BL, Harris JP. Right atrial thrombi in children with cancer and indwelling catheters. J Pediatr 1996; 128: 841–846

87. Talbott GA, Winters WD, Bratton SL, O'Rourke PP. A prospective study of femoral catheter-related thrombosis in children. Arch Pediatr Adolesc Med 1995; 149: 288–291

88. Krafte-Jacobs B, Sivit C, Mejia R, Pollack M. Catheter related femoral venous thrombosis in critically ill children. Crit Care Med 1994; 22: A159

89. Shefler A, Gillis J, Lam A, O'Connell AJ, Schell D, Lammi A. Inferior vena cava thrombosis as a complication of femoral vein catheterisation. Arch Dis Child 1995; 72: 343–345

90. Ross P, Ehrenkranz R, Kleinman CS, Seashore JH. Thrombus associated with central venous catheters in infants and children. J Pediatr Surg 1989; 24: 253–256

91. Leiby JM, Purcell H, De Maria JJ, Kraut EH, Sagone AL, Metz EN. Pulmonary embolism as a result of Hickman catheter-related thrombosis. Am J Med 1989; 86: 228–231

92. Goldstein AM, Weber JM, Sheridan RL. Femoral venous access is safe in burned children: An analysis of 224 catheters. J Pediatr 1997; 130: 442–446

93. Krafte-Jacobs B, Sivit CJ, Mejia R, Pollack MM. Catheter-related thrombosis in critically ill children: Comparison of catheters with and without heparin bonding. J Pediatr 1995; 126: 50–54

94. Schmidt-Sommerfield E, Snyder G, Rossi TM, Lebenthal E. Catheter-related complications in 35 children and adolescents with gastrointestinal disease on home parenteral nutrition. J Parenter Enter Nutr 1990; 14: 148–151

95. Martelle RR, Linde LM. Cerebrovascular accidents with tetralogy of Fallot. Am J Dis Child 1961; 101: 206–209

96. Rosenthal TN, Friedman AH, Kleinman CS, Kopf GS, Rosenfeld LE, Hellenbrand WE. Thromboembolic complications after Fontan operations. Circulation 1995; 92: 287–293

97. Jahangiri M, Ross DB, Redington AN, Lincoln C, Shinebourne EA. Thromboembolism after the Fontan procedure and its modifications. Ann Thorac Surg 1994; 58: 1409–1414

98. Cromme-Dijkhuis AH, Henkes CMA, Bijleveld CMA, Hillege HL, Bom VJJ, Meer van der J. Coagulation factor abnormalities as possible thrombotic risk factors after Fontan operations. Lancet 1990; 336: 1087–1090

99. Monagle P, Cochrane A, McCrindle B, Benson L, Williams W, Andrew M. Thromboembolic complications after Fontan procedures: The role of prophylactic anticoagulation. J Thorac Cardiovasc Surg 1998; 115: 493–498

100. Roubey RAS. Autoantibodies to phospholipid-binding plasma proteins: a new view of lupus anticoagulants and other "antiphospholipid" autoantibodies. Blood 1994; 84: 2854–2867

101. Oosting JD, Derksen RHWM, Bobbink IWG, Hackeng TM, Bouma BN, De Groot PG. Antiphospholipid antibodies directed against a combination of phospholipids with prothrombin, protein C or protein S: an explanation for their pathogenic mechanism? Blood 1993; 81: 2618–2625

102. Scheven von E, Athreya BH, Rose CD, Goldsmith DP, Morton L. Clinical characteristics of antiphospholipid antibody syndrome in children. J Pediatr 1996; 129: 339–345

103. Montes de Oca MA, Babron MC, Blétry O, Broyer M, Courtecuisse V, Fontaine JL, Loirat C, Méry JP, Reinert P, Wechsler B, Levy M. Thrombosis in systemic lupus erythematosus: a French collaborative study. Arch Dis Child 1991; 66: 713–717

104. Nuss R, Hays T, Chudgar U, Manco-Johnson M. Antiphospholipid antibodies and coagulation regulatory protein abnormalities in children with pulmonary emboli. J Pediatr Hematol Oncol 1997; 19: 202–207

105. Griffin JH, Evatt B, Zimmerman TS, Kleiss AJ. Deficiency of protein C in congenital thrombotic disease. J Clin Invest 1981; 68: 1370–1373

106. Allaart CF, Poort SR, Rosendaal FR, Reitsma PH, Bertina RM, Briët E. Increased risk of venous thrombosis in carriers of hereditary protein C deficiency defect. Lancet 1993; 341: 134–138

107. Greffe BS, Marlar RA, Manco-Johnson MJ. Neonatal protein C: molecular composition and distribution in normal infants. Thromb Res 1989; 56: 91–98

108. Comp PhC, Esmon CT. Recurrent venous thromboembolism in patients with a partial deficiency of protein S. N Engl J Med 1984; 311: 1525–1528

109. Thaler E, Lechner K. Antithrombin III deficiency and thromboembolism. Clin Hematol 1981; 10: 369–390

110. De Stefano V, Leone G, De Carolis MP, Ferrelli R, De Carolis S, Pagano L, Tortorolo G, Bizzi B. Antithrombin III in fullterm and preterm newborn infants: Three cases of neonatal diagnosis of AT III congenital defect. Thromb Haemost 1987; 57: 329–331

111. Koster T, Rosendaal FR, Ronde F de, Briët E, Vandenbroucke JP, Bertina RM. Venous thrombosis due to poor anticoagulant response to activated protein C: Leiden thrombophilia study. Lancet 1993; 342: 1503–1506

112. Voorberg J, Roelse J, Koopman R, Buller H, Berends F, ten Cate JW, Mertens K, Mourik van JA. Association of idiopatic venous thromboembolism with single point-mutation at Arg506 of factor V. Lancet 1994; 343: 1535–1536

113. Heyboer H, Brandjes DPM, Büller HR, Sturk A, Ten Cate JW. Deficiencies of coagulation-inhibiting and fibrinolytic proteins in outpatients with deep-vein thrombosis. N Engl J Med 1990; 323: 1512–1516

114. Malm J, Laurell M, Nilsson IM, Dahlbäck B. Thromboembolic disease – critical evaluation of laboratory investigation. Thromb Haemost 1992; 68: 7–13

115. Monagle P, Andrew M, Halton J, Marlar R, Jardine L, Vegh P, Johnston M, Webber C, Massicotte MP. Homozygous protein C deficiency: Description of a new mutation and successful treatment with low molecular weight heparin. Thromb Haemost 1998; 79: 756–761

116. Nowak-Göttl U, Kries von R, Göbel U. Neonatal symptomatic thromboembolism in Germany: two year survey. Arch Dis Child 1997; 76: 163–167

117. Sifontes MT, Nuss R, Jacobson LJ, Griffin JH, Manco-Johnson MJ. Thrombosis in otherwise well children with the factor V Leiden mutation. J Pediatr 1996; 128: 324–328

118. Gurgey A, Mesci L, Renda Y, Olcay L, Kocak N, Erdem G. Factor V R 506 Q mutation in children with thrombosis. Am J Hematol 1996; 53: 37–39

119. Kodish E, Potter C, Kirschbaum NE, Foster PA. Activated protein C resistance in a neonate with venous thrombosis. J Pediatr 1995; 127: 645–648

120. Petäjä J, Jalanko H, Holmberg C, Kinnunen S, Syrjälä M. Resistance to activated protein C as an underlying cause of recurrent venous thrombosis during relapsing nephrotic syndrome. J Pediatr 1995; 127: 103–105

121. Kohlhase B, Veilhaber H, Kehl HG, Kececioglu D, Koch HG, Nowak-Göttl U. Thromboembolism and resistance to activated protein C in children with underlying cardiac disease. J Pediatr 1996; 129: 677–179

122. Koeleman BPC, Reitsma PH, Allaart CF, Bertina RM. Activated protein C resistance as an additional risk factor for thrombosis in protein C-deficient families. Blood 1994; 84: 1031–1035

123. Rosendaal FR. Thrombosis in the young: Epidemiology and risk factors. A focus on venous thrombosis. Thromb Haemost 1997; 78: 1–6

124. Manco-Johnson MJ. Disorders of hemostasis in childhood: Risk factors for venous thromboembolism. Thromb Haemost 1997; 78: 710–714

125. Boven HH van, Reitsma PH, Rosendaal FR, Bayston TA, Chowdhury V, Bauer KA, Scharrer I, Conard J, Lane DA. Factor V Leiden (FV R506Q) in families with inherited antithrombin deficiency. Thromb Haemost 1996; 75: 417–421

126. Meer FJM van der, Koster T, Vandenbroucke JP, Briët E, Rosendaal FR. The Leiden Thrombophilia Study (LETS). Thromb Haemost 1997; 78: 631–635

127. Poort SR, Rosendaal FR, Reitsma PH, Bertina RM. A common genetic variation in the 3′untranslated region of the prothrombin gene is associated with elevated plasma prothrombin levels and an increase in venous thrombosis. Blood 1996; 88: 3698–3703

128. Nowak-Göttl U, Debus O, Findeisen M, Kassenböhmer R, Koch HG, Pollmann H, Postler C, Weber P, Vielhaber H. Lipoprotein (a): Its role in childhood thromboembolism. J Pediatr 1997; 99: 865

129. Mudd SH, Levy HL, Skorby F. Disorders of transsulfuration. In: Scriver CR, Beaudet AI, Sly WS, Valle DL, eds. The metabolic and molecular bases of inherited disease. New York: McGraw-Hill, 1995:1279–1327

130. Mandel H, Brenner B, Berant M, Rosenberg N, Lanir N, Jacobs C, Fowler B, Seligsohn U. Coexistence of hereditary homocystinuria and Factor V Leiden-Effect on thrombosis. N Engl J Med 1996; 334: 763–768

131. Heyer den M, Koster T, Blom HJ, Bos GMJ, Briët E, Reitsma PH, Vandenbroucke JP, Rosendaal FR. Hyperhomocysteinemia as a risk factor for deep-vein thrombosis. N Engl J Med 1996; 334: 759–762

132. McBride WJ, Gadowski GR, Keller MS, Vane DW. Pulmonary embolism in pediatric trauma patients. J Trauma 1994; 37: 913–915

133. Prewitt R. Hemodynamic management in pulmonary embolism and acute hypoxemia respiratory failure. Crit Care Med 1990; 18: 61–69

134. Michelson AD, Bovill E, Andrew M. Antithrombotic therapy in children. Chest 1995; 108: 506–522

135. Hirsh J. Heparin. N Engl J Med 1991; 324: 1565–1574

136. David M, Manco-Johnson MJ, Andrew M. Diagnosis and treatment of venous thromboembolism in children and adolescents. On behalf of the Subcommittee on Perinatal Haemostasis of the Scientific and Standardization Committee of the ISTH. Thromb Haemost 1995; 74: 791–792

137. Potter C, Cox Gill J, Scot JP, McFarland JG. Heparin-induced thrombocytopenia in a child. J Pediatr 1992; 121: 135–138

138. Oriot D, Wolfe M, Wood C, Brun P, Sidi D, Devictor D, Tohernia G, Huault G. Severe thrombocytopenia induced by heparin in an infant with acute myocarditis. Arch Fr Pediatr 1990; 47: 357–359

139. Warkentin TE, Beng HC, Greinacher A. Heparin-induced thrombocytopenia: towards consensus. Thromb Haemost 1998; 79: 1–7

140. Andrew M. Indications and drugs for anticoagulation therapy in children. Thromb Res 1996; 81: 61–73

141. Doyle JJ, Koren G, Cheng MY, Blanchette VS. Anticoagulation with sodium warfarin in children: effect of loading regimen. J Pediatr 1988; 113: 1095–1097

142. Hirsh J. Oral anticoagulant drugs. N Engl J Med 1991; 324: 1865–1875

143. Owens JP, Mirtallo JM, Murphy CC. Oral anticoagulation in patients with short bowel syndrome. DICP 1990; 24: 585–589

144. Boneu B, Buchanan MR, Caranobe C, Gabaig AM, Dupouy D, Sie P, Hirsh J. The disappearance of a low molecular weight heparin fraction (CY 216) differs from standard heparin in rabbits. Thromb Res 1987; 46: 845–853

145. Andersson LO, Barrowcliffe TW, Holmer E, Johnson EA, Sims GEC. Anticoagulant properties of heparin fractionated by affinity chromatography on matrix-bound antithrombin III and by gel filtration. Thromb Res 1976; 9: 575–583

146. Johnson EA, Kirkwood TBL, Stirling Y, Perez-Requejo JL, Ingram GIC, Bangham DR, Brozovic M. Four heparin preparations: Anti-Xa potentiating effects of heparin after subcutaneous injection. Thromb Haemost 1976; 35: 586–591

147. Lensing AWA, Prins MH, Davidson BL, Hirsh J. Treatment of deep venous thrombosis with low molecular weight heparins. Arch Intern Med 1995; 155: 601–607

148. Hirsh J, Levine MN. Low molecular weight heparin. Blood 1992; 79: 1–17

149. Ginsberg JS. Management of venous thromboembolism. N Engl J Med 1996; 335: 1816–1828

150. A Cooperative Study. Urokinase-streptokinase embolism trial. JAMA 1974; 229: 1606–1613

151. Charbonnier B, Meyer G, Stem M, Sors H, Brochier ML. Thrombolytic treatment of acute pulmonary embolism. Herz 1989; 14: 157–171

152. Marder VJ, Sherry S. Thrombolytic therapy: current status. N Engl J Med 1988; 318: 1585–1595

153. Andrew M, Paes B, Milner R, Johnston M, Mitchell L, Tollefsen D, Powers P. Development of the human coagulation system in the full-term infant. Blood 1987; 70: 165–172

154. Andrew M, Paes B, Johnston M. Development of the hemostatic system in the neonate and young infant. Am J Pediatr Hematol Oncol 1990; 12: 95–104

155. Andrew M, Vegh P, Johnston M, Bowker J, Ofosu F, Mitchell L. Maturation of the hemostatic system during childhood. Blood 1992; 80: 1998–2005

156. Andrew M, Paes B, Milner R, Johnston M, Mitchell L, Tollefsen D, Castle V, Powers P. Development of the human coagulation system in the healthy premature infant. Blood 1988; 72: 1651–1657

157. Kothari SS, Varma S, Wasir HS. Thrombolytic therapy in infants and children. Am Heart J 1994; 127: 651–657

158. Benavent A, Estellés A, Aznar J, Martinez-Sales V, Gilabert J, Fornas E. Dysfunctional plasminogen in full term newborn – study of active site plasmin. Thromb Haemost 1984; 51: 67–70

159. Andrew M, Brooker L, Leaker M, Paes B, Weitz J. Fibrin clot lysis by thrombolytic agents is impaired in newborns due to low plasminogen concentration. Thromb Haemost 1992; 68: 325–330

160. Zureikat GY, Martin GR, Silverman NH, Newth CJL. Urokinase therapy for a catheter related right atrial thrombus and pulmonary embolism in a 2-month-old infant. Pediatr Pulmonol 1986; 2: 303–306

161. Beitzke A, Zobel G, Zenz W, Gamillscheg A, Stein JI. Catheter-directed thrombolysis with recombinant tissue plasminogen activator for acute pulmonary embolism after Fontan operation. Pediatr Cardiol 1996; 17: 410–412

162. Pyles LA, Pierpont MEM, Steiner ME, Hesslein PS, Smith II CM. Fibrinolysis by tissue plasminogen activator in a child with pulmonary embolism. J Pediatr 1990; 116: 801–804

163. Pritchard SL, Culham JAG, Rogers PCJ. Low-dose fibrinolytic therapy in infants. J Pediatr 1985; 106: 594–598

164. Delaplane D, Scott JP, Riggs TW, Silverman BL, Hunt CE. Urokinase therapy for a catheter-related right atrial thrombus. J Pediatr 1982; 100: 149–152

165. Rehan VK, Cronin CM, Bowman JM. Neonatal portal vein thrombosis successfully treated by regional streptokinase infusion. Eur J Pediatr 1994; 153: 456–459

166. Curnow A, Idowu J, Behrends E, Toomey F. Urokinase therapy for silastic catheter induced intravascular thrombi in infants and children. Arch Surg 1985; 120: 1237–1240

167. Doyle E, Britto J, Freeman J, Munro F, Morton NS. Thrombolysis with low dose tissue plasminogen activator. Arch Dis Child 1992; 67: 1483–1484

168. Levy M, Benson LN, Burrows PE, Bentur Y, Strong DK, Smith J, Johnson D, Jacobson S, Koren G. Tissue plasminogen activator for the treatment of thromboembolism in infants and children. J Pediatr 1991; 118: 467–472

169. Beaufils F, Schlegel N, Loirat C, Marrote R, Pillion G, Mathieu H. Urokinase treatment of pulmonary artery thrombosis. Complicating pediatric nephrotic syndrome. Crit Care Med 1985; 13: 132–134

170. Leaker M, Massicotte MP, Brooker LA, Andrew M. Thrombolytic therapy in pediatric patients: A comprehensive review of the literature. Thromb Haemost 1996; 76: 132–134

171. Leaker M, Massicotte MP, Brooker LA, Andrew M. Thrombolytic therapy in pediatric patients: Ten year experience in a single institution. Thromb Haemost

172. Gorlach G, Hager KJ, Mulch J, Scheld HH, Boldt H, Hehrlein FW. Surgical therapy of pulmonary thrombosis due to candidiasis in a premature infant. J Cardiovasc Surg 1986; 27: 341–343

173. Moreno-Cabral RJ, Breitweser JA. Pulmonary embolectomy in the neonate. Chest 1983; 84: 502–504

174. Putnam JB, Lemmer JH, Rocchini AP, Bove EL. Embolectomy for acute pulmonary artery occlusion following Fontan procedure. Ann Thorac Surg 1988; 45: 335–336

175. Becker DM, Philbrick JT, Selby JB. Inferior vena cava filters. Indications, safety, effectiveness. Arch Intern Med 1992; 152: 1985–1994

176. Khong PL, John PR. Technical aspects of insertion and removal of an inferior vena cava IVC filter for prophylactic treatment of pulmonary embolus. Pediatr Radiol 1997; 27: 239–241

177. Tracy T, Posner MP, Drucker DEM, Greenfield LJ, Langham MR, Mendez-Picon G, Krummel TM, Salzberg AM. Use of the Greenfield filter in adolescents for deep vein thrombosis and pulmonary embolism. J Pediatr Surg 1988; 23: 529–532

178. Decousus H, Leizorovicz A, Parent A, Page Y, Tardy B, Girard P, Laporte S, Faivre R, Charbonnier B, Barral FG, Huet Y, Simmonneau G. A clinical trial of vena caval filters in the prevention of pulmonary embolism in patients with proximal deep-vein thrombosis. N Engl J Med 1998; 338: 409–415

179. Jones DRB, MacIntyre IMC. Venous thromboembolism in infancy and childhood. Arch Dis Child 1975; 50: 153–155

180. Egli F, Elmiger P, Stalder G. Thromboembolism in the nephrotic syndrome. Pediatr Res 1974; 8: 903

181. Hoyer PF, Gonda S, Barthels M, Krohn HP, Brodehl J. Thromboembolic complications in children with nephrotic syndrome. Acta Paediatr Scand 1986; 75; 804–810

182. Hsu D, Addoniziol, Hordof A, Gensony W. Acute pulmonary embolism in pediatric patients awaiting heart transplantation. J. Am Coll Cardiol 1991; 17: 1621

183. Marraro G, Uderzo C, Marchi P, Gastagnini G, Vaj PL, Masera G. Acute respiratory failure and pulmonary thrombosis in leukemic children. Cancer 1991; 67: 696–702

184. Raman TK, Blake JA, Harris TM. Pulmonary embolism in Landry-Guillain-Barre-Strohl syndrome. Chest 1971; 60: 555–557

185. Piat JH, Hoffman HJ. Cor pulmonale: A lethal complication of ventriculoatrial CSF diversion. Child's Nerv Syst 1989; 5: 29–31

186. Sanerkin NG, Edwards P, Jacobs J. Pulmonary thrombo-embolic phenomena in the newborn. J Pathol Bacteriol 1966; 91: 569–574

187. Uderzo C, Marraro G, Riva A, Bonanomi E, Vaj PL, Marchi PF, Locasciulli A, Masera G. Pulmonary thromboembolism in leukaemic children undergoing bone marrow transplantation. Bone Marrow Transplant 1993; 11: 201–203

188. Nguyên LT, Laberge JM, Guttman FM, Albert D. Spontaneous deep vein thrombosis in childhood and adolescence. J Pediatr Surg 1986; 21: 640–643

189. Zimmerman RL, Novek S, Chen JTT, Roggli V. Pulmonary thrombosis in a 10-year-old child with minimal change disease and nephrotic syndrome. Am J Clin Pathol 1994; 101: 230–236

190. Olson TM, Driscoll DJ, Edwards WD, Puga FJ, Danielson GK. Pulmonary microthrombi. Caveat for successful modified Fontan operation. J Thorac Cardiovasc Surg 1993; 106: 739–744

191. Rosenthal DN, Bulbul ZR, Friedman AH, Hellenbrand WE, Kleinman CS. Thrombosis of the pulmonary artery stump after distal ligation. J Thorac Cardiovasc Surg 1995; 110: 1563–1565

192. Svane S. Primary thrombosis of pulmonary artery in a child with tetralogy of Fallot. Br Heart J 1977; 39: 815–819

193. Fink SM, Bockman DE, Howell CG, Falls DG, Kanto WP. Bypass circuits as the source of thromboemboli during extracorporeal membrane oxygenation. J Pediatr 1989; 115: 621–624

194. Eberhard DA. Two-year-old boy with Proteus syndrome and fatal pulmonary thromboembolism. Pediatr Pathol 1994; 14: 771–779

195. Machin GA, Kent S. Pulmonary thromboembolism from a large hemangioma in a 4 weeks-old infant. Pediatr Pathol 1989; 9: 73–78

196. Landing BH, Nadorra R, Hyman CB, Ortega JA. Pulmonary lesions of thalassemia major. Perspec Pediatr Pathol 1987; 11: 82–96

197. Werder EA, Waibel P, Sege D, Flury R. Severe thrombosis during oestrogen treatment for tall stature. Eur J Pediatr 1990; 149: 389–390

198. Conte FA, Grumbach MM. Estrogen use in children and adolescents: a survey. Pediatr 1978; 62: 1091–1097

199. Ament J, Newth CJ. Deep venous lines and thromboembolism. Pediatr Pulmonol 1995; 20: 347–348

200. Gosseye S, Obbergh L van, Weynand B, Scheiff JM, Moulin D, De Ville de Goyet J, Otte JB. Platelet aggregates in small lung vessels and death during liver transplantation. Lancet 1991; 338: 532–534

201. Brandstetter Y, Weinhouse E, Splaingard ML, Tang TT. Cor pulmonale as a complication of methylmalonic acidemia and homocystinuria (Cbl-C type). Am J Med Gen 1990; 36: 167–171

202. Wesley JR, Keens TG, Miller SW, Platzker ACG. Pulmonary embolism in the neonate: Occurrence during the course of total parenteral nutrition. J Pediatr 1978; 93: 113–115

203. Risseeuw-Appel IM, Dekker I, Hop WC, Hahlen K. Minimal effects of E-coli and Erwinia asparaginase on the coagulation system in childhood acute lymphoblastic leukemia: a randomized study. Medical & Pediatric Oncology; 1994; 24 (4): 335–343

204. Mitchell L, Hoogendoorn H, Giles AR, Vegh P, Andrew M. Increased endogenous thrombin generation in children with acute lymphoblastic leukemia: Risk of thrombotic complications in l'asparaginase-induced antithrombin III deficiency. Blood 1994; 83: 386–391

205. Peters M, ten Cate H, Sturk A. Acquired protein S deficiency might be associated with a prethrombotic state during estrogen treatment for tall stature. Thromb Haemost 1992; 68: 371–372

206. Peters M, Plaat BEC, ten Cate H, Wolters HJ, Weening RS, Brandjes DPM. Enhanced thrombin generation in children with sickle cell disease. Thromb Haemost 1994; 71: 169–172

Index

Thomas Grumme / Wolfgang Kluge /
Konrad Kretzschmar / Andreas Roesler

Cerebral and Spinal Computed Tomography

3rd completely revised and enlarged edition.
1998. 279 pages, more than 1200 illustrations. Hardback.
£ 99,50   ISBN 0-632-04855-7

The third edition of this tried and tested standard volume shows that computed tomography (CT) still rates highly in the modern diagnosis of disorders of the central nervous system.
The new edition contains the following features:
- The excellent didactic principles remain unchanged.
- The illustrative material has been completely updated and expanded.
- The comparative tables for differentiating the various kinds of tumours have been completely revised.
- Greater attention has been paid to the differential diagnosis of lumbosciatica.
- Modern examination methods such as spiral CT and the 3D reconstruction technique, as well as interventional procedures, are introduced.
- Postoperative and post-traumatic problems are described in detail.
- A whole new chapter has been devoted to the subject of AIDS.
- In view of the increasing importance of magnetic resonance imaging (MRI) in the diagnosis of disorders of the central nervous system, the relative diagnostic capabilities and expressiveness of CT versus MRI have been carefully compared.

Practitioners and learners will now have a work at their disposal that uniquely combines diversity of information with ease of use.

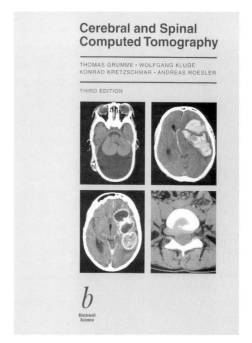

The german edition "Zerebrale und Spinale CT" (3-89412-288-9) is available through
Blackwell Wissenschafts-Verlag GmbH, Kurfürstendamm 57, 10707 Berlin
Fax: 030/32 79 06-44, Phone: 030/32 79 06-27/28

The english edition is available through:

Blackwell Science

Prices are subject to change

Osney Mead, Oxford OX2 0EL, UK · Tel: 44 1865 206206 · Fax: 44 1865 206096
Telex: 83355 MEDBOK G · web site: http://www.blackwell-science.com

Ernst Groechenig

Cor pulmonale
Treatment of Pulmonary Hypertension

1999. XIV, 160 pages, 41 figures, 17 x 24 cm. Paperback. ISBN 0-632-05424-7

Pulmonary hypertension and cor pulmonale are severe diseases whose incidence is considerably underestimated.

The many functions of the heart, lungs and blood vessels play an important role in the development of and recovery from these two diseases. The author provides a concise summary of the important anatomical, physiological and pathological features of these three organ systems.

Coverage ranges from ventilatory physiology and general aspects of cardiac diseases to disorders of coagulation.

Particular attention is paid to the newer drug treatments in a well-referenced section.

The book is appropriate for all medical staff involved with these clinical syndromes. *Family physicians, internists, respiratory physicians, cardiologists, cardiac and thoracic surgeons and radiologists* will all find important new information for their daily practice. Numerous clear illustrations explain the complex interrelationships.

Medical students will profit from the comprehensive presentation of this complex topic because most of the internal medicine text books give only scant coverage of pulmonary hypertension and cor pulmonale.

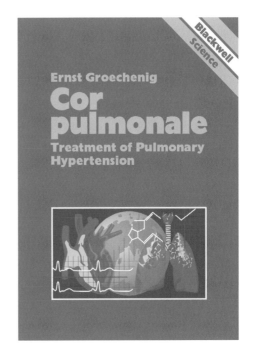

The german edition (3-89412-403-2) is available through
Blackwell Wissenschafts-Verlag GmbH, Kurfürstendamm 57, 10707 Berlin
Fax: 030/32 79 06-44, Phone: 030/32 79 06-27/28

The english edition is available through:

Blackwell Science

Osney Mead, Oxford OX2 0EL, UK · Tel: 44 1865 206206 · Fax: 44 1865 206096
Telex: 83355 MEDBOK G · web site: http://www.blackwell-science.com